American Heart Association®

Learn and Live SM

PALS
Provider Manual

Senior Science Editor
Mary Fran Hazinski, RN, MSN

Editors
Arno L. Zaritsky, MD
Vinay M. Nadkarni, MD
Robert W. Hickey, MD
Stephen M. Schexnayder, MD
Robert A. Berg, MD

Past Editors of the PALS Text and Instructor's Manual
Leon Chameides, MD
Arno L. Zaritsky, MD
Deborah L. Burkett, EdD
Mary Fran Hazinski, RN, MSN
Deborah Henderson, RN, MA
Robert C. Luten, MD
James McCrory, MD
Vinay M. Nadkarni, MD
Linda Quan, MD
James S. Seidel, MD, PhD

Illustrator
Anne Jorunn Pedersen

Special Contributors
Terry Adirim, MD
Dianne L. Atkins, MD
Tom P. Aufderheide, MD
Dana Braner, MD
Cindy J. Brownlee, RN, CCRN
Lisa A. Carlson, RN, MS, CPNP
Arthur Cooper, MD
Richard O. Cummins, MD, MPH, MSc
Jay Deshpande, MD
Kathleen Doobinin, MD
Cindy Doyle, RN
Harald Eikland
Mary E. Fallat, MD
John M. Field, MD
Wayne H. Franklin, MD
Jim Gerard
Michael J. Gerardi, MD
William E. Hauda II, MD
Thomas A. Hazinski, MD
Harriet Hawkins, RN, CCRN
John Kattwinkel, MD
Robert Kerns, MD
Steven P. Laffey, MD
Richard Levitan, MD

ISBN 0-87493-322-6

Special Contributors (continued)

Thomas G. Martin, MD, MPH
Mark Mattes, JD
Bohdan Minczak, MD
Thomas Nakagawa, MD
Steven R. Neish, MD
Susan Niermeyer, MD
Jeffrey Perlman, MD
Rhonda M. Phillipi, RN
Gail Rasmussen, MD
Ricardo Samson, MD
Anthony J. Scalzo, MD
L.R. "Tres" Scherer III, MD
Charles L. Schleien, MD
Glen A. Sinks, RN, MSN, EMT-P
Edward R. Stapleton, EMT-P
Mark E. Swanson, MD
Daniel Timmel, MSW
Robert K. Waddell II, EMT-P

Subcommittee on Pediatric Resuscitation 1997-2002

Robert W. Hickey, MD, Chair, 2001-2002
Robert A. Berg, MD, Chair, 1998-2001
Vinay M. Nadkarni, MD, Chair, 1995-1998
Terry Adirim, MD
Dianne L. Atkins, MD
Cindy J. Brownlee, RN, CCRN
G. Patricia Cantwell, MD
Waldemar Carlo, MD, Special Consultant
Lisa A. Carlson, RN, MS, CPNP
Leon Chameides, MD, Special Consultant
Ashraf Coovadia, MD, ILCOR Liaison
Amy Davis, RN, MSN
Jay Deshpande, MD
Kathleen Dracup, RN, DNSc Special Consultant

Mary E. Fallat, MD, Special Consultant
Marianne Gausche, MD, Special Consultant
Michael J. Gerardi, MD, ACEP Liaison
John Kattwinkel, MD, Special Consultant
Steven R. Neish, MD, AAP Liaison
Susan Niermeyer, MD
Martin H. Osmond, MD, CM, HSF Liaison
Jeffrey Perlman, MD, NRP Liaison
Rhonda M. Phillippi, RN
Barbara Phillips, MD, ERC Liaison
Linda Quan, MD
Gail Rasmussen, MD
Amelia Gorete Reis, MD, ILCOR Liaison
Sally Reynolds, MD
Anthony J. Scalzo, MD, Toxicology Consultant
L. R. "Tres" Scherer III, MD, ACS liaison
Stephen M. Schexnayder, MD
Charles L. Schleien, MD
Thomas E. Terndrup, MD
James Tibballs, MD, ILCOR Liaison
Patrick Van Reempts, MD, PhD, ERC Liaison
Robert K. Waddell II, EMSC Liaison
Arno L. Zaritsky, MD, Product Development Consultant
David Zideman, MD, ERC Liaison

Reviewers

Susan Fuchs, MD
Ronald A. Dieckmann, MD
Jo Haag, RN, MSN
Barbara Phillips, MD
Mark Ralston, MD
Amelia Gorete Reis, MD
Ricardo Samson, MD
Thomas E. Terndrup, MD
Timothy S. Yeh, MD

Contents

Contents

Contents

Contents

Chapter 11
Children With Special Healthcare Needs

Chapter 12
Toxicology

Chapter 13
Neonatal Resuscitation

Chapter 14
Rapid Sequence Intubation

Chapter 15
Sedation Issues for the
PALS Provider

Chapter 16
Coping With Death and Dying

Contents

Preface

More than a dozen years ago, at the start of a crisp fall day following an overnight shift in the ED, I ran my first code. The patient was a small, thin boy who had just begun to walk. I imagine that, like all children, this child's progress from lying, to sitting, to standing was accompanied by a sense of wonder and glee as his visual horizon grew and his world expanded. The newfound ability to walk and explore an increasingly visible and interactive world must have occupied his dreams and energized his waking hours.

This liberation, which is a source of pride for most parents, was a source of frustration for this child's parents, and they had reacted in an almost incomprehensible way. As we undressed him and his bruises slowly came into focus, they seized my attention indelibly. With sudden, unremitting, painful clarity I recognized the pattern of abuse. They had beaten him fatally.

Years later I cannot remember the name of this child, yet I can remember the way his clothes were gathered on the hospital floor.

The death of a child is always accompanied by a sense of emotional turmoil and the frightening possibility that the world is without meaning or measure. I suppose this is what people have in mind when they ask me "How can you do what you do? You must see horrible things."

Yet those of us who take care of children know better. We know that children are a rejuvenating wellspring of love and wonder, and caring for them nurtures us as well as them. We know that our work results in more laughter, more discovery, more sleepovers, more birthday parties, more cupcakes, more dances, more graduations, and eventually more of us. It is my belief that nowhere are the stakes higher or the rewards greater than in the care of critically ill children. It is our duty and our privilege to do our best. Those of us who have dedicated our lives to caring for ill children have done so because we understand these things.

The many contributors to this textbook have drawn upon this knowledge to partner with you during an incredibly challenging circumstance—the resuscitation and stabilization of a critically ill child. It is our shared goal to perform our best and give our children the greatest chance possible to lead healthy, fulfilling lives.

To help meet this shared goal, the AHA Subcommittee on Pediatric Resuscitation has dramatically revised the pediatric advanced life support course. Over 500 international experts reviewed more than 25,000 journal articles to update the science, presented in the *ECC Guidelines 2000.** The new science has been incorporated into new materials designed to meet the specific needs of targeted healthcare providers. This was accomplished by developing a modular course consisting of "core content" and "supplemental" modules.

Core content modules contain material that is essential for the resuscitation of any ill or injured children and therefore represents a common learning objective for all course participants. Supplemental modules are targeted to meet the needs of specific groups of targeted healthcare providers. Supplemental module topics include children with special healthcare needs, toxicology, the newly born, trauma and spinal immobilization, coping with death, procedural sedation, and rapid sequence intubation. Additional modules addressing anaphylaxis, complex heart disease, seizures, and other topics are under development. Although this new material has expanded the length of the textbook, we anticipate that the increased flexibility will allow learners to participate in a course that is more likely to meet their specific needs.

To actively engage the PALS participant we have expanded the use of case-based scenarios. Chapters now begin and end with a series of cases and questions to help the learner focus on key concepts within the context of real-life situations.

---

*American Heart Association in collaboration with International Liaison Committee on Resuscitation. Guidelines 2000 for Cardiopulmonary Resuscitation and Emergency Cardiac Care: International Consensus on Science. *Circulation*. 2000;102(suppl I).

Experienced healthcare providers may wish to review this material first; for many this review will be sufficient. PALS participants requiring additional explanation will find it in the body of the chapter. Another change to the course is the addition of video instruction to many of the modules. Video instruction, as an educational tool, is efficient, consistent, and dynamic. If a picture conveys a thousand words, a video clip of respiratory distress conveys 10,000 words. Similarly, the *Coping with Death* videotape captures the heart-wrenching emotions surrounding the death of a child in a manner impossible with pen and paper

These changes in resuscitation science and educational material are possible because of contributions from hundreds of international experts and the hard work of present and past members of the Pediatric Subcommittee.

The Subcommittee would like to thank the many healthcare providers who, like you, have taken the PALS Provider Course and who strive to deliver the best care possible to our children.

Robert W. Hickey, MD
Chair, Subcommittee on
    Pediatric Resuscitation

Acknowledgments

Anne Pederson and Harald Eikland created new illustrations for this text. We appreciate their extraordinry efforts and good humor throughout the process.

Special thanks are due to members of the AHA staff whose dedication helped keep this mission alive. We especially thank Mary Ann McNeely and F. G. Stoddard for their uncompromising dedication to quality. As director of product development Mary Ann brings to her work grace under pressure, warmth, and strength. She can see the mission in every product, and she epitomizes the very best of AHA. As ECC editor-in-chief F. G. brings a perspective to his work that is cultured, literary, scientific, and humane. We value his esprit de corps.

A very special thanks is due to Mary Fran Hazinski, whose labors on this text, the *PALS Instructor's Manual* and *Toolkit*, and the entire compass of ECC are heroic and monumental. Her keen intelligence and sharp eye inform every facet of this book. She is a generous, supportive colleague and an inspirational leader.

Note on Medication Doses

Emergency Cardiovascular Care is a dynamic science. Advances in treatment and drug therapies occur rapidly. Readers are advised to check for changes in recommended dose, indications, and contraindications in the following sources: *Currents in Emergency Cardiovascular Care,* the *ECC Handbook of Emergency Cardiovascular Care for Healthcare Providers,* and the package insert product information sheet for each drug.

Level of Evidence and Class of Recommendation

The resuscitation councils and experts who participated in the international Guidelines 2000 Conference used the tools and principles of evidence-based medicine for all proposed guidelines. The process required a search for evidence, an evaluation of the methodologic level of evidence, and then an integration of all the evidence into a final, summary "class of recommendation." The following tables convey the definitions used for this process.

Evidence Level	Definition
1. Positive RCTs ($P<0.05$)	A prospective, randomized, controlled trial (RCT); conclusions: new treatment significantly better (or worse) than control treatment.
2. Neutral RCTs (NS)	An RCT; conclusions: new treatment no better than control treatment.
3. Prospective, nonrandom	Nonrandomized, *prospective*, observational study; 1 group used new treatment; must have a control group for comparison.
4. Retrospective, nonrandom	Nonrandomized, *retrospective*, observational study; 1 group used new treatment; must have a control group for comparison.
5. Case series	Series of patients received new treatment in past or will receive in future; watch to see what outcomes occur; no control group.
6. Animal studies (A and B)	Studies using animals or mechanical models; A-level animal studies are higher quality than B-level studies.
7. Extrapolations	Reasonable extrapolations from existing data or data gathered for other purposes; quasi-experimental designs.
8. Rational conjecture, common sense	Fits with common sense; has face validity; applies to many non–evidence-based guidelines that "made sense." No evidence of harm.

Integration of many articles across all evidence levels with

- **Critical appraisal**
- **Experts' consensus discussions**
- **Input from Evidence Evaluation Conference**
- **Input from Guidelines 2000 Conference**

Class of Recommendation	Criteria for Class	Clinical Definition
Class I **Definitely recommended**	Supported by **excellent** evidence, with at least 1 **prospective, randomized, controlled trial.**	**Class I** interventions are always acceptable, safe, and effective. Considered definitive care, standard of care.
Class IIa **Acceptable and useful**	Supported by **good to very good** evidence. Weight of evidence and expert opinion strongly in favor.	**Class IIa** interventions are acceptable, safe, and useful. Considered *intervention of choice* by majority of experts.
Class IIb **Acceptable and useful**	Supported by **fair** to **good** evidence. Weight of evidence and expert opinion not strongly in favor.	**Class IIb** interventions are also acceptable, safe, and useful. Considered *optional* or *alternative interventions* by majority of experts.
Indeterminate **Promising, evidence lacking, immature**	Preliminary research stage. Evidence: no harm but no benefit. Evidence insufficient to support a final class decision.	**Indeterminate:** describes treatments of promise but limited evidence. AHA-ILCOR accepts some indeterminates but only by expert consensus.
Class III **May be harmful; no benefit documented**	Not acceptable, not useful, **may be harmful.**	**Class III** refers to interventions with **no** evidence of **any** benefit; often some evidence of harm.

The Chain of Survival and Emergency Medical Services for Children

Introductory Case Scenario

A 2-year-old toddler is found floating in the family swimming pool. His father shouts for help (the mother is inside the house) and pulls the child out of the water. The father notes that the child is pale and does not respond to touch or voice. The father opens the child's airway using a jaw thrust and notes that the child is not breathing.

- What measures might have prevented this emergency?

- What is your initial assessment of this toddler's status?

- What actions should be performed next by rescuers at the scene?

- When should the emergency medical services (EMS) system be activated?

- What are the 4 critical links in the pediatric Chain of Survival?

Learning Objectives

After completing this chapter the PALS provider should be able to

- State why *prevention* of illness and injury is the most effective component of the Chain of Survival to improve the healthcare status of children

- Describe the epidemiology and prevention of common childhood injuries and emergencies

- State how and when to activate the EMS system

- Identify the key elements (links) of the pediatric Chain of Survival

- Identify how and why the sequence of links in the pediatric Chain of Survival differs slightly from the sequence of links in the adult Chain of Survival

Introduction

The functional survival of critically ill and injured children is influenced by the provision of timely and appropriate pediatric emergency care in both the prehospital and hospital environments. The EMS system delivers prehospital care. EMS systems were initially created for out-of-hospital cardiac emergencies in adults in developed nations. Pediatric EMS concerns were often of secondary importance, so the equipment, training, experience, and expertise of prehospital providers were often less well developed to meet the needs of children.

Specific EMS needs of pediatric patients have now been identified.[1-4] In addition, the EMS system now must meet the needs of a growing number of children with special healthcare needs. These children have chronic physical, developmental, behavioral, or emotional conditions that require services not typically needed by normally developing children.[5-7]

In the United States death rates for victims treated in the EMS system are higher for children than for adults, especially in areas where tertiary pediatric care is unavailable.[8-15]

To improve pediatric out-of-hospital care, EMS personnel should be optimally trained and equipped to care for pediatric victims, medical dispatchers should use emergency protocols appropriate for children, and emergency departments that provide care for children should be appropriately staffed and equipped.[3,4]

Emergency departments that provide care for acutely ill or injured children should have an ongoing agreement with a pediatric tertiary care service through which patients can receive postresuscitation care in a pediatric intensive care unit (PICU) under the supervision of trained personnel. Similar emergency preparedness procedures should be developed and practiced in physician offices and hospitals.

An EMS-C (emergency medical services for children) system must therefore be developed in every community and locale. The EMS-C system is responsible for a broad spectrum of services including prevention, early recognition of problems, initial stabilization of infants and children, and rehabilitative care (see FYI on the next page).

Current pediatric basic life support (PBLS) and advanced life support (PALS) guidelines delineate a series of skills performed sequentially to assess, support, or restore effective ventilation and circulation to the child with respiratory or cardiorespiratory arrest (Figure 1). Although this process is often taught as a sequence of distinct steps to enhance skills retention, several actions

Following identification of the need for specialized EMS programs to improve the prehospital care of children, federal funding for emergency medical services for children (EMS-C) programs was established in 1984. The Maternal and Child Health Bureau (MCHB) provides grants to states to improve EMS services for children. The program was launched in 1985 and is administered by the MCHB, Health Resources and Services Administration, Public Health Service, and US Department of Health and Human Services. Since then all states have received federal funds to develop programs and improve emergency medical services for children. These programs have contributed to the quality of pediatric EMS care and have strengthened educational programs, referral protocols, and quality-improvement monitoring.

The goals of the EMS-C programs are as follows:

If a child has a serious or life-threatening injury or illness anywhere in the United States:

1. The child will receive state-of-the-art emergency medical care

2. The pediatric service is well integrated into an emergency medical services system backed by optimum resources

3. The EMS-C component of the EMS system will provide a spectrum of services from primary prevention of illness and injury to identification of problems, as well as acute care and rehabilitation

From Seidel JS, Henderson DP, eds. *Emergency Medical Services for Children: A Report to the Nation.* Washington, DC: National Center for Education in Maternal Child Health; 1991.

---

may be accomplished simultaneously (eg, begin CPR and phone EMS) if multiple rescuers are present. The appropriate actions in a given emergency are determined by the epidemiology of the emergency and factors such as the interval since arrest, how the victim responded to previous resuscitative interventions, and whether special resuscitation circumstances exist.

Epidemiology of Common Infant, Child, and Adolescent Injuries and Emergencies Requiring Resuscitation

In adults most sudden, nontraumatic cardiopulmonary arrests are *cardiac* in origin. The most common terminal cardiac rhythm is ventricular fibrillation (VF). In research studies *nontraumatic, witnessed arrest with a presenting rhythm of VF or pulseless ventricular tachycardia (VT)* is the gold standard of out-of-hospital adult arrest used to compare outcomes among prehospital systems and in-hospital centers.[16] For these victims the time from collapse to attempted defibrillation is the single greatest determinant of survival.[17-22] Bystander CPR also increases survival after sudden, witnessed adult cardiopulmonary arrest.[23,24] Thus, the adult Chain of Survival prioritizes early activation of EMS, bystander CPR, and rapid defibrillation.

In children the incidence, precise etiology, and outcome of cardiac arrest and resuscitation are difficult to ascertain because most reports contain an insufficient number of patients or use inconsistent inclusion and exclusion criteria or inconsistent definitions that prevent generalization of study conclusions to all children.[25] The causes of pediatric cardiopulmonary arrest are heterogeneous and include sudden infant death syndrome (SIDS), trauma, asphyxia, submersion, and sepsis.[26-32] Thus, there is no single gold standard pediatric cardiac arrest stereotype for research.[33]

Most out-of-hospital cardiac arrests in infants and children occur in or around the home, where children are under the supervision of parents or childcare providers. In the home SIDS, trauma, submersion, poisoning, choking, severe asthma, and pneumonia are the most

---

FIGURE 1. AHA pediatric Chain of Survival. Link 1: Prevention of injury or arrest. Link 2: Early and effective CPR. Link 3: Early EMS activation. Link 4: Early ALS, including stabilization, transport, and rehabilitation.

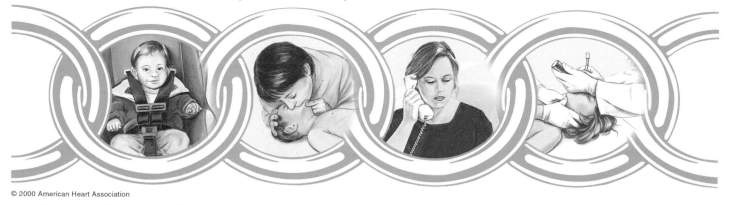

common causes of arrest. In industrialized nations trauma is the leading cause of death from the age of 6 months through young adulthood.[34] In general, pediatric out-of-hospital arrest is characterized by progression from hypoxia and hypercarbia to respiratory arrest and bradycardia and then asystolic cardiac arrest.[29,32,35] VT or VF has been reported in ≤15% of pediatric victims of out-of-hospital arrest[36-38] even when the rhythm is assessed by first responders.[39,40] The prevalence of shockable rhythms may be higher in subsets of patients with risk factors such as congenital heart disease, myocarditis, or toxin or drug ingestion predisposing to arrhythmias. Survival from out-of-hospital cardiopulmonary arrest ranges from 3% to 17% in most studies, and survivors are often neurologically devastated. With respiratory arrest alone, neurologically intact survival rates of ≥50% have been reported for resuscitation of children.[41,42]

Prompt, effective chest compressions and rescue breathing have been shown to improve return of spontaneous circulation and to increase the chance of neurologically intact survival in children with cardiac arrest.[32,36] No other intervention has been definitively shown to improve survival or neurologic outcome. Approximately 5% to 10% of newly borns require some degree of active resuscitation at birth, including stimulation to breathe,[43] and approximately 1% to 10% born in-hospital may require assisted ventilation.[43,44]

Worldwide more than 5 million neonatal deaths occur annually, with asphyxia at birth responsible for approximately 19% of these deaths.[45] Implementation of relatively simple resuscitation techniques could save the lives of an estimated 1 million infants per year.[46,47] Organized, rapid delivery of out-of-hospital BLS and ALS has improved the outcome of drowning victims in cardiac arrest, perhaps the best-studied scenario of out-of-hospital cardiac arrest.[48]

Because most pediatric cardiac arrests are secondary to progressive respiratory failure, immediate CPR ("phone fast" rather than "phone first") is emphasized as the default approach in the pediatric Chain of Survival. Effective BLS should be provided for infants and children as quickly as possible. In some circumstances, however, primary arrhythmic cardiac arrest (ie, VF or pulseless VT) should be suspected. One example is the sudden collapse of a child, especially if the child has a history of underlying cardiac disease or a history of arrhythmias. In these circumstances it may be important to immediately activate the EMS system before beginning CPR.

Whenever multiple rescuers are present for the victim of any age, the first links in the Chain of Survival should be accomplished simultaneously. One rescuer should begin CPR while the other activates the emergency medical response system.

To simplify the message to the lay public, the adult Chain of Survival and resuscitation sequence ("phone first") and adult BLS techniques are generally used for victims 8 years of age and older in the out-of-hospital setting. Again, trained BLS and ALS providers should be aware of exceptions to the "phone first" approach in a victim this age (≥8 years). For example, immediate provision of bystander CPR is associated with improved early return of spontaneous circulation and neurologically intact survival for submersion victims of all ages.[48,49] Other victims 8 years of age and older who may benefit from immediate CPR include those with respiratory or cardiac arrest caused by trauma or respiratory arrest caused by drug overdose.

Whenever resuscitation is attempted or the need for it contemplated, the rescuer should determine if the physician, family, and child (as appropriate) have made a decision to limit resuscitative efforts or withhold resuscitation attempts. Legal issues and regulations regarding requirements for these no-CPR directives vary from country to country and, in the United States, from state to state. It is always important for families to inform EMS providers when such directives exist. For more information about the ethical issues of resuscitation, see Chapter 17.

Prevention of Common Infant, Child, and Adolescent Injuries and Emergencies Requiring Resuscitation

The first critical link in the pediatric Chain of Survival is prevention of the injury or illness (see Figure 2). Prevention efforts are most effective if they attempt to limit the most frequent injuries or illnesses for which effective prevention strategies are available. The leading cause of death in infants 1 month to 1 year of age is SIDS.

Critical Concepts:
Comparison of the Pediatric and Adult Chains of Survival

Pediatric links	Adult links
— Prevention	— Early EMS activation
— Early CPR	— Early CPR
— Early EMS activation	— Early defibrillation
— Early ALS	— Early ALS

Every healthcare professional should know how to activate resuscitation personnel and equipment resources in his/her work environment by dialing 911 or other local emergency response numbers.

FIGURE 2. AHA pediatric Chain of Survival. Link 1: Prevention of injury or arrest.

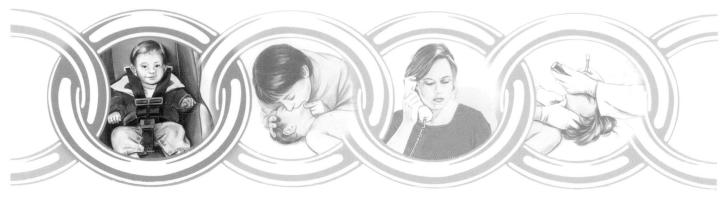

In Americans aged 1 to 44 years, injury is the leading cause of death. Injury is responsible for more childhood deaths than all other causes combined.[50,51] Internationally injuries are the leading cause of death for children 1 to 14 years of age as well as for young adults 15 to 24 years of age.[34,52] The 6 most common types of fatal childhood injuries amenable to prevention strategies are motor vehicle passenger injuries, pedestrian injuries, bicycle injuries, submersion, burns, and firearm injuries (Figure 3).[3,53] Prevention of these common fatal injuries would substantially reduce infant and child disability and deaths.

The Science of Injury Control

Prevention of deaths requires identification and elimination of risk factors for death. If you can identify and reduce risk factors for any cause of death in a community, you will reduce the number of deaths from that cause. Injury control attempts either to prevent the injury from occurring or to minimize its effects. Injury control operates in 3 phases: prevention, minimization of damage, and postinjury care. In planning injury prevention strategies, 3 principles deserve emphasis. First, passive injury prevention strategies are generally preferred because they are more likely to be used than active strategies, which require repeated, conscious effort. For example, seat belt–shoulder harnesses that automatically engage with closure of the car door (passive restraint) may ultimately protect more occupants of motor vehicles than restraints that require occupants to engage the locking mechanism

FIGURE 3. International injury deaths for children 1 to 14 years of age. From Fingerhut LA, Cox CS, Warner M. International comparative analysis of injury mortality: findings from the International Collaborative Effort (ICE) on injury statistics. Centers for Disease Control and Prevention, National Center for Health Statistics, No. 303, October 7, 1998.

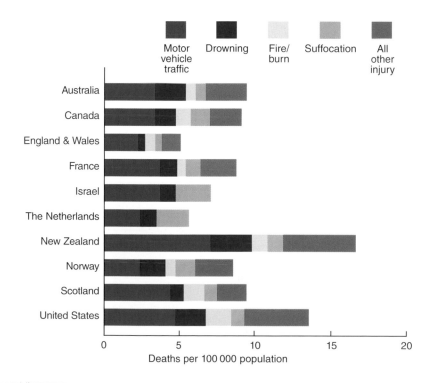

Foundation Facts: Injury Versus Accident

The term *injury* is emphasized rather than the term *accident* because an injury is often preventable. The term *accident* implies that nothing can be done to prevent the episode.

(active restraint) every time they ride in the car. Second, specific instructions (eg, keep water heater temperature lower than 120°F) are more likely to be followed than general advice (eg, reduce the temperature of hot tap water in your home). Third, individual education reinforced by community-wide educational programs will be more effective than isolated educational sessions.[54,55]

The Subcommittee on Pediatric Resuscitation has developed a safety checklist to help parents and childcare providers make their home and work environments as safe as possible for infants and children. This checklist can be used to inspect a home, childcare center, or any place where children spend time. The checklist is published in the following AHA publications: *BLS for Healthcare Providers, Fundamentals of BLS for Healthcare Providers,* the *BLS Instructor's Manual,* Appendix C. These

Foundation Facts:
Pediatric Chain of Survival— Reducing the Risk of SIDS and Injury

- SIDS is the most common cause of death in infants 6 months of age and younger. SIDS deaths have fallen dramatically throughout the world following educational campaigns to teach parents and childcare providers to put infants "back to sleep" (on their back or propped on their side rather than on their stomach) and avoiding the use of soft, fluffy bedding.

- Motor vehicle–related trauma is the most common cause of death in children from 6 months through young adulthood. Use of appropriate child seat restraints and lap–shoulder harnesses can prevent nearly half of motor vehicle–related child occupant deaths.

publications can be purchased from the AHA ECC distributors. The checklist is also posted on the AHA ECC website (**www.americanheart.org/cpr**). Healthcare providers are encouraged to use the checklist and to provide it to parents and childcare providers.

Reducing the Risk of SIDS

SIDS is the sudden death of an infant, typically between the ages of 1 month and 1 year, that is unexpected from the infant's history and unexplained by other causes when a postmortem examination is performed. SIDS probably represents a variety of conditions caused by several mechanisms, including rebreathing asphyxia with decreased arousal and possibly blunted response to hypoxemia or hypercarbia.[56] Many factors have been associated with an increased risk of SIDS, including prone sleeping position, winter months, lower family income, male gender, a mother who smokes cigarettes or is addicted to drugs, a history of apparent life-threatening events, and low birth weight.

SIDS occurs much more frequently in infants who sleep prone (on their stomach) than in infants who sleep supine (on their back) or on their side.[57-59] The prone position, particularly on a soft surface, is thought to contribute to rebreathing asphyxia.[56] This type of asphyxia occurs when air is trapped close to the infant's mouth and nose, resulting in rebreathing (breathing of expired air) and thus depletion of oxygen and accumulation of CO_2 in inspired air.

The supine sleeping position has not been associated with an increase in any significant adverse events, such as vomiting or aspiration.[57] The side position may be used, but infants placed in this position should be propped to prevent them from rolling to the prone position. In addition, infants should not sleep on soft surfaces such as lambs wool, fluffy comforters, or other objects that might trap exhaled air near the face. Investigators in Australia, New Zealand, and several European countries documented a significant reduction in the

incidence of SIDS when parents and childcare providers were taught to place healthy infants to sleep on their back (supine) or on their side.[60] This "back to sleep" public education campaign was introduced in the United States in 1992 and has been associated with a marked (more than 50%) reduction in SIDS deaths.[26]

Prevention of Motor Vehicle Injuries

Motor vehicle–related trauma accounts for nearly half of all pediatric injuries and deaths.[34,47,50] Contributing factors include failure to use proper passenger restraints, inexperienced adolescent drivers, and alcohol abuse. Proper use of age-appropriate child seat restraints and lap-shoulder harnesses could prevent an estimated 65% to 75% of serious injuries and fatalities to passengers younger than 4 years and 45% to 55% of all pediatric motor vehicle passenger injuries and deaths.[50,61]

Further development of passive restraint devices is needed, including adjustable shoulder harnesses, automatic lap and shoulder belts, and air bags. The benefits of air bags continue to far outweigh the risks. Since 1987 airbags have saved more than 5000 lives in the United States alone. Most of the 74 US children with fatal airbag-related injuries reported through April 1999 were improperly restrained for their age or not restrained at all. Within a few years cars will be equipped with so-called "smart airbags" that will automatically adjust rate/speed/force of inflation based on the weight of the passenger in the seat in front of the airbag.

Adolescent drivers are responsible for a disproportionate number of motor vehicle–related injuries. Surprisingly, adolescent driver education classes have increased the number of adolescent drivers at risk with no improvement in safety.[62-65] Approximately 50% of motor vehicle fatalities involving adolescents also involve alcohol. Although intoxication rates decreased for drivers of all age groups from 1987 to 1999, drunk drivers are still responsible

Foundation Facts: Child Passenger Safety

The following child passenger safety recommendations are from the American Academy of Pediatrics, the Centers for Disease Control and Prevention, and the National Highway Traffic Safety Administration:

1. Children should ride in rear-facing infant seats until they weigh at least 20 pounds (9 kg), are at least 1 year of age, and have good head control. These seats should be secured in the *back* seat of the automobile.

   ■ Never place a rear-facing safety seat in the front passenger seat of a car with a passenger-side airbag.

   ■ Convertible seats can be used for children younger than 1 year and weighing less than 20 pounds (9 kg) if the seats are placed in the reclined and rear-facing position.

2. A child who is older than 1 year and weighs 20 to 40 pounds (9 to 18 kg) can be placed in a convertible car safety seat used in the upright and forward-facing position as long as the child fits well in the seat. The harness straps should be positioned at or above the child's shoulders. These seats should also be placed in the *back* seat of the automobile.

3. Belt-positioning booster seats should be used for children weighing 40 to 80 pounds (18 to 36 kg) until they are at least 58 inches (4 feet, 10 inches or 148 cm) tall. These belt-positioning seats ensure that the lap and shoulder belts restrain the child over bones rather than soft tissues. The lap belt should be low and snug across the child's hips. The shoulder harness should cross from the child's clavicle across the sternum to the hip. The shoulder harness should not cross the child's neck.

4. Children may be restrained in automobile lap shoulder belts when they weigh 40 to 80 pounds (18 to 36 kg) and are at least 58 inches (4 feet, 10 inches or 148 cm) tall. A properly fitting lap-shoulder belt will lie low across the child's hips and flat across the shoulder and sternum, away from the neck and face. The child's legs should be long enough that the knees bend at the edge of the seat.

5. Children 12 years old and younger should not sit in the front seat of cars equipped with passenger-side air bags.[66,67]

   Note: Voluntary checkpoints for child-restraint devices sponsored by such organizations as Safe Kids and the National Highway Traffic Safety Administration have documented that most child-restraint devices in use are improperly installed in a manner that would significantly compromise their ability to protect the child. To ensure effective use of any child-restraint device, the device used must be appropriate for the age and size of the child, the child must be restrained properly in the device, and the device must be properly secured in the vehicle.

for a large proportion of all motor vehicle crashes and pose a significant risk to children.[50,68-72]

Prevention of Pedestrian Injuries

Pedestrian injuries are a leading cause of death among children 5 to 9 years of age in the United States.[47,53] Pedestrian injuries typically occur when a child darts into the street, crossing between intersections.[50] Although educational programs aimed at improving children's street-related behavior hold promise, roadway interventions, including adequate lighting, construction of sidewalks, and roadway barriers, must also be pursued in areas of high pedestrian traffic.

Prevention of Bicycle Injuries

Bicycle crashes are responsible for approximately 200 000 injuries and more than 600 deaths in children and adolescents in the United States every year.[47,73] Head injuries cause most bicycle injury–related morbidity and mortality.[74] It is estimated that bicycle helmets reduce the severity of head and brain injuries by approximately 85%. A successful bicycle helmet education program includes an ongoing, communitywide, multidisciplinary approach that provides focused information about the protection provided by a helmet and the need to wear the helmet whenever riding a bicycle. Such programs should ensure the acceptability, accessibility, and affordability of helmets.[73,75]

Prevention of Submersion and Drowning

Internationally submersion is responsible for approximately 15% of injury deaths in children 1 to 14 years of age.[34] It is a significant cause of disability and death in children younger than 4 years in the United States.[47,50,53,76,77]

Childcare providers should be aware of water hazards for children of all ages. Young children and children with seizure disorders should never be left unattended in bathtubs or near swimming pools, ponds, or beaches. Some submersion injuries and deaths in swimming pools may be prevented by completely surrounding the pool with appropriate fencing, including gates with secure latching mechanisms.[76,78] A house wall is not an effective barrier to the pool if it has a door opening to the pool area.

Children older than 5 years should learn to swim. No one should ever swim alone, and even supervised children should wear personal flotation devices when playing in rivers, streams, or lakes.

Alcohol is a significant risk factor for submersion injuries and deaths in adolescents.

Adolescent education, limiting access to alcohol, and the use of personal flotation devices on waterways should be encouraged.

Prevention of Burn Injuries

Fires, burns, and suffocation are a leading cause of injury death worldwide.[34] Approximately 80% of fire- and burn-related deaths result from house fires.[61,78-82] Most fire-related deaths occur in private residences, usually in homes without working smoke detectors.[61,79,80,83] *Smoke detectors are the most effective intervention for preventing death from burns and smoke inhalation.* When used correctly, smoke detectors can reduce fire-related death and severe injury by 86% to 88%.[80,83] Smoke detectors should be placed near or on the ceiling outside the doors to sleeping or napping rooms and on each floor at the top of the stairway. Families, schools, and childcare centers should develop and practice a fire evacuation plan. Continued improvements in flammability standards for furniture, bedding, and home builders' materials should further reduce the incidence of fire-related injuries and deaths.

Prevention of Firearm Injuries

Firearms, particularly handguns, are responsible for a large number of injuries and deaths in infants, children, and adolescents. Firearm-related injuries and deaths may be labeled as unintentional, homicide, or suicide.[26] Firearm homicide remains the leading cause of death among African-American adolescents and young adults and the second-highest cause of death among all adolescents and young adults in the United States, Norway, Israel, and France.[34,84,85] Firearms are used in an increasing proportion of child and adolescent suicides. Mortality (ratio of deaths to injury) from firearm injuries is highest in young children, whether the injury is unintentional or related to homicide or suicide.[86]

Most guns used in childhood unintentional shootings, school shootings, and suicides are from the home. Thirty-four percent of high school students surveyed reported easy access to guns, and an increasing number of children carry guns to school.[87-89] The mere presence of a gun in the home is associated with an increased likelihood of adolescent suicide.[90,91] Guns should be stored locked and unloaded, with ammunition stored separately from the gun. The use of trigger locks should be encouraged. The development and marketing of "smart" guns that can be fired by only the gun owner may particularly reduce the frequency of unintentional and suicide injuries.[92] But any strategy designed to reduce firearm-related deaths must be validated.

Prevention of Choking (Foreign-Body Airway Obstruction)

More than 90% of deaths from foreign-body aspiration in children occur in those younger than 5 years; 65% of victims are infants. With the development of consumer product safety standards regulating the minimum size of toys and toy parts for young children,[93,94] the incidence of foreign-body aspiration has decreased significantly. But toys, balloons, small objects, and foods (eg, hot dogs, round candies, nuts, seeds, grapes, and popcorn) may still cause foreign-body airway obstruction (FBAO)[95] and should be kept away from infants and small children. Children should not be permitted to eat while playing, because running and other play activities increase the risk of choking.

Early and Effective BLS and EMS Activation

Immediate bystander CPR (Figure 4) is crucial to survival from both respiratory and cardiac arrest. In both adult[18,23,24] and pediatric[32,35,47,48] studies, bystander CPR is linked to improved return of spontaneous circulation and neurologically intact survival. The greatest impact of bystander CPR will probably be on children with noncardiac (respiratory) causes of out-of-hospital arrest.[48,96] Two studies have described the outcomes of children who were successfully resuscitated solely by reported bystander CPR before arrival of EMS personnel.[32,36] A third study[48] documents the success of attempted "resuscitation" (including a variety of actions ranging from stimulation only and rescue breathing only to traditional ventilations and compressions) for pediatric submersion victims.

The true frequency of successful prehospital resuscitation is unknown but is likely underestimated because victims resuscitated by bystanders are often excluded from studies of out-of-hospital cardiac arrest. Unfortunately bystander CPR typically is provided for approximately ≤30% of pediatric victims of out-of-hospital arrest.[32,35] For further information about the effects of CPR and the relative merits of rescue breathing and chest compressions, see Chapter 3.

All the links in the Chain of Survival are connected. It is difficult to evaluate the effect of EMS system activation or specific EMS interventions in isolation. Local EMS and in-hospital emergency response team response intervals, dispatcher training, and protocols may dictate the most appropriate sequence of EMS activation and early life support interventions for a given situation.

Foundation Facts: Prevention of Foreign-Body Airway Obstruction (Choking)

High-risk objects for children less than 5 years of age

- Small toys
- Balloons
- Small objects
- Foods (eg, hot dogs, round candies, nuts, seeds, grapes, and popcorn)

FIGURE 4. AHA pediatric Chain of Survival. Link 2: Early and effective CPR. Link 3: Early EMS activation.

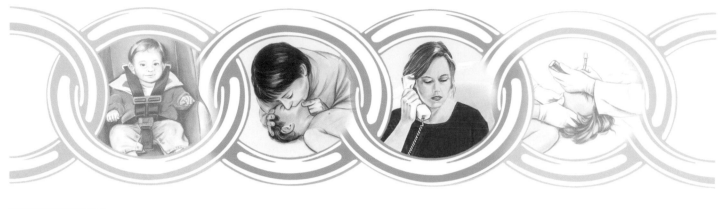

©2002 American Heart Association

It is important to remember that the phone first or phone fast sequence applies only to the lone rescuer. When multiple rescuers are present, EMS can be activated and CPR performed simultaneously—one rescuer remains with the victim of any age and begins CPR while another activates the EMS response system. It is unknown how frequently 2 or more lay responders are present during initial evaluation of a pediatric cardiopulmonary emergency.

Although rescuer exposure during CPR carries a theoretical risk of infectious disease transmission, the risk is very low.[97] Most out-of-hospital cardiac arrests in children occur at home, where it is likely that family members and care providers have already been exposed to that disease or are aware of the disease and keep appropriate barrier devices available. Surveys of family members indicate that risk of infection is not a concern that would prevent them from providing CPR to a loved one.

Advanced healthcare providers, family members, and lay rescuers of infants and children at high risk for cardiopulmonary emergencies should be taught a sequence of rescue actions tailored to the potential victim's specific condition.[98,99] Hospitals, medical facilities, and many businesses and building complexes have established emergency medical response systems onsite. Such systems notify rescuers of the location of an emergency and the type of response needed. If the cardiopulmonary emergency occurs in a facility with an established medical response system, that system should be known and notification of the system should be practiced.

Access to EMS Services

Entry into the EMS or emergency response system occurs when someone phones the EMS dispatcher or activates the EMS response team. The accessibility of this critical contact and the speed and quality of the dispatcher's response vary widely throughout the United States.

In the prehospital setting the universal emergency access number 911 is an excellent concept, but 911 is not yet universally available in the United States. "Enhanced 911" service is an improvement over the simple 911 access number. Enhanced 911 provides immediate computerized identification of the telephone number and location of the caller so that the dispatcher can send appropriate help regardless of the quality of information provided by the caller.

Currently about 25% of calls to 911 are from cellular phones. Federal legislation has mandated that in the next several years 911 calls from cellular phones be traceable.

EMS Dispatchers

EMS dispatcher protocols and training vary widely. The use of dispatcher protocols reduces the variability of information provided by dispatchers and ensures that succinct, accurate emergency information is provided to every caller. Protocols must be developed and implemented so that dispatchers can properly instruct callers in pediatric CPR, relief of FBAO, and essential first aid until EMS personnel arrive.[100,101] EMS services are sometimes underused in emergencies.[102,103]

EMS Response and Early ALS (Figure 5)

Preparation and Education

Approximately 10% of out-of-hospital EMS patients in both rural and urban areas are children less than 14 years of age.[104,105] Thus, it is mandatory that EMS personnel develop and maintain expertise in assessment and stabilization of infants and young children. If such experience cannot be maintained in the field, EMS personnel must arrange for pediatric-focused educational experiences.[1,8,106]

The optimal type of training required to ensure skilled provider performance is unclear. A nationwide survey of EMS training programs in 1993 documented that 97% of the programs included pediatric intubation in their curricula.[107]

FIGURE 5. AHA pediatric Chain of Survival. Link 4: Early ALS, including stabilization, transport, and rehabilitation.

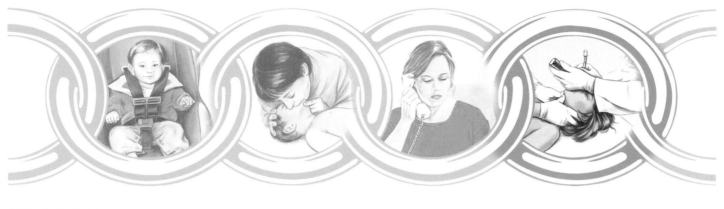

Methods of teaching intubation, however, varied widely. Paramedics can become proficient in intubating children in the operating room, but field intubation may require unique modification of these skills.[107] Many programs use only manikins for training; some use animal models. In retrospective studies, increased accuracy and a reduced complication rate for intubation have been associated with increased training (including supervised time spent in the operating room as well as in the field),[32,108] use of minimal requirements for ongoing experience, and use of paralytic agents.[32,109,110] In some EMS systems the success rate for pediatric intubation is relatively low and the complication rate high.[111]

In the only pediatric prospective, randomized, controlled trial in which bag-mask ventilation was compared with tracheal intubation in the prehospital setting, bag-mask ventilation was generally as effective as tracheal intubation. For the subgroup with respiratory failure, bag-mask ventilation was associated with an improved survival rate.[111] It is important to note that the transport times for this EMS study system were short; all providers received detailed training in bag-mask ventilation and tracheal intubation, but individual ALS providers had infrequent opportunities to perform pediatric intubation. Only approximately 5% of the nearly 3000 paramedics trained performed a single intubation in the 3-year study period.

Paramedics in 1-tiered systems typically do not have many opportunities to perform pediatric intubation because the need for intubation is infrequent among all pediatric EMS calls. In multitiered EMS systems the second tier of prehospital providers may have sufficient training and ongoing experience to perform intubation safely and effectively.[32] Dedicated critical care or interhospital transport personnel (including helicopter transport personnel) also may have a high success rate with tracheal intubation.[110,112] Many creative and innovative techniques for improved teaching and retention of resuscitative interventions are under study.[113]

This data shows that healthcare providers caring for infants and children require adequate initial training and ongoing experience for critical ALS interventions. EMS systems must also establish methods to monitor success, outcomes, and potential complications of interventions performed (quality-improvement monitoring). EMS response systems should ensure proper initial and ongoing training and continuous monitoring of the safety and effectiveness of critical ALS interventions.

ALS Equipment, Protocols, and Communication in the Prehospital, Physician Office, Transport, and Hospital Environments

All emergency response vehicles must contain specific equipment and supplies for provision of appropriate pediatric emergency care. Lists of suggested supplies and equipment are included in the Appendix to this chapter, Tables 1 and 2.

Communication between the EMS provider and the hospital should be guided by protocol so that critical information is not omitted during an emergency. These protocols should be in place before they are needed.

Pediatric physician offices and ambulatory and urgent care centers in which acutely ill and injured children are treated may not have the necessary equipment for pediatric emergency care.[114] To assist pediatricians in the development of community (and office) readiness for emergency care, the American Academy of Pediatrics has published guidelines for the role of the primary care provider in EMS for children.[115] A list of suggested supplies and equipment for the primary care office is included in the Appendix to this chapter, Table 3.

If possible, children with critical illness or multisystem trauma should be transported rapidly to trauma centers with pediatric expertise.[116-119] The value of aeromedical transport compared with ground transport of children with multiple trauma is unclear and should be evaluated by individual EMS systems.[120,121] Depending on the characteristics of each EMS system, it is likely that one mode of transport will be favored over the other.

Interfacility transfer agreements, provision of PICU transport team services, and educational outreach by PICUs to community hospitals may also improve outcome (see Chapter 9: "Postarrest Stabilization and Transport").[122] Ideally the appropriate level of ALS expertise, equipment, and support should accompany the patient throughout resuscitation, stabilization, recovery, and rehabilitation (see the Appendix to this chapter, Tables 4 and 5).

Rehabilitation should begin when the child enters the EMS system and continue until the child has reached his/her full potential. The goal of rehabilitation is to achieve an optimal level of function by restoring or enhancing impaired or residual biologic function.

To improve outcomes for critically ill and injured infants, children, and young adults, all EMS-C components must be integrated into existing EMS systems. All responders must be educated to activate EMS appropriately and provide first aid and BLS until help arrives.[2,123]

Summary Points

The pediatric Chain of Survival begins with injury prevention as the most effective way to ensure a good outcome. Early and effective CPR should be provided, followed by rapid activation of the EMS response team to bring trained providers and ALS equipment and expertise to the victim. ALS should be coordinated to provide appropriate resuscitation, stabilization, transport, and rehabilitative care.

Initial priority is given to support of oxygenation and ventilation unless special resuscitation circumstances are known or suspected. AHA healthcare providers should know how to activate and respond to pediatric emergencies within the scope of their care.

■ The 4 links in the AHA Pediatric Chain of Survival are prevention of illness or injury (prevent the arrest), early CPR, early EMS activation, and early ALS.

■ The outcome of pediatric cardiac arrest is dismal; prevention will likely save more lives than resuscitation attempts.

■ Simple strategies can prevent many of the major causes of fatal injuries in children.

■ The lone rescuer should begin CPR and phone EMS after about 1 minute (phone fast) for most causes of pediatric cardiopulmonary arrest and for adult (8 years of age and older) victims of submersion, injury, or drug overdose. The lone rescuer should phone first if the child collapses suddenly or has a history of heart disease or the suspected cause of the arrest is cardiac.

■ Early CPR is essential for pediatric victims of out-of-hospital arrest, particularly when the arrest is likely caused by respiratory failure or even respiratory failure and shock.

■ EMS systems must be equipped to care for children and trained to provide appropriate care. Appropriate quality-improvement monitoring is required for treatments such as prehospital intubation.

Case Scenarios
Case Scenario 1

The parents of a 2-month-old boy find him pale, limp, and blue in his crib. He is surrounded by a soft comforter and is lying prone (on his stomach), with no obvious injury or evidence of emesis. He was previously healthy, receiving no medications, and had taken his bottle normally about 4 hours before being placed in the crib. He is unresponsive to verbal or tactile stimulation and does not appear to be breathing.

Acceptable Actions: Interventions

The following actions are generally *acceptable* for assessment and management of the infant in this scenario:

■ Complete a rapid cardiopulmonary assessment, confirm unresponsiveness, shout for help, open the airway, confirm lack of normal or adequate breathing, deliver 2 effective breaths, and then check for signs of circulation. If no signs of circulation are present, begin chest compressions.

■ If you are alone with the infant, perform CPR for approximately 1 minute, then activate the EMS system (phone 911).

Rationale for Acceptable Actions

■ *Rapid cardiopulmonary assessment:* You must be able to rapidly recognize the emergency and confirm that the infant is unresponsive.

■ *Early activation of EMS by phoning 911* is ideal when a second rescuer is present. Arrest in infants and children is most frequently respiratory in origin, so the lone rescuer should provide approximately 1 minute of CPR *before* leaving the infant to activate the EMS system. This sequence differs from the phone-first approach advocated for adults. In adults with sudden cardiac arrest, time to defibrillation is crucial, so EMS must be activated first.

■ If this infant had a history of heart disease, it would be appropriate for the lone rescuer to phone first (activate the EMS system before beginning CPR) to hasten the arrival of a defibrillator with ACLS personnel and equipment.

■ The 4 major links in the pediatric Chain of Survival are

— Prevention

— Early and effective CPR

— Early EMS activation

— Early ALS, including stabilization, transport, and rehabilitation

Acceptable Actions: Risk Reduction

Many factors are associated with an increased risk of SIDS: prone sleeping position, winter months, lower family income, male gender, a mother who smokes cigarettes or is addicted to drugs, and low birth weight. To reduce the risk of SIDS:

- Place healthy infants on their back to sleep

- Do not place infants on soft, fluffy sleeping surfaces

- Remove objects that might trap air near the infant's face from the crib

Reducing risk will not *eliminate* SIDS. But these measures have been linked to a *reduced incidence* of SIDS.

Case Scenario 1 Progression

After approximately 1 minute of CPR and simultaneous activation of EMS, the following information is provided to EMS: the location of the emergency, the telephone number from which the call is being made, what happened, the number of victims, the condition of the victim(s), and the nature of the aid being given. EMS personnel arrive and note that the infant has occasional spontaneous breaths and a pulse of 60 bpm. They provide oxygen and assisted bag mask ventilation as they prepare to transport the infant to the hospital.

Case Scenario 2

A 3-year-old child is sitting unrestrained in the rear seat of a motor vehicle when it crashes. The child is ejected from the car and thrown 10 feet onto the pavement. The car appears to be leaking radiator fluid or coolant, but the fluid is not in contact with the child. The child was momentarily unresponsive but breathing. He is now responsive, moaning, and clutching his right thigh. The adolescent driver of the car, who was wearing a seat belt, is awake and walking without pain or problem. You and several other witnesses rush to the child's side.

Acceptable Actions

The following actions are generally performed to prevent motor vehicle injury and reduce the risk of further injury at the scene of an automobile crash:

- *Activate* appropriate fire, police, and EMS services. If several rescuers are present, EMS can be activated while scene safety is ensured.

- *Ensure scene safety:*
  — Ensure that the child and rescuers are out of the line of traffic and that traffic is diverted.
  — Minimize explosion hazards.

- *Avoid unnecessary movement of the injured victim:*
  — Do not move the child unless the scene is unsafe for the victim or rescuers. There is no evidence in this scenario to suggest that the scene is unsafe.
  — Carefully move the child or other victims away from the scene if there is a risk of fire or other dangers. Immobilize the victim's spine during any movement.

- Once the scene is safe, *assess the child's responsiveness and begin to assess and support the ABCs of CPR:*
  — If the child becomes unresponsive, open and maintain the airway; immobilize the cervical spine because the mechanism of injury may cause head or neck injury.
  — Evaluate breathing and circulation and provide support as necessary.

Rationale for Acceptable Actions

- *Be sure that the EMS system is activated,* particularly if multiple rescuers are present.

- *Ensure scene safety.* If victims are in or near a burning building, in the water, or near electrical wires or other flammable hazards, the rescuer must first ensure that both the victim and rescuers are safe. In this case the leaking coolant posed no apparent hazard. If the car were burning, it would be necessary to move victims located in or near the car.

- *Avoid unnecessary movement of the victim.* Movement of trauma victims increases the risk of spinal cord injury.

- *Assess and support the ABCs with spine immobilization.* Use a jaw thrust rather than a head tilt–chin lift to open the airway in a trauma victim.

Acceptable Actions: Risk Reduction

Prevention of motor vehicle injury: Motor vehicle–related trauma accounts for nearly half of all pediatric injuries and deaths in the United States. Contributing factors include failure to use proper passenger restraints, inexperienced adolescent drivers, excessive speed, and alcohol abuse. Proper use of child seat restraints and lap-shoulder harnesses will prevent an estimated 50% of all pediatric motor vehicle passenger injuries and deaths.

Case Scenario 2 Progression

While a bystander activates the EMS system by cell phone and provides appropriate information, you ask additional bystanders to divert traffic around and away from the crash. You approach the child and confirm that he is responsive and breathing adequately. You and another bystander immobilize the child (including the head, neck, torso, and femur).

EMS personnel arrive within 4 minutes and confirm that police, fire, and rescue vehicles have been dispatched. EMS rescuers confirm that the leaking fluid from the car is not a significant hazard at this time and that responding personnel have diverted traffic. Using universal precautions, EMS personnel rapidly evaluate the child and stabilize him for transport, carefully immobilizing his spine during this process.

Review Questions

1. **Of the 4 links in the pediatric Chain of Survival, which link is *most likely* to have the *greatest* effect on reducing morbidity and mortality in infants and children?**

   a. prevention

   b. early CPR

   c. early EMS activation

   d. early ALS, including stabilization, transport, and rehabilitation

   The correct answer is a. All 4 links in the pediatric Chain of Survival are important, but prevention most effectively reduces morbidity and mortality in infants and children.

   Answer b is incorrect because survival from pulseless cardiac arrest remains low despite provision of basic and advanced life support.

   Answers c and **d** are incorrect also. Although early EMS activation and early ALS are important, prevention of the cause of arrest and immediate restoration of oxygenation and ventilation are more likely to reduce childhood disability and death.

2. **A 3-month-old full-term infant is put to bed after a normal feeding. The infant is placed prone (on his stomach) on a flat surface free of fluffy covers. When his caretaker checks on him, he appears limp, cyanotic, and apneic. What is the *most important* risk factor for SIDS that *parents* can modify *after* the infant is born?**

   a. male gender

   b. winter months

   c. prone sleeping position

   d. low birth weight

   The correct answer is c. The supine sleeping position ("back to sleep") and avoidance of soft, fluffy sleeping surfaces and objects that might trap exhaled air near the infant's face have *reduced the frequency* of SIDS. Unfortunately these measures will not eliminate SIDS or prevent it in every infant. SIDS is probably multifactorial; some SIDS deaths will occur despite use of the supine sleeping position and avoidance of fluffy sleeping surfaces.

   Answers a and **b** are incorrect because male gender and winter months, both risk factors for SIDS, cannot be modified.

   Answer d is also incorrect. Although prenatal care can prevent low birth weight in some infants, it cannot prevent it in all infants, and low birth weight cannot be modified after birth.

3. **You are a healthcare provider accompanying a 3-year-old patient to the Radiology Department. The child needs a lateral neck x-ray to evaluate croup and respiratory distress. The radiology technician leaves the room, and you are alone with the child. As the child rests supine on the x-ray table, he becomes acutely distressed with cyanosis, retractions, and nasal flaring. The pulse oximeter indicates oxyhemoglobin desaturation to less than 60%, and the child becomes unresponsive to verbal or painful stimuli. You shout for help. What should you do *next*?**

   a. leave the patient to phone 911 or the hospital emergency activation number

   b. use universal precautions, open the airway, and check breathing; if there is no breathing or no adequate breathing, attempt rescue breathing

   c. check the pulse oximeter for malfunction and call a respiratory therapist to prepare a nasal cannula

   d. open the airway but do not provide rescue breathing unless a bag and mask are available

   The correct answer is b. Whenever you are alone with a patient in acute respiratory failure in the hospital, you should shout for help (which was done in the scenario) and begin the ABCs of CPR.

   Answer a is incorrect because leaving the patient to activate the emergency response team will delay the immediate support of airway and breathing that this child needs.

   Answer c is incorrect because the patient exhibits clinical signs and symptoms of hypoxemia. Checking the equipment is reasonable in many cases, but this patient requires immediate support of breathing.

   Answer d is incorrect because this child needs immediate support of breathing.

4. **You are alone when you see your neighbors' 13-year-old daughter floating facedown in their swimming pool. She is unresponsive, limp, and cyanotic when you pull her from the water. You did not see her enter the water. Which of the following best summarizes the first steps you should take to maximize this adolescent's chance of survival?**

   a. shout for help, open her airway with a jaw thrust while keeping her cervical spine immobilized, check breathing, and provide 2 rescue breaths if she is not breathing adequately

   b. carefully lay her on the ground, leave her to phone 911, and then return, open her airway, and continue the steps of CPR

   c. immediately begin cycles of 5 chest compressions and 1 ventilation

   d. shout for help, and if no one arrives, open her airway with a head tilt–chin lift, check breathing, and provide 2 rescue breaths if she is not breathing adequately

The correct answer is a. This victim is 13 years old. Although she falls within the *age* category for the adult sequence of BLS actions, which generally directs the lone rescuer to phone first before beginning the steps of CPR, submersion is a special resuscitation situation for victims of *all* ages. All submersion victims need immediate rescue breathing if they are not breathing when they are removed from the water. Whenever you rescue a submersion victim and the submersion was not witnessed, you should presume that head and neck injuries (eg, a diving injury) are present. You should immobilize the cervical spine and open the airway using a jaw thrust.

Answer b is incorrect because you should immediately check breathing and provide rescue breathing if the victim is not breathing adequately. You should not follow the typical adult sequence of resuscitation for submersion victims.

Answer c is incorrect because, first, you should not begin chest compressions unless there are no signs of circulation after you have delivered 2 rescue breaths. Second, a compression-ventilation ratio of 5:1 is recommended for children 1 to 8 years of age, but a ratio of 15:2 is recommended for children 8 years of age and older and for adults, particularly for prehospital BLS.

Answer d is incorrect because you should not use a head tilt–chin lift to open the airway. The victim may have a head or neck injury. You should treat all submersion victims as though they have a head or neck injury unless you witnessed submersion without trauma.

References

1. Seidel JS, Henderson DP, ed. *Emergency Medical Services for Children: A Report to the Nation.* Washington, DC: National Academy Press; 1991.

2. Durch J, Lohr KN. *Emergency Medical Services for Children.* Washington, DC: National Academy Press; 1993.

3. Care of children in the emergency department: guidelines for preparedness. *Ann Emerg Med.* 2001;37:423-427.

4. Care of children in the emergency department: guidelines for preparedness. *Pediatrics.* 2001;107:777-781.

5. Newacheck PW, Strickland B, Shonkoff JP, Perrin JM, McPherson M, McManus M, Lauver C, Fox H, Arango P. An epidemiologic profile of children with special health care needs. *Pediatrics.* 1998;102:117-123.

6. McPherson M, Arango P, Fox H, Lauver C, McManus M, Newacheck PW, Perrin JM, Shonkoff JP, Strickland B. A new definition of children with special health care needs. *Pediatrics.* 1998;102:137-140.

7. Committee on Pediatric Emergency Medicine, American Academy of Pediatrics. Emergency preparedness for children with special health care needs. *Pediatrics.* 1999;104:e53.

8. Seidel JS. Emergency medical services and the pediatric patient: are the needs being met? II: training and equipping emergency medical services providers for pediatric emergencies. *Pediatrics.* 1986;78:808-812.

9. Seidel JS. EMS-C in urban and rural areas: the California experience. In: Haller JA Jr, ed. *Emergency Medical Services for Children: Report of the 97th Ross Conference on Pediatric Research.* Columbus, Ohio: Ross Laboratories; 1989.

10. Applebaum D. Advanced prehospital care for pediatric emergencies. *Ann Emerg Med.* 1985;14:656-659.

11. Zaritsky A, French JP, Schafermeyer R, Morton D. A statewide evaluation of pediatric prehospital and hospital emergency services. *Arch Pediatr Adolesc Med.* 1994;148:76-81.

12. Graham CJ, Stuemky J, Lera TA. Emergency medical services preparedness for pediatric emergencies. *Pediatr Emerg Care.* 1993;9:329-331.

13. Cook RT Jr. The Institute of Medicine report on emergency medical services for children: thoughts for emergency medical technicians, paramedics, and emergency physicians. *Pediatrics.* 1995;96:199-206.

14. Makhmudova NM, Urinbaev MZ, Pak MA, Abukov MI, Faizieva NP. Organization of emergency medical services for the children in Tashkent [in Russian]. *Sov Zdravookhr.* 1990;55-59.

15. Foltin GL. Critical issues in urban emergency medical services for children. *Pediatrics.* 1995;96:174-179.

16. Cummins RO, Chamberlain D, Hazinski MF, Nadkarni V, Kloeck W, Kramer E, Becker L, Robertson C, Koster R, Zaritsky A, Bossaert L, Ornato JP, Callanan V, Allen M, Steen P, Connolly B, Sanders A, Idris A, Cobbe S. Recommended guidelines for reviewing, reporting, and conducting research on in-hospital resuscitation: the in-hospital 'Utstein style.' American Heart Association. *Circulation.* 1997;95:2213-2239.

17. Cummins RO. From concept to standard-of-care? Review of the clinical experience with automated external defibrillators. *Ann Emerg Med.* 1989;18:1269-1275.

18. Larsen MP, Eisenberg MS, Cummins RO, Hallstrom AP. Predicting survival from out-of-hospital cardiac arrest: a graphic model. *Ann Emerg Med.* 1993;22:1652-1658.

19. White RD, Vukov LF, Bugliosi TF. Early defibrillation by police: initial experience with measurement of critical time intervals and patient outcome. *Ann Emerg Med.* 1994;23:1009-1013.

20. Ladwig KH, Schoefinius A, Danner R, Gurtler R, Herman R, Koeppel A, Hauber P. Effects of early defibrillation by ambulance personnel on short- and long-term outcome of cardiac arrest survival: the Munich experiment. *Chest.* 1997;112:1584-1591.

21. Stiell IG, Wells GA, Field BJ, Spaite DW, De Maio VJ, Ward R, Munkley DP, Lyver MB, Luinstra LG, Campeau T, Maloney J, Dagnone E. Improved out-of-hospital cardiac arrest survival through the inexpensive optimization of an existing defibrillation program: OPALS study phase II. Ontario Prehospital Advanced Life Support. *JAMA.* 1999;281:1175-1181.

22. White RD, Hankins DG, Bugliosi TF. Seven years' experience with early defibrillation by police and paramedics in an emergency medical services system. *Resuscitation.* 1998;39:145-151.

23. Van Hoeyweghen RJ, Bossaert LL, Mullie A, Calle P, Martens P, Buylaert WA, Delooz H. Quality and efficiency of bystander CPR. Belgian Cerebral Resuscitation Study Group. *Resuscitation.* 1993;26:47-52.

24. Bossaert L, Van Hoeyweghen R. Bystander cardiopulmonary resuscitation (CPR) in out-of-hospital cardiac arrest. The Cerebral Resuscitation Study Group. *Resuscitation.* 1989;17(suppl):S55-S69.

25. Nadkarni V, Hazinski MF, Zideman D, Kattwinkel J, Quan L, Bingham R, Zaritsky A, Bland J, Kramer E, Tiballs J. Pediatric resuscitation: an advisory statement from the Pediatric Working Group of the International Liaison Committee on Resuscitation. *Circulation.* 1997;95:2185-2195.

26. Hoyert DL, Kochanek KD, Murphy SL. Deaths: final data for 1997. *Natl Vital Stat Rep.* 1999;47:1-104.

27. Slonim AD, Patel KM, Ruttimann UE, Pollack MM. Cardiopulmonary resuscitation in pediatric intensive care units. *Crit Care Med.* 1997;25:1951-1955.

28. Richman PB, Nashed AH. The etiology of cardiac arrest in children and young adults: special considerations for ED management. *Am J Emerg Med.* 1999;17:264-270.

29. Kuisma M, Suominen P, Korpela R. Paediatric out-of-hospital cardiac arrests: epidemiology and outcome. *Resuscitation.* 1995; 30:141-150.

30. Kuisma M, Maatta T, Repo J. Cardiac arrests witnessed by EMS personnel in a multitiered system: epidemiology and outcome. *Am J Emerg Med.* 1998;16:12-16.

31. Finer NN, Horbar JD, Carpenter JH. Cardiopulmonary resuscitation in the very low birth weight infant: the Vermont Oxford Network experience. *Pediatrics.* 1999; 104:428-434.

32. Sirbaugh PE, Pepe PE, Shook JE, Kimball KT, Goldman MJ, Ward MA, Mann DM. A prospective, population-based study of the demographics, epidemiology, management, and outcome of out-of-hospital pediatric cardiopulmonary arrest. *Ann Emerg Med.* 1999; 33:174-184.

33. Zaritsky A. Outcome following cardiopulmonary resuscitation in the pediatric intensive care unit. *Crit Care Med.* 1997;25:1937-1938.

34. Fingerhut LA, Cox CS, Warner M. International comparative analysis of injury mortality: findings from the ICE on injury statistics. International Collaborative Effort on Injury Statistics. *Adv Data.* 1998;1-20.

35. Young KD, Seidel JS. Pediatric cardiopulmonary resuscitation: a collective review. *Ann Emerg Med.* 1999;33:195-205.

36. Hickey RW, Cohen DM, Strausbaugh S, Dietrich AM. Pediatric patients requiring CPR in the prehospital setting. *Ann Emerg Med.* 1995;25:495-501.

37. Appleton GO, Cummins RO, Larson MP, Graves JR. CPR and the single rescuer: at what age should you "call first" rather than "call fast"? *Ann Emerg Med.* 1995;25:492-494.

38. Mogayzel C, Quan L, Graves JR, Tiedeman D, Fahrenbruch C, Herndon P. Out-of-hospital ventricular fibrillation in children and adolescents: causes and outcomes. *Ann Emerg Med.* 1995;25:484-491.

39. Dieckmann RA, Vardis R. High-dose epinephrine in pediatric out-of-hospital cardiopulmonary arrest. *Pediatrics.* 1995;95:901-913.

40. Losek JD, Hennes H, Glaeser PW, Smith DS, Hendley G. Prehospital countershock treatment of pediatric asystole. *Am J Emerg Med.* 1989;7:571-575.

41. Friesen RM, Duncan P, Tweed WA, Bristow G. Appraisal of pediatric cardiopulmonary resuscitation. *Can Med Assoc J.* 1982;126: 1055-1058.

42. Zaritsky A, Nadkarni V, Getson P, Kuehl K. CPR in children. *Ann Emerg Med.* 1987;16: 1107-1111.

43. Saugstad OD. Practical aspects of resuscitating asphyxiated newborn infants. *Eur J Pediatr.* 1998;157(suppl 1):S11-S15.

44. Palme-Kilander C. Methods of resuscitation in low-Apgar-score newborn infants:a national survey. *Acta Paediatr.* 1992;81:739-744.

45. *The World Health Report: Report of the Director-General.* Geneva, Switzerland: World Health Organization; 1995.

46. Kattwinkel J, Niermeyer S, Nadkarni V, Tibballs J, Phillips B, Zideman D, Van Reempts P, Osmond M. An advisory statement from the Pediatric Working Group of the International Liaison Committee on Resuscitation. *Pediatrics.* 1999;103:e56.

47. Childhood injuries in the United States. Division of Injury Control, Center for Environmental Health and Injury Control, Centers for Disease Control. *Am J Dis Child.* 1990; 144:627-646.

48. Kyriacou DN, Arcinue EL, Peek C, Kraus JF. Effect of immediate resuscitation on children with submersion injury. *Pediatrics.* 1994;94: 137-142.

49. Rosen P, Stoto M, Harley J. The use of the Heimlich maneuver in near drowning: Institute of Medicine report. *J Emerg Med.* 1995; 13:397-405.

50. *1999 Injury Facts.* Itasca, Ill: National Safety Council; 1999.

51. Peters KD, Kochanek KD, Murphy SL. Deaths: final data for 1996. *Natl Vital Stat Rep.* 1998;47:1-100.

52. Danseco ER, Miller TR, Spicer RS. Incidence and costs of 1987-1994 childhood injuries: demographic breakdowns. *Pediatrics.* 2000; 105:E27.

53. From the Centers for Disease Control. Fatal injuries to children—United States, 1986. *JAMA.* 1990;264:952-953.

54. Guyer B, Ellers B. Childhood injuries in the United States: mortality, morbidity, and cost. *Am J Dis Child.* 1990;144:649-652.

55. Cushman R, James W, Waclawik H. Physicians promoting bicycle helmets for children: a randomized trial. *Am J Public Health.* 1991; 81:1044-1046.

56. Brooks JG. Sudden infant death syndrome. *Pediatr Ann.* 1995;24:345-383.

57. Positioning and sudden infant death syndrome (SIDS): update. American Academy of Pediatrics Task Force on Infant Positioning and SIDS. *Pediatrics.* 1996;98:1216-1218.

58. American Academy of Pediatrics AAP Task Force on Infant Positioning and SIDS: Positioning and SIDS. *Pediatrics.* 1992; 89:1120-1126.

59. Willinger M, Hoffman HJ, Hartford RB. Infant sleep position and risk for sudden infant death syndrome: report of meeting held January 13 and 14, 1994, National Institutes of Health, Bethesda, MD. *Pediatrics.* 1994; 93:814-819.

60. Mitchell EA, Scragg R. Observations on ethnic differences in SIDS mortality in New Zealand. *Early Hum Dev.* 1994;38:151-157.

61. Injury prevention: meeting the challenge. The National Committee for Injury Prevention and Control. *Am J Prev Med.* 1989;5:1-303.

62. Patel DR, Greydanus DE, Rowlett JD. Romance with the automobile in the 20th century: implications for adolescents in a new millennium. *Adolesc Med.* 2000;11:127-139.

63. Harre N, Field J. Safe driving education programs at school: lessons from New Zealand. *Aust N Z J Public Health.* 1998;22:447-450.

64. Brown RC, Gains MJ, Greydanus DE, Schonberg SK. Driver education: position paper of the Society for Adolescent Medicine. *J Adolesc Health.* 1997;21:416-418.

65. Robertson LS. Crash involvement of teenaged drivers when driver education is eliminated from high school. *Am J Public Health.* 1980; 70:599-603.

66. Giguere JF, St-Vil D, Turmel A, Di Lorenzo M, Pothel C, Manseau S, Mercier C. Airbags and children: a spectrum of C-spine injuries. *J Pediatr Surg.* 1998;33:811-816.

67. Bourke GJ. Airbags and fatal injuries to children. *Lancet.* 1996;347:560.

68. Margolis LH, Kotch J, Lacey JH. Children in alcohol-related motor vehicle crashes. *Pediatrics.* 1986;77:870-872.

69. O'Malley PM, Johnston LD. Drinking and driving among US high school seniors, 1984-1997. *Am J Public Health.* 1999;89:678-684.

70. Lee JA, Jones-Webb RJ, Short BJ, Wagenaar AC. Drinking location and risk of alcohol-impaired driving among high school seniors. *Addict Behav.* 1997;22:387-393.

71. Quinlan KP, Brewer RD, Sleet DA, Dellinger AM. Characteristics of child passenger deaths and injuries involving drinking drivers. *JAMA.* 2000;283:2249-2252.

72. Margolis LH, Foss RD, Tolbert WG. Alcohol and motor vehicle-related deaths of children as passengers, pedestrians, and bicyclists. *JAMA.* 2000;283:2245-2248.

73. DiGuiseppi CG, Rivara FP, Koepsell TD, Polissar L. Bicycle helmet use by children:

74. Thompson RS, Rivara FP, Thompson DC. A case-control study of the effectiveness of bicycle safety helmets. *N Engl J Med*. 1989; 320:1361-1367.

75. DiGuiseppi CG, Rivara FP, Koepsell TD. Attitudes toward bicycle helmet ownership and use by school-age children. *Am J Dis Child*. 1990;144:83-86.

76. Byard RW, Lipsett J. Drowning deaths in toddlers and preambulatory children in South Australia. *Am J Forensic Med Pathol*. 1999; 20:328-332.

77. Sachdeva RC. Near drowning. *Crit Care Clin*. 1999;15:281-296.

78. Fergusson DM, Horwood LJ. Risks of drowning in fenced and unfenced domestic swimming pools. *N Z Med J*. 1984;97:777-779.

79. Forjuoh SN, Coben JH, Dearwater SR, Weiss HB. Identifying homes with inadequate smoke detector protection from residential fires in Pennsylvania. *J Burn Care Rehabil*. 1997;18:86-91.

80. Marshall SW, Runyan CW, Bangdiwala SI, Linzer MA, Sacks JJ, Butts JD. Fatal residential fires: who dies and who survives? *JAMA*. 1998;279:1633-1637.

81. Rice DP, E.J. MacKenzie and Associates. *Cost of Injury in the United States: A Report to Congress*. Atlanta, Ga: Division of Injury, Epidemiology, and Control, Center for Environmental Health and Injury Control, Centers for Disease Control; 1989.

82. Hall J, Quincy M, Karter M. National Safety Council Tabulations of National Center for Health Statistics Mortality Data. 1999.

83. *An Evaluation of Residential Smoke Detector Performance Under Actual Field Conditions*. Washington, DC: Federal Emergency Management Agency; 1980.

84. Fingerhut LA, Ingram DD, Feldman JJ. Firearm homicide among black teenage males in metropolitan counties. Comparison of death rates in two periods, 1983 through 1985 and 1987 through 1989. *JAMA*. 1992;267:3054-3058.

85. Fingerhut LA. Firearm mortality among children, youth, and young adults 1–34 years of age, trends and current status: United States, 1985-90. *Adv Data*. 1993;1-20.

86. Beaman V, Annest JL, Mercy JA, Kresnow MJ, Pollock DA. Lethality of firearm-related injuries in the United States population. *Ann Emerg Med*. 2000;35:258-266.

87. Callahan CM, Rivara FP. Urban high school youth and handguns: a school-based survey. *JAMA*. 1992;267:3038-3042.

88. Cohen LR, Potter LB. Injuries and violence: risk factors and opportunities for prevention during adolescence. *Adolesc Med*. 1999;10: 125-135.

89. Simon TR, Crosby AE, Dahlberg LL. Students who carry weapons to high school: comparison with other weapon-carriers. *J Adolesc Health*. 1999;24:340-348.

90. Brent DA, Perper JA, Allman CJ, Moritz GM, Wartella ME, Zelenak JP. The presence and accessibility of firearms in the homes of adolescent suicides: a case-control study. *JAMA*. 1991;266:2989-2995.

91. Svenson JE, Spurlock C, Nypaver M. Pediatric firearm-related fatalities: not just an urban problem. *Arch Pediatr Adolesc Med*. 1996;150:583-587.

92. Rivara FP, Grossman DC, Cummings P. Injury prevention: second of two parts. *N Engl J Med*. 1997;337:613-618.

93. Reilly JS. Prevention of aspiration in infants and young children: federal regulations. *Ann Otol Rhinol Laryngol*. 1990;99:273-276.

94. Harris CS, Baker SP, Smith GA, Harris RM. Childhood asphyxiation by food: a national analysis and overview. *JAMA*. 1984;251: 2231-2235.

95. Rimell FL, Thome A Jr, Stool S, Reilly JS, Rider G, Stool D, Wilson CL. Characteristics of objects that cause choking in children. *JAMA*. 1995;274:1763-1766.

96. Kuisma M, Alaspaa A. Out-of-hospital cardiac arrests of non-cardiac origin. Epidemiology and outcome. *Eur Heart J*. 1997;18:1122-1128.

97. Mejicano GC, Maki DG. Infections acquired during cardiopulmonary resuscitation: estimating the risk and defining strategies for prevention. *Ann Intern Med*. 1998;129:813-828.

98. Hazinski MF. Is pediatric resuscitation unique? Relative merits of early CPR and ventilation versus early defibrillation for young victims of prehospital cardiac arrest. *Ann Emerg Med*. 1995;25:540-543.

99. Montgomery WH, Brown DD, Hazinski MF, Clawsen J, Newell LD, Flint L. Citizen response to cardiopulmonary emergencies. *Ann Emerg Med*. 1993;22:428-434.

100. Dieckmann RA. Pediatrics in the EMS: the effect of dispatch center and base hospitals on the quality of field care. *Pediatr Emerg Care*. 1990;6:76-77.

101. Clawson JJ. Telephone treatment protocols: reach out and help someone. *J Emerg Med Serv*. 1986;11:43-46.

102. Knolle LL, McDermott RJ, Ritzel DO. Knowledge of access to and use of the emergency medical services system in a rural Illinois county. *Am J Prev Med*. 1989;5:164-169.

103. White-Means SI, Thornton MC, Yeo JS. Sociodemographic and health factors influencing black and Hispanic use of the hospital emergency room. *J Natl Med Assoc*. 1989;81:72-80.

104. Seidel JS, Henderson DP, Ward P, Wayland BW, Ness B. Pediatric prehospital care in urban and rural areas. *Pediatrics*. 1991;88: 681-690.

105. Tsai A, Kallsen G. Epidemiology of pediatric prehospital care. *Ann Emerg Med*. 1987;16:284-292.

106. Sinclair LM, Baker MD. Police involvement in pediatric prehospital care. *Pediatrics*. 1991;87:636-641.

107. Stratton SJ, Underwood LA, Whalen SM, Gunter CS. Prehospital pediatric endotracheal intubation: a survey of the United States. *Prehospital Disaster Med*. 1993; 8:323-326.

108. Brownstein DR, Quan L, Orr R, Wentz KR, Copass MK. Paramedic intubation training in a pediatric operating room. *Am J Emerg Med*. 1992;10:418-420.

109. Ma OJ, Atchley RB, Hatley T, Green M, Young J, Brady W. Intubation success rates improve for an air medical program after implementing the use of neuromuscular blocking agents. *Am J Emerg Med*. 1998; 16:125-127.

110. Sing RF, Rotondo MF, Zonies DH, Schwab CW, Kauder DR, Ross SE, Brathwaite CC. Rapid sequence induction for intubation by an aeromedical transport team: a critical analysis. *Am J Emerg Med*. 1998;16:598-602.

111. Gausche M, Lewis RJ, Stratton SJ, Haynes BE, Gunter CS, Goodrich SM, Poore PD, McCollough MD, Henderson DP, Pratt FD, Seidel JS. Effect of out-of-hospital pediatric endotracheal intubation on survival and neurological outcome: a controlled clinical trial. *JAMA*. 2000;283:783-790.

112. Thomas SH, Harrison T, Wedel SK. Flight crew airway management in four settings: a six-year review. *Prehosp Emerg Care*. 1999; 3:310-315.

113. ECC advisory statement: innovations in CPR training. A statement for BLS providers and instructors from the American Heart Association Emergency Cardiac Care Committee, the BLS and Program Administration Subcommittees, and the Education Working Group. *Curr Emerg Card Care*. 1996;7:9-11.

114. Seidel JS, Henderson DP, Lewis JB. Emergency medical services and the pediatric patient. III: resources of ambulatory care centers. *Pediatrics*. 1991;88:230-235.

115. Singer J, Ludwig S. *Emergency Medical Services for Children: the Role of the Primary Care Provider. Committee on Pediatric Emergency Medicine, American Academy of Pediatrics*. Elk Grove Village, Ill: American Academy of Pediatrics; 1992.

116. Seidel JS, Gausche M. Standards for emergency departments. In: Dieckmann RA, ed. *Pediatric Emergency Care Systems: Planning and Management*. Baltimore, Md: Williams and Wilkins; 1992.

117. Pettigrew AH. Pediatric intensive care systems in northern and central California. In: Haller JA, ed. *Emergency Medical Services for Children: Report of the 97th Ross Conference on Pediatric Research*. Columbus, Ohio: Ross Laboratories; 1989.

118. Pollack MM, Alexander SR, Clarke N, Ruttimann UE, Tesselaar HM, Bachulis AC. Improved outcomes from tertiary center pediatric intensive care: a statewide comparison of tertiary and nontertiary care facilities. *Crit Care Med*. 1991;19:150-159.

119. Dykes EH, Spence LJ, Young JG, Bohn DJ, Filler RM, Wesson DE. Preventable pediatric trauma deaths in a metropolitan region. *J Pediatr Surg*. 1989;24:107-110.

120. Koury SI, Moorer L, Stone CK, Stapczynski JS, Thomas SH. Air vs ground transport and outcome in trauma patients requiring urgent operative interventions. *Prehosp Emerg Care*. 1998;2:289-292.

121. Moront ML, Gotschall CS, Eichelberger MR. Helicopter transport of injured children: system effectiveness and triage criteria. *J Pediatr Surg*. 1996;31:1183-1186.

122. Rivara FP, Thompson RS, Thompson DC, Calonge N. Injuries to children and adolescents: impact on physical health. *Pediatrics*. 1991;88:783-788.

123. Guidelines 2000 for Cardiopulmonary Resuscitation and Emergency Cardiac Care: International Consensus on Science. Part 9: pediatric basic life support. *Circulation*. 2000;102(suppl I):I-253-I-290.

TABLE 1. Suggested Pediatric Equipment for Prehospital BLS Units

Equipment*	Priority†
Assessment and Diagnostic	
Universal precautions equipment (gloves, face shields/masks, protective eyewear)	1
AED (if operator is trained and authorized to use)	1
Blood pressure cuffs	2
Stethoscope	1
Airway Management	
Portable oxygen with delivery devices and regulator	1
Manual resuscitator with reservoir—child, adult‡	1
Oxygen delivery devices (masks and nasal cannulas)	1
Masks	
Pocket mask with 1-way valve	1
Masks for manual resuscitator—neonatal, infant, child, adult	1
Nonrebreathing masks	1
Airways	
Oropharyngeal airways	1
Nasopharyngeal airways—sizes 18F to 34F or 4.5 to 8.5 mm	1
PTL, LMA, CombiTube or equivalent device (if trained and authorized to use)	3
Suction	
Bulb suction device	1
Portable suction device	1
Fixed/powered suction device	1
Suction catheters—tonsil tip and flexible (6F through 14F)	1
Immobilization Devices	
Backboard	1
Cervical immobilization device(s)—infant, child, adolescent, adult§	1
Extremity splints	2
Medications (if trained and authorized to use)	
Autoinjectable epinephrine	1
Bronchodilator(s) nebulizer supplies	1
Other	
Burn dressings	2
Sterile scissors	3
Obstetric pack	1
Thermal blanket	2
Water-soluble lubricant	1
Infant car seat	2
Glasgow Coma Scale reference	3
Pediatric Trauma Score reference	3
Small stuffed toy	3
Computer with CD-ROM capability (at base station)	3
EMS-C CD-ROM training discs//	3

*Equipment should be available for servicing the entire spectrum of pediatric ages/sizes from the newly born to the adolescent. Age-appropriate size for selected equipment is listed in Table 5.

†Priority levels: 1, **Essential item** for almost all settings; should be **immediately available** for healthcare providers with a duty to respond if within the responder's scope of practice. 2, **Highly recommended** item for the stated setting; should be **available within 15 minutes;** availability can vary based on local needs and protocols. 3, **Recommended but optional** item for the stated setting; often **needed within 30 minutes;** availability can vary based on local needs and protocols.

‡Ventilation bags (ie, manual resuscitators) used for resuscitation should be self-refilling. Child and adult bags are suitable for supporting adequate tidal volumes for the entire pediatric age range. A child-sized bag has a volume of 450 to 750 mL. An adult-sized bag has a volume of at least 1000 mL.

§A cervical immobilization device can immobilize the neck of an infant, a child, or an adult. This device may consist of towel rolls, or it may be a commercially available device made specifically for cradling the neck. Spinal immobilization of small infants may be better achieved by the use of towels and tape rather than by a rigid collar, which may not fit properly (see Chapter 10: "Trauma Resuscitation and Spinal Immobilization.").

//Contact EMSC Clearinghouse, 2070 Chain Bridge Road, Suite 450, Vienna, VA 22182 (703-902-1203 or -1272), emsc@circsol. com or info@emscnrc.com; or visit the EMS-C website: **www.ems-c.org.**

Additional resources include Seidel et al. Committee on Ambulance Equipment and Supplies, National Emergency Medical Services for Children Resource Alliance. *Ann Emerg Med.* 1996;28:699-701.

TABLE 2. Suggested Pediatric Equipment for Prehospital ALS Units

Equipment*	Priority†
ALS units should have all the equipment in the BLS list (Table 1) plus the following items:	
Assessment and Diagnostic	
ECG monitor/defibrillator with appropriately sized paddles and electrodes	1
Pulse oximeter	1
Glucometer or blood glucose testing equipment	2
Thermometer—suitable for hypothermic and hyperthermic measurements (25°C to 44°C)	3
Vascular Doppler monitor	3
Airway Management	

Tracheal tubes‡§
    Uncuffed sizes 2.5 to 6.0
    Cuffed sizes 3.0 to 8.0
	
	1
	1

Tracheal tube, meconium suction adaptor	1
Magill forceps—pediatric, adult‡	1
Stylets for tracheal tubes—pediatric, adult‡	1
Intubation ancillary items (tube holder or tape, bite block, spare batteries or bulbs, water-soluble lubricant, 10-mL syringes)‡	1

Laryngoscope with‡
    Straight blades (No. 0, 1, 2)
    Curved blades (No. 2, 3, 4)
	
	1
	1

Exhaled CO_2 detector (or other device to confirm intubation)—pediatric, adult‡	1
Nasogastric tubes 6F to 16F	 2
Vascular Access and Medication Administration	
Intravenous catheters 14 to 24 gauge	 1
Intraosseous needles† 15 to 18 gauge	 1
Ancillary IV equipment (fluid administration tubing with calibrated chamber, 3-way stopcocks, T connectors, site prep and antiseptic materials, rubber arm bands, catheter securing devices, tape, sharps container, bandaging materials)	1
Intravenous fluids that meet local standard of practice	1
Microdrip IV devices	2

Medication administration supplies
    18- to 25-gauge needles, 1- to 60-mL syringes
    20- to 25-gauge needles
	
	1

Umbilical vein catheters	2
Butterfly needles—19- to 25-gauge	2
Pharmacology	
Resuscitation drugs that meet local standard of practice	1
Other	
Drug dose tape or chart//	1
Communication access to medical control physician	1

*Equipment should be available for servicing the entire spectrum of pediatric ages/sizes from the newly born to the adolescent. Age-appropriate size for selected equipment is listed in Table 5.

†Priority levels: 1, **Essential item** for almost all settings; should be **immediately available** for healthcare providers with a duty to respond if within the responder's scope of practice. 2, **Highly recommended** item for the stated setting; should be **available within 15 minutes;** availability can vary based on local needs and protocols. 3, **Recommended but optional** item for the stated setting; often **needed within 30 minutes;** availability can vary based on local needs and protocols.

‡These items are required only if the skill is part of the local scope of practice of EMS providers.

§The Subcommittee on Pediatric Resuscitation recommends uncuffed sizes 2.5 to 6.0 plus several cuffed tubes, especially from 4.5 to 6.0. It may not be necessary or practical to stock very small or very large sizes of cuffed tubes for initial stabilization of children.

//This item may be a chart giving drug doses in milliliters or milligrams per kilogram or precalculated doses based on weight, or it may be a tape that generates the drug dose based on the patient's height or length.

Additional resources include Seidel et al. Committee on Ambulance Equipment and Supplies, National Emergency Medical Services for Children Resource Alliance. *Ann Emerg Med.* 1996;28:699-701.

TABLE 3. Suggested Pediatric Emergency Equipment for Physician Offices

Equipment*	Priority†
Assessment and Diagnostic	
Universal precautions equipment (gloves, face mask, eye protection)	1
Portable ECG monitor/defibrillator	1 or 2, based on patient age/risk
Blood pressure cuffs	1
Sphygmomanometer or noninvasive blood pressure monitor	1
Pulse oximeter	2
Airway Management	
Pocket mask with 1-way valve	1
Oropharyngeal airways	1
Nasopharyngeal airways	1
Oxygen masks—infant, child, adult	1
Oxygen source, portable or fixed, with flowmeter (to deliver >15 L/min)	1
Manual resuscitator device	1
Masks for manual resuscitator—neonatal, infant, child, adult	1
Suction catheters—Yankauer tip and flexible (8F to 14F)	1
Suction devices, portable or fixed/powered	1

Intubation equipment
  Tracheal tubes—uncuffed 2.5 to 6.0 and cuffed 5.0 to 8.0
  Exhaled CO_2 detector
  Laryngoscope batteries and bulbs
  Laryngoscope handle with straight blades (No. 0, 1, 2)
    and curved blades (No. 2, 3, 4)
  Magill forceps—pediatric, adult
  Stylets for tracheal tubes—pediatric, adult
	3

Vascular Access and Medication Administration	
Intraosseous needle—15- and 18-gauge	2
Intravenous catheters—14- to 24-gauge	2
Isotonic fluids (normal saline or lactated Ringer's solution)	2
Ancillary IV equipment (fluid administration sets, site prep and antiseptic materials, rubber arm bands, catheter securing devices, tape, sharps container)	2
Pediatric drip chambers and tubing	2
Pharmacology	

Epinephrine
  1:10 000
  1:1000
	1

Lidocaine	1
Bronchodilator nebulizer supplies	1
Miscellaneous Equipment	
Cardiac arrest board	2
Feeding tubes or umbilical catheters—3.5F, 5F	2
Foley urine catheters—8F, 10F	3
Nasogastric tubes—10F, 14F	2

*Equipment should be available for servicing the entire spectrum of pediatric ages/sizes from the newly born to the adolescent. Age-appropriate size for selected equipment is listed in Table 5.

†Priority levels: 1, **Essential item** for almost all settings; should be **immediately available** for healthcare providers with a duty to respond if within the responder's scope of practice. 2, **Highly recommended** item for the stated setting; should be **available within 15 minutes;** availability can vary based on local needs and protocols. 3, **Recommended but optional** item for the stated setting; often **needed within 30 minutes;** availability can vary based on local needs and protocols.

Additional resources include Altieri M, Bellet J, Scott H. Preparedness for pediatric emergencies encountered in the practitioner's office. *Pediatrics.* 1990;85: 710-714.

Heath BW, Coffey JS, Malone P, Courtney J. Pediatric office emergencies and emergency preparedness in a small rural state. *Pediatrics.* 2000;106:1391-1396.

Schweich PJ, DeAngelis C, Duggan AK. Preparedness of practicing pediatricians to manage emergencies. *Pediatrics.* 1991;88:223-229.

TABLE 4. Suggested Pediatric Equipment for Emergency Departments

Equipment*	Priority†
Assessment and Diagnostic	
ECG monitor/defibrillator capable of pediatric doses (with monitoring electrodes and hands-free pediatric pads or paddles)	1
Universal precautions equipment (gloves, face mask, eye protection)	1
Blood pressure cuffs	1
Glucometer or blood glucose testing equipment	1
Thermometer—suitable for hypothermic and hyperthermic measurements (25°C to 44°C)	1
Doppler, vascular (with gel)	2
Pulse oximeter	1
Sphygmomanometer	1
Doppler blood pressure device	1
Airway Management	
Oropharyngeal airways	1
Nasopharyngeal airways	1
Laryngeal mask airway—sizes 1, 1.5, 2, 2.5, 3, 4, 5	2
Pocket mask with 1-way valve	1
Manual resuscitator device	1
Masks for manual resuscitators—neonatal, infant, child, adult	1

Tracheal tubes
    Uncuffed sizes 2.0 to 8.0
    Cuffed sizes 3.0 to 8.0
	1

Meconium suction adapter for tracheal tube	1
Stylets—infant, pediatric, adult	1
Magill forceps—pediatric, adult	1

Laryngoscope with
    Straight blades (No. 0, 1, 2, 3)
    Curved blades (No. 2, 3, 4)
	1

Nasogastric tube—6F to 16F	1
Chest tubes	1
Tracheostomy tubes—sizes 00 to 6	1
Oxygen supply source, portable or fixed unit, with flow regulator	1
Oxygen delivery devices (masks and nasal cannulas)	1
Suction catheters—tonsil tip and flexible (6F through 14F)	1

Suction devices
    Bulb syringe
    Portable and fixed/powered
	1
	1

Alternative airway, needle cricothyrotomy, and jet insufflation setup	1
Exhaled CO_2 detector (or other device/method to confirm and monitor tracheal tube placement)—pediatric, adult	1

Equipment*	Priority†
Vascular Access	
Peripheral IV cannulation devices—butterfly needles, catheter-over-needle devices	1
Central vein access kits with 3F, 4F, and 5F catheters	2
Intraosseous needles—15- to 18-gauge	1

Umbilical vein catheters
    Sizes 3.5F and 5F
    Size 5F feeding tube may be used
	1

IV fluid and blood warmer	2
Pharmacology	
Adenosine	1
Atropine sulfate	1
Amiodarone	1
Calcium chloride Or calcium gluconate	1 1
Dobutamine	1
Dopamine	1

Epinephrine
    1:1000 (ECC: minimum of 10 mg or multidose)
    1:10 000
	1

Glucose, 10% and 25%	1
Inhaled bronchodilator(s)	1
Lidocaine	1
Magnesium sulfate	1
Naloxone	1
Neuromuscular blocking agent(s)	1
Phenytoin or equivalent	1
Potassium chloride	1
Procainamide	1

Sodium bicarbonate
    8.4%
    4.2%
	1
	1

Acetylcysteine	2
Activated charcoal	2
Aminophylline	2
β-Blocker	2
Corticosteroids	2
Cyanide poisoning kit (amyl nitrite, sodium nitrite, sodium thiosulfate)	2
Diphenhydramine	2
Digibind	2
Digoxin	2
Flumazenil	2
Furosemide	2
Glucagon	2

TABLE 4. (continued)

Equipment*	Priority†
Insulin	2
Ipecac	2
Mannitol	2
Methylene blue	2
Milrinone (amrinone/inamrinone)	2
Morphine	2
Prostaglandin E_1	1
Sedatives/anticonvulsants	2
Sodium nitroprusside	2
Dextrose 25% and 50%	1
Analgesics	2
Antibiotics (parenteral)	2
Antipyretics	2
Specialized Pediatric Trays	
Tube thoracotomy with water seal drainage capability	1
Lumbar puncture Spinal needles, 20-, 22-, and 25-gauge	2
Urinary catheterization with Foley catheters 5F to 12F 5F to 16F Pediatric catheters	2
Obstetric pack	1
Newborn kit With umbilical vessel cannulation supplies With meconium aspirator	1
Venous cutdown	1
Needle cricothyrotomy tray	1
Surgical airway kit; may include Tracheostomy tray Cricothyrotomy tray Needle jet kit	1
Other	
Thermocontrol materials	1
Pediatric dose chart or tape	1
Device(s) for immobilization of cervical spine	1
Pediatric restraint devices	1
Infant and standard scales	1
Infant formula and oral rehydrating solutions	2
Heating source (infrared lamps or overhead warmer)	1
Towel rolls, blanket rolls, or equivalent	1
Resuscitation board	1
Sterile linen (available within hospital for burn care)	2
Medical photography capability	2

*Equipment should be available for servicing the entire spectrum of pediatric ages/sizes from the newly born to the adolescent. Age-appropriate size for selected equipment is listed in Table 5.

†Priority levels: 1, **Essential item** for almost all settings; should be **immediately available** for healthcare providers with a duty to respond if within the responder's scope of practice. 2, **Highly recommended** item for the stated setting; should be **available within 15 minutes;** availability can vary based on local needs and protocols. 3, **Recommended but optional** item for the stated setting; often **needed within 30 minutes;** availability can vary based on local needs and protocols.

Additional resources include Seidel et al. Committee on Pediatric Equipment and Supplies for Emergency Departments, National Emergency Medical Services for Children Resource Alliance. *Ann Emerg Med.* 1998;31:54-57.

American Academy of Pediatrics. Guidelines for pediatric emergency care facilities (RE9536). *Pediatrics.* 1995;96:526-537.

Emergency care guidelines. American College of Emergency Physicians. September 1996.

Equipment for ambulances. American College of Emergency Physicians and the National Association of Emergency Medical Technicians. September 1994.

Pediatric equipment guidelines. American College of Emergency Physicians. April 1994.

TABLE 5. Pediatric Resuscitation Supplies* Based on Color-Coded Resuscitation Tape

Equipment	Newborn/ Small infant (3-5 kg)	Infant (6-9 kg)	Toddler (10-11 kg)	Small Child (12-14 kg)	Child (15-18 kg)	Child (19-22 kg)	Large Child (24-30 kg)	Adult (≥32 kg)
Resuscitation bag	Infant	Child	Child	Child	Child	Child	Child/adult	Adult
O$_2$ mask	Newborn	Newborn	Pediatric	Pediatric	Pediatric	Pediatric	Adult	Adult
Oral airway	Infant/small child	Infant/small child	Small child	Child	Child	Child/small adult	Child/small adult	Medium adult
Laryngoscope blade (size)	0-1 straight	1 straight	1 straight	2 straight	2 straight or curved	2 straight or curved	2-3 straight or curved	3 straight or curved
Tracheal tube (mm)	Premature infant 2.5 Term infant 3.0-3.5 uncuffed	3.5 uncuffed	4.0 uncuffed	4.5 uncuffed	5.0 uncuffed	5.5 uncuffed	6.0 cuffed	6.5 cuffed
Tracheal tube length (cm at lip)	10-10.5	10-10.5	11-12	12.5-13.5	14-15	15.5-16.5	17-18	18.5-19.5
Stylet (F)	6	6	6	6	6	14	14	14
Suction catheter (F)	6-8	8	8-10	10	10	10	10	12
BP cuff	Newborn/ infant	Newborn/ infant	Infant/child	Child	Child	Child	Child/adult	Adult
IV catheter (G)	22-24	22-24	20-24	18-22	18-22	18-20	18-20	16-20
Butterfly (G)	23-25	23-25	23-25	21-23	21-23	21-23	21-22	18-21
Nasogastric tube (F)	5-8	5-8	8-10	10	10-12	12-14	14-18	18
Urinary catheter (F)	5-8	5-8	8-10	10	10-12	10-12	12	12
Defibrillation/ cardioversion external paddles	Infant paddles	Infant paddles until 1 yr or 10 kg	Adult paddles when ≥1 yr or ≥10 kg	Adult paddles	Adult paddles	Adult paddles	Adult paddles	Adult paddles
Chest tube (F)	10-12	10-12	16-20	20-24	20-24	24-32	28-32	32-40

*Adapted from the Broselow Pediatric Resuscitation Tape, with permission from Armstrong Medical Industries, Lincolnshire, Ill. Modified from Hazinski MF, ed. *Manual of Pediatric Critical Care.* St. Louis, Mo: Mosby–Year Book; 1999.

Recognition of Respiratory Failure and Shock

Introductory Case Scenario

A 3-year-old toddler is brought to the Emergency Department (ED) 2 hours after drinking some type of lamp oil. EMS personnel found a tachypneic, anxious-appearing toddler and transported him to the ED after attaching a partial non-rebreathing face mask.

On arrival in the ED the toddler continues to appear tachypneic, anxious, and somewhat agitated. He makes an expiratory grunting sound with each breath and is using accessory muscles with nasal flaring. His respiratory rate is 48 breaths/min, heart rate is 156 bpm, blood pressure is 124/80 mm Hg, and oxyhemoglobin saturation by pulse oximeter is 92% on nonrebreathing face mask. Axillary temperature is 97.5°F. The child is warm and well perfused, with brisk capillary refill (less than 2 seconds) and pink color centrally. Auscultation of the lungs reveals decreased distal air movement with bilateral, scattered moist crackles during inspiration and an expiratory grunting sound with each breath.

- What is your rapid cardiopulmonary assessment of this child?

- On the basis of your cardiopulmonary assessment, what are your treatment priorities?

- What components of the exam indicate that this child may be at risk for respiratory failure?

- What supplemental test(s) would you like to perform?

Learning Objectives

After completing this chapter the PALS provider should be able to

- Define respiratory failure

- Define shock

- Define cardiopulmonary failure and cardiac arrest

- List the components of rapid cardiopulmonary assessment

- List examination findings consistent with respiratory compromise

- List examination findings consistent with circulatory compromise

- State the criteria for defining decompensated shock in children of different ages

Anticipating Cardiac Arrest: Defining Respiratory Failure and Shock

Cardiac arrest (also referred to as *cardiopulmonary* arrest) is the cessation of cardiac mechanical activity. It is characterized by unresponsiveness, apnea, and the absence of a palpable central pulse (ie, no signs of circulation). Pediatric cardiac arrest frequently represents the terminal event of progressive shock or respiratory failure rather than sudden collapse secondary to an arrhythmia. The progression from shock or respiratory failure to cardiac arrest associated with each of these causes may vary, making development of a uniform treatment approach difficult.

The causes of cardiac arrest are heterogeneous and vary with age, the underlying health of the child, and the location of the event. In the out-of-hospital setting, conditions such as trauma, sudden infant death syndrome (SIDS), submersion, poisoning, choking, severe asthma, and pneumonia are common causes of arrest. In the hospital common causes of cardiac arrest are sepsis, respiratory failure, drug toxicity, metabolic disorders, and arrhythmias. These in-hospital causes often complicate an underlying condition. The ED represents a transition from the out-of-hospital setting to the in-hospital setting. In the ED cardiac arrest may be seen in children with underlying conditions typical for the hospital setting and in children with conditions seen more often in the out-of-hospital setting.

Most out-of-hospital cardiac arrest in infants and children occurs at or near home. SIDS is a leading cause of death in infants under 6 months of age, although its frequency has decreased in recent years with the "back to sleep" campaign, which instructs parents to place infants on their back to sleep. From 6 months of age through adolescence, trauma is the predominant cause of death. Regardless of the initiating event or disease process, the final common pathway for cardiac arrest is the development of cardiopulmonary failure (Figure 1). Once cardiac arrest ensues, the outcome is dismal.[1-5] Because the outcome of cardiac arrest is poor, it is important for the clinician to recognize symptoms of respiratory failure or shock and initiate therapy promptly. This chapter provides information on detecting respiratory failure and shock, anticipating cardiac arrest in infants and children, and establishing priorities in care.

Respiratory distress is characterized by signs of increased work of breathing, including tachypnea or hyperpnea, nasal flaring, the use of accessory muscles of respiration, and inspiratory retractions. Tachycardia is typically present. You can identify signs of respiratory distress and institute supportive care on the basis of clinical examination alone. Note that respiratory distress may serve as a compensated state in which the patient maintains adequate gas exchange by increasing the breathing rate (tachypnea) and/or depth (hyperpnea) prior to the development of respiratory failure. As the child tires or the respiratory function or effort deteriorates, clinical signs of respiratory failure develop.

Respiratory failure is a clinical state characterized by inadequate oxygenation, ventilation, or both. Defining strict criteria for respiratory failure is difficult because the baseline (ie, premorbid) respiratory function of an individual infant or child may be abnormal. For example, an infant with cyanotic congenital heart disease and an arterial oxygen saturation of 75% is not necessarily in respiratory failure, although that degree of hypoxemia would be a sign of respiratory failure in a child with normal baseline cardiopulmonary physiology. Thus, respiratory failure may be functionally characterized as a clinical state that *requires intervention* to prevent respiratory or cardiac arrest. Respiratory failure may be caused by intrinsic lung or airway disease, airway obstruction, or inadequate respiratory *effort* (eg, apnea or shallow, slow respirations). When respiratory *effort* is inadequate, respiratory failure may occur *without* respiratory distress.

Strict definitions of respiratory failure traditionally emphasize arterial blood gas analysis, ie, hypoxemia (low PaO_2), hypercarbia (high $PaCO_2$), and acidosis (pH less than 7.35).[6] This approach is problematic for several reasons. Most important, arterial blood gas analysis may not be available (eg, during transport) or may delay initiation of therapy. Second, a single blood gas analysis may provide limited information, and evaluation of patient trends and response to therapy are often more valuable. Third, interpretation of the results of arterial

FIGURE 1. The pathway of various precipitating conditions and events which, if left untreated or inadequately treated, lead to cardiopulmonary failure in infants and children. Children with cardiopulmonary failure may progress to death or early cardiovascular recovery. Death may occur rapidly from an inability to restore cardiovascular function or later from multiple organ dysfunction syndrome (MODS). Similarly, early cardiovascular recovery may lead to either complete recovery or MODS of varying severity.

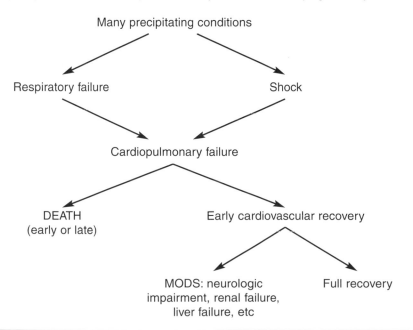

Cardiorespiratory arrest or *cardiopulmonary arrest* (may also be referred to as *cardiac arrest*): The absence of detectable cardiac activity, clinically recognized by the absence of a response to stimulation and movement, absence of breathing, and absence of pulses or other signs of circulation.

Respiratory arrest: The absence of breathing (ie, apnea).

Respiratory failure: The clinical state of inadequate oxygenation, ventilation, or both. Respiratory failure is often accompanied by *respiratory distress* (ie, increased respiratory effort, rate, and work of breathing) but may result from inadequate respiratory effort and no signs of distress.

Shock: Inadequate tissue perfusion resulting in oxygen and substrate delivery that is insufficient to meet tissue metabolic demands. *Decompensated shock* is defined by the presence of hypotension (ie, systolic blood pressure is less than the 5th percentile for age).

blood gas analysis requires consideration of the patient's clinical appearance and must be modified based on the patient's underlying condition.

For example, an infant with bronchopulmonary dysplasia (a form of chronic lung disease) may have chronic hypoxemia and hypercarbia, so diagnosis of acute respiratory failure in this infant relies heavily on clinical examination and evaluation of the arterial pH. At baseline the infant will compensate for the chronic hypercarbia, and arterial pH will be normal or nearly normal. Uncompensated respiratory acidosis will be apparent if the child's respiratory status (ie, hypercarbia) is significantly worse than the baseline status.

This chapter emphasizes the recognition of children at risk for respiratory failure, based on *clinical* evaluation of the child. If a child with potential respiratory failure fails to improve after initial therapy or if further clinical deterioration is observed, more aggressive therapy should be considered, because respiratory failure is likely present. Arterial blood gas analysis may be used to confirm the clinical impression or to evaluate the child's response to therapy, but it is not required to identify *potential* respiratory failure.

Shock is a clinical state characterized by inadequate tissue perfusion resulting in delivery of oxygen and metabolic substrates that is insufficient to meet tissue metabolic demands. Shock typically produces signs of inadequate organ and tissue perfusion and function, such as oliguria and lactic acidosis. Other clinical signs of shock are determined by the type of shock present and are summarized later in this chapter. Shock may occur with normal, increased, or decreased cardiac output and normal, increased, or decreased blood pressure.[7,8] For example, a patient with carbon monoxide intoxication may have increased cardiac output

and excellent organ perfusion with normal blood pressure, yet be in shock; this is because the red blood cells are unable to release oxygen efficiently to the tissues, causing lactic acidosis to develop. The severity of shock can be characterized as compensated or decompensated.

Compensated shock is defined as a clinical state of tissue perfusion that is inadequate to meet metabolic demand in the presence of blood pressure within the normal range. *Decompensated shock* has the additional feature of hypotension, ie, *systolic* blood pressure (SBP) less than the 5th percentile for age. Although cardiac output is often reduced in decompensated shock, it may occur with a high cardiac output, such as that seen in a patient with septic shock. Once decompensated shock develops, organ perfusion is typically severely compromised, and urgent treatment is required to prevent rapid progression to cardiac arrest.

Respiratory failure and shock may begin as clinically distinct problems, but these often progress to a state of *cardiopulmonary failure* in the final moments preceding cardiac arrest. Cardiopulmonary failure is characterized by insufficient oxygen delivery to meet tissue metabolic demand *and* inadequate oxygenation or ventilation.

Oxygen Delivery

Respiratory failure may include a state of inadequate oxygenation. Shock is defined by inadequate substrate delivery to meet tissue metabolic demands, and oxygen is the major substrate of aerobic metabolism. For these reasons it is important to understand the determinants of oxygen delivery. *Oxygen delivery* is the amount of oxygen delivered to the entire body per minute. It is the product of arterial oxygen content and cardiac output (or cardiac index, which is the cardiac output indexed to the child's body surface area):

Oxygen delivery = Arterial oxygen content × Cardiac output (× constant)

Arterial oxygen content is determined by the hemoglobin concentration and its saturation with oxygen as seen in the equation at the foot of this page.

The normal arterial oxygen content is approximately 18 to 20 mL of oxygen per deciliter (100 mL) of blood.

Cardiac output is the product of heart rate and ventricular stroke volume:

Cardiac output = Heart rate × Stroke volume

Stroke volume is the quantity of blood ejected from the heart with each contraction.

Several factors determine oxygen delivery to the tissues, and uncompensated changes in these factors can reduce oxygen delivery and result in shock. Oxygen delivery to the tissues falls if either arterial oxygen content or cardiac output falls without a commensurate and compensatory increase in the other component. For example, arterial oxygen content typically is reduced in respiratory failure. If cardiac output can increase sufficiently, oxygen delivery to the tissues may be maintained at normal or near-normal levels. However, if cardiac output cannot increase in proportion to the fall in oxygen content, oxygen delivery to the tissues falls dramatically because both cardiac output and oxygen content are impaired. Moreover, the increased work of breathing that often occurs in patients with respiratory failure adds to the patient's metabolic demand and increases the likelihood of shock developing.

Arterial oxygen content itself may be affected by changes in cardiac output, especially when there is significant respiratory compromise with impaired oxygenation (see FYI box). Any fall in cardiac output (such as that which occurs in some forms of shock or with some arrhythmias) is likely to decrease oxygen delivery.

| Arterial oxygen content (mL of oxygen per dL of blood) | = | Hemoglobin concentration (g/dL) | × | 1.34 mL oxygen | × | Oxyhemoglobin saturation | + | (Pao$_2$ × 0.003) |

FYI: Dissolved Oxygen Constitutes a Small but Potentially Important Portion of Oxygen Content

Under normal conditions the quantity of oxygen dissolved in the liquid component of blood ($PaO_2 \times 0.003$) represents only a small portion (1% to 2%) of the total arterial oxygen content. But this dissolved oxygen can be important in patients with severe anemia. For example, in a child with leukemia and severe anemia (hemoglobin = 3 g/dL) with PaO_2 of 100 mm Hg (oxyhemoglobin saturation of 100%), the arterial oxygen content is 4.32 mL/100 mL of blood. If 100% oxygen is given and PaO_2 increases to 550 mm Hg, the dissolved oxygen increases from 0.3 mL/100 mL of blood to 1.65 mL/100 mL of blood, resulting in a net increase in arterial oxygen content of almost 40% by this simple procedure. In summary, with no change in cardiac output, delivery of 100% oxygen to a patient with severe anemia can substantially increase arterial oxygen content and oxygen delivery. This increase in oxygen delivery is often sufficient to stabilize the patient until cross-matched blood is available.

Shock is defined by a *mismatch* between oxygen delivery and tissue metabolic demand. As a result cardiac output and oxygen delivery must be evaluated in terms of their adequacy in meeting tissue requirements (demands) rather than simply their relationship to normative data. In other words, it is less important to know if cardiac output and oxygen delivery are "low," "normal," or "high" when compared with normative data than it is to know if cardiac output and oxygen delivery are *adequate* to meet metabolic demands and maintain aerobic metabolism.

Metabolic demand is increased by fever, pain, injury, sepsis, and other inflammatory conditions. When tissue oxygen requirements exceed oxygen delivery, anaerobic metabolism leads to accumulation of lactic acid. The latter is often readily measured in the hospital and if elevated helps confirm the clinical suspicion of shock.

Clinical signs of shock and respiratory failure result from end-organ dysfunction caused by tissue hypoxia and acidosis (Table 1). These signs include tachycardia, altered levels of consciousness (irritability or lethargy), oliguria, hypotonia, weak central (proximal) pulses with weak or absent peripheral pulses, cool extremities, and prolonged capillary refill despite a warm ambient temperature. Bradycardia, hypotension, and irregular respirations are late, ominous signs.

TABLE 1. Conditions Requiring Rapid Cardiopulmonary Assessment and Potential Cardiopulmonary Support

Respiratory rate >60 breaths/min
Heart rate*
  Newborn: <80 bpm or >200 bpm
  0-1 year: <80 bpm or >180 bpm
  1-8 years: <60 bpm or >180 bpm
  >8 years: <60 bpm or >160 bpm
Poor perfusion with weak or absent
  distal pulses
Increased work of breathing
  (retractions, nasal flaring, grunting)
Cyanosis or a decrease in oxyhemoglobin saturation
Altered level of consciousness
  (unusual irritability, lethargy, or
  decreased response to parents
  or painful stimulus)
Seizures
Fever with petechiae
Multiple trauma
Burns totaling >10% of body surface
  area

*bpm indicates beats per minute

Factors Influencing Respiratory Function

Normal spontaneous ventilation is accomplished with minimal work, resulting in quiet breathing. The normal respiratory rate is inversely related to age; it is rapid in the neonate, then decreases in older infants and children. The neonatal respiratory rate is typically ≤ 40 to 60 breaths/min; the respiratory rate in a 1-year-old is approximately 24 breaths/min. The normal respiratory rate in an 18-year-old is approximately 12 breaths/min during quiet breathing. Higher respiratory rates would be expected in the presence of any condition causing an increase in metabolic demand and thus CO_2 production, such as excitement, anxiety, exercise, pain, or fever.

Normalized tidal volume (ie, the volume of each breath per kilogram of body weight) remains fairly constant throughout life (approximately 4 to 6 mL/kg). Adequacy of tidal volume is assessed clinically by observation of chest wall excursion and auscultation of the lungs, noting the quality of air movement, particularly in distal lung fields.

Minute ventilation is conceptually similar to cardiac output; it is the product of *tidal volume* (similar to stroke volume) and *respiratory rate* (similar to heart rate). Hypoventilation (ie, low minute ventilation) may result from small tidal volumes (ie, each breath is shallow) or from too few breaths taken each minute. Note that hypoventilation may occur with an increased respiratory rate if the tidal volumes are small (just as cardiac output can be low despite the presence of tachycardia if stroke volume is reduced).

Abnormal respiratory rates can be classified as too fast (tachypnea), too slow (bradypnea), or absent (apnea). Breathing effort is characterized by the presence of increased work of breathing, a normal breathing effort, or an abnormal breathing pattern. Tachypnea with normal effort ("quiet tachypnea") often represents a compensatory response to metabolic acidosis.

FYI: Increased Cardiac Output Can Improve Arterial Oxygen Saturation in Patients With Intrapulmonary Shunts

When a patient has parenchymal lung disease leading to ventilation-perfusion mismatch, the patient's arterial oxygen saturation and therefore oxygen content and delivery may be affected by changes in cardiac output as well as by changes in pulmonary function. This is illustrated in Figure 2.

Figure 2A shows oxygen saturation at different points of the circulation in a patient with low cardiac output and severe pulmonary disease. The oxygen saturation depicted on the far left side of Figure 2A represents mixed venous oxygen saturation (as measured in the pulmonary artery). This patient has severe pulmonary disease with an intrapulmonary shunt of 50% (ie, $Q_p/Q_s = 0.5$), where Q_p is the apparent pulmonary blood flow and Q_s is the apparent systemic blood flow. Note that the values of Q_p and Q_s are calculated based on the assumption that all pulmonary blood

flow participates in normal gas exchange at the alveolus, so that if there is shunting through collapsed alveoli, the apparent pulmonary blood flow is less than the actual. In addition, the initial cardiac output in the top picture is low. When cardiac output is low, oxygen extraction in the peripheral tissues is increased, leading to low mixed venous oxygen saturation (40%). Practically speaking, an intrapulmonary shunt of 50% means that half the blood going through the lungs returns to the left atrium with the same oxygen saturation it had when it entered the pulmonary artery. The other half of the blood is fully saturated (pulmonary venous blood oxygen saturation is 100%) as illustrated by the lower and upper branches of Figure 2A. Net arterial oxygen saturation is 70% after the blood mixes in the left heart.

Figure 2B illustrates the effect of increased cardiac output on arterial oxygen saturation in the same patient with severe pulmonary

disease. The intrapulmonary shunt remains unchanged at 50%. In this case, however, improved cardiac output leads to better organ blood flow, so that less oxygen must be extracted in the peripheral tissues and mixed venous oxygen saturation is higher. The improvement in mixed venous oxygen saturation improves arterial oxygen saturation as noted in the figure.

Thus, patients with severe disturbances in oxygenation, such as those seen in acute respiratory distress syndrome (ARDS) or pneumonia, may benefit from therapies designed to increase cardiac output independent of any change in pulmonary status. These therapies may include use of inotropes, vasodilators, and/or increased preload by fluid volume administration. Blood administration may be particularly useful because it increases oxygen-carrying capacity as well as ventricular preload.

Causes of Respiratory Failure

Acute respiratory failure can result from any airway, pulmonary, or neuromuscular disease that impairs oxygen exchange (oxygenation) or elimination of CO_2 (ventilation).[6] The resultant hypoxemia, hypercapnia, and respiratory acidosis reflect the severity of respiratory failure.

The pediatric patient has a high oxygen demand per kilogram of body weight because the child's metabolic rate is high. Oxygen consumption in infants is 6 to 8 mL/kg per minute compared with 3 to 4 mL/kg per minute in adults.[8,9] Therefore, in the presence of apnea or inadequate alveolar ventilation, hypoxemia and potential tissue hypoxia can develop more rapidly in the child than in the adult.

FIGURE 2. The effects of improving cardiac output on arterial oxygen saturation in a patient with severe parenchymal lung disease. See text for detailed explanation.

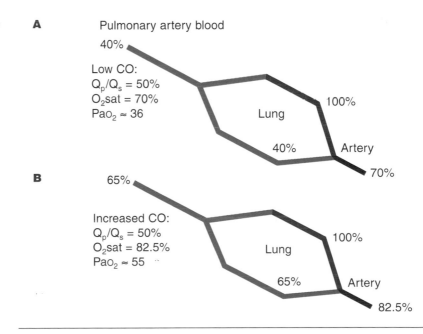

An illness leading to respiratory distress or failure may cause hypoxemia and potential tissue hypoxia by several mechanisms:

■ The disease process directly interferes with the exchange of oxygen or CO_2 or both (eg, pneumonia or ARDS).

■ Mismatch of ventilation and perfusion causes shunting of pulmonary blood through the lung, leading to hypoxemia and (to a lesser extent) hypercarbia (eg, asthma, bronchiolitis, or aspiration pneumonia).

■ The disease process decreases lung compliance or increases airway resistance or both, resulting in increased work of breathing and increased oxygen consumption that exceeds delivery (eg, pneumonia, ARDS, or asthma).

Ventilatory function (ie, adequacy of CO_2 elimination) can be compromised by increased airway resistance, decreased lung compliance, and injury to the lung parenchyma. Ventilatory function also may be compromised by depression of central control of ventilation. Causes of depressed respiratory effort typically result from central nervous system injury, compromised brain perfusion, or drug intoxication. Causes include severe hypoxemia, hypothermia, medication effects, metabolic derangements (eg, hypoglycemia), or seizures. Although cervical spine injuries are relatively uncommon in infants and children, high spinal injury (C4 and above) may cause apnea by disrupting the innervation of the diaphragm. Respiratory rate and effort must be carefully monitored in patients with drug intoxication or head injury because apnea is relatively common in these patients.

Evaluation of Respiratory Performance

Infants and children at risk for respiratory arrest may initially demonstrate one or more of the following signs and symptoms:

■ Increased respiratory rate, increased respiratory effort or diminished breath sounds

■ Diminished level of consciousness or response to parents or response to pain

■ Poor skeletal muscle tone

■ Cyanosis

The assessment of respiratory function requires careful evaluation of

■ Respiratory rate

■ Respiratory mechanics (eg, quality of breath sounds, use of accessory muscles)

■ Level of consciousness

■ Color of the skin and mucous membranes

Respiratory Rate

Respiratory rate is often best evaluated by observing the patient before you touch or examine him/her, because anxiety and agitation commonly alter the baseline respiratory rate. Tachypnea is often the first manifestation of respiratory distress in infants. Tachypnea without other signs of respiratory distress ("quiet tachypnea") is typically an attempt to maintain a normal pH by increasing minute ventilation, (ie, to generate a compensatory respiratory alkalosis). Quiet tachypnea commonly results from nonpulmonary diseases such as metabolic acidosis associated with shock, diabetic ketoacidosis, some congenital cardiac abnormalities, inborn errors of metabolism, salicylate poisoning, chronic diarrhea, or chronic renal insufficiency.

A slow or irregular respiratory rate in an acutely ill infant or child is an ominous clinical sign. Possible causes include fatigue, central nervous system depression, and hypothermia. Clinical conditions causing increased work of breathing may eventually lead to respiratory muscle fatigue and outright respiratory failure due to inadequate respiratory effort or respiratory rate. Changes in respiratory rate must be evaluated in light of other clinical findings.

A decrease in respiratory rate from a rapid to a more "normal" rate may indicate an overall improvement if accompanied by improvements in mental status and lessened signs of air hunger. Decreasing

respiratory rate or an irregular respiratory rhythm in a child with deteriorating level of consciousness, however, is often associated with worsening respiratory failure. Thus, *a decreasing respiratory rate or an irregular respiratory rhythm may indicate deterioration rather than improvement in the child's clinical condition.* Assessment of the child's level of consciousness and responsiveness will reveal if the child is improving or deteriorating.

Foundation Facts:
Signs of Altered Respiratory Mechanics

Evaluate work of breathing noting the following:

■ *Retractions:* Occur during inspiratory phase. Retractions accompanied by inspiratory stridor suggest upper airway obstruction. Retractions accompanied by grunting or labored respirations suggest decreased lung compliance (ie, parenchymal lung disease). Retractions may be accompanied by head bobbing or abdominal breathing.

■ *Grunting:* Occurs during expiratory phase—a sign of small airway or alveolar collapse or both

■ *Stridor:* High-pitched sound during inspiration—suggests *extrathoracic* airway obstruction

■ *Wheezing or prolonged exhalation:* Suggests *intrathoracic* airway obstruction, especially of small airways

■ *Diminished distal air entry:* Suggests abnormalities such as airflow obstruction, parenchymal lung disease, or poor respiratory effort resulting in poor breath sounds and chest excursion. Careful auscultation helps determine if the patient's tidal volume is adequate.

Respiratory Mechanics

Increased breathing effort results from conditions that increase resistance to airflow or decrease lung compliance (ie, cause the lungs to be stiffer). Decreased lung compliance often results from alveolar diseases such as pneumonia and ARDS. Increased work of breathing often produces nasal flaring and intercostal, subcostal, and suprasternal inspiratory retractions. As work of breathing increases, a greater proportion of the cardiac output must be delivered to the respiratory muscles, which increases oxygen demand and produces more CO_2 that must be exhaled (see Chapter 4).

Terms used to describe abnormal respiratory mechanics are included in Foundation Facts: "Signs of Altered Respiratory Mechanics." Head bobbing, grunting, stridor, and prolonged exhalation are signs of significant alteration in respiratory mechanics. Bobbing of the head with each breath is a sign of increased respiratory effort. Severe chest retractions accompanied by abdominal distention during inspiration are called "seesaw" respirations and usually indicate upper airway obstruction. Seesaw respirations may also be called *abdominal breathing* because the chest wall retracts and the abdomen expands when the diaphragm contracts. This inefficient form of ventilation with low tidal volume may cause fatigue in a short time.

Grunting is produced by premature glottic closure accompanying late expiratory contraction of the diaphragm. Infants and children grunt to increase airway pressure, thereby maintaining patency of their small airways and alveoli (ie, preserving or increasing functional residual capacity—the volume of gas in the lungs at the end of exhalation). Grunting occurs in patients with alveolar collapse and loss of lung volume associated with pulmonary edema, pneumonia, or atelectasis.

Stridor (an inspiratory, high-pitched sound) is a sign of upper airway (*extrathoracic*) obstruction. Causes of upper airway obstruction include congenital or acquired abnormalities (eg, a large tongue, laryngo-malacia, vocal cord paralysis, or airway hemangioma, tumor, or cyst), infections (eg, croup, bacterial tracheitis, or epiglottitis), upper airway edema (eg, allergic reaction), and aspiration of a foreign body.

Prolonged forced exhalation, usually accompanied by wheezing, is a sign of *intrathoracic* airway obstruction, usually at the bronchial or bronchiolar level. Causes of prolonged exhalation include bronchiolitis, asthma, pulmonary edema, or the presence of an intrathoracic foreign body.

Careful assessment of the child's respiratory mechanics enables identification of the likely cause of respiratory problems.

Altered respiratory mechanics and clinical presentations of respiratory failure are summarized in Foundation Facts: "Presentation of Respiratory Failure." See Chapter 4, Figures 2 and 4.

Air Entry

Tidal volume and effectiveness of ventilation are clinically assessed by evaluation of chest expansion and auscultation of breath sounds. Chest expansion during inspiration should be symmetric. The expansion may be subtle during spontaneous quiet breathing but should be readily observed during positive-pressure ventilation (such as during bag-mask ventilation or

Foundation Facts:
Presentation of Respiratory Failure

Four general types of respiratory problems lead to respiratory failure. All 4 types of respiratory problems produce alteration in respiratory mechanics and additional clinical signs:

- **Upper airway obstruction:** The major clinical signs occur during the *inspiratory* phase of the respiratory cycle. The child may have stridor, hoarseness, or a change in voice or cry. Inspiratory retractions, use of accessory muscles, and nasal flaring are present. The respiratory rate is often only mildly elevated.

- **Lower airway obstruction:** The major clinical signs occur during the *expiratory* phase of the respiratory cycle. The child often has wheezing and a prolonged expiratory phase requiring increased effort. The respiratory rate is usually elevated, particularly in infants. Retractions become prominent when the lower airway obstruction impairs both inspiration and exhalation, requiring increased respiratory effort.

- **Parenchymal lung disease:** The child's lungs become stiff, requiring increased respiratory effort during both inspiration and exhalation. Therefore, retractions are common, and hypoxemia is often marked due to alveolar collapse or reduced oxygen diffusion caused by pulmonary edema fluid and inflammatory debris in alveoli. Tachypnea is common and often quite marked. The patient frequently attempts to counteract alveolar and small airway collapse by increased efforts to maintain an elevated end-expiratory pressure; this is usually manifested by *grunting* respirations.

- **Abnormal control of ventilation:** The breathing pattern is abnormal; often the parent will state that the child is "breathing funny." There may be periods of increased effort followed by decreased effort, or the child's respiratory rate or effort may be continuously inadequate. The net effect is hypoventilation, which results from a host of conditions such as injury to the brain or brainstem or drug overdose.

mechanical ventilation). Decreased chest expansion may result from inadequate effort, airway obstruction, atelectasis, pneumothorax, hemothorax, pleural effusion, mucous plug, or foreign-body aspiration.

Breath sounds should be equal and easily heard bilaterally. Typically the chest wall in an infant or a child is thin, and the chest is relatively small, so breath sounds are readily transmitted and heard from one hemithorax to the other. This may lead to an overestimation of air exchange and tidal volume. The intensity and pitch of breath sounds must be evaluated; both should be equal over all lung fields. A decrease in intensity or a change in pitch of breath sounds may indicate pathology, such as atelectasis, pneumothorax, or effusion.

Breath sounds should be auscultated over the anterior and posterior chest as well as in the axillary areas. The axillary areas are particularly important because they are farthest from the conducting airways and therefore provide a better means to evaluate distal air entry. Transmitted airway sounds from the larger conducting airways are less likely to be transmitted to the distal airways.

Skin Color and Temperature

Skin color and temperature should be consistent over the trunk and extremities if the child has good oxygenation and perfusion and is in a warm environment. Mucous membranes, nail beds, and the palms of the hands and soles of the feet will be pink if cardiorespiratory function is normal. As perfusion deteriorates, the hands and feet are typically affected first, becoming cool, pale, or dusky. Subsequently the skin over the trunk or extremities may become mottled if hypoxemia or perfusion worsens.

Central cyanosis may be apparent in a child with hypoxemia, but the appearance of this clinical sign is affected by several factors. For central cyanosis to be clinically apparent, approximately 5 g

of reduced hemoglobin per deciliter of blood must be present *in the skin capillaries*. Thus, cyanosis may not be apparent in an anemic child despite the presence of marked hypoxemia, because hemoglobin saturation would have to fall to extremely low levels (less than 37% in a child with a hemoglobin level of 8 g/dL) to create 5 g of reduced hemoglobin per deciliter. In addition, the appearance of cyanosis depends on the rate of blood flow in the skin and the degree of oxygen extracted by the tissues. Thus a polycythemic child (eg, a child with uncorrected cyanotic heart disease and a high hemoglobin concentration) is more likely to demonstrate cyanosis in the presence of hypoxemia than the child with a normal or low hemoglobin concentration. Cyanosis is most likely to occur when low arterial oxygen saturation is combined with low cardiac output. For these reasons central cyanosis is not considered an early or reliable indication of hypoxemia.

The ambient temperature should be considered when the child's skin color and temperature are evaluated. If the child is exposed to a cool environmental temperature, peripheral vasoconstriction may produce mottling or pallor with cool skin and delayed capillary refill (particularly in the extremities).[8] When the child is warmed, however, the color should improve, and the extremities should again feel warm with brisk capillary refill. In summary, the capillary refill time must be evaluated in the context of ambient temperature and other clinical findings.[9]

Pulse oximetry should be used to monitor hemoglobin oxygen saturation if a child is at risk for developing hypoxemia. Arterial blood gases should be analyzed if respiratory impairment (particularly hypercarbia or acidosis) is suspected.

Factors Influencing Cardiovascular Function

Shock is present when perfusion of the vital organs is inadequate to meet organ

tissue metabolic demand.[10-12] The failure to deliver adequate metabolic substrate and remove metabolites leads to anaerobic metabolism, accumulation of lactic acid, and irreversible cellular damage. Death may then rapidly result from cardiovascular collapse or later from multiple organ system dysfunction. Shock most often results from inadequate circulating blood volume or cardiovascular dysfunction.

Critical Concepts: Classification of Shock

Shock is classified by *etiology*:

- *Hypovolemic:* inadequate intravascular volume relative to the vascular space. Hypovolemic shock is the most common type of shock occurring in children.

- *Cardiogenic:* myocardial dysfunction. Cardiogenic shock may be associated with hypovolemia or inappropriate distribution of blood flow, and it is present in all forms of prolonged shock regardless of etiology.

- *Distributive:* inappropriate distribution of blood flow. Distributive shock is characteristic of sepsis and anaphylaxis.

Shock is also classified according to its effect on *blood pressure*:

- *Compensated:* systolic blood pressure in normal range

- *Decompensated:* systolic blood pressure less than 5th percentile for age

Shock may be classified according to its effect on *cardiac output*. But regardless of whether cardiac output is low, normal, or high, when shock is present, cardiac output is inadequate to meet metabolic demands.

FYI. Factors Affecting Stroke Volume

The pumping function of the heart is determined by 3 components: preload, contractility, and afterload. Figure 3 illustrates the relationship between these parameters. Each of these parameters may be manipulated to improve stroke volume and thus cardiac output. Optimal use of fluid and vasoactive drug therapy requires an understanding of these determinants of stroke volume.

Ventricular *preload* is the amount of stretch on the ventricular muscle before the onset of contraction. Increased preload increases muscle contraction via the Frank-Starling relationship—the greater the stretch, the greater the resultant stroke volume. Preload is better represented by the *volume* of blood in the

ventricle (ie, the end-diastolic volume) than by the central venous or left atrial *pressure* (ie, ventricular end-diastolic pressure). Although filling pressures are related to preload, the relationship is complex and may be influenced by such external factors as the use of positive end-expiratory pressure and ventricular compliance.

Afterload refers to the sum of forces that oppose or impede ventricular ejection. Afterload is typically approximated by the systemic or pulmonary vascular resistance. Figure 4 illustrates the importance of afterload. As afterload (ie, systemic vascular resistance [SVR]) is increased in a patient with a normal ventricle, the healthy ventricle maintains stroke volume with a resultant increase in blood pressure. This results from the following relationship:

$CO \approx MAP \div SVR$, where CO is cardiac output, MAP is mean arterial pressure, and SVR is systemic vascular resistance.

If heart rate remains constant, then stroke volume (SV) is directly proportional to CO. Substituting SV for CO yields $MAP \propto SVR \times SV$. Thus, if SV is maintained and SVR increases, MAP must increase (ie, blood pressure increases). Conversely, as seen in the lower line in Figure 4, if the patient has poor ventricular function, an increase in SVR decreases SV. Note that in this case there may be little change in MAP, illustrating that blood pressure is often a poor indicator of stroke volume in patients with poor ventricular function such as cardiogenic shock.

FIGURE 3. The relationship between the 3 factors affecting ventricular stroke volume. *Preload* is the amount of stretch on the muscle fiber. Clinically this represents the myocardial muscle stretch before contraction and is most closely related to the filling *volume* (not the filling pressure) of the heart chamber. The filling volume is that volume contained in the ventricle at the end of diastole. *Contractility* is the strength and efficiency of muscle contraction. Contractility is influenced by the metabolic state of the myocardium and the presence of factors that increase the force of contraction, such as catecholamine inotropes. The sum of the forces opposing or impeding ventricular ejection is the *afterload*. Clinically afterload is determined by the elasticity of the vascular bed and resistance to flow within the arteries and arterioles. Clinically, systemic vascular resistance is equal to the afterload of the left ventricle, and pulmonary vascular resistance is equal to the afterload of the right ventricle.

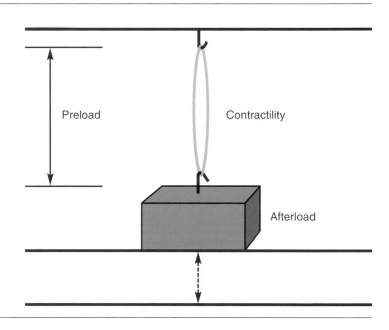

Causes and Classification of Shock

Shock Classification Based on Etiology

Shock may be characterized according to its cause or its effect on the child's

physiologic status. When shock is characterized by etiology, the terms *hypovolemic, cardiogenic,* and *distributive* shock are used. Any method of classification represents an oversimplification because etiologies often overlap the classification system.

Hypovolemic shock is characterized by inadequate intravascular volume in relation to the vascular space. Hypovolemia is the leading cause of shock in children worldwide. It often results from dehydration or hemorrhage but may also be caused by "third spacing" of fluids from the

FIGURE 4. The relationship between stroke volume (SV) and systemic vascular resistance (SVR). The upper curve shows changes in SV in a patient with normal ventricular contractility and function. As SVR increases from point A to B, blood pressure (MAP) increases because the healthy ventricle maintains SV (and thus CO) constant. Further increases in SVR eventually depress SV, moving the patient to point C. The lower curve illustrates the relation between SVR and SV in a patient with poor ventricular function. As SVR increases, SV falls proportionately. Note that the reciprocal changes between SV and SVR may cause little to no change in MAP as the patient moves from point A′ to C′. Conversely, note that reducing SVR (moving from C′ to A′ by using a vasodilator) may improve SV with no change in MAP.

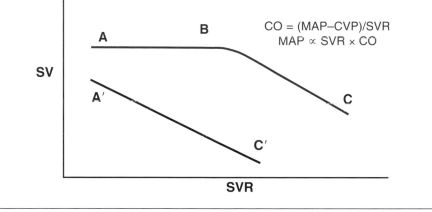

$$CO = (MAP–CVP)/SVR$$
$$MAP \propto SVR \times CO$$

vascular to the extravascular compartment due to increased capillary permeability. This intravascular to extravascular movement of fluid may be observed in children with inflammatory conditions such as burns or sepsis. Relative hypovolemia occurs when systemic vasodilation increases the vascular capacity, such as occurs in sepsis and anaphylaxis.

Cardiogenic shock is characterized by myocardial dysfunction. Typically intravascular volume is adequate or increased, but inadequate myocardial function limits stroke volume and cardiac output. If the patient has been ill with poor oral intake or vomiting, the patient with cardiogenic shock may also be hypovolemic.

Distributive shock is characterized by inappropriate distribution of blood volume. This form of shock may be caused by sepsis or anaphylaxis.

Although the etiologic classification of shock is useful to help clarify the focus of therapy, it is important to recognize that any child with severe or sustained shock, regardless of the etiology, develops some degree of myocardial dysfunction. Many children with shock require fluid administration even in the absence of documented fluid loss, and some will require pharmacologic therapy to increase cardiac output or redistribute it.

Shock Classification Based on Physiologic Status

Shock is also characterized by its effect on the patient's physiologic status and thus can be labeled as *compensated* or *decompensated*. Compensated shock is defined by the presence of *systolic* blood pressure within the normal range with signs and symptoms of inadequate tissue and organ perfusion (eg, lactic acidosis, oliguria, altered level of consciousness). Decompensated shock is present when signs of shock are associated with systolic hypotension.

Finally, shock may be characterized by the patient's cardiac output. Although shock is often associated with low cardiac output, cardiac output may be increased in septic and anaphylactic shock.[10,13-15]

As previously noted, high cardiac output does not ensure adequate tissue oxygen delivery. For this reason clinical evaluation of the patient should determine whether cardiac output is *adequate* or *inadequate* to meet tissue metabolic requirements. Inadequacy of cardiac output is indicated by the presence of lactic acidosis.

When shock is associated with a low flow (low cardiac output) state, such as that which occurs with hypovolemic or cardiogenic shock, compensatory mechanisms of the sympathetic nervous system divert blood flow from the skin, mesenteric, and renal circulations. The skin becomes cool and mottled or pale due to high systemic vascular resistance, and urine output falls. Initially arterial blood pressure is maintained and cardiac output is distributed to vital organs (the heart and brain) by increasing systemic vascular resistance.

Septic, anaphylactic, and other forms of distributive shock characteristically are associated with high cardiac output. But cardiac output is unevenly distributed, so some tissue beds remain inadequately perfused whereas other tissue beds (skeletal muscle and skin) receive blood flow well in excess of their metabolic demand. Low systemic vascular resistance increases skin blood flow and causes bounding peripheral pulses. The ischemic tissue beds (often the splanchnic vascular bed) generate lactic acid, leading to acidosis. Therefore, despite the presence of high cardiac output, shock and metabolic acidosis develop because blood flow is inappropriately distributed.

Early signs of sepsis are often subtle and thus may be difficult to recognize. Based on the Consensus Terminology published by the Society of Critical Care Medicine and the American College of Chest Physicians, *sepsis* is diagnosed when the child demonstrates 2 or more of the following criteria: fever or hypothermia, tachycardia, tachypnea with respiratory alkalosis, and a change in white blood cell count (leukocytosis, leukopenia, or an increase in immature or band forms of white blood cells) plus the presence of suspected infection.[14,16,17] *Severe sepsis* is present when signs of sepsis are observed in association with evidence of inadequate organ perfusion and function (eg, altered mental status, oliguria, or lactic acidosis).[14,16,17] Thus, evaluation of systemic perfusion and analysis of blood gases should allow identification of sepsis before decompensated shock develops. *Septic shock* is defined by the presence of hypotension despite fluid administration or when normotension is maintained only with vasoactive drug support.[17,18]

Evaluation of Cardiovascular Performance

The relationship between various hemodynamic parameters that determine cardiac output and oxygen delivery is shown in Figure 5. Cardiac output is the volume of blood ejected by the heart each minute (heart rate × stroke volume). Stroke volume is the volume of blood ejected by the ventricles with each contraction. Mean arterial blood pressure is the product of flow (cardiac output) and resistance (systemic vascular resistance). Of the variables affecting and affected by cardiac output, only the heart rate and blood pressure can be easily measured (Figure 5). Stroke volume and systemic vascular resistance must be indirectly assessed by examining the quality of pulses and evaluating tissue perfusion.

Heart Rate

Table 2 lists normal heart rates in infants and children. Sinus tachycardia is a common response to many types of stress (eg, anxiety, pain, fever, hypoxia, hypercapnia, hypovolemia, or cardiac impairment). The development of sinus tachycardia mandates evaluation to determine if it is a sign of shock.

In comparison with older children and adults, the stroke volume in neonates, infants, and small children is small, and cardiac output is more dependent on heart rate than stroke volume. The typical

FIGURE 5. Hemodynamic relationships. Stroke volume is determined by the pumping function of the ventricle, which is derived from the contractility, afterload, and preload of the ventricle. Cardiac output is the product of stroke volume and heart rate. Cardiac output is also determined by the driving pressure (ie, mean blood pressure) and vascular resistance. Net oxygen delivery to the tissue is the product of cardiac output and oxygen content. Note that the only clinically measurable determinants of tissue perfusion (ie, oxygen delivery) are heart rate, blood pressure, and arterial oxygen saturation.

Boxes enclose variables commonly manipulated by therapy.

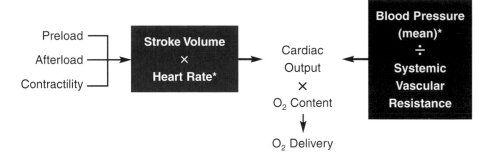

*A clinical parameter that is easily assessed or measured.

physiologic response to a fall in cardiac output is tachycardia; in neonates, however, ischemia or hypoxia may cause a paradoxical bradycardia.

Monitoring the change in heart rate in response to therapy or interventions also may be helpful. In adults an increase in heart rate of more than 30 bpm in response to changing from a recumbent to standing position is a sensitive indicator of hypovolemia.[19] Similar data is not available for infants and children, but the usefulness of postural changes in evaluating heart rate is likely applicable in adolescents. Improved

detection of dehydration in children can be obtained by evaluating multiple potential signs of poor perfusion and level of hydration (eg, delayed capillary refill, absent tears, dry mucous membranes, and ill general appearance in children with dehydration[20]).

A very rapid heart rate in infants and children may be caused by an underlying cardiac condition that produces supraventricular tachycardia, atrial flutter, or ventricular tachycardia. Regardless of the reason, a very rapid heart rate increases myocardial oxygen demand while simul-

TABLE 2. Normal Heart Rates (bpm) in Children*

Age	Awake Rate	Mean	Sleeping Rate
Newborn to 3 mo	85-205	140	80-160
3 mo to 2 y	100-190	130	75-160
2 y to 10 y	60-140	80	60-90
>10 y	60-100	75	50-90

*bpm indicates beats per minute

From Gillette PC, Garson A Jr, Porter CJ, McNamara DG. Dysrhythmias. In: Adams FG, Emmanouilides GC, Reimenschenider TA, eds. *Moss' Heart Disease in Infants, Children and Adolescents.* 4th ed. Baltimore, Md: Williams and Wilkins; 1989:725-741.

taneously impairing myocardial oxygen delivery because the left ventricle is perfused during diastole and diastole is shortened with severe tachycardia. A very rapid rate may impair diastolic filling of the atria and ventricles, leading to low stroke volume. In combination these factors may lead to cardiogenic shock.

When tachycardia fails to maintain adequate cardiac output and oxygen delivery, tissue hypoxia and hypercapnia produce acidosis. As acidosis and inadequate substrate delivery continue, myocardial function decreases. If urgent interventions are not initiated, bradycardia and cardiac arrest may follow.

Blood Pressure

Compensatory mechanisms to maintain cardiac output include tachycardia and increased cardiac contractility; the latter results in more complete emptying of the ventricle with each contraction. When these compensatory mechanisms fail, hypotension develops and decompensated shock is present. As previously noted, cardiac output and systemic vascular resistance determine mean blood pressure. When cardiac output falls, normal blood pressure can be maintained *only* if compensatory vasoconstriction occurs.

Tachycardia persists until cardiac reserve is depleted. Figure 6 depicts an idealized model of the cardiovascular response to hemorrhagic shock. Initially cardiac output is maintained as blood volume is lost because the venous system contracts to maintain venous return with a smaller total blood volume and the heart rate increases to compensate for a fall in stroke volume. Eventually cardiac output begins to fall as blood volume is depleted. Mean blood pressure is initially maintained by an increase in systemic vascular resistance. Hypotension is a late and often sudden sign of cardiovascular decompensation. Therefore, even mild hypotension must be treated quickly and vigorously because it signals decompensation and cardiac arrest may be imminent.

Normal blood pressure values according to age are provided in Table 3. The median (50th percentile) *systolic* blood pressure for children 1 to 10 years of age may be approximated by the following formula:

90 mm Hg + (2 × age in years)

According to the *ECC Guidelines 2000,* hypotension (ie, decompensated shock) is characterized by the following limits of *systolic* blood pressure (SBP):

- For term neonates (0 to 28 days): SBP less than 60 mm Hg

- For infants 1 to 12 months: SBP less than 70 mm Hg

- For children 1 to 10 years of age: SBP less than 70 mm Hg + (2 × age in years)

- For children more than 10 years of age: SBP less than 90 mm Hg

Note that these blood pressure thresholds overlap normal values, including the 5% of normal children who have an SBP less than the 5th percentile for age. An observed fall of 10 mm Hg in SBP from baseline should prompt careful serial evaluations for additional signs of shock.

Foundation Facts

Accurate blood pressure measurement requires the use of a proper-sized cuff. Current recommendations require the use of a cuff bladder that equals 40% of the mid-upper arm circumference.[21] Additional information can be obtained from measuring the diastolic blood pressure and calculated pulse pressure. *Pulse pressure* is the difference between systolic and diastolic blood pressure. Normally diastolic blood pressure is two thirds of systolic blood pressure (ie, pulse pressure is one third of systolic pressure). For example, if systolic blood pressure is 90 mm Hg, normal diastolic blood pressure should be about 60 mm Hg. When systemic vascular resistance is increased, as expected in hypovolemic and cardiogenic shock, pulse pressure narrows. Conversely, when systemic vascular resistance is low, as expected in septic shock, pulse pressure widens.

FIGURE 6. Hemodynamic response to hemorrhage. Model for cardiovascular response to hypovolemia from hemorrhage (based on normative data).[22] CO indicates cardiac output; MAP, mean arterial pressure; CVP, central venous pressure; SVR, systemic vascular resistance; HR, heart rate; and SV, stroke volume.

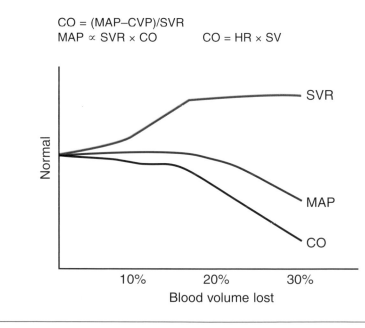

$$CO = (MAP{-}CVP)/SVR$$
$$MAP \propto SVR \times CO \qquad CO = HR \times SV$$

The presence of hypotension in a patient with multisystem trauma traditionally was assumed to indicate a blood volume loss ≥20% and the need for urgent volume replacement and blood transfusion, but minimal data supports this assumption. Moreover, hypotension in a traumatized child also may occur secondary to reversible causes such as tension pneumothorax or pericardial tamponade or may result from a neurologic insult (eg, spinal cord injury or massive brain or brainstem injury), resulting in loss of sympathetic nervous system control of peripheral vascular tone.

Systemic Perfusion

Because sinus tachycardia is a nonspecific sign of circulatory compromise and hypotension is a late sign of shock, recognition of early compensated shock requires evaluation of indirect signs of blood flow and systemic vascular resistance. This is best accomplished by noting the presence and volume of peripheral pulses and assessing end-organ perfusion and function.

Evaluation of Pulses

The carotid, axillary, brachial, radial, femoral, dorsalis pedis, and posterior tibial pulses should be readily palpable in healthy infants and children, although they may be difficult to palpate in obese infants or if the ambient temperature is cold. A discrepancy in the volume between peripheral and central pulses may be caused by vasoconstriction associated with a cold ambient temperature or may be an early sign of decreased cardiac output.

The palpable pulse volume (strength of the pulse) is normally related to stroke volume and pulse pressure (the difference between systolic and diastolic pressures). When cardiac output decreases as a result of a fall in stroke volume (low cardiac output shock), systemic vascular resistance increases, narrowing pulse pressure. The net result is that the distal pulse feels "thready"; as cardiac output continues to fall, it finally becomes impossible to feel. In contrast, early septic shock is typically a high-output state and is characterized

TABLE 3. Normal Blood Pressures in Children*

Age	Systolic (mm Hg)	Diastolic (mm Hg)
Birth (12 h, <1000 g)	39-59	16-36
Birth (12 h, 3 kg)	50-70	25-45
Neonate (96 h)	60-90	20-60
Infant (6 mo)	87-105	53-66
Toddler (2 y)	95-105	53-66
School age (7 y)	97-112	57-71
Adolescent (15 y)	112-128	66-80

*Blood pressure ranges taken from the following sources: *Neonate:* Versmold H, et al. Aortic blood pressure during the first 12 hours of life in infants with birth weight 610 to 4220 g. *Pediatrics.* 1981;67:107. 10th to 90th percentile ranges used. *Children:* Horan MJ. Task Force on Blood Pressure Control in Children: report of the Second Task Force on Blood Pressure in Children. *Pediatrics.* 1987;79:1. 50th to 90th percentile ranges indicated.

Reproduced from Hazinski MF. Children are different. In: Hazinski MF, ed. *Nursing Care of the Critically Ill Child.* 2nd ed. St Louis, Mo: Mosby Year Book; 1992.

by a wide pulse pressure with normal or increased stroke volume leading to bounding pulses. Loss of *central* pulses is a premorbid sign requiring very rapid intervention.

Skin

Decreased skin perfusion can be an early sign of shock. When the child is well perfused and the ambient temperature is warm, the hands and feet should be warm and dry and the palms pink to the distal phalanx. When cardiac output decreases, cooling of the skin begins peripherally (in the fingers and toes) and extends proximally (toward the trunk).[23] Sluggish, delayed, or prolonged capillary refill (a refill time of more than 2 seconds after blanching) is caused by shock, a rising fever, or a cold ambient temperature.[8,9,23] Note that a rise in body temperature is often characterized by dermal vasoconstriction as the temperature control mechanisms attempt to increase core temperature.

When capillary refill is evaluated, lift the extremity slightly above the level of the heart to ensure assessment of arteriolar capillary (and not venous stasis) refill.

Interpret capillary refill in the context of other signs of shock because it is a relatively insensitive and nonspecific indicator of shock when assessed alone.

Mottling, pallor, delayed capillary refill, and peripheral cyanosis often indicate poor skin perfusion. Acrocyanosis, however, may be normal in newborn or polycythemic patients. Severe vasoconstriction produces a gray or ashen color in newborns and pallor in older children.

Brain

The clinical signs of brain hypoperfusion are determined by severity and duration of ischemia.[24] When the ischemic insult is sudden, few signs of neurologic compromise precede loss of consciousness: muscular tone is lost, and generalized seizures and pupillary dilation may be observed.

When the onset of the ischemic insult is more gradual, neurologic symptoms are typically more insidious. Altered consciousness occurs with confusion, irritability, and lethargy. Agitation may alternate with lethargy.

After 2 months of age an infant should normally focus on the faces of his/her parents. Failure to recognize or make eye contact with parents may be an early, ominous sign of cortical hypoperfusion or cerebral dysfunction. Failure to respond to a painful stimulus is also an ominous sign in a previously normal child. Parents may be the first to recognize these signs, but they may be unable to describe them other than to say something is wrong. Listen to the parents!

More profound hypoperfusion produce greater changes in the level of consciousness. As the level of consciousness declines, the child's neurologic response may be characterized by the **AVPU** description:

- **A**lert
- Responsive to **V**oice
- Responsive to **P**ain
- **U**nresponsive

With progressive decline in the level of consciousness, deep tendon reflexes may be depressed, pupils may be small but reactive, and breathing patterns may be altered. Hypotonia and intermittent flexor or extensor posturing may occur with prolonged cerebral hypoperfusion or extreme hypoxemia (PaO_2 less than 30 mm Hg).

Kidneys

Urine output is directly proportional to renal blood flow and glomerular filtration rate. Although urine output is a good indicator of renal function, it is not very helpful in the initial evaluation of renal perfusion, because it is often difficult for parents to estimate recent urine production, and the quantity of urine in the bladder may represent urine production over various time periods. Normal urine output averages 1 to 2 mL/kg per hour in children. Urine flow of less than 1 mL/kg per hour in a child or less than 30 mL/h in adolescents in the absence of known renal disease is often a sign of poor renal perfusion or hypovolemia. An indwelling urinary catheter facilitates accurate and continuous determination of urine flow.

Table 4 summarizes the characteristic clinical signs and hemodynamic changes in different types of shock. The table does not include unusual causes of shock, such as carbon monoxide poisoning or severe left ventricular output obstruction from aortic stenosis.

Rapid Cardiopulmonary Assessment

Assessment and management of the seriously ill or injured child begins with rapid cardiopulmonary assessment. This assessment is the foundation of pediatric advanced life support and is designed to quickly identify potential or actual respiratory failure and shock and the effects of these problems on end-organ perfusion and function. This identification will enable planning of appropriate interventions. Laboratory tests are useful adjuncts in determining the severity of physiologic derangements, but they are not essential to the initial evaluation.

Every clinician who works with children should be able to recognize respiratory and circulatory failure and impending cardiac arrest based on a rapid cardiopulmonary assessment (see Critical Concepts: "Elements of Rapid Cardiopulmonary Assessment"). Assessment by a trained provider requires less than 30 seconds to complete.

The rapid cardiopulmonary assessment uses the same ABC approach used in CPR but adds assessment of mental status:

- **A**irway: The rescuer must determine if the airway is (1) patent; (2) maintainable with head positioning, suctioning, or adjuncts; or (3) unmaintainable and requiring interventions such as intubation, removal of a foreign body, or needle cricothyrotomy. If airway intervention is needed, note the presence of inspiratory sounds (eg, stridor) and the work of breathing.

- **B**reathing: Evaluation of breathing focuses on determination of respiratory rate and assessment of inspiratory breath sounds, work of breathing, adequacy of tidal volume, and resultant chest expansion. The evaluation should focus on determining if minute ventilation is adequate or inadequate to sustain oxygenation and ventilation and thus heart rate and circulation.

- **C**irculation: Qualitative examination of the systemic circulation provides indirect evidence of the efficacy/effectiveness of cardiac output. The heart rate, presence and quality of peripheral and central pulses, capillary refill time (considered in the context of ambient

Critical Concepts: Assessment for Shock

Assessment of circulation for *shock* includes the following parameters:

- *Heart rate:* fast or slow. A very fast heart rate may be the cause of shock or may be a sign of stress.

- *Blood pressure:* assess systolic and diastolic pressure and calculate pulse pressure

- *Systemic perfusion:*
  — Pulse location—palpable peripherally and centrally? If absent peripherally, decompensated shock is present

  — Pulse volume—note if thready or bounding

  — Skin temperature—color, capillary refill

  — CNS function—evaluate response to environment; AVPU scale

  — Urine output—reflects renal perfusion and often reflects splanchnic perfusion

temperature), and skin perfusion as well as end-organ function are assessed using criteria discussed previously.

■ **D**isability is assessed by noting the patient's interaction with his/her environment, response to stimulation, muscle tone, and pupillary response.

Examination of the ill infant or child does not end when the rapid cardiopulmonary assessment is completed. The patient's condition is often dynamic, and *repeated* assessments are necessary to evaluate trends in his/her condition and response to therapy. It may be necessary to interrupt the rapid cardiopulmonary

assessment to provide life-saving therapy, such as opening the airway or assisting ventilation in an apneic patient.

Priorities in Management

Based on the rapid cardiopulmonary assessment, the child's physiologic status is categorized as

■ Stable

■ Respiratory distress

■ Respiratory failure (may have increased or inadequate respiratory effort)

■ Shock

— Compensated

— Decompensated

■ Cardiopulmonary failure

When clinical signs of distress are subtle and respiratory or circulatory failure is suspected, frequent sequential assessments must be made. Supplemental laboratory studies, such as pulse oximetry, arterial blood gas analysis, and chest x-ray may be useful. When inadequate ventilation, oxygenation, or perfusion threatens cardiopulmonary stability, intervention(s) followed by reassessment should be performed promptly and continued until the child's condition is stable.

TABLE 4. Summary of Clinical and Cardiovascular Signs of Shock

Clinical Signs	Hypovolemic Shock	Distributive (Septic) Shock	Cardiogenic Shock
Respiratory rate	⇑	⇑ to ⇑⇑	⇑⇑
Respiratory effort	Normal	Normal to ⇑	⇑⇑
Breath sounds	Normal	Normal (crackles with pneumonia, ARDS)	Abnormal: rales or grunting
Heart rate	⇑	⇑ to ⇑⇑	⇑⇑
Pulse quality	Thready	Early—bounding Late—thready	Thready
Pulse pressure	Narrow	Widened	Narrow
Skin perfusion: color, temperature, capillary refill	Pink, cool distally, normal to prolonged capillary refill	Pink, often warm in early shock, normal to prolonged capillary refill	Mottled gray or blue, cool to cold, prolonged capillary refill
Level of consciousness	Usually normal unless severe hypovolemia	Lethargic or confused/agitated Coma occurs late	Lethargic to coma
Urine output	Decreased	Decreased	Markedly decreased
Cardiovascular Factors			
Stroke volume	Low	Normal to increased	Markedly diminished
Preload	Low	Low	Often high
Afterload (SVR)	High	Low	High
Acidosis	Mild to moderate	Mild to marked	Moderate to marked

Specific clinical or cardiovascular signs that help distinguish the type of shock are highlighted in shaded cells.

Critical Concepts: Elements of Rapid Cardiopulmonary Assessment

Evaluation of General Appearance

- General color ("looks good" vs "looks bad")
- Mental status, responsiveness
- Activity, movement, muscle tone
- Age-appropriate response (to parents, healthcare providers, painful procedures)
  Note: A decreased response to painful stimulus is abnormal.

Examination of Airway, Breathing, and Circulation

Airway

- Clear
- Maintainable with noninvasive assistance (positioning, suction, bag-mask ventilation)
- Not maintainable without invasive intervention/intubation

Breathing

- Respiratory rate
- Respiratory effort and mechanics
- Air entry/tidal volume
- Skin color

Classification of Respiratory Status

- Respiratory distress: increased effort/work of breathing
- Respiratory failure: inadequate gas exchange resulting in inadequate oxygenation and/or ventilation (may be present with or without respiratory distress)

Circulation

- Cardiovascular function
  - Evaluation of responsiveness (AVPU scale)
    Alert
    Voice (responsive to voice)
    Pain (responsive to pain)
    Unresponsive

  - Heart rate
    "Normal" heart rate decreases as the child ages
    Increased heart rate may be a nonspecific sign of distress
    (Heart rate ranges for sinus tachycardia and supraventricular tachycardia [SVT] overlap)
    Consider diagnosis of SVT for HR >220 bpm for an infant and >180 bpm for a child
  - Pulses, capillary refill, skin perfusion
    Peripheral pulses may be diminished in shock
    Evaluate temperature, capillary refill, color of skin
  - Blood pressure
    Lower limit (5th percentile) SBP for 1 to 10 years of age: 70 mm Hg + (2 × age)
    Compensated shock: signs of shock without hypotension
    Decompensated shock: signs of shock with hypotension
- End-organ function, perfusion
  - Brain: see above evaluation of responsiveness
  - Skin: see above evaluation of temperature, capillary refill, color
  - Kidneys: normal urine output is 1 to 2 mL/kg per hour (will decrease when renal perfusion is compromised)

Classification of Circulatory Status

- Compensated (early): tachycardia, poor systemic perfusion
- Decompensated (late): weak central pulses, altered mental status, hypotension
- Septic shock: fever or hypothermia, tachycardia and tachypnea, leukocytosis or leukopenia or increased bands

Assessment in Special Resuscitation Circumstances

Trauma

- Airway and breathing problems common
- Use PALS approach *plus*
  - Airway assessment and support with cervical spine immobilization
  - Breathing assessment and support, often including management of pneumothorax
  - Circulation assessment and support, often including control of bleeding
- Identify and treat life-threatening injuries

Toxicology

- Airway obstruction, breathing depression, and circulatory dysfunction common
- Use PALS approach *plus*
  - Airway assessment and support—watch for reduced airway protective mechanisms
  - Breathing assessment and support—watch for respiratory depression
  - Circulation assessment and support—watch for arrhythmias, hypotension, and coronary ischemia
- Identify and treat reversible complications
- Identify toxin and administer antidote

Classification of Cardiopulmonary Physiologic Status

- Stable
- Respiratory distress
- Respiratory failure
- Shock (compensated vs decompensated)
- Cardiopulmonary failure

A child with respiratory distress or compensated shock should be approached promptly and efficiently, yet thoughtfully and gently to minimize fear and oxygen demand. Administer supplemental oxygen in a nonthreatening manner whenever possible. Support the infant's head in a neutral position. Allow older patients to assume a position of maximal comfort to minimize work of breathing and optimize airway patency. Maintain the patient's normal ambient and body temperature and withhold oral intake if there is any concern that the patient's condition may deteriorate or that invasive interventions (eg, intubation or bag-mask ventilation) will be needed.

If signs of respiratory failure are present, establish a patent airway and ensure adequate ventilation with maximum supplemental oxygen (see Chapter 4). When signs of shock are present, establish vascular access rapidly (see Chapter 6) and provide volume expansion and medications as needed (see Chapter 5).

When cardiopulmonary failure is detected, give initial priority to ventilation and oxygenation. If circulation and perfusion fail to improve rapidly, provide therapy for shock (see Chapters 5 and 7).

Summary

A large number of respiratory and circulatory conditions can lead to cardiorespiratory failure. If cardiorespiratory failure is not rapidly corrected, cardiac arrest may develop, with poor outcome. Therefore, early recognition of children at risk for respiratory failure and decompensated shock is necessary to prevent progression to cardiac arrest.

This chapter summarizes the signs and symptoms of children with respiratory or circulatory conditions that may lead to respiratory failure or shock. Initial evaluation using a consistent approach—the rapid cardiopulmonary assessment—will rapidly identify children at risk. The child's clinical signs and symptoms determine his/her physiologic status and guide appropriate

intervention. Appropriate interventions for shock and respiratory failure are described in the remainder of this text. For summary information that will be useful during the PALS Provider Course, see the Appendix. This appendix contains summary poster information about recognition and initial stabilization of respiratory failure and shock.

- *Cardiorespiratory arrest,* or *cardiopulmonary arrest,* is the absence of response to stimulation, absence of adequate breathing, and absence of pulses or other signs of circulation

- *Respiratory arrest* is the absence of breathing (ie, apnea)

- *Respiratory failure* is the clinical state of inadequate oxygenation, ventilation, or both

- *Respiratory distress* is the presence of increased respiratory effort, rate, and work of breathing

- *Shock* is characterized by inadequate tissue perfusion and substrate (particularly oxygen) delivery. *Compensated shock* is present when there are signs of shock with blood pressure within the normal range. *Decompensated shock* is present when there are signs of shock with hypotension (in children 1 to 10 years of age, systolic blood pressure less than 70 mm Hg plus [2 × age in years]).

- *Oxygen delivery* is arterial oxygen content × cardiac output. If arterial oxygen content falls without a commensurate increase in cardiac output, oxygen delivery will fall. A fall in cardiac output will produce a fall in oxygen delivery.

- *Arterial oxygen content* is oxygen bound to hemoglobin plus the dissolved oxygen. The oxygen bound to hemoglobin is the product of hemoglobin concentration in grams per deciliter × 1.34 mL oxygen/g × oxyhemoglobin saturation. The dissolved oxygen is PaO_2 in mm Hg × 0.003 mL O_2/mm Hg. Normal arterial oxygen content is 18 to 20 mL/dL of

blood. Under normal conditions the dissolved oxygen constitutes an inconsequential portion of total oxygen content, although an increase in dissolved oxygen can substantially increase oxygen content in the severely anemic patient.

- Cardiac output is a product of heart rate and stroke volume. Children are very dependent on an adequate heart rate to maintain adequate cardiac output. If there is a decrease in heart rate or stroke volume without a commensurate and compensatory increase in the other factor, cardiac output will fall. Shock may be present with normal, high, or low cardiac output, but if shock is present, cardiac output is inadequate.

- Minute ventilation is tidal volume × respiratory rate. If either tidal volume or respiratory rate decreases without a commensurate and compensatory increase in the other component, hypoventilation can develop.

- Respiratory failure can result from any airway, pulmonary, or neuromuscular disease that impairs oxygen exchange or elimination of carbon dioxide. The resultant hypoxemia, hypercapnia, and acidosis reflect the severity of respiratory failure.

- Pediatric patients have a high oxygen demand per kilogram of body weight because their metabolic rate is high. Any increase in oxygen demand or decrease in oxygen delivery can cause tissue hypoxia and acidosis.

- Infants and children at risk for respiratory arrest may demonstrate increased respiratory rate, increased respiratory effort, diminished level of consciousness, poor skeletal muscle tone, or cyanosis.

- The provider evaluates respiratory function by evaluating respiratory rate, respiratory mechanics, level of consciousness, and color of skin and mucous membranes.

- A slow or irregular respiratory rate in the acutely ill or injured child is ominous. A decreasing respiratory rate or irregular respiratory rhythm may indicate deterioration in the child's condition.

- Evaluation of respiratory mechanics includes evaluation of work of breathing and monitoring for signs such as retractions, grunting, stridor, wheezing or prolonged exhalation, or diminished distal air entry.

- Respiratory failure may develop from upper airway obstruction, lower airway obstruction, parenchymal lung disease, or abnormal control of ventilation.

- Shock may be classified by etiology (hypovolemic, cardiogenic, or distributive) or its effect on blood pressure (compensated or decompensated).

- Cardiac output is the volume of blood ejected by the heart per minute (heart rate × stroke volume). Stroke volume is the volume of blood ejected by the ventricles with each contraction. Mean arterial blood pressure is proportional to flow (cardiac output) and resistance (systemic vascular resistance). Of the variables affecting and affected by cardiac output, only heart rate and blood pressure can be easily measured, so the provider must be able to evaluate indirect signs of organ perfusion and oxygen delivery.

- Providers must be skilled in performing rapid cardiopulmonary assessment to identify signs of respiratory failure or shock and initiate treatment.

Case Scenarios

1. For case scenarios involving recognition of respiratory failure, see Chapter 4: "Airway, Ventilation, and Management of Respiratory Distress and Failure."

2. For case scenarios involving recognition of shock, see Chapter 7: "Case Scenarios in Shock."

Review Questions

1. **Which of the following statements best describes the *most common* factors that contribute to the development of cardiopulmonary arrest in infants and children?**

   a. cardiopulmonary arrest is usually the first symptom of underlying cardiovascular disease in infants and children

   b. cardiopulmonary arrest in infants and children is most often precipitated by sudden onset of ventricular arrhythmias

   c. cardiopulmonary arrest in infants and children is most often the result of congenital heart block or other abnormalities of the conduction system (eg, long QT syndrome) or anomalous coronary arteries

   d. cardiopulmonary arrest in infants and children is most often the end result of deterioration in respiratory and circulatory function

   The correct answer is d. This explains why rapid cardiopulmonary assessment and identification of respiratory failure and shock are important to prevent arrest.

   Answer a is incorrect because cardiopulmonary arrest is not typically the first symptom of underlying heart disease. Many children with heart disease present with congestive heart failure or hypoxemia long before they present with sudden cardiac arrest.

   Answer b is incorrect because the sudden onset of ventricular arrhythmias is the leading cause of sudden cardiac arrest in adults but is not the most common cause of cardiopulmonary arrest in infants and children.

   Answer c is incorrect because although congenital heart block and conduction abnormalities and anomalous coronary arteries can cause cardiopulmonary arrest, they are not the most common cause of cardiopulmonary arrest in children.

2. **An 18-month-old child has ingested his aunt's narcotic analgesic. He is brought to the ED because his mother describes him as lethargic and "not breathing right." Which of the following are the first things you should assess during your rapid cardiorespiratory assessment of this child?**

   a. determine heart rate and blood pressure to see if he is in compensated or decompensated shock

   b. determine the strength of peripheral pulses to see if shock of any kind is present

   c. evaluate his arterial blood gases to determine the need for intubation

   d. evaluate airway and breathing by assessing respiratory rate, air movement, and color of skin and mucous membranes

   The correct answer is d. Your first priority should be support of airway and breathing.

   Answer a is incorrect because evaluation of heart rate and blood pressure should be accomplished only *after* you assess the child's airway and breathing.

   Answer b is incorrect because you should assess the child's airway and breathing before you assess the strength of pulses and signs of circulation.

   Answer c is incorrect because evaluation of arterial blood gases should be performed after assessment of airway and breathing and initial evaluation of circulation.

3. **You are evaluating a responsive 2-year-old toddler who presents with fever, irritability, mottled color, cool extremities, and a prolonged capillary refill time. Her heart rate is 160 bpm, respiratory rate is 45 breaths/min, and BP is**

82/46 mm Hg. Which of the following most accurately describes this child's condition, using the terminology taught in the PALS course and in this text?

a. decompensated shock associated with inadequate tissue perfusion

b. decompensated shock associated with inadequate tissue perfusion and significant hypotension

c. compensated shock requiring no intervention

d. compensated shock associated with inadequate tissue perfusion

The correct answer is d. The child definitely is in shock. *Compensated* shock is present because blood pressure is adequate (ie, hypotension is *not* present), but signs of inadequate tissue and organ perfusion (eg, irritability, mottled color, cool extremities) *are* observed. To determine whether blood pressure is adequate in children 1 to 10 years of age, estimate the lower limit (5th percentile) of adequate systolic blood pressure using the following formula: 70 mm Hg + (2 × age in years). A systolic blood pressure below the number yielded by this formula indicates hypotension. With this formula the lower limit of adequate systolic blood pressure for a 2-year-old child is 74 mm Hg. In this case the child's SBP was 82 mm Hg, indicating adequate blood pressure and thus *compensated* shock.

Answers a and **b** are incorrect because decompensated shock is defined by the presence of hypotension. In this case decompensated shock would be present if the child's systolic blood pressure fell below 74 mm Hg.

Answer c is incorrect because compensated shock should be treated promptly. Failure to treat compensated shock may result in deterioration to decompensated shock or cardiac arrest.

4. **You are evaluating a lethargic and pale 8-month-old with a history of vomiting and diarrhea. The infant has a respiratory rate of 57 breaths/min with no retractions and good breath sounds. Her heart rate is 170 bpm, with weak pulses; capillary refill time is 5 seconds. Which of the following diagnoses is most consistent with this infant's presentation?**

a. cardiorespiratory failure

b. SVT with poor perfusion

c. hypovolemic shock

d. very mild dehydration

The correct answer is c. The toddler has evidence of shock with tachycardia, weak pulses, and prolonged capillary refill. Hypovolemic shock is the most likely type of shock because the toddler has a history of vomiting and diarrhea.

Answer a is incorrect because the infant has no signs of respiratory failure. Although the toddler is tachypneic, this can be explained by the presence of shock (with respiratory compensation for metabolic acidosis). The toddler has no retractions or other signs of respiratory distress and has good breath sounds.

Answer b is incorrect because although signs of shock are present, the infant's heart rate is not high enough to be caused by SVT. In an infant you would suspect SVT if the heart rate were greater than 220 bpm.

Answer d is incorrect because very mild dehydration is not associated with signs of shock. When signs of shock are present, moderate or severe dehydration is present.

References

1. Young KD, Seidel JS. Pediatric cardiopulmonary resuscitation: a collective review. *Ann Emerg Med.* 1999;33:195-205.

2. Sirbaugh PE, Pepe PE, Shook JE, Kimball KT, Goldman MJ, Ward MA, Mann DM. A prospective, population-based study of the demographics, epidemiology, management, and outcome of out-of-hospital pediatric cardiopulmonary arrest [published correction appears in *Ann Emerg Med.* 1999;33:358]. *Ann Emerg Med.* 1999;33:174-184.

3. Zaritsky A, Nadkarni V, Getson P, Kuehl K. CPR in children. *Ann Emerg Med.* 1987;16:1107-1111.

4. Eisenberg M, Bergner L, Hallstrom A. Epidemiology of cardiac arrest and resuscitation in children. *Ann Emerg Med.* 1983;12:672-674.

5. O'Rourke PP. Outcome of children who are apneic and pulseless in the emergency room. *Crit Care Med.* 1986;14:466-468.

6. Downes JJ, Fulgencio T, Raphaely RC. Acute respiratory failure in infants and children. *Pediatr Clin North Am.* 1972;19:423-445.

7. Perkin RM, Levin DL, Webb R, Aquino A, Reedy J. Dobutamine: a hemodynamic evaluation in children with shock. *J Pediatr.* 1982;100:977-983.

8. Gorelick MH, Shaw KN, Baker MD. Effect of ambient temperature on capillary refill in healthy children. *Pediatrics.* 1993;92:699-702.

9. Baraff LJ. Capillary refill: is it a useful clinical sign? [editorial]. *Pediatrics.* 1993;92:723-724.

10. Hazinski MF, Barkin RM. Shock. In: Barkin RM, ed. *Pediatric Emergency Medicine: Concepts and Clinical Practice.* St. Louis, Mo: Mosby Year Book, Inc; 1992.

11. Perkin RM, Levin DL. Shock in the pediatric patient, part II: therapy. *J Pediatr.* 1982;101:319-332.

12. Perkin RM, Levin DL. Shock in the pediatric patient, part I. *J Pediatr.* 1982;101:163-169.

13. Ceneviva G, Paschall JA, Maffei F, Carcillo JA. Hemodynamic support in fluid refractory pediatric septic shock. *Pediatrics.* 1998;102:e19.

14. Hazinski MF, Iberti TJ, MacIntyre NR, Parker MM, Tribett D, Prion S, Chmel H. Epidemiology, pathophysiology and clinical presentation of gram-negative sepsis. *Am J Crit Care.* 1993;2:224-235.

15. Parker MM, McCarthy KE, Ognibene FP, Parrillo JE. Right ventricular dysfunction and dilatation, similar to left ventricular changes, characterize the cardiac depression of septic shock in humans. *Chest.* 1990;97:126-131.

16. Bone RC, Balk RA, Cerra FB, Dellinger RP, Fein AM, Knaus WA, Schein RM, Sibbald WJ. Definitions for sepsis and organ failure and guidelines for the use of innovative therapies in sepsis: the ACCP/SCCM Consensus Conference Committee. American College of Chest Physicians/Society of Critical Care Medicine. *Chest*. 1992;101:1644-1655.

17. Carcillo JA et al. Clinical practice parameters for the hemodynamic support of pediatric and neonatal septic shock. *Crit Care Med*. 2002; 30(6). In press.

18. Abraham E, Matthay MA, Dinarello CA, Vincent JL, Cohen J, Opal SM, Glauser M, Parsons P, Fisher CJ Jr, Repine JE. Consensus conference definitions for sepsis, septic shock, acute lung injury, and acute respiratory distress syndrome: time for a reevaluation. *Crit Care Med*. 2000;28:232-235.

19. McGee S, Abernethy WB III, Simel DL. Is this patient hypovolemic? *JAMA*. 1999;281: 1022-1029.

20. Gorelick MH, Shaw KN, Murphy KO. Validity and reliability of clinical signs in the diagnosis of dehydration in children. *Pediatrics*. 1997;99:e6.

21. Update on the 1987 Task Force Report on High Blood Pressure in Children and Adolescents: a working group report from the National High Blood Pressure Education Program. National High Blood Pressure Education Program Working Group on Hypertension Control in Children and Adolescents. *Pediatrics*. 1996;98(pt 1):649-658.

22. Schwaitzberg SD, Bergman KS, Harris BH. A pediatric trauma model of continuous hemorrhage. *J Pediatr Surg*. 1988;23:605-609.

23. Joly HR, Weil MH. Temperature of the great toe as an indication of the severity of shock. *Circulation*. 1969;39:131-138.

24. Plum F, Posner JB. *The Diagnosis of Stupor and Coma*. 3rd ed. Philadelphia, Pa: FA Davis; 1980.

Basic Life Support for the PALS Healthcare Provider

Introductory Case Scenario 1

A 2-year-old child is transported to your care 2 hours after he fell down a flight of stairs. He briefly lost consciousness after the fall. On arrival in the ED the child appears anxious but is in no distress and shows no obvious signs of injury. His vital signs, oxygen saturation on room air, and capillary refill time are normal. During the initial evaluation he has a brief (20 seconds) tonic-clonic seizure, which is followed by apnea and cyanosis, with no response to verbal or tactile stimulation.

- What is your rapid cardiopulmonary assessment of this child?

- On the basis of your cardiopulmonary assessment, what are your treatment priorities?

- How do you activate the emergency response team in your area of practice?

- How do you perform the steps of CPR for the child less than 8 years of age?

Introductory Case Scenario 2

You are called to examine a 3-month-old infant with a history of fever and irritability. His parents are concerned because they had difficulty arousing him after his nap. The infant is not moving and is unresponsive to painful stimuli. His airway is patent, but he only gasps occasionally. You deliver 2 rescue breaths. After the breaths there is still no breathing, coughing, or movement, and you cannot palpate his pulses. The infant's skin is cool and appears pale and cyanotic.

- What is your rapid cardiopulmonary assessment of this child?

- On the basis of your cardiopulmonary assessment, what are your treatment priorities?

- How do you activate the emergency response team in your area of practice?

- How do you perform the steps of CPR for an infant (less than approximately 1 year of age)?

Learning Objectives

After completing this chapter the PALS provider should be able to

- Describe the priorities of BLS treatment for infants and children

- List the sequence of actions you should perform when you encounter an infant (newborn to 1 year of age) or child (1 to 8 years of age) in respiratory or cardiac arrest

- Describe and demonstrate the ABCs of CPR for infants and children

- State the sequence of interventions for foreign-body airway obstruction (FBAO) in infants and children

---

FIGURE 1. Cardiopulmonary resuscitation and life support for infants and children should be an integral part of the Chain of Survival in every community, linking injury prevention, early and effective CPR, early access to emergency medical response prepared for the needs of children, and early and effective ALS, including stabilization, transport, and eventual access to rehabilitation.

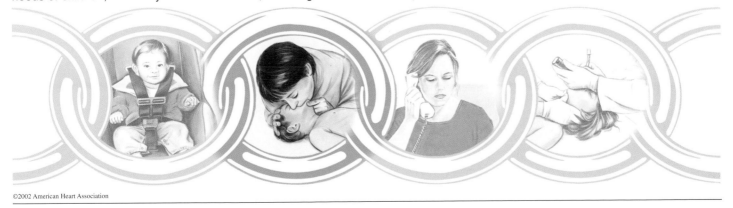

Many children who require resuscitation have underlying conditions that predispose them to development of cardiopulmonary failure.[1] The epidemiology of pediatric cardiopulmonary arrest, issues of prevention, and activation of the emergency medical response systems are presented in Chapter 1: "The Chain of Survival and Emergency Medical Services for Children."

Critical Concepts:
The "Phone First" vs "Phone Fast" Approach to EMS Activation

If you and another rescuer find an unresponsive child, you should begin CPR while the other rescuer activates the emergency response system. Simultaneous rather than sequential actions are performed.

When you are alone and the cause of the emergency is known, you can provide a targeted response sequence tailored to the most likely cause of the emergency. When the cause of the emergency is not known, the response should be based on the age of the victim:

Infants and Children From Birth to 8 Years

Provide CPR first and then phone fast because a respiratory cause of arrest is more common than a cardiac cause of arrest (rescue breathing is required)

Exception: Apparent sudden cardiac collapse

Children Older Than 8 Years and Adults

Phone first and then provide CPR because a cardiac cause of arrest is more common than a respiratory cause of arrest (defibrillation plus CPR is required)

Exception: Unresponsiveness with respiratory compromise (submersion, trauma, drug overdose)

Sudden cardiopulmonary arrest in infants and children is much less common than sudden cardiac arrest in adults.[2,3] Unlike cardiac arrest in adults, cardiac arrest in infants and children is typically preceded by a period of cardiorespiratory deterioration, and *noncardiac* causes of arrest predominate over *cardiac* causes (see Critical Concepts: "The 'Phone First' vs 'Phone Fast' Approach to EMS Activation").[2]

The etiology of cardiac arrest in infants and children varies according to the age, setting, and underlying health of the child. For these reasons the sequence of CPR and activation of EMS for infants and children differs from that for adults (Figure 1).

This chapter briefly reviews the healthcare provider skills sequence (ABCs) of CPR in infants and children 1 to 8 years of age. CPR techniques used for children 8 years of age and older and adults are also reviewed briefly in this section. Pediatric BLS and ALS interventions tend to "blur at the margins" of the age definitions of infant, child, and adult because no single anatomic or physiologic characteristic consistently distinguishes the infant victim from the child victim from the adult victim of cardiac arrest (see Foundation Facts: "Pediatric BLS Definitions Based on Approximate Age").

Pediatric BLS includes assessments and motor skills designed to support or restore effective oxygenation, ventilation, and circulation to the child in respiratory or cardiac (cardiopulmonary) arrest. Early and effective BLS can be performed by any trained bystander, and it can substantially improve the victim's chance of survival.

Prompt access to ALS is also required when cardiopulmonary arrest is imminent or present. Although BLS requires no advance adjuncts, the healthcare provider should use universal precautions and adjuncts that are readily available, such as a barrier device or ventilation bag and mask.

BLS for Children With Special Healthcare Needs

Children with special healthcare needs have chronic physical, developmental, behavioral, or emotional conditions and require health and related services of a type or amount not usually required by typically developing children.[4-6] These children may need emergency care for acute, life-threatening complications unique to their chronic condition,[6] such as obstruction of a tracheostomy, failure of support technology (eg, ventilator failure), or progression of underlying disease.

Approximately half of EMS calls for children with special healthcare needs, however, are unrelated to the child's chronic condition. Instead, the calls are for more typical emergencies, such as trauma,[7] which require no treatment beyond the normal EMS standard of care.

Emergency care of children with special healthcare needs can be complicated by lack of specific medical information about the child's baseline condition, medical plan of care, current medications, and any "do not attempt resuscitation" orders. The American Academy of Pediatrics and the American College of Emergency Physicians have developed a standardized form, the Emergency Information Form (EIF),[6] which is available on the internet (**www.pediatrics.org/cgi/content/full/10 4/4/e53**). Parents and childcare providers should have access to this information and should be familiar with signs of deterioration in the child and any existing advance directives.[7,8]

If the physician, parents, and child (as appropriate) have made a decision to limit resuscitative efforts or to withhold resuscitation attempts, a physician order specifying the limits of resuscitative efforts must be written for use in the hospital setting. In most countries a separate order must be written for the out-of-hospital setting. Legal issues, regulations, and requirements for these out-of-hospital

Foundation Facts:
Pediatric BLS Definitions Based on Approximate Age

No single anatomic or physiologic characteristic consistently distinguishes the infant victim from the child victim from the adult victim of cardiac arrest.

Age Definitions

In PALS the term *newly born* is used to describe the infant in the first minutes to hours after birth. The term focuses attention on the needs of the infant at and immediately after birth. The terms *newborn* or *neonate* do not clearly refer to the first hours of life.

The term *neonate* describes infants in the first 28 days (first month) of life.[9]

The term *infant* comprises the neonatal period and up to 12 months or approximately 1 year. For the purposes of BLS, the term *infant* is defined by the approximate size of the young child who can receive effective chest compression given with 2 fingers or 2 thumbs with encircling hands. By consensus the age cutoff for infants is 1 year. Note, however, that this definition is not based on physiologic differences between infants younger than 12 months and children slightly older than 12 months.

To simplify BLS education, the term *child*
has been used in the ECC Guidelines to designate victims 1 to 8 years of age. Cardiac compression can usually be provided with one hand for victims between the ages of 1 and 8 years. Variability in the size of the victim or the size and strength of the rescuer, however, can require the use of the 2-finger or 2 thumb–encircling hands techniques for a small toddler or the 2-handed adult compression technique in a large child 6 to 7 years of age.[10,11]

Anatomic and Physiologic Differences Affecting Cardiac Arrest and Resuscitation

Respiratory failure or arrest is a common cause of cardiac arrest in infants, children, and young adults. The pediatric BLS guidelines emphasize that the lone rescuer should provide CPR—including opening of the airway and delivery of rescue breathing—*immediately before* activating the local EMS system. This emphasis on immediate support of oxygenation and ventilation is based on knowledge of the important role of respiratory failure in cardiac arrest and the frequency of hypoxic, hypercarbic arrest in young victims.

no-CPR directives vary from country to country and in the United States from state to state. It is always important for families to inform the local EMS system when advance directives are established for out-of-hospital care.

The ABCs of CPR
Rapid Assessment

The actual steps of CPR begin when the victim is found unresponsive. The steps of CPR form a logical sequence of assessment and intervention in which the rescuer provides only as much support as the victim needs (see Figure 2). An initial visual survey can be quickly accomplished as the rescuer approaches the victim, looking for movement, crying, or respirations and evaluating muscle tone and color.

To simplify teaching, the skills of CPR are taught as a sequence of distinct steps. But evaluation and intervention for the infant and child are often simultaneous processes, especially when several rescuers are present (eg, in the hospital setting or when 2 EMS responders are present). The sequence and priorities of action may be modified by the cause of the arrest, the time elapsed since the resuscitation attempt was initiated, and the infant's or child's response to previous resuscitative interventions.

FIGURE 2. The steps of CPR for infants and children. CPR includes both assessment and support steps, performed in sequence. The rescuer provides only the support the victim needs.

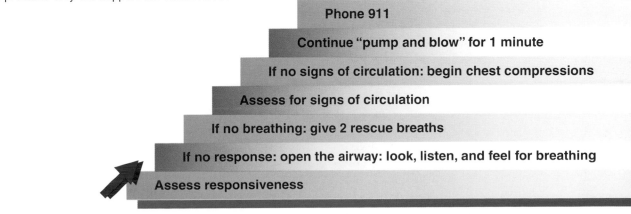

Phone 911

Continue "pump and blow" for 1 minute

If no signs of circulation: begin chest compressions

Assess for signs of circulation

If no breathing: give 2 rescue breaths

If no response: open the airway: look, listen, and feel for breathing

Assess responsiveness

FIGURE 3. International pediatric BLS algorithm.

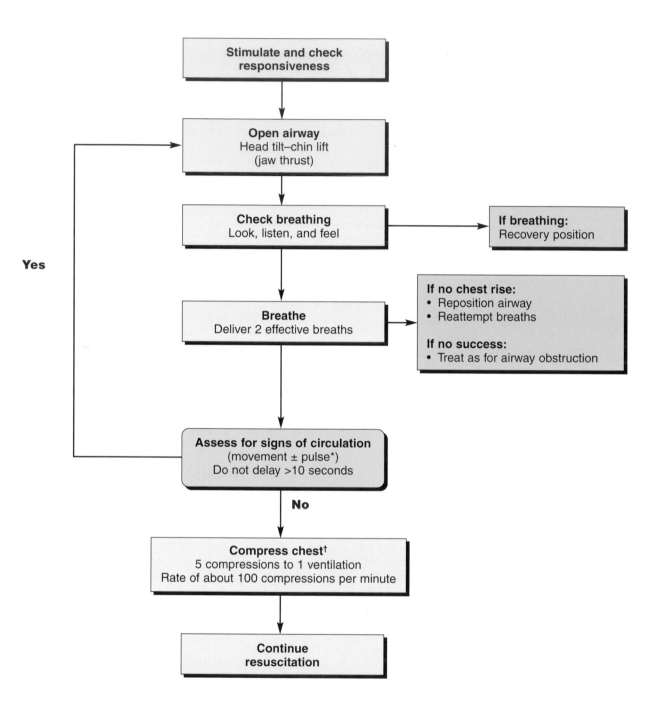

Stimulate and check
responsiveness

Open airway
Head tilt–chin lift
(jaw thrust)

Check breathing
Look, listen, and feel

If breathing:
Recovery position

Breathe
Deliver 2 effective breaths

If no chest rise:
• Reposition airway
• Reattempt breaths

If no success:
• Treat as for airway obstruction

Yes

Assess for signs of circulation
(movement ± pulse*)
Do not delay >10 seconds

No

Compress chest†
5 compressions to 1 ventilation
Rate of about 100 compressions per minute

Continue
resuscitation

*Pulse check should be taught to healthcare providers but is not expected of laypersons.
†Continue rescue breathing and cardiopulmonary resuscitation as indicated. Activate emergency medical services as soon as possible, based on local and regional availability, training of responder, and circumstances of arrest.

Ensure the Safety of Rescuer and Victim

When a rescuer prepares to help a victim of an emergency in the prehospital setting, he/she must first verify the safety of the scene. The rescuer who becomes injured or incapacitated because the scene is unsafe cannot help the victim. When the rescuer has determined that it is safe to approach the victim, he/she should then decide whether the victim should be moved. The lay rescuer should move an injured victim *only* if it is necessary to ensure the safety of the victim or rescuer (eg, the victim is inside a burning building).

Healthcare providers should follow universal precautions, including the use of gloves and protective shields, and should consider the use of barrier devices during procedures in which they may be exposed to droplets of blood, saliva, or other body fluids. These precautions reduce the very small risk of infectious disease transmission during CPR. Between 1960 and 1998 only 15 reports of CPR-related infection were published, and no reports were published from 1998 to 2001. No reports of transmission of human immunodeficiency virus (HIV), hepatitis B virus (HBV), hepatitis C virus (HCV), or cytomegalovirus have been found in the literature.[12]

Stimulate and Check Responsiveness

The steps of CPR are initiated when the rescuer determines that the child is *unresponsive* (Figure 3). To check for responsiveness, gently stimulate the child and ask loudly "Are you all right?" Do not move or shake the victim with head or neck trauma because such handling may aggravate a spinal cord injury.

If the child is *unresponsive* and you are the *only rescuer* present, shout for help and be prepared to provide CPR for approximately 1 minute before leaving the child to activate the EMS response system. If a second rescuer is present, that person should activate the EMS response system as soon as the emergency is identified. If

trauma is suspected, the second rescuer should activate the EMS system and then help immobilize the child's cervical spine, preventing movement of the neck (extension, flexion, and rotation) and torso. If the child must be positioned for resuscitation or moved for safety reasons, rescuers should support the child's head and torso and turn as a unit.

The rescuer who phones EMS should be prepared to provide the following information:

1. Location of the emergency, including address and names of streets or landmarks
2. Telephone number from which the call is being made
3. Nature of the emergency (eg, auto crash or submersion)
4. Number of victims
5. Condition of victims
6. Nature of aid being given
7. Any other information requested

The caller should hang up *only* when instructed to do so by the dispatcher.

Airway

Hypoxemia and respiratory arrest may cause or contribute to acute deterioration and cardiopulmonary arrest in children. In addition, when the victim loses consciousness, the tongue often obstructs the upper airway and interferes with effective ventilation. Thus, establishing and maintaining a patent airway and support of adequate ventilation are the most important components of BLS for young victims.

Position the Victim

If the child is unresponsive, turn the child as a unit into the supine (face up) position and place the child on a flat, hard surface, such as a sturdy table, the floor, or the ground. If head or neck trauma is present or suspected, move the child only if necessary. Carefully turn the head and torso as a unit. If the victim is an infant and no trauma is suspected, you can carry the child supported by your forearm (your

forearm supports the long axis of the infant's torso, with the infant's legs straddling your elbow and wrist and the hand supporting the infant's head and neck) while beginning the steps of CPR.

Open the Airway

The tongue is the most common cause of airway obstruction in the unconscious pediatric victim. When the victim loses consciousness, the muscles of the jaw and neck relax, and the tongue falls back against the throat, blocking the airway. In infants and children the head often has a prominent occiput that promotes neck flexion and produces further airway obstruction when the infant is unresponsive and supine (see Figure 4A and B).[13-16] Therefore, once the infant or child is found unresponsive, open the airway with a maneuver designed to lift the tongue away from the back of the pharynx, creating an open airway.[17] This may be accomplished by using a head tilt–chin lift or a jaw thrust.[18-21]

Control of the airway is required as long as the victim remains unresponsive, and it must be provided throughout resuscitation, transport, and stabilization. If trauma is suspected, simultaneous spinal immobilization is also needed.

Head Tilt–Chin Lift Maneuver

If the victim is unresponsive *and trauma is not suspected*, open the child's airway by tilting the head back and lifting the chin (Figure 5A and B). *If injury to the head or neck is suspected, do not use the head tilt–chin lift maneuver. Instead use the jaw-thrust maneuver (see below) to open the airway.*

To perform the head tilt–chin lift maneuver:

■ Place one hand on the child's forehead and gently tilt the head back into a neutral position. The neck will be slightly extended.

■ At the same time, place the fingertips of your other hand under the bony part of the child's lower jaw, near the point

FIGURE 4. Obstruction of the airway relieved by positioning. **A,** In an unresponsive supine infant the prominent occiput may induce flexion of the neck, and the airway can become obstructed. Airway obstruction also can be caused by the tongue falling back against the throat. **B,** Position the infant with the neck in a neutral position so that the tragus of the ear is level with the top of the shoulder. This position will keep the airway open.

A

B

FIGURE 5. Opening the airway with the head tilt–chin lift. Gently lift the chin with one hand and push down on the forehead with the other hand. **A,** Infant. **B,** Child.

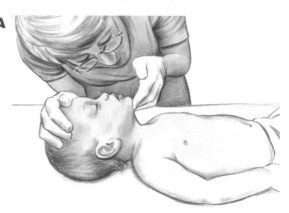

A

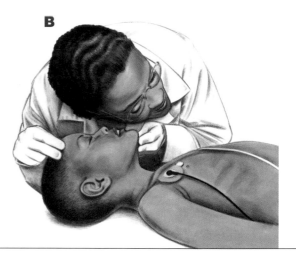

B

of the chin. Lift the mandible upward and outward to open the airway.

- Be careful not to close the lips and mouth or push on the soft tissues under the chin because such maneuvers may obstruct rather than open the airway.

- If secretions, vomitus, or a foreign body is visible, remove it.

Jaw-Thrust Maneuver

Spinal cord injuries in infants and children are uncommon, but they can be devastating. The incidence of overt spinal cord injury producing motor deficits can be determined at the time of admission to the hospital. But it is impossible to know what portion of these injuries occurred at the moment of trauma and which, if any, of these injuries represent aggravation of incomplete injury by movement *after*

Critical Concepts:
Opening the Airway—
Special Circumstances

- When a head or neck injury is suspected, use the *jaw-thrust* maneuver with spinal immobilization instead of the head tilt–chin lift. Maintain airway control and cervical spine immobilization throughout resuscitation, transport, and stabilization.

- When bag-mask ventilation will be performed, use the *jaw-thrust*.

- When FBAO is suspected and the victim is not responsive, use the *tongue–jaw lift*.

trauma. To limit the risk of aggravating a potential cervical spine injury, open the airway with a jaw thrust while you immobilize the cervical spine. Be sure, however, that you open the airway adequately because hypoventilation is known to develop after serious injury, and inadequate oxygenation and ventilation are associated with increased morbidity in patients with head injuries.

The jaw-thrust maneuver is also used to open the airway when bag-mask ventilation is performed.

To perform the jaw-thrust maneuver[18-21]:

- If you will be performing simultaneous bag-mask (or mouth-to-mask) ventilation or cervical spine immobilization, position yourself at the victim's head. If you are alone and anticipate the

FIGURE 6. Opening the airway with the jaw thrust. Lift the angles of the jaw. This moves the jaw and tongue forward and opens the airway without bending the neck.

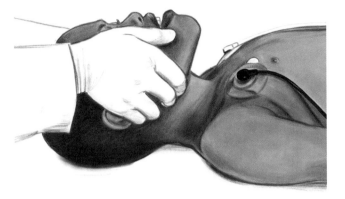

FIGURE 7. Recovery position.

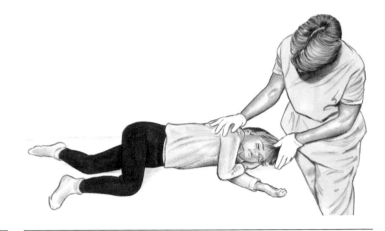

need for mouth-to-mouth or mouth-to–face shield ventilation, you will need to perform the jaw thrust from the victim's side.

■ Place 2 or 3 fingers under each side of the lower jaw at its angle and lift the jaw upward and outward. Your elbows may rest on the surface on which the victim is lying (Figure 6).

■ The lone rescuer positioned at the head of the bed can perform simultaneous immobilization of the head and neck and opening of the airway by lifting the jaw with 2 fingers of each hand while using the remaining fingers and both hands to hold the head and neck immobile. Ideally a second rescuer is available for this purpose (see "BLS in Special Situations—BLS for the Trauma Victim").

■ If secretions, vomitus, blood, dental fragments, or a foreign body is visible, remove it.

Tongue–Jaw Lift Maneuver

The tongue-jaw lift is used to open the airway to look for an obstructing foreign body in an unresponsive victim. To perform the tongue-jaw lift:

■ Verify that the victim is unresponsive.

■ Insert your thumb in the victim's mouth and position 2 or 3 fingers under the jaw. Grasp the tongue and lower jaw between your thumb and fingers and lift upward and outward.

■ Inspect the mouth briefly. If secretions, vomitus, blood, dental fragments, or a foreign body is visible, remove it.

The tongue–jaw lift maneuver is recommended only when the victim is *unrespon-*

> ## Critical Concepts:
> ### Airway Management in Suspected Head or Neck Trauma
>
> When head or neck trauma is present, it is important to immobilize the victim's cervical spine *and* open the airway adequately with a jaw-thrust maneuver. The head tilt–chin lift is not recommended for opening the airway of the victim with a possible cervical spine injury because movement of the neck may worsen the injury. The rescuer should maintain the neck in a neutral position. Note that the prominent occiput of the child predisposes the neck to slight flexion when the child is placed on a flat surface, so a spine board with an occipital well should be used. Alternatively blankets can be placed beneath the child's torso to lift the torso above the board and maintain the neck in a neutral position (see Chapter 10 for more information).[22,23]

sive and FBAO is suspected. This maneuver is illustrated in the section "Relief of Foreign-Body Airway Obstruction (Choking)" later in this chapter. In addition to the tongue-jaw lift, healthcare providers are taught a sequence of actions to attempt for relief of suspected FBAO in the unresponsive victim.

Breathing

Check Breathing

After opening the airway the rescuer must determine if the child is breathing adequately. **Look** for a rise and fall of the chest and abdomen, **listen** at the child's nose and mouth for exhaled breath sounds, and **feel** for exhaled air flow from the child's mouth for no more than 10 seconds.

It may be difficult to determine whether the victim is breathing.[24,25] Healthcare providers must be able to differentiate ineffective and inadequate gasping or obstructed breathing efforts from *effective* or *adequate* breathing.[26,27] If you are not confident that respirations are *adequate,* proceed with rescue breathing.

Recovery Position

If the child is breathing adequately and there is no evidence of trauma, turn the child to the side in a recovery position (Figure 7) to help maintain a patent airway. Although many recovery positions can be used in the management of pediatric patients,[28-31] no single recovery position can be universally endorsed on the basis of scientific studies of children. There is consensus that an ideal recovery position should help maintain a patent airway and cervical spine stability, minimize risk for aspiration, limit pressure on bony prominences and peripheral nerves, enable the rescuer to observe the child's respiratory effort and appearance (including color), and provide access to the patient for interventions.

If head or neck trauma is suspected, keep the victim supine with cervical spine immobilization. The victim should not be placed in the recovery position if ongoing rescue breathing or other CPR is required.

To place the victim in a **recovery position**:

- Move the victim's head, shoulders, and torso simultaneously.

- Turn the victim onto his/her side.

- Limit pressure on bony prominences and peripheral nerves.

- Monitor the victim's respiratory effort and appearance.

- You may bend the victim's leg and move the knee forward to stabilize the victim.

Rescue Breathing

If the victim is not breathing adequately, maintain a patent airway with a head tilt–chin lift or jaw thrust with spinal immobilization. If a mask with a 1-way valve, barrier device, or bag-mask device is immediately available, use it during rescue breathing. But do not delay rescue breathing to locate such a device.

Under direct vision carefully remove any obvious airway obstruction and deliver rescue breaths. Regardless of the technique used, provide rescue breaths with a volume sufficient to make the child's chest rise visibly:

- Provide 2 effective slow breaths (1 to 1½ seconds each) to the victim, pausing briefly after the first breath to allow exhalation.

- Use ventilation adjuncts and oxygen when available (eg, bag mask).

- Be sure the chest rises with each breath.

Rescue breaths provide essential support for a nonbreathing infant or child. Because size and lung compliance vary widely in children, it is impossible to make precise recommendations about the pressure or volume of breaths to deliver during rescue breathing. Although the goal of assisted ventilation is delivery of adequate oxygen and removal of CO_2 with the smallest risk of iatrogenic injury, measurement of oxygen and CO_2 levels during pediatric BLS is not practical.

The volume of each rescue breath should be sufficient to cause the chest to rise visibly without causing excessive gastric inflation.[32] *If the child's chest does not rise during rescue breathing, ventilation is probably ineffective.* Because the small airway of the infant or child may provide high resistance to air flow, particularly in the presence of large or small airway obstruction, a relatively high pressure may be required to deliver an adequate volume of air to ensure chest expansion.

If air enters freely and the chest rises, the airway is clear. If air does not enter freely or the chest does not rise, either the airway is obstructed or greater volume or pressure is needed to provide adequate rescue breaths. Improper opening of the airway is the most common cause of airway obstruction and inadequate ventilation during resuscitation. If air does not enter freely and the chest does not rise during initial ventilation attempts, reposition the airway and reattempt ventilation.[32]

If there is no head or neck injury, you may need to move the child's head through a range of positions to open the airway and provide effective rescue breathing. If neck or spine trauma is suspected and ventilations are ineffective, be sure that the jaw thrust is lifting the jaw effectively.

Gastric inflation can interfere with effective rescue breathing and may increase risk of

FYI: 2 vs 5 Initial Rescue Breaths

The current ILCOR consensus recommendations suggest that between 2 and 5 rescue breaths should be delivered initially to ensure that at least 2 effective ventilations are provided.[33,34] *There is no data to support the choice of any single number of initial breaths to be delivered to the unresponsive, nonbreathing victim.* Both hypoxia and hypercarbia are present in most pediatric victims of cardiac arrest. If the rescuer is unable to establish effective ventilation with 2 rescue breaths, additional breaths may be beneficial for improving oxygenation and restoring an adequate heart rate for an apneic, bradycardic infant or child. The rescuer should ensure that at least 2 breaths delivered are effective and produce visible chest rise.

regurgitation of gastric contents.[32] Slow delivery of rescue breaths may minimize gastric inflation. If the victim is *unconscious or unresponsive and has no gag reflex,* application of cricoid pressure will also reduce gastric inflation (see Chapter 4: "Airway, Ventilation, and Management of Respiratory Distress and Failure"). Healthcare providers may insert a nasogastric or an orogastric tube to decompress the stomach if gastric inflation develops during resuscitation. Ideally this is done after tracheal intubation to avoid stimulation of the gag reflex and potential aspiration before the airway is secured.

If there is no chest rise or inadequate chest rise with initial breaths, reposition the victim and try to reopen the airway and again deliver rescue breaths. If there is still no chest movement and no obvious reason for failure of rescue breathing, treat the victim for a presumed FBAO (see FBAO, below).

FIGURE 8. Mouth-to–mouth-and-nose rescue breathing for an infant. Place your mouth over the infant's nose and mouth. If you cannot cover both the nose and mouth, cover only the nose to provide rescue breathing.

FIGURE 9. Mouth-to-mouth rescue breathing for a child. While keeping the child's airway open, cover the child's mouth with your mouth and pinch the child's nose closed.

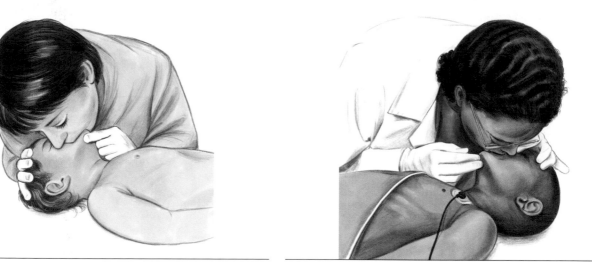

Rescue Breathing Without Barrier Devices

Rescue Breathing Techniques for Infants

If the victim is less than 1 year of age, use the mouth-to–mouth-and-nose technique (see Figure 8) to provide rescue breathing when no barrier device or bag-mask manual resuscitator is available. Other techniques may be used, including mouth-to-nose or mouth-to-mouth breathing. To provide mouth-to–mouth-and-nose or mouth-to-nose or mouth-to-mouth breathing for an infant:

- Open the victim's airway.

- Inhale deeply.

- Place your mouth over the infant's mouth and nose to create a seal.

- Blow into the infant's mouth and nose simultaneously, delivering the breaths slowly over 1 to 1½ seconds each. Inhale and then deliver a second breath in the same manner. Be sure the chest rises with each breath.

- *If you are unable to create a seal around the infant's mouth and nose,* use either mouth-to-nose or mouth-to-mouth ventilation (see below). For mouth-to-nose ventilation, place your mouth over the infant's nose and proceed with rescue breathing. It may be necessary to close the infant's mouth during mouth-to-nose ventilation to prevent the rescue breaths from escaping through the infant's mouth. A chin lift will help maintain airway patency by moving the tongue forward and may help keep the mouth closed.

Rescue Breathing Techniques for Children

For child victims use the mouth-to-mouth technique (Figure 9) to provide rescue breathing when no bag-mask or barrier device is available. To perform mouth-to-mouth rescue breathing:

- Open the victim's airway.

- Inhale deeply.

- Pinch the victim's nose tightly with the thumb and forefinger of your hand (the one on the victim's forehead). Cover the victim's mouth with your mouth, making a seal.

- Blow into the victim's mouth, giving a slow breath (over 1 to 1½ seconds). Inhale and deliver a second breath in the same manner.

- Make sure that the chest rises visibly with each rescue breath.

Rescue Breathing With a Barrier Device

Mouth-to-mouth breathing is a safe and effective technique that has saved many lives. Despite decades of experience indicating its safety for victims and rescuers alike, some potential rescuers may hesitate to perform mouth-to-mouth rescue breathing because of concerns about transmission of infectious diseases. For several reasons this concern appears to be less of an issue for those who attempt resuscitation of infants and children.

First, most *out-of-hospital* emergencies in children occur at home, so they will receive CPR from a primary caretaker who is aware of their infectious status. Second, although adults who work with children are exposed to pediatric infectious agents daily, any exposure during rescue breathing is brief. As of March 2000 there have been no reports of disease transmission during CPR training and no reports of spread of HIV (the virus that causes AIDS), HBV, HCV, or cytomegalovirus during performance of CPR.[12]

The use of barrier devices may improve aesthetics for the rescuer but has not been shown to reduce the risk of disease transmission.[12,35] The Occupational Safety

Critical Concepts:
Tips for Successful Rescue Breaths

- Each rescue breath should be sufficient to cause the chest to rise visibly.

- The most common cause of airway obstruction is improper airway opening; if the rescue breaths are ineffective, reopen the airway.

- Minimize gastric inflation in the unresponsive victim with no gag reflex by delivering slow breaths and using cricoid pressure.

- A rescuer with a small mouth may have difficulty covering both the nose and open mouth of a large infant.[36-45] Under these conditions mouth-to-nose ventilation may be effective.[36,38]

- It is important to pause between the 2 initial breaths. This pause allows the rescuer to inhale between breaths, maximizes oxygen content, and minimizes concentration of CO_2 in the delivered breaths.[46] If the rescuer fails to take this replenishing breath, the second rescue breath delivered will be low in oxygen and high in CO_2.

and Health Administration (OSHA) recommends that barrier devices (or bag-mask devices) be available in the healthcare facility and the workplace and that employees use these devices when performing CPR. The AHA recommends the use of barrier or bag-mask devices during rescue breathing by rescuers with a duty to respond. A barrier device is *not required* to provide CPR.

Regardless of whether a barrier device is available, the key actions of the rescuer remain the same:

1. Open the airway with the head tilt–chin lift (or jaw thrust if the victim has a head or neck injury).

2. Provide rescue breaths (1 to 1½ seconds each).

When you use a barrier device, position the face shield or face mask over the victim's mouth and ensure an adequate air seal. *Deliver rescue breaths through the barrier device with just enough force to make the chest rise visibly.*

There are 2 types of barrier devices: face shields and face masks. The most critical step in using a face shield or mask is achieving a good seal around the mouth and nose. A good seal prevents leakage of air during rescue breaths.

Rescue Breathing With a Face Shield

In rescue breathing with a face shield the rescuer places a clear plastic or silicone sheet on the victim's face to keep the rescuer's mouth from touching the victim's mouth. The opening of the face shield is placed over the victim's mouth. Some face shields have a short (1- to 2-inch) tube that can be inserted into the victim's mouth over the tongue. To perform rescue breathing, pinch the victim's nose closed and seal your mouth around the center opening or tube of the face shield. Provide 2 slow breaths (2 seconds each) through the 1-way valve or filter in the center of the face shield. When you lift your mouth off the shield, the victim's exhaled air will escape between the shield and the victim's face.

Keep the face shield on the victim's face while performing chest compressions. If the victim begins to vomit during rescue efforts, remove the face shield.

The major disadvantages of face shields are proximity of the rescuer to the victim's face and the possibility of contamination if the victim vomits. Many face shields have no exhalation valve, and often air leaks around the shield. Because the efficacy of face shields in prevention of infection has not been documented, healthcare professionals and those with a duty to respond should also be instructed in the use of mouth-to-mask rescue breathing

or bag-mask ventilation. Face shields should be used only as a substitute for mouth-to-mouth breathing. They should be replaced with mouth-to-mask or bag-mask devices at the first opportunity.

Rescue Breathing With a Mask

In mouth-to-mask rescue breathing the rescuer places a transparent mask with or without a 1-way valve on the victim's face to separate the rescuer's mouth from the victim's mouth. The 1-way valve directs the rescuer's breath into the victim while diverting the victim's exhaled air away from the rescuer. Some masks have an oxygen inlet that permits administration of supplemental oxygen. Oral airways and cricoid pressure may be used with mouth-to-mask and any other form of rescue breathing in the unconscious or unresponsive victim who has no gag reflex.

Effective use of the mask barrier device requires instruction and supervised practice. Effective mouth-to-mask ventilation can be easier to perform than mouth-to–face shield ventilation because the rescuer can use both hands to open the airway and to seal the mask to the victim's face. These barrier devices, however, may increase resistance to gas flow, so the rescuer must ensure that the chest rises visibly with each breath.[47,48]

The proper technique for mouth-to-mask rescue breathing is determined by the number of rescuers, their experience, and the equipment available. The 2 most common techniques for using the mouth-to-mask device are the cephalic and lateral techniques. The *cephalic* technique is used when 2 or more rescuers are present or when a lone rescuer is providing rescue breathing without chest compressions. When trauma is not suspected, the *lateral* technique is ideal for 1-rescuer CPR because the rescuer can provide both rescue breathing and chest compressions from that position.

Cephalic Technique (Figure 10A). Position yourself directly above the victim's head and do the following:

FIGURE 10. Use of a mask in rescue breathing for a child. **A,** Cephalic technique using a bag-mask. **B,** Lateral mouth-to-mask technique. Press the mask firmly against the child's face while holding the airway open. Use the index finger and thumb of one hand to hold the mask against the bridge of the victim's nose. Also use this hand to tilt the head back. Use the thumb of the other hand to press the mask to the chin. Use the fingers of that same hand to lift the jaw up to the mask.

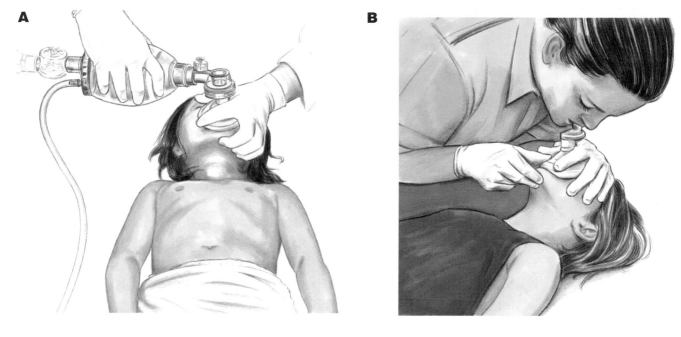

A   **B**

- Apply the mask to the victim's face, using the bridge of the nose as a guide for correct positioning.

- Place your thumbs and the base of the thumbs along the lateral edges of the mask.

- Place the index fingers of both hands below the victim's mandible and lift the jaw into the mask as you tilt the head back. Position your other fingers under the angle of the jaw.

- Create a tight seal between the face and mask by lifting the jaw into the mask and pressing the mask against the face.

- Provide 2 slow rescue breaths (1 to 1½ seconds each), ensuring that the chest rises adequately with each breath.

The "E-C clamp technique" is an alternative method of the cephalic technique. Use the thumb and first finger of each hand to hold the mask against the face. Use the remaining fingers to lift the mandible and face up to the mask and to tilt the head to extend the neck. This technique

is described in more detail in the section "Bag-Mask Ventilation."

With either variation of the cephalic technique the rescuer uses both hands to hold the mask and open the airway. In victims with suspected cervical spine injury the rescuer uses a jaw thrust to lift the mandible at the angles of the jaw *without* tilting the head.

Lateral Technique (Figure 10B). Position yourself at the victim's side in a location that will facilitate both rescue breathing and chest compressions:

- Apply the mask to the victim's face, using the bridge of the nose as a guide for correct positioning.

- Seal the mask by placing the index finger and thumb of your hand that is closer to the top of the victim's head along the nasal border of the mask and placing the thumb of your other hand along the lower margin of the mask.

- Place the remaining fingers of the hand that is closer to the victim's feet

along the bony margin of the jaw and lift the jaw with a head tilt–chin lift.

- Compress firmly and completely around the outside edge of the mask to provide a tight seal between the mask and the victim's face.

- Provide 2 slow rescue breaths and observe for chest rise.

Bag-Mask Ventilation

Ventilation with a bag-mask device requires more skill than mouth-to-mouth or mouth-to-mask ventilation and should be performed only by personnel who have received proper training. All healthcare providers who provide BLS for infants and children should be skilled in delivering effective oxygenation and ventilation with a manual resuscitator (bag) and mask. Training should focus on selection of an appropriately sized mask and bag, opening the airway and securing the mask to the face, delivering adequate ventilation, and assessing the effectiveness of ventilation. Periodic demonstration of proficiency is recommended.

Neonatal-size (250 mL) ventilation bags may be inadequate to support effective tidal volume and the longer inspiratory times required by full-term neonates and infants.[47,49] For this reason resuscitation bags used for ventilation of full-term newly born infants, infants, and children should have a minimum volume of 450 to 500 mL. Studies involving infant manikins showed that effective infant ventilation can be achieved with pediatric (and larger) resuscitation bags.[50]

Regardless of the size of the manual resuscitator used, *the rescuer should use only the force and tidal volume necessary to cause the chest to rise visibly.* Excessive ventilation volumes and airway pressures may have harmful effects. They may compromise cardiac output by raising intrathoracic pressure, distending alveoli or the stomach or both, impeding ventilation, and increasing risk of regurgitation and aspiration.[51] In patients with small-airway obstructions (eg, asthma and bronchiolitis), excessive tidal volume and ventilation rate can result in air trapping, barotrauma, air leak, and severely compromised cardiac output. In the patient with a head injury or cardiac arrest, excessive ventilation volume and rate may result in hyperventilation with potentially adverse effects on neurologic outcome.

The goal of ventilation with a bag and mask should be to approximate normal ventilation and achieve physiologic oxygen and CO_2 levels while minimizing risk of iatrogenic injury.

Types and characteristics of ventilation bags (manual resuscitators) are reviewed in Chapter 4: "Airway, Ventilation, and Management of Respiratory Distress and Failure."

Selection of Bag and Mask

Select a bag and mask of appropriate size. The mask must completely cover the victim's mouth and nose without covering the eyes or overlapping the chin. The bag must have a minimum volume of 450 to 500 mL.

E-C Clamp Technique

In the E-C clamp technique the thumb and forefinger form a "C" shape to tightly seal the mask onto the face while the remaining fingers of the same hand form an "E" shape to lift the jaw, pulling the face toward the mask. To perform bag-mask ventilation with the E-C clamp technique:

■ Kneel at the victim's head. If the victim has no head or neck injury, tilt the victim's head back and place a towel or pillow beneath the head of the child or the torso of the infant. If the victim has a head or neck injury, open the airway with the jaw-thrust technique without head tilt. If another rescuer is present, have that person immobilize the victim's cervical spine.

■ Apply the mask to the victim's face, using the bridge of the nose as a guide for correct positioning. Lift the jaw, using the last 3 fingers (fingers 3, 4, and 5) of your other hand. Position these 3 fingers under the angle of the mandible to lift the jaw up and forward. (These 3 spread fingers appear to form the letter "E" [see Figure 11A and B]). When you lift the jaw, you also lift the tongue away from the posterior pharynx, preventing the tongue from obstructing the pharynx. Do not put pressure on the soft tissues under the jaw because this may compress the airway.

■ Place the thumb and forefinger of the same hand in a "C" shape over the mask and exert downward pressure. Create a tight seal between the mask and the victim's face using the hand holding the mask and lifting the jaw. If you are alone, maintain the E-C clamp with one hand and compress the ventilation bag with the other hand. Be sure that the chest rises visibly with each breath.

FIGURE 11. Use of a bag-mask device by one rescuer, E-C clamp technique. Using the thumb and index finger of one hand, form a C shape over the mask. Using the third, fourth, and fifth fingers, form an E along the jaw. Lift the jaw with the 3 fingers (the E) to keep the airway open (jaw thrust). Press down on the mask with your thumb and index finger (the C) to hold the mask in place. **A,** Infant. **B,** Child.

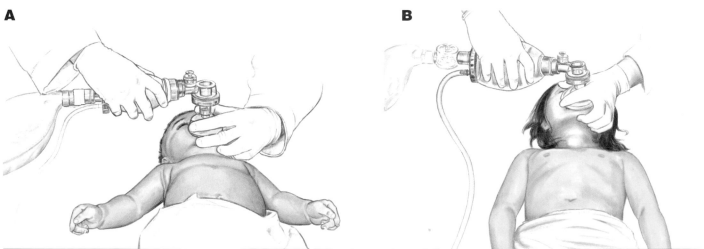

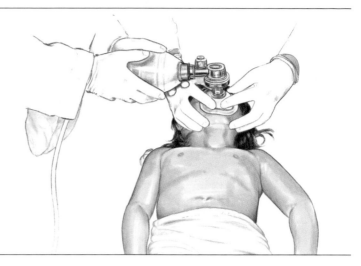

FIGURE 12. Use of a bag-mask device by 2 rescuers. One rescuer opens the airway (with a head tilt–chin lift plus a jaw thrust or a jaw thrust only) and holds the mask in place. This rescuer creates a tight seal between the mask and the victim's face and looks for the chest to rise. The second rescuer squeezes the bag. If a third rescuer is present and the victim is unresponsive with no gag reflex, a third rescuer may apply cricoid pressure to compress the esophagus and prevent gastric inflation.

Two-Rescuer Bag-Mask Ventilation

Superior bag-mask ventilation can be achieved with 2 rescuers (Figure 12). If the victim has significant airway obstruction or poor lung compliance, 2 rescuers may be required. One rescuer uses both hands to open the airway and maintain a tight E-C clamp mask-to-face seal while the other rescuer compresses the ventilation bag.[52] Both rescuers should observe the chest to ensure that it rises visibly with each breath. If a third rescuer is present and the victim is unconscious *with no gag reflex*, the third rescuer can apply cricoid pressure during ventilation to compress the esophagus and prevent gastric inflation.

Ventilation Through a Tracheostomy or Stoma

Some pediatric victims, particularly those with special healthcare needs and chronic respiratory failure, may have a tracheostomy. Anyone responsible for the care of a child with a tracheostomy should be taught to ensure that the airway is patent and to provide CPR with the artificial airway. If CPR is required, provide rescue breathing and manual ventilation through the tracheostomy tube. Rescue breathing may be provided by mouth to tube, mouth to stoma, or bag to stoma. If the upper airway is patent, it may be necessary to close the victim's mouth and pinch the nose to prevent leakage of air when the rescuer provides rescue breaths into the tracheostomy tube or stoma. As with any form of rescue breathing, the key sign of effective ventilation is adequate bilateral chest expansion.

If the tracheostomy tube becomes obstructed, preventing delivery of effective ventilation, remove and replace the tube. If a clean tube is unavailable, provide ventilations at the tracheostomy stoma until the site can be intubated with a tracheostomy tube or tracheal tube. If the upper airway is patent, it may be possible to provide some bag-mask ventilation through the nose and mouth with a conventional bag and mask while occluding the superficial tracheal stoma site. (See Chapter 11: "Children With Special Healthcare Needs.")

Ventilation With Oxygen

Healthcare providers should administer oxygen to all seriously ill or injured patients with respiratory insufficiency, shock, or trauma as soon as it is available. In these patients inadequate pulmonary gas exchange or inadequate cardiac output limits oxygen delivery to the tissues.

During cardiac arrest a number of factors contribute to severe progressive tissue hypoxia and the need for supplementary oxygen administration. At best, mouth-to-mouth ventilation provides 16% to 17% oxygen with a maximum alveolar oxygen tension of 80 mm Hg.[53] Even optimal external chest compressions provide only a fraction of normal cardiac output, so blood flow and oxygen delivery to the brain and body are substantially lower than normal. In addition, CPR is associated with right-to-left pulmonary shunting due to ventilation-perfusion mismatch. Preexisting pulmonary conditions may further compromise oxygenation. The combination of low blood flow and low oxygenation contributes to metabolic acidosis and organ failure. For all these reasons oxygen should be administered to children with cardiopulmonary arrest or compromise

FYI: **The Uncommon Use of Reduced Inspired-Oxygen Concentration**

Occasionally an infant may require *reduced* inspired-oxygen concentration or manipulation of oxygenation and ventilation to control pulmonary blood flow (eg, the neonate with congenital heart disease/single-ventricle physiology or persistent pulmonary hypertension). A review of these unique situations is beyond the scope of this manual, but healthcare providers should be aware of these situations when providing resuscitation.

even if measured arterial oxygen tension is high. Whenever possible, humidify the administered oxygen to prevent drying and thickening of pulmonary secretions; dried secretions may contribute to obstruction of natural or artificial airways.

Circulation

Pulse Check and Signs of Circulation

Cardiac arrest results in the absence of *signs of circulation*, including the absence of a central pulse. The pulse check continues to be the gold standard relied on by *healthcare providers* for evaluating circulation. Data is limited regarding the specificity and sensitivity of the pulse check in pediatric victims of cardiac arrest.[54] Three studies have documented the inability of *lay rescuers* to find and count a pulse in healthy infants.[55-57] Healthcare providers also may have difficulty reliably separating venous from arterial pulsation during CPR.[58] For these reasons the pulse check has been eliminated from the recommendations for *lay rescuer* CPR. It remains a recommended assessment for healthcare providers.

Critical Concepts:
Signs of Circulation Checked by Healthcare Providers

After delivery of 2 rescue breaths the healthcare provider checks for the following:

■ Breathing (must be *adequate*— agonal respirations are not adequate)

■ Coughing

■ Movement

■ Pulse confidently felt within 10 seconds (in an infant: brachial pulse; in a child: carotid pulse)

If a pulse is felt but the heart rate is less than 60 bpm in an infant or a child with poor perfusion, provide chest compressions.

Healthcare providers should use the pulse check as one of several signs of circulation. The other signs of circulation are breathing, coughing, or movement in response to rescue breaths. If the rescuer is uncertain if signs of circulation, including a pulse, are present, he/she should begin chest compressions. The risk of performing unnecessary chest compressions is low because the reported complication rate from chest compressions in infants and children is low.[59-66]

Healthcare professionals should assess signs of circulation by performing a pulse check while simultaneously evaluating the victim for adequate breathing, coughing, or movement in response to the 2 initial rescue breaths. Apnea or agonal respirations (occasional slow, irregular gasps) are not adequate methods of ventilation. This assessment for signs of circulation should take no more than 10 seconds.

If you do not confidently detect a pulse or other signs of circulation or if the heart rate is less than 60 bpm in an infant or a child with signs of poor perfusion, provide chest compressions. It is important to note that unresponsive, apneic infants and children may have a slow heart rate or no heart rate at all. If you do not confidently feel a pulse within a few seconds, be prepared to begin chest compressions.

The brachial pulse is the recommended pulse to assess in infants. Healthcare providers should learn to palpate the brachial pulse,[55] although the femoral pulse may be used as an alternative (Figure 13A and B). The brachial pulse is on the inside of the upper arm, between the infant's elbow and shoulder. Press your index and middle fingers gently on the inside of the upper arm for no more than 10 seconds in an attempt to feel the pulse.

Attempted palpation of the carotid pulse in infants is not recommended for several reasons. The short, chubby neck of infants makes rapid location of the carotid artery difficult. In addition, it is easy to compress the airway and stimulate a vagal response

Foundation Facts:
No Pulse Check for Lay Rescuers

The validity of the pulse check by laypersons has been evaluated with adult manikin simulation[67] in unconscious adult patients undergoing cardiopulmonary bypass,[68] unconscious mechanically ventilated adult patients,[69] and conscious adult "test persons."[70,71] These studies suggest that the pulse check as performed by laypersons has limited accuracy, sensitivity, and specificity. In these studies the error rate for palpation of pulses averaged 35%.

while attempting to palpate a carotid pulse. A check of the apical pulse is not recommended because precordial activity represents an *impulse* rather than a pulse. The infant's or child's precordium may be quiet, and a precordial impulse may not be palpated despite the presence of satisfactory cardiac function and a strong central pulse.[55]

Healthcare providers should learn to locate and palpate the carotid artery in children and adults.[72] The carotid artery is the recommended pulse to assess because it is the most accessible central artery in children and adults. The carotid artery lies on the side of the neck between the trachea and the strap (sternocleidomastoid) muscles. To feel the artery, locate the victim's larynx (Adam's apple) with 2 or 3 fingers of one hand while maintaining an open airway with the other hand. On the side closer to the rescuer, slide the fingers into the groove between the trachea and the sternocleidomastoid muscles, and gently palpate the area over the artery (see Figure 14A and B) for no more than 10 seconds.

If signs of circulation are present but spontaneous breathing is absent, provide rescue breathing at a rate of 20 breaths/min

FIGURE 13. Palpation of central pulse in infant. **A,** Palpation of brachial pulse. **B,** Palpation of femoral pulse.

A

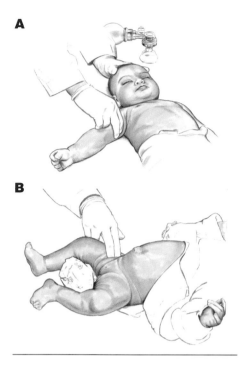

B

FIGURE 14. Palpation of carotid pulse in child. **A,** Locate the child's Adam's apple with 2 or 3 fingers of one hand while maintaining head tilt with the other hand. **B,** Slide 2 or 3 fingers into the groove on the side of the neck closer to the rescuer, between the trachea and the sternocleidomastoid muscles, and gently palpate the artery.

A   **B**

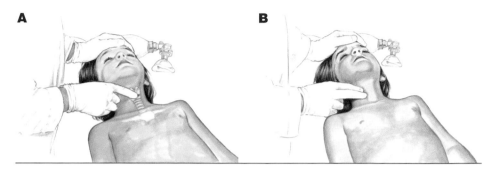

(once every 3 seconds) until spontaneous breathing resumes or advanced airway and ventilation support can be provided. In the prehospital setting the lone rescuer should activate the EMS system after providing approximately 20 breaths (about 1 minute of rescue support). If adequate breathing resumes and there is no suspicion of head or neck trauma, turn the child onto the side into a recovery position until EMS rescuers arrive (see Figure 7).

Indications for Chest Compressions

If signs of circulation are absent or if the heart rate is less than 60 bpm in the infant or child with signs of poor perfusion, begin a series of compressions coordinated with ventilations. Profound bradycardia in the presence of poor perfusion is an indication for chest compressions because an inadequate heart rate with poor perfusion indicates that cardiac arrest is imminent. Cardiac output in infants and children largely depends on heart rate.

If there are no signs of circulation in the out-of-hospital setting and the victim is

1 to 8 years of age or older and an AED is available, attach the AED. The child 1 to 8 years of age weighs approximately 20 to 55 pounds (9 to 25 kg). In the hospital attach a monitor/defibrillator/pacer, assess the ECG rhythm, and deliver a shock if needed.

Use of AEDs

In the prehospital setting AEDs are commonly used for adults in sudden collapse. When attached to the victim with adhesive electrodes, the AED evaluates the victim's ECG to determine if a "shockable" rhythm is present, charges to an appropriate dose, and when activated by the rescuer, delivers a shock. AEDs use voice prompts to assist the operator.

Several manufacturers now market AEDs that accommodate both adult electrode pads and pediatric cable-pad systems that attenuate the delivered energy to a dose more appropriate for children under the age of 8 years. Clinical experience with these devices has yet to be published. Data from two recent, large studies of the effectiveness of the AED rhythm analysis algorithms in pediatric patients have been published since the ECC Guidelines 2000 were drafted.[73,74]

The following conclusions are part of an advisory statement that has been prepared to revise the ECC Guidelines 2000 recommendation for use of AEDs in children under the age of 8 years.[75]

- AEDs may be used for children 1 to 8 years of age with no signs of circulation. Ideally the device should deliver a child dose. The arrhythmia detection algorithm used in the device should demonstrate high specificity for pediatric shockable rhythms (ie, will not recommend shock delivery for non-shockable rhythms): *Class IIb.*

- Currently there is insufficient evidence to support a recommendation for or against the use of AEDs in infants <1 year of age.

- For a single rescuer responding to a child without signs of circulation, 1 minute of CPR continues to be recommended before any other action, such as activating EMS or attaching an AED.

- Defibrillation is recommended for documented VF/pulseless VT: *Class I.*

The steps for AED use are as follows (also see Figure 15):

- POWER ON the AED (turn it on).

- Attach the AED pads/electrodes to the victim's chest (right upper sternal border, left chest under the arm at the level of the left nipple).

- "Clear" the victim and analyze the rhythm.

- If a shock is indicated, "clear" the victim and deliver a shock.

FIGURE 15. Algorithm for prehospital use of AEDs in children 1 to 8 years of age or older.

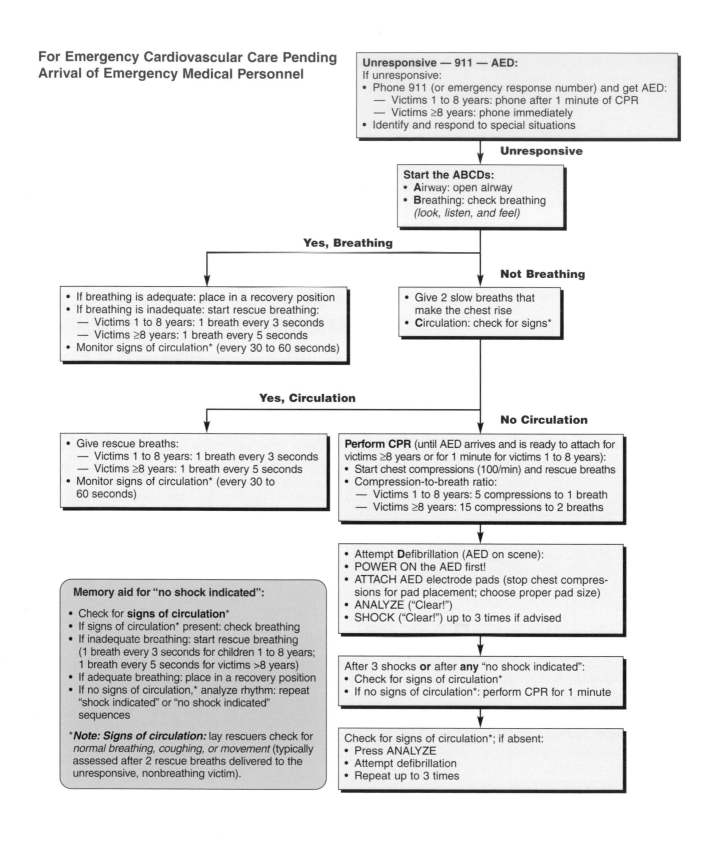

For Emergency Cardiovascular Care Pending Arrival of Emergency Medical Personnel

Unresponsive — 911 — AED:
If unresponsive:
• Phone 911 (or emergency response number) and get AED:
— Victims 1 to 8 years: phone after 1 minute of CPR
— Victims ≥8 years: phone immediately
• Identify and respond to special situations

Unresponsive

Start the ABCDs:
• **A**irway: open airway
• **B**reathing: check breathing
(look, listen, and feel)

Yes, Breathing

• If breathing is adequate: place in a recovery position
• If breathing is inadequate: start rescue breathing:
— Victims 1 to 8 years: 1 breath every 3 seconds
— Victims ≥8 years: 1 breath every 5 seconds
• Monitor signs of circulation* (every 30 to 60 seconds)

Not Breathing

• Give 2 slow breaths that make the chest rise
• **C**irculation: check for signs*

Yes, Circulation

• Give rescue breaths:
— Victims 1 to 8 years: 1 breath every 3 seconds
— Victims ≥8 years: 1 breath every 5 seconds
• Monitor signs of circulation* (every 30 to 60 seconds)

No Circulation

Perform CPR (until AED arrives and is ready to attach for victims ≥8 years or for 1 minute for victims 1 to 8 years):
• Start chest compressions (100/min) and rescue breaths
• Compression-to-breath ratio:
— Victims 1 to 8 years: 5 compressions to 1 breath
— Victims ≥8 years: 15 compressions to 2 breaths

• Attempt **D**efibrillation (AED on scene):
• POWER ON the AED first!
• ATTACH AED electrode pads (stop chest compressions for pad placement; choose proper pad size)
• ANALYZE ("Clear!")
• SHOCK ("Clear!") up to 3 times if advised

Memory aid for "no shock indicated":

• Check for **signs of circulation***
• If signs of circulation* present: check breathing
• If inadequate breathing: start rescue breathing (1 breath every 3 seconds for children 1 to 8 years; 1 breath every 5 seconds for victims >8 years)
• If adequate breathing: place in a recovery position
• If no signs of circulation,* analyze rhythm: repeat "shock indicated" or "no shock indicated" sequences

***Note: Signs of circulation:** lay rescuers check for *normal breathing, coughing, or movement* (typically assessed after 2 rescue breaths delivered to the unresponsive, nonbreathing victim).

After 3 shocks **or** after **any** "no shock indicated":
• Check for signs of circulation*
• If no signs of circulation*: perform CPR for 1 minute

Check for signs of circulation*; if absent:
• Press ANALYZE
• Attempt defibrillation
• Repeat up to 3 times

■ Repeat shocks up to a total of 3; after 3 shocks or whenever the AED indicates *"no shock indicated,"* check the airway, breathing, and circulation and provide the steps of CPR as indicated for 1 minute, then reanalyze rhythm and provide more shocks if needed.

It is important to note that basic life support with rescue breathing and chest compressions remains the initial treatment of choice for victims of all ages in cardiac arrest associated with asphyxia (eg, after submersion).

All healthcare providers should be trained in the use of an AED, including special resuscitation circumstances (see Critical Concepts: "Special Circumstances That Can Influence AED Use") and AED troubleshooting. Healthcare providers who routinely care for children at risk for arrhythmias and cardiac arrest (eg, in-hospital settings) should continue to use defibrillators capable of appropriate energy adjustment.

Potential Complications From Chest Compressions

Complications associated with chest compressions are uncommon in infants and children. Although rib fractures and injuries to the bony thorax have been attributed to resuscitative efforts in adults,[63] almost all rib fractures observed after resuscitative efforts in infants and children can be attributed to preceding trauma, abuse, or underlying bone disease.[59-66] Despite prolonged and aggressive resuscitation, significant iatrogenic injuries attributable to CPR are reported in less than 3% of infant and child victims.

Technique of Chest Compressions

Chest compressions are serial, rhythmic compressions of the chest that cause blood to flow to the vital organs (the heart, lungs, and brain) in an attempt to keep them viable until ALS can be provided. Chest compressions provide circulation as a result of changes in intrathoracic pressure or direct compression of the heart.[76-80] Chest compressions for infants and children should be provided with ventilations.[81,82]

To provide chest compressions, press the lower half of the sternum to a relative depth of approximately one third to one half the anterior-posterior diameter of the chest at a rate of at least 100 compressions per minute for the infant and approximately 100 compressions per minute for the child. Be sure to avoid compressing the xiphoid process.

The rationale for use of a relative depth of compression with de-emphasis of an absolute depth of compression in inches is provided in FYI: "Rationale for a Relative Rather Than an Absolute Compression Depth in Infants and Children." The difference between a compression rate and the number of compressions delivered per minute during CPR is summarized in

Foundation Facts: "Difference Between Compression *Rate* per Minute and Number of Compressions *Delivered* per Minute."

Healthcare providers should evaluate the effectiveness of compressions during CPR. Chest compressions should produce palpable pulses in a central artery (eg, the carotid, brachial, or femoral artery). Although pulses palpated during chest compression may actually represent *venous* pulsations rather than *arterial* pulses,[58] pulse assessment by the healthcare provider during CPR remains the quickest and most practical method of assessing chest compression efficacy.

Adjuncts may be used to evaluate the effectiveness of chest compressions. Continuous exhaled (end-tidal) CO_2 detectors can assist

Critical Concepts:
Special Circumstances That Can Influence AED Use

1. *Children less than 1 year of age:* AED use is a Class Indeterminate recommendation. AEDs may be used for children 1 to 8 years of age (see text).

2. *Victim in standing water:* Remove the victim from the water and dry the victim's chest.

3. *Victim with implanted defibrillator/pacemaker:* Do not place an electrode pad directly over an implanted

device (the device may block current and reduce delivery of current to the heart).

4. *Victim with a transdermal medication patch:* Do not place an electrode pad directly over a medication patch. If the patch is in the way, remove the patch and wipe the victim's skin before attaching the AED.

FYI: Rationale for a Relative Rather Than an Absolute Compression Depth in Infants and Children

For the infant or child, a relative depth of compression of one third to one half the depth of the chest is recommended. The use of relative rather than absolute depth of compressions in newly born infants, infants, and children was determined by consensus, not scientific evidence. This relative depth was offered to simplify teaching after many rescuers reported difficulty estimating absolute

depth of compression in inches or centimeters during performance of compressions. In the newly born, adequate compressions are thought to be provided if the chest is compressed to one third its depth because the anterior-posterior diameter of the chest of the newly born infant is less in than that of the older infant or child.

Foundation Facts:
Difference Between Compression *Rate* per Minute and Number of Compressions *Delivered* per Minute

The compression rate is the speed of compressions. You will compress at a rate that, if uninterrupted, would result in delivery of at least 100 compressions per minute. You will actually deliver fewer than 100 compressions per minute because you must interrupt compressions to deliver rescue breaths.

The compression rate can be likened to the speed you drive (miles per hour) in a car. Imagine driving at 40 miles per hour with the need to stop at a stoplight every fifth mile. At the end of an hour you will have driven fewer than 40 miles because that rate of speed was interrupted by frequent stops. If you compress at a rate of at least 100

compressions per minute but you stop every fifth compression to deliver a rescue breath, the actual number of compressions delivered will be determined not only by the rate of compressions but by the time it takes you to open the airway, deliver the breath, and then prepare to resume chest compressions (likened to the time you stop the car at stoplights).

Some rescuers are more efficient than others and will be able to deliver the rescue breath and resume chest compressions quickly whereas other rescuers will require more time to deliver the rescue breath (so fewer compressions will be delivered).

FYI: Compression Duty Cycle

When the compression phase is somewhat shorter than the relaxation phase of each chest compression, improved blood flow has been observed in a very young infant animal model of CPR.[83] During actual CPR, however, the rescuer is compressing at a rate of at least 100 times per minute (nearly 2 compressions per second), so it is not practical to attempt to judge or manipulate compression and relaxation ratios. In addition, details regarding such manipulation would increase the complexity of CPR instruction. For these reasons provide compressions for infants and children using approximately equal compression and relaxation phases.

---

the healthcare provider in evaluating blood flow resulting from chest compressions. If chest compressions produce inadequate cardiac output and pulmonary blood flow, exhaled CO_2 will remain extremely low (less than approximately 10 mm Hg) throughout resuscitation. If cardiac output and pulmonary blood flow improve during chest compressions, exhaled CO_2 may rise during resuscitation.

If an arterial catheter is in place during resuscitation (eg, during chest compressions provided to a patient in the intensive care unit [ICU] with an arterial monitor in place), the depth of chest compressions can be guided by the displayed arterial waveform to a target pressure; the rescuer should increase the force of compressions if an inadequate pulse pressure is depicted by the arterial waveform. The downward (compression) and upward (relaxation) time during each compression should be approximately equal (see FYI: "Compression Duty Cycle").

You should usually perform CPR where the victim is found, but efforts must be

made to optimize the effectiveness of chest compressions. To facilitate optimal chest compressions, the child should be supine on a hard, flat surface. If cardiac arrest occurs in a hospital bed, place firm support (a resuscitation board) beneath the patient's back. For optimal support, use a resuscitation board that extends from the shoulders to the waist and across the full width of the bed. The use of a wide board is particularly important when providing chest compressions to larger children. If the board is too small, it will be pushed deep into the mattress during compressions, dispersing the force and compromising the effectiveness of compressions. Spine boards, preferably with head wells, can be used in ambulances and mobile life support units.[22,84] They provide a firm surface for CPR in the emergency vehicle or on a wheeled stretcher and may also be useful for extricating and immobilizing victims.

Infants with no signs of head or neck trauma may be successfully carried on the rescuer's forearm during resuscitation.

Use the palm of one hand to support the infant's back while the fingers of the other hand compress the sternum. This maneuver effectively lowers the infant's head, allowing the head to tilt back slightly into a neutral position that maintains airway patency. If the infant is carried during CPR, the hard surface behind the back is created by the rescuer's forearm, which supports the length of the infant's torso while the infant's head and neck are supported by the rescuer's hand. Take care to keep the infant's head no higher than the rest of the body. Use the other hand to perform chest compressions. You can lift the infant to provide ventilation (see Figure 16).

Chest Compression in the Infant (Less Than 1 Year of Age)

Two Thumb–Encircling Hands Technique

The 2 thumb–encircling hands technique is the preferred technique for 2 or more healthcare providers when physically feasible. Perform compressions with this technique as follows:

FIGURE 16. Chest compression for infant supported on rescuer's forearm.

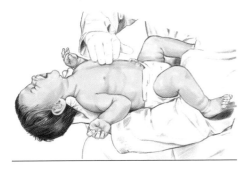

1. Stand at the infant's feet or side.

2. Place your thumbs side by side over the lower half of the infant's sternum, ensuring that the thumbs do not compress on or near the xiphoid process.[78,85-88] The thumbs may overlap when the infant is very small. Encircle the infant's chest and support the infant's back with the fingers of both hands. Both thumbs should be located on the lower half of the infant's sternum, approximately 1 finger's width below the intermammary line. The intermammary line is an imaginary line located between the nipples, over the breastbone.

3. With your hands encircling the chest, use both thumbs to depress the sternum approximately one third to one half the depth of the infant's chest. This will correspond to a depth of approximately ½ to 1 inch (1¼ to 2½ cm), but these measurements are not exact (see Figure 17A). Deliver compressions in a smooth fashion, with approximately equal time in the compression and relaxation phases. Be sure that after each compression you completely release the pressure on the sternum and allow the sternum to return to the normal position without lifting your thumbs off the chest wall.

4. Compress the sternum at a *rate of at least 100 times per minute* (this corresponds to a rate that is slightly less than 2 compressions per second during the groups of 5 compressions).

5. After 5 compressions, pause briefly for the second rescuer to open the airway with a head tilt–chin lift (or if trauma is suspected, with a jaw thrust) and deliver 1 effective breath (the chest should rise with the breath). Compressions and ventilations should be coordinated to avoid simultaneous delivery and to ensure adequate ventilation and chest expansion, especially when the airway is unprotected.[89] Once the airway is secured, compressions and ventilations can be asynchronous.

6. Continue compressions and ventilations in a ratio of 5 compressions to 1 ventilation. This ratio is recommended for infants and children whether there are 1 or 2 rescuers. Note that for resuscitation of newly born infants, a ratio of 3:1 is recommended; for resuscitation of adults a ratio of 15:2 is recommended (see "Compression-Ventilation Ratios").

Two-Finger Compression Technique

The 2-finger chest compression technique is the preferred technique for the lone rescuer. Perform the 2-finger compression technique as follows:

1. Place the 2 fingers of one hand over the lower half of the sternum[85-88] approximately 1 finger's width below the intermammary line, avoiding compressing on or near the xiphoid process.[10] The intermammary line is an imaginary line located between the nipples, over the breastbone (see Figure 17B).

2. Press down on the sternum, depressing it approximately one third to one half the depth of the infant's chest. This will correspond to a depth of about ½ to 1 inch (1¼ to 2½ cm), but these measurements are not exact. After each compression completely release the pressure on the sternum and allow the sternum to return to the normal position without lifting your fingers off the chest wall.

3. Deliver compressions in a smooth fashion, with approximately equal time in the compression and relaxation phases.

4. Compress the infant's sternum at *a rate of at least 100 times per minute*. This corresponds to a rate of slightly less than 2 compressions per second during the groups of 5 compressions.

5. After 5 compressions open the airway with a head tilt–chin lift (or if trauma is present, use the jaw thrust) and give 1 effective breath. Be sure that the chest rises with the breath.

6. Coordinate compressions and ventilations to avoid simultaneous delivery and ensure adequate ventilation and chest expansion, especially when the airway is unprotected.[89] You may use your other hand (the one not compressing the chest) to maintain the infant's head in a neutral position during the 5 chest compressions. This may help

FIGURE 17. Chest compression technique for infants. **A,** Two thumb–encircling hands technique is preferred when 2 healthcare providers are present. The first provider performs bag-mask ventilation while the second provides chest compressions. **B,** Two-finger chest compression technique is appropriate for the lone rescuer or if the rescuer is unable to compress the chest sufficiently with the 2 thumb–encircling hands technique.

A

B

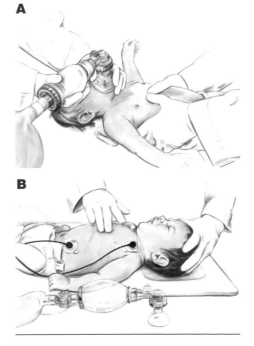

you provide ventilation without the need to reposition the head after each set of 5 compressions. To maintain a neutral head position, place your other (noncompressing) hand behind the infant's chest. This will elevate the chest, ensuring that the head is in a neutral position relative to the chest. Alternatively, if there is no sign of head or neck trauma, you can place your other (noncompressing) hand on the infant's forehead to maintain head tilt (refer to Figure 18). As a third option, if signs of head or neck trauma are present, place your other (noncompressing) hand on the infant's forehead to maintain stability without performing a head tilt. Continue compressions and ventilations in a ratio of 5:1 (for 1 or 2 rescuers).

Chest Compression for the Child (Approximately 1 to 8 Years of Age)

Chest compressions and ventilations for the infant or child are performed at a ratio of 5:1 whether 1 or 2 rescuers are present. Perform chest compressions in the child using the following steps:

1. Place the heel of one hand over the lower half of the sternum between the nipple line and the bottom of the sternum. Be sure that you do not compress on or near the xiphoid process. Lift your fingers to avoid pressing on the child's ribs (see Figure 18).

2. Depress the sternum approximately one third to one half the depth of the child's chest. This corresponds to a compression depth of approximately 1 to 1½ inches (2½ to 4 cm), but these measurements are not exact. After the compression, release the pressure on the sternum, allowing it to return to the normal position, but do not lift your hand from the surface of the chest. If you are unable to depress the sternum sufficiently with the heel of 1 hand, use the 2-hand adult technique to compress the sternum, but continue to use the child compression rate and compression-ventilation ratio.

FIGURE 18. One-hand chest compression technique for child.

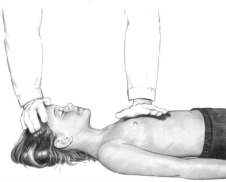

3. Deliver compressions in a smooth fashion, with approximately equal time in the compression and relaxation phases.

4. Compress the sternum *at a rate of approximately 100 times per minute.* This corresponds to a rate of slightly less than 2 compressions per second during the groups of 5 compressions.

5. After 5 compressions open the airway and give 1 effective rescue breath. Be sure the chest rises with the breath.

6. Return your hand immediately to the correct position on the sternum and give 5 chest compressions. Continue compressions and breaths in a ratio of 5:1 (for 1 or 2 rescuers).

Chest Compression for Children 8 Years of Age and Older

For children 8 years of age and older, use the adult 2-handed method of chest compression to achieve an adequate depth of compression as follows:

1. Place the heel of one hand on the lower half of the sternum (between the nipples). Place the heel of your other hand on top of the first hand. Avoid pressing on the xiphoid process.

2. Interlock the fingers of both hands and lift the fingers to avoid pressure on the child's ribs. Position yourself vertically above the victim's chest, and with your arm straight, press down on the sternum to depress it approximately 1½ to 2 inches (4 to 5 cm). Release the pressure completely after

each compression, allowing the sternum to return to its normal position, but do not remove your hands from the surface of the chest.

3. Deliver compressions in a smooth fashion, with approximately equal time in the compression and relaxation phases.

4. Compress the sternum *at a rate of approximately 100 times per minute.* This corresponds to a rate of slightly less than 2 compressions per second during the groups of 15 compressions.

5. If the airway is *not secured* (ie, no tracheal intubation), pause after each series of 15 compressions to open the airway and give 2 effective rescue breaths (or allow a colleague to deliver 2 effective rescue breaths). Be sure that the chest rises with the breath.

   If the airway *is secured (ie, tracheal intubation),* compressions and ventilations can be asynchronous. Deliver compressions at a rate of approximately 100 per minute and ventilations at a rate of approximately 12 per minute (see below). Be sure the chest rises with each breath.

6. If you interrupt compressions to deliver ventilations, after the 2 breaths return your hands immediately to the correct position on the sternum and give 15 chest compressions.

Coordination of Compressions and Rescue Breathing

External chest compressions for infants and children should always be accompanied by rescue breathing. When 2 rescuers are providing CPR for an infant or a child with an unsecured airway, the rescuer providing compressions should pause after every fifth compression to allow the second rescuer to provide 1 effective ventilation (inspiration). Chest compression can be initiated at the end of inspiration, and it will facilitate expiration. This pause is necessary to ensure adequate lung inflation until the airway is secured (intubated).

FYI: Simultaneous Compression and Ventilation

Although the technique of simultaneous compression and ventilation may augment coronary perfusion pressure in some settings,[90-93] it may produce barotrauma and decrease ventilation and is not recommended. Priority is given to ensuring adequate ventilation and avoiding potentially harmful excessive barotrauma in children.[92]

Once the airway is secured (the trachea is intubated), the pause for ventilation is no longer necessary. But coordination of compressions and ventilations is still encouraged for resuscitation of the newly born because it may facilitate adequate ventilation even after tracheal intubation. All rescuers should ensure that ventilation is effective throughout resuscitative efforts for infants and children.

Reassess the victim after 20 cycles of compressions and ventilations (slightly longer than 1 minute) and every few minutes thereafter for any sign of resumption of spontaneous breathing or signs of circulation. The number 20 is easy to remember, so it is used to provide a guideline interval for reassessment rather than an indication of the absolute number of cycles delivered in exactly 1 minute. In the delivery room more frequent assessments of heart rate—approximately every 30 seconds—are recommended for the newly born.

In infants it may be difficult for the lone rescuer to coordinate delivery of rapid compressions and ventilations in a 5:1 ratio with a compression rate of at least 100 compressions per minute.[94-96] To minimize interruptions in chest compressions, if no trauma is present the rescuer can maintain airway patency during compressions by using the hand that is not performing compressions to maintain a head tilt (see Figures 17B and 18).

Effective chest expansion should be visible with each breath you provide. In children head tilt alone is often inadequate to maintain airway patency. If the chest does not rise during rescue breaths and you are a lone rescuer, use the hand performing chest compressions to perform a chin lift (or jaw thrust) to open the airway each time you deliver rescue breaths. After the breath is delivered, visualize the approximate position of your hand on the sternum during the previous sequence of compressions and return your hand to that position. This will minimize the time needed to perform ventilations and resume compressions. If trauma is present, use the hand that is not performing compressions to maintain head stability during chest compressions.

If the chest does not rise during mouth-to-mask ventilation, be sure the airway is open and that there is a good seal between the victim's face and the mask. Ensure that adequate tidal volume is provided and allow time between compressions for delivery of effective tidal volume. If the trachea has been intubated, verify tube placement and patency and replace the tube if it is not in the trachea.

Compression-Ventilation Ratios

Research data has not yet established ideal compression-ventilation ratios for infants and children. From an educational standpoint it would be desirable to recommend a single universal compression-ventilation ratio for victims of all ages. But there is insufficient evidence to justify changing the current recommendations for compression-ventilation ratios in infants and children to a universal ratio.

Studies of monitored rescuers have shown that a compression-ventilation ratio of 15:2 generally delivers more compressions per minute, and a ratio of 5:1 generally delivers more ventilations per minute.[94,97] The actual number of interventions (compressions and ventilations) delivered per minute will vary from rescuer to rescuer and will depend on the compression rate, amount of time the rescuer spends opening the airway and providing ventilation,

and rescuer fatigue (see Foundation Facts: "Difference Between Compression *Rate* per Minute and Number of Compressions *Delivered* per Minute").[94,98,99]

There is consensus among resuscitation councils that pediatric guidelines should continue to recommend a compression-ventilation ratio of 3:1 for newly born infants and 5:1 for infants and children up to 8 years of age. A compression-ventilation ratio of 15:2 is now recommended for children 8 years of age and older and adults for 1- or 2-rescuer CPR until the airway is secure.

A compression-ventilation ratio of 3:1 is recommended for newly-born infants. The compression rate should be fast enough to deliver approximately 90 compressions and 30 ventilations per minute (120 events per minute). The higher number of ventilations delivered with this compression-ventilation ratio is appropriate for newly born infants because inadequate ventilation is the most common cause of neonatal cardiopulmonary distress and arrest.

A compression-ventilation ratio of 5:1 is used in pediatric resuscitation because this ratio provides more ventilations per minute than the 15:2 ratio used in adult resuscitation. The higher number of ventilations delivered with this ratio is appropriate for pediatric resuscitation because most children who develop cardiorespiratory arrest are hypoxic and hypercarbic, so delivery of a greater number of ventilations, establishment of adequate oxygenation, and ventilation are important.

Emerging evidence in *adult* victims of cardiac arrest suggests that provision of longer sequences of uninterrupted chest compressions (a compression-ventilation ratio greater than 5:1) may be easier to teach and retain.[100] In addition, data from animals suggests that longer sequences of uninterrupted chest compressions may improve coronary perfusion.[101,102] Finally, longer sequences of compressions may allow more efficient second-rescuer interventions in the out-of-hospital EMS setting and will result in delivery of more compressions per minute than a 5:1 ratio.[95]

Therefore, a compression-ventilation ratio of 15:2 is recommended for 1- and 2-rescuer CPR in children 8 years of age and older and adults until the airway is secure.

"Partial" CPR: Is Something Better Than Nothing?

Clinical studies have established that outcomes are dismal when the pediatric victim of cardiac arrest remains in cardiac arrest until the arrival of EMS personnel.[103,104] In comparison, excellent outcomes are typical when the child is successfully resuscitated before the arrival of EMS personnel.[105-111] Some of these patients were apparently resuscitated with "partial CPR," which is chest compressions or rescue breathing only.

In some published surveys healthcare providers have expressed reluctance to perform mouth-to-mouth ventilation for strangers in cardiopulmonary arrest.[112-114] This reluctance has also been expressed by some surveyed potential lay rescuers,[106,115] although reluctance has not been expressed about resuscitation of infants and children.

The effectiveness of partial or "compression-only" or "no ventilation" CPR has been studied in adult animal models of acute VF sudden cardiac arrest and in some clinical trials of adult out-of-hospital cardiac arrest. Some evidence suggests that positive-pressure ventilation may not be essential during the initial 6 to 12 minutes of an *acute adult VF* cardiac arrest.[116-123] Spontaneous gasping and passive chest recoil may provide some ventilation during that time without the need for active rescue breathing.[119,122] In addition, cardiac output during chest compression is only about 25% of normal output, so the ventilation required to maintain optimal ventilation-perfusion relationships may be minimal.[124,125] *It does not appear that these observations can be applied to resuscitation of infants and children.*

Preliminary evidence suggests that both chest compressions and active rescue breathing are necessary for optimal resuscitation of the asphyxial arrests most commonly encountered in children.[81,82] For pediatric cardiac arrest, the lay rescuer should provide immediate chest compressions and rescue breathing. If the lay rescuer is unwilling or unable to provide rescue breathing or chest compressions, it is better to provide either chest compressions or rescue breathing than no bystander CPR.

Circulatory Adjuncts and Mechanical Devices for Chest Compression

The use of mechanical devices to provide chest compressions during CPR is not recommended for children. These devices have been designed and tested for use in adults, and their safety and efficacy in children have not been studied. Active compression-decompression CPR (ACD-CPR) has been shown to increase cardiac output compared with standard CPR in adult animal models.[126,127] ACD-CPR maintains coronary perfusion during compression and decompression in humans[128,129] and provides ventilation if the airway is patent.[128,130] In clinical trials ACD-CPR has produced variable results.[131-135] Although ACD-CPR is considered an optional technique for adult CPR, it cannot be recommended for use in children because it has not been studied in this age group.

Interposed abdominal compression CPR (IAC-CPR) has been shown to increase blood flow in laboratory and computer models[136-138] of *adult* CPR. IAC-CPR has been shown to improve the hemodynamics of CPR and return of spontaneous circulation for *adult* patients in some clinical in-hospital settings,[139,140] with no evidence of excessive harm. The technique is slightly more complex than standard CPR, however, and it requires an additional rescuer. IAC-CPR has been recommended as an alternative technique for trained adult healthcare providers in the in-hospital setting, but it cannot be recommended for use in children because it has not been studied in this age group.

Relief of Foreign-Body Airway Obstruction (Choking)

BLS providers should be able to recognize and relieve severe or complete FBAO. Three maneuvers to remove foreign bodies are suggested: back blows, chest thrusts, and abdominal thrusts. There is consensus that lack of protection of the upper abdominal organs by the rib cage puts infants at risk for iatrogenic trauma from abdominal thrusts,[141] so abdominal thrusts are not recommended for relief of FBAO in infants.

Epidemiology and Recognition of FBAO

Most reported cases of FBAO in adults are caused by impacted food and occur while the victim is eating. Most reported episodes of choking in infants and children occur during eating or play, when parents or childcare providers are present. The choking event is therefore commonly witnessed, and the rescuer usually intervenes when the victim is conscious/responsive.

More than 90% of deaths from foreign-body aspiration in the pediatric age group occur in children younger than 5 years; 65% of victims are infants.[142] With the development of consumer product safety standards regulating the minimum size of toys and toy parts for young children, the incidence of foreign-body aspiration has decreased. But toys, balloons, or small objects and especially foods (eg, hot dogs, round candies, nuts, and grapes) may still be aspirated.[142-144]

Signs of severe or complete FBAO in infants and children include the *sudden* onset of respiratory distress associated with weak or silent coughing, inability to speak, stridor (a high-pitched, noisy sound or wheezing), and increasing respiratory difficulty. These signs and symptoms of airway obstruction may also be caused by infections such as epiglottitis and croup, which produce airway edema. But signs of FBAO typically develop very abruptly, with no other signs of illness or infection such as fever, signs of congestion, hoarseness, drooling, lethargy, or limpness. In contrast, *infectious* causes of airway obstruction typically develop more gradually or are associated with other signs of illness or infection. If the child has an *infectious* cause of airway obstruction, the Heimlich maneuver, back blows, and chest thrusts will *not* relieve the airway obstruction. The child with infectious airway obstruction should be taken immediately to an emergency facility.

Priorities for Teaching Relief of Severe or Complete FBAO

When FBAO produces signs of severe or *complete* airway obstruction, you must act quickly to relieve the obstruction. The child may signal distress with the universal choking sign (Figure 19). If partial obstruction is present and the child is coughing forcefully, do not interfere with the child's spontaneous coughing and breathing efforts. Attempt to relieve the obstruction only if the cough is or becomes ineffective (loss of sound), respiratory difficulty increases and is accompanied by stridor, or the victim becomes unresponsive.

If a *responsive infant* demonstrates signs of complete FBAO, deliver a combination of back blows and chest thrusts until the object is expelled or the victim becomes unresponsive. Although the data in this age group is limited, Heimlich abdominal thrusts are not recommended because they may damage the relatively large and unprotected liver. Reports of gastric rupture and abdominal injury associated with the Heimlich maneuver have contributed to this concern.[145,146]

If a *responsive child* (1 to 8 years of age) demonstrates signs of severe or complete FBAO, provide a series of Heimlich subdiaphragmatic abdominal thrusts.[147,148] These thrusts increase intrathoracic pressure, creating artificial "coughs" that can force air and the foreign body out of the airway.

Epidemiologic data[144,149] does not distinguish between FBAO fatalities in which the victims are responsive when first encountered and those in which the victims

FIGURE 19. Universal choking sign in a child.

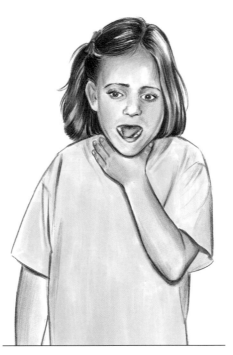

are unresponsive when initially encountered, so it is impossible to determine how many victims of choking are unresponsive when they are first encountered by rescuers. Most resuscitation experts think that the incidence of FBAO in victims who are *unresponsive* at the time of discovery is very low. For this reason there is continued emphasis on teaching lay rescuers the skills to relieve FBAO in *responsive victims*. All rescuers should perform abdominal thrusts for responsive adults and children with complete FBAO and alternating back blows and chest thrusts for responsive infants with complete FBAO until the object is expelled or the victim becomes unresponsive. Only healthcare providers will be taught a unique set of skills to attempt to relieve FBAO in the unresponsive victim.

Relief of FBAO in the Responsive Infant or Child

Relief of FBAO in the Responsive Infant: Back Blows and Chest Thrusts

To clear a foreign-body obstruction from the airway of a responsive infant, deliver

alternating back blows (Figure 20A) and chest thrusts (Figure 20B) until the object is expelled or the infant becomes unresponsive.

Perform the sequence of alternating back blows and chest thrusts seated or kneeling with the infant held on your lap as follows:

1. Hold the infant prone, with the infant's body resting on your forearm and the infant's head slightly lower than the chest. Support the infant's head by firmly supporting the jaw with your hand. Take care to avoid compressing the soft tissues of the infant's throat. Rest your forearm on your thigh to support the infant.

2. Deliver up to 5 back blows forcefully in the middle of the back between the

Critical Concepts:
Signs of Severe or Complete Airway Obstruction

In a responsive, choking infant or child the following signs of severe or complete airway obstruction require immediate action:

■ Universal choking sign: the child may clutch his/her neck with the thumb and index finger (Figure 19)

■ Inability to speak or cry audibly

■ Weak, ineffective coughs

■ High-pitched sounds or no sounds during inhalation

■ Increased difficulty breathing with distress

■ Cyanosis

Note: You do *not* need to act if the victim can cough forcefully and speak. Do not interfere at this point because a strong cough is the most effective way to remove a foreign body. Stay with the victim and monitor his/her condition. If the partial obstruction persists, seek healthcare support.

infant's shoulder blades, using the heel of your other hand. Deliver each blow with sufficient force to attempt to dislodge the foreign body (Figure 20A).

3. After delivering up to 5 back blows, place the hand that was delivering the back blows on the infant's back, supporting the occiput of the infant's head with the palm of that hand. This will temporarily cradle the infant between your 2 forearms, with the palm of one hand supporting the face and jaw while the palm of the other hand supports the occiput.

4. Turn the infant supine as a unit onto that second hand and arm while carefully supporting the head and neck. Hold the infant in the supine position with your forearm resting on your thigh. Keep the infant's head lower than the trunk and continue to hold the occiput of the infant's head with your hand.

5. Provide up to 5 quick downward chest thrusts in the same location as chest compressions: the lower third of the sternum, approximately 1 finger's width below the intermammary line. Deliver the chest thrusts at a rate of approximately 1 per second, each with the intention of creating enough of an "artificial cough" to dislodge the foreign body (Figure 20B).

6. Continue alternating back blows and chest thrusts until the object is expelled or the infant becomes unresponsive. If the infant becomes unresponsive, see "Relief of FBAO in the Unresponsive Infant or Child."

Relief of FBAO in the Responsive Child: Abdominal Thrusts (Heimlich Maneuver)

Use abdominal thrusts to relieve complete FBAO in the responsive child.[150-154] The child may be standing or sitting. Perform the following steps:

1. Stand or kneel behind the victim, arms directly under the victim's axillae, encircling the victim's chest.

2. Place the flat, thumb side of one fist against the victim's abdomen in the midline slightly above the navel and well below the tip of the xiphoid process.

3. Grasp the fist with the other hand and exert a series of up to 5 quick inward and upward thrusts (see Figure 21). Do not compress the xiphoid process

or the lower margins of the rib cage because force applied to these structures may damage internal organs.[141,155,156]

4. Deliver each thrust as a separate, distinct movement, with the intent to relieve the obstruction. Continue the series of up to 5 thrusts until the foreign body is expelled or the patient becomes unresponsive.

Relief of FBAO in the Unresponsive Infant or Child

There are several cautions you must remember when you attempt to relieve FBAO in the unresponsive infant or child (see Critical Concepts: "Cautions During Attempts to Relieve FBAO in Infants and Children"). First, maneuvers to relieve FBAO for the unresponsive infant or child should be performed only when the infant or child has become unresponsive—do not attempt to open the airway of a *responsive* victim. Second, blind finger sweeps should *not* be performed in infants and children because the finger may actually push the foreign body back into the airway, causing further obstruction or injury to the supraglottic area.[157,158]

When the infant or child with FBAO becomes unresponsive/unconscious, you should first look in the airway. Open the victim's mouth by grasping both the tongue and lower jaw between the thumb and finger and lifting (tongue-jaw lift).[17] This action draws the tongue away from the back of the throat and may itself partially relieve the obstruction (see Figure 22A and B). If you see the obstructing object, carefully remove it, but do not perform a blind finger sweep.

Relief of FBAO in the Unresponsive Infant

If the infant victim becomes unresponsive, you will still use back blows and chest thrusts. Perform the unresponsive obstructed airway sequence for the unresponsive infant as follows:

1. Open the victim's airway with a *tongue-jaw lift* and look for an object in the

FIGURE 20. Maneuvers to relieve complete FBAO in the responsive infant. Alternate 5 back blows (**A**) and 5 chest thrusts (**B**) until the object is expelled or the infant becomes unresponsive.

A   **B**

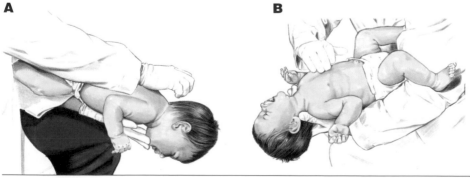

FIGURE 21. Abdominal thrusts to relieve complete FBAO in the responsive child. The rescuer kneels or stands behind the victim and performs the abdominal thrusts until the object is expelled or the child becomes unresponsive.

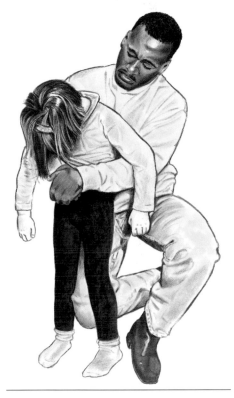

mouth and pharynx. If you see an object, remove it. Do not perform a blind finger sweep.

2. Open the airway with a head tilt–chin lift and attempt to provide rescue breaths. If the breaths are not effective, reposition the head and reattempt ventilation.

3. If the breaths are still not effective, perform up to 5 back blows and 5 chest thrusts.

4. Repeat steps 1 through 3 (Figures 20A and B) until the object is dislodged and the airway is patent or until attempts have lasted approximately 1 minute. If the infant remains unresponsive after approximately 1 minute of rescue efforts, activate the EMS system.

5. If rescue breaths are effective, check for signs of circulation and continue

CPR as needed, or place the infant in a recovery position if the infant demonstrates adequate spontaneous breathing.

Relief of FBAO in the Unresponsive Child

If the child victim becomes unresponsive, you will still use abdominal thrusts. Perform the obstructed airway sequence for the unresponsive child as follows:

1. Open the victim's airway using a *tongue-jaw lift* and look for an object in the mouth and pharynx. If an object is visible, remove it. Do not perform blind finger sweeps.

2. Open the airway with a head tilt–chin lift and attempt to provide rescue breaths. If breaths are not effective, reposition the head and reattempt ventilation.

3. If the breaths are still not effective, kneel beside the victim or straddle the victim's hips and prepare to perform abdominal thrusts (Heimlich maneuver) as follows:

   a. Place the heel of one hand on the child's abdomen in the midline slightly above the navel and well below the rib cage and xiphoid process. Place the other hand on top of the first.

   b. Press both hands onto the abdomen with a quick inward and upward thrust (Figure 23). Direct each thrust upward in the midline and not to either side of the abdomen. If necessary, perform a series of up to 5 thrusts. Each thrust should be a separate and distinct movement of sufficient force to dislodge the obstruction.

4. Repeat steps 1 through 3 until the object is dislodged and the airway is patent or until attempts have lasted approximately 1 minute. If the child remains unresponsive after approximately 1 minute of rescue efforts, activate the EMS system.

FIGURE 22. Tongue-jaw lift technique in an unresponsive victim with suspected FBAO. The tongue and jaw of the infant (**A**) and child (**B**) are lifted up to open the mouth and airway and enable the rescuer to look inside the mouth. Remove a foreign body if you see it, but do not perform a blind finger sweep.

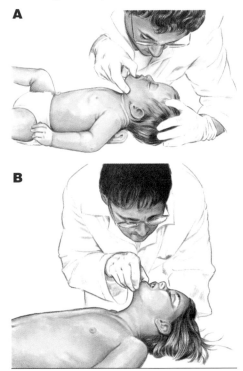

5. If rescue breaths are effective, check for signs of circulation and provide additional steps of CPR as needed, or place the child in a recovery position if the child demonstrates adequate spontaneous breathing.

BLS in Special Situations

BLS for the Trauma Victim

The principles of resuscitation of the seriously injured child are the same as those for any pediatric patient with potential cardiorespiratory deterioration. Some aspects of pediatric trauma care require emphasis, however, because inadequate volume resuscitation is a major cause of preventable pediatric trauma death.[159-161] The special aspects of pediatric trauma resuscitation are addressed in Chapter 10.

Cautions During Attempts to Relieve FBAO in Infants and Children

- Do NOT interfere if the infant or child is coughing forcefully.

- Do NOT perform a tongue-jaw lift or attempt to reach in the mouth of a *responsive* choking victim.

- Do NOT press on the xiphoid process (extreme lower margin of the rib cage) when performing abdominal thrusts.

- Do NOT perform *blind* finger sweeps in infants and children.

FIGURE 23. Abdominal thrusts performed for the supine, unresponsive child.

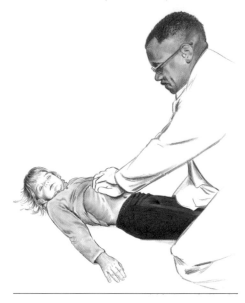

FIGURE 24. Simultaneous opening of the airway with the jaw-thrust technique while immobilizing the cervical spine. The rescuer is positioned above the victim's head, so a second rescuer will be needed to perform ventilation and chest compressions if needed.

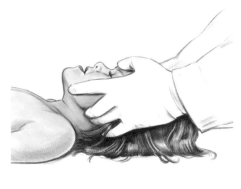

Ideally a qualified surgeon should be involved early in the course of resuscitation. In regions with developed EMS systems, children with multisystem trauma should be rapidly transported to trauma centers with pediatric expertise.

BLS support requires meticulous attention to airway, breathing, and circulation from the moment of injury. The *most common error during pediatric trauma resuscitation is the failure to open and maintain the airway with cervical spine immobilization.* During initial assessment use the jaw–thrust maneuver to open the airway. The head tilt–chin lift is contraindicated because it may worsen existing cervical spinal injury. Although the incidence of secondary cervical spinal injury from such movement is unknown, it is prudent to avoid movement of the head and neck when cervical spine injury is suspected.

The rescuer must use both hands to perform the jaw thrust. The rescuer is most often positioned at the victim's head (Figure 24). This position will allow you to open the airway with a jaw thrust while immobilizing the cervical spine. From this position you can provide mouth-to-mask ventilation or bag-mask ventilation using the E-C clamp technique to hold the mask. To immobilize the cervical spine, use only the amount of manual control necessary to prevent cranial-cervical motion.

The lone rescuer will need to perform the jaw thrust from the victim's side if rescue breathing using a mouth-to-mouth technique or mouth-to–barrier device technique is required or if chest compressions are needed (Figure 25A and B). To provide rescue breathing, the lone rescuer can hold the airway open using both hands to perform the jaw thrust and can provide mouth-to-mouth ventilation by using his/her cheek to obstruct the child's nose.

The trauma victim's airway may become obstructed by soft tissues, blood, or dental fragments. You must anticipate and treat these causes of airway obstruction. As noted, airway control includes spinal immobilization, which is continued during transport and stabilization in an ALS facility.

It may be difficult to immobilize the cervical spine of an infant or young child in a neutral position. When a young child is placed supine on a firm surface, the large occiput tends to encourage neck flexion.[22,23,162] Spinal immobilization of young children is ideally accomplished by using a backboard with a recess for the head. If such a board is unavailable, the effect of a head recess can be simulated by placing a layer of towels or sheets ½ to 1 inch high (1 to 2.5 cm) on the board to elevate the torso (from shoulders to buttocks) and maintain the neck in neutral alignment.[22,84,163,164] The neck and airway should be in a neutral position when the head rests on the backboard.

Semirigid cervical collars are available in a wide range of sizes to help immobilize the cervical spine. The child's head and neck should be further immobilized with linen rolls and tape, with secondary immobilization of the child on a spine board.

If 2 rescuers are present, the first rescuer opens the airway with a jaw-thrust maneuver while the second rescuer ensures that the cervical spine is absolutely stabilized in a neutral position. Avoid traction or movement of the neck, which may convert a partial injury to a complete spinal cord injury. Once the airway is controlled, immobilize the cervical spine with a semirigid cervical collar and a spine board, linen rolls, and tape. Throughout immobilization and during transport, support oxygenation and ventilation.[165] A more thorough discussion of spine immobilization and trauma care is presented in Chapter 10.

FIGURE 25. Jaw-thrust maneuver by the lone rescuer. The rescuer uses both hands to lift the jaw and open the airway without tilting the head or neck. **A,** Front view of rescuer's hands lifting the jaw. **B,** Lateral view of rescuer's hands lifting the jaw. To provide rescue breathing while maintaining the jaw thrust, the lone rescuer can place his/her cheek against the victim's nostrils, sealing them, while performing mouth-to-mouth breathing.

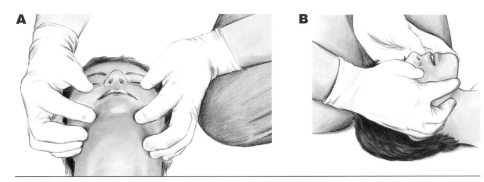

BLS for the Submersion Victim

Submersion is a leading cause of death in children worldwide. *The duration and severity of hypoxia sustained during submersion is the single most important determinant of outcome. CPR, particularly rescue breathing, should be attempted as soon as the unresponsive submersion victim is pulled from the water.* If possible, rescue breathing should be provided even while the victim is still in the water if the rescuer's safety can be ensured.

Many infants and children submerged for brief periods of time will respond to stimulation or rescue breathing alone.[104] If the child does not have signs of circulation (breathing, coughing, or movement) after initial rescue breaths are provided, begin chest compressions.

In 1994 the Institute of Medicine reviewed the AHA recommendations for resuscitation of submersion victims and supported the emphasis on initial establishment of effective ventilation.[145] There is no evidence that water acts as a foreign body, obstructing the airway, and time should not be wasted attempting to remove water from the victim's lungs with maneuvers such as abdominal thrusts. Such maneuvers will delay critically important support of ventilation and oxygenation.[145]

Family Presence During Resuscitation

Most family members would like to be present during the attempted resuscitation of a loved one, according to surveys in the United States and the United Kingdom.[167-172] Parents and those who care for chronically ill children are often knowledgeable about and comfortable with medical equipment and emergency procedures. Family members with no medical background report that being at the side of a loved one and saying goodbye during the final moments of life is extremely comforting.[166,167,173] Parents or family members often fail to ask if they can be present, but healthcare providers should offer the opportunity whenever possible.[166,170,174,175]

Family members present during resuscitation report that their presence helped them adjust to the death of their loved one,[167,169] and most indicate they would do so again.[167] Standardized psychological examinations administered after the experience suggest that family members present during resuscitation show less anxiety and depression and more constructive grief behavior than family members not present during resuscitation.[171]

When family members are present during resuscitative efforts, resuscitation team members should be sensitive to their presence. One member of the healthcare team should remain with the family to answer questions, clarify information, and offer comfort.[176]

In the prehospital setting, family members are typically present during resuscitation of a loved one. Although prehospital care providers may be completely involved with the resuscitative effort, brief explanations and the opportunity to remain with the loved one can be comforting. Some EMS systems provide follow-up visits to family members after an unsuccessful resuscitation attempt.

Termination of Resuscitative Efforts

Despite the best efforts of healthcare providers, most children who experience a cardiac arrest do not survive and never demonstrate return of spontaneous circulation. Return of spontaneous circulation is unlikely if the child fails to respond to effective BLS and ALS and 2 or more doses of epinephrine.[1,2,106] Special resuscitation circumstances, local resources, and underlying conditions and prognoses create a complex decision matrix for the resuscitation team. In general, in the absence of recurring or refractory VF or VT, history of a toxic drug exposure, or a primary hypothermic injury, the resuscitation team should discontinue resuscitative efforts after approximately 30 minutes, especially if there is no return of spontaneous circulation. For further discussion, see Chapter 17: "Ethical and Legal Aspects of CPR in Children."

Use of Audio and Visual CPR Performance Aids for BLS Interventions

CPR is a complex psychomotor task that is difficult to teach, learn, remember, and perform. Not surprisingly, observed CPR performance is often poor (inadequate compression depth, inadequate compression rate, etc). The use of audio and visual CPR performance aids during training can improve acquisition of CPR psychomotor skills. The use of audio prompts (eg, a metronome or an audiotape with the appropriate cadence of "compress-compress-compress-compress-compress-breathe") improves CPR performance in both clinical and laboratory settings.[96,101,177-179] Use of these devices should be considered in areas where CPR is performed.

Summary Points

The epidemiology and outcome of pediatric cardiopulmonary arrest and the priorities, techniques, and sequence of pediatric resuscitation assessments and interventions differ from those for adults. The ABCs of CPR for infants and children form a critical link in the Chain of Survival and emphasize oxygenation and ventilation as initial steps in resuscitation. Special resuscitation circumstances may alter these interventions (eg, traumatic injury, newly born victim). The rescuer should be aware of resuscitation skills and techniques that are appropriate for victims of different ages, as summarized in the Table.

■ The outcome of cardiac arrest in infants and children is poor. Healthcare providers should prevent arrest when possible by reducing risk of sudden infant death, trauma, and submersion.

■ Cardiopulmonary arrest in infants and children is most often the result of progressive respiratory failure or shock. Respiratory arrest often precedes cardiac arrest. If the infant or child develops respiratory arrest, it may be possible to prevent cardiac arrest if the rescuer intervenes and provides rescue breathing.

■ Ideally EMS is activated simultaneously with initiation of CPR. If this is not possible when a lone rescuer finds an unresponsive infant or child, the rescuer should perform approximately 1 minute of CPR and then phone 911 or the emergency response system ("phone fast").

■ If the lone rescuer encounters an infant or child who collapses suddenly and the rescuer has reason to believe that sudden cardiac arrest has occurred, the rescuer should phone 911 (or the emergency response system) and then return to the victim to perform CPR.

■ Open the airway. Use the head tilt–chin lift if trauma is not suspected. Use the jaw thrust without head tilt if a spinal injury is suspected.

■ Use universal precautions whenever possible.

■ Healthcare providers must be proficient in bag-mask ventilation.

■ Healthcare providers should perform a pulse check while checking for other signs of circulation (breathing, coughing, or movement, or response to stimulation).

■ If an AED is available in the prehospital setting and the victim of cardiac arrest is 8 years of age or older, attach the AED.

■ The ratio of 5 compressions to 1 ventilation is recommended for both 1- and 2-rescuer CPR for the infant or child victim.

■ The compression rate for 1- and 2-rescuer CPR is at least 100 compressions per minute for infant victims and approximately 100 compressions per minute for child victims.

■ The ABCs of CPR for infants and children are as follows:

  1. Assess responsiveness.

  2. If the victim is unresponsive, open the airway.

  3. Assess breathing (look, listen, and feel).

  4. If the victim is not breathing, provide rescue breathing.

  5. Check for signs of circulation (breathing, coughing, movement, or pulse).

  6. If there are no signs of circulation, provide chest compressions.

■ For victims in respiratory arrest but with signs of circulation, initially provide 2 slow rescue breaths, then deliver 1 breath every 3 seconds (20 breaths/min)

■ Forceful or excessive ventilation during CPR may cause gastric inflation, regurgitation, and aspiration. Cricoid pressure may be helpful in certain circumstances.

Case Scenarios

Introductory Case Scenario 1

A 2-year-old child falls down a flight of stairs and experiences a brief loss of consciousness. His parents transport him to your care 2 hours after his fall. On arrival the toddler appears anxious but is in no distress and shows no obvious signs of injury. His vital signs, oxygen saturation on room air, and capillary refill time are normal. During the initial evaluation he has a brief (20 seconds) tonic-clonic seizure, followed by apnea and cyanosis, with no response to verbal or tactile stimulation.

Initial Assessment

■ Perform a rapid and thorough cardiopulmonary assessment and identify arrest (respiratory and cardiorespiratory arrest) or prearrest conditions (respiratory distress or failure and shock).

■ This child demonstrates unresponsiveness, so you will need to initiate the steps of CPR. The child also demonstrates apnea and cyanosis; these are consistent with respiratory arrest.

Acceptable Actions

The following actions are generally *acceptable* for assessment and management of the toddler in this scenario:

■ Perform a rapid cardiopulmonary assessment to identify respiratory arrest.

■ Perform the steps of CPR as needed. The priorities of BLS treatment for infants and children (less than 8 years of age) are the ABCs: Airway-Breathing-

BLS Healthcare Provider Resuscitation Interventions for Victims of All Ages

CPR/Rescue Breathing	Adult and Older Child	Child (≈1-8 y)	Infant (<1 y)	Newly Born
Establish unresponsiveness, activate EMS				
Open airway (Head tilt–chin lift or jaw thrust)	Head tilt–chin lift (If trauma is present, use jaw thrust)	Head tilt–chin lift (If trauma is present, use jaw thrust)	Head tilt–chin lift (If trauma is present, use jaw thrust)	Head tilt–chin lift (If trauma is present, use jaw thrust)
Check for breathing: (look, listen, feel) If victim is breathing: place in recovery position. If victim is not breathing: give 2 effective slow breaths. **Initial**	2 effective breaths at 2 seconds per breath (unless oxygen available)	2 effective breaths at 1-1½ seconds per breath	2 effective breaths at 1-1½ seconds per breath	2 effective breaths at approximately 1 second per breath
Subsequent	12 breaths/min (approximate)	20 breaths/min (approximate)	20 breaths/min (approximate)	30-60 breaths/min (approximate)
FBAO	Abdominal thrusts	Abdominal thrusts	Back blows and chest thrusts (no abdominal thrusts)	Back blows and chest thrusts (no abdominal thrusts)
Signs of circulation: Check for breathing, coughing, or movement, pulse. If signs of circulation are present: provide airway and breathing support. If signs of circulation are absent: begin chest compressions interposed with breaths.	**Pulse check** Carotid	**Pulse check** Carotid	**Pulse check** Brachial or femoral	**Pulse check** Umbilical
Compression landmarks	Lower half of sternum	Lower half of sternum	Lower half of sternum (1 finger's width below intermammary line)	Lower half of sternum (1 finger's width below intermammary line)
Compression method	Heel of one hand, other hand on top	Heel of one hand	Two thumb–encircling hands for 2-rescuer trained providers or 2-finger technique	Two thumb–encircling hands for 2-rescuer trained providers or 2-finger technique
Compression depth	Approximately 1½ to 2 inches (4-5 cm)	Approximately ⅓ to ½ depth of chest	Approximately ⅓ to ½ depth of chest	Approximately ⅓ depth of chest
Compression rate	Approximately 100/min	Approximately 100/min	At least 100/min	Approximately 120 events/min (90 compressions/ 30 breaths)
Compression-ventilation ratio	15:2 (1 or 2 rescuers, unprotected airway) 12 to 15 breaths/min (2 rescuers, protected airway) administered asynchronous with chest compressions (about 1 breath every 4 to 5 seconds)	5:1 (1 or 2 rescuers)	5:1 (1 or 2 rescuers)	3:1 (1 or 2 rescuers)

Circulation. The spine must be immobilized because this child has a history of trauma.

■ Activate the emergency response system in your workplace.

Rationale for Acceptable Actions

■ *Perform a rapid and thorough cardiopulmonary assessment and determine the need for CPR.* The child is unresponsive, so you begin the steps of CPR. CPR and life support for infants and children should be an integral part of the Chain of Survival in every community, linking

— Injury prevention

— Early and effective CPR

— Early access to emergency medical response prepared for the needs of children

— Early and effective ALS, including stabilization, transport, and eventual access to rehabilitation

■ *Begin the steps of CPR and provide support of airway, breathing, and circulation as needed.* You should shout for help and initiate the ABCs of CPR while someone else activates the emergency medical response system. This toddler demonstrates respiratory arrest, so he requires immediate intervention. Healthcare providers and those with a duty to respond should use universal precautions. In addition, *spinal immobilization* is required because the toddler may have suffered a head or neck injury.

— Open the airway with a jaw-thrust maneuver and check breathing.

— The toddler is not breathing adequately (he is apneic and cyanotic), so you should provide 2 rescue breaths that make the chest rise.

— After you deliver 2 effective rescue breaths, check for signs of circulation, including breathing, coughing, and movement in response to the rescue breaths, and a carotid pulse.

If the child has no signs of circulation (including no carotid pulse), you should begin chest compressions.

— If chest compressions are indicated, place the heel of one hand on the lower half of the sternum to deliver compressions at a rate of approximately 100 compressions per minute. Provide cycles of ventilations and compressions in a ratio of 5 compressions to 1 ventilation.

■ Activate the emergency response system in your workplace. All PALS providers should know how to access an ALS response in the environment in which they provide care for children. If you are alone, activate the emergency response system after you provide about 1 minute of rescue support.

Unacceptable Actions

The following actions are inappropriate in the clinical situation depicted in this case scenario:

■ Failing to perform a rapid cardiopulmonary assessment. A rapid initial assessment of the toddler will indicate that the toddler is not responsive and CPR is needed.

■ Delaying initiation of CPR. Any delay can result in hypoxia.

■ Failing to immobilize the cervical spine when the airway is opened. This child suffered a fall that could produce head, neck, and spinal cord injuries, so the cervical spine must be immobilized to reduce the risk of secondary injury.

Case Scenario 1 Progression and Conclusion

This toddler responded to delivery of rescue breaths with oxygen. You provided this support while maintaining cervical spine immobilization. No chest compressions were necessary because the child maintained a pulse during the respiratory arrest episode. The local hospital transport team arrived and transported the child to the hospital, where he made a complete recovery from his head injury.

Introductory Case Scenario 2

You are called to examine a 3-month-old infant with a history of fever and irritability. His parents are concerned because they had difficulty arousing him from his nap. You note that the infant is unresponsive, with no movement or response to painful stimuli, so you shout for help in the examination room. You open the infant's airway and note that he makes only an occasional gasp. You immediately provide 2 breaths using a bag and mask. After the 2 breaths you see no breathing, coughing, or movement. The infant's pulses are faint, his heart rate is 56 bpm, and his skin is cool, pale, and cyanotic.

Initial Assessment

■ Perform a rapid and thorough cardiopulmonary assessment and determine the need for CPR.

■ This infant has respiratory arrest and requires immediate support of airway and breathing and possible support of circulation.

Acceptable Actions

The following actions are generally *acceptable* for assessment and management of the infant in this scenario:

■ Perform a rapid and thorough cardiopulmonary assessment and determine that this infant is in respiratory arrest and requires immediate support of airway and breathing and possible support of circulation.

■ Perform the steps of CPR as needed. The priorities of BLS treatment for infants and children to 8 years of age are the ABCs: Airway-Breathing-Circulation. This child has respiratory arrest and needs evaluation and immediate support of airway and breathing. In addition he demonstrates profound bradycardia with pulses and requires chest compressions until the heart rate increases to ≥60 bpm with good perfusion.

- Reassess the infant after effective ventilation (and chest compressions) have been provided for about 1 minute.

- Activate the emergency response system appropriate for your location.

Rationale for Acceptable Actions

- Perform a rapid and thorough cardiopulmonary assessment and determine the need for CPR.

- When you assess infants and children with cardiorespiratory distress, look for arrest and prearrest conditions that require immediate intervention: respiratory distress or failure, shock, respiratory arrest, or cardiopulmonary arrest.

- This child has respiratory arrest of unknown etiology with impending cardiopulmonary arrest. An occasional gasp is not normal or adequate breathing. Lack of adequate breathing, cough, and movement in response to stimulation suggests absence of circulation. This infant, however, has a slow heart rate (56 bpm), indicating a bradycardia probably caused by hypoxia.

- *Perform the steps of CPR as needed.* The priorities of BLS treatment for infants and children less than 8 years old are the ABCs: Airway-Breathing-Circulation.

  — *Airway.* Open the airway with a head tilt–chin lift. Spinal immobilization is not indicated if the infant is found in bed with no signs of injury.

  — *Breathing.* This infant has respiratory arrest and needs support of breathing at a rate of approximately 20 breaths/min. Use a barrier device if one is available. In the healthcare setting a bag and mask (manual resuscitator) should be used with oxygen.

  — *Circulation.* Check for signs of circulation (breathing, coughing, or movement in response to the 2 rescue breaths) and a brachial pulse.

- Although this infant has palpable pulses, the heart rate is less than 60 bpm with signs of poor perfusion (cyanosis and cool skin), so chest compressions are required.

- If 2 healthcare providers are present, use the 2 thumb–encircling hands technique to compress the lower half of the sternum about one third to one half the depth of the chest. If the healthcare provider is alone, use the 2-finger technique to compress the lower half of the sternum, avoiding pressure over the xiphoid process.

- Deliver compressions at a rate of at least 100 compressions per minute in a ratio of 5 compressions to 1 ventilation.

- If the heart rate is ≥60 bpm in an infant with respiratory arrest or less than 60 bpm with good perfusion, chest compressions are not indicated. The rescuer should provide 1 rescue breath about every 3 seconds (or about 20 breaths/min).

- *Reassess the infant after effective ventilation and chest compressions (if indicated) have been provided for about 1 minute.* In this infant you would expect the heart rate to increase once effective oxygenation and ventilation are provided, so you should recheck for signs of circulation and pulse rate in approximately 1 minute to see if the heart rate has risen sufficiently to allow you to stop chest compressions.

- *Activate the emergency response system appropriate for your location.* All PALS providers should know how to access an ALS response in the environment in which they provide care for children.

Key Unacceptable Actions

The following actions are inappropriate in this case scenario:

- Failure to perform a rapid cardiopulmonary assessment. A rapid initial assessment of the infant's responsiveness will indicate that the infant is not responsive and CPR is needed.

- Delay in initiation of CPR. Any delay can result in development or worsening of hypoxia and reduction of the infant's chance of survival.

- Failure to provide chest compressions. This infant has palpable pulses, but they are too slow to support adequate circulation and oxygen delivery, so chest compressions are required.

- Failure to reassess the infant after about 1 minute of rescue support.

- Failure to ensure that the emergency response system/EMS is activated.

Case Scenario 2 Progression and Resolution

This infant developed septic shock with cardiopulmonary failure and required support of ventilation and volume resuscitation. After a stormy course in the PICU, the infant recovered completely.

Review Questions

1. **A mother approaches you carrying her 3-month-old infant in her arms. She says, "He was crying, but I think he stopped breathing on the way here." As you take the infant from her, what should be your *first* step in the BLS sequence of action?**

   a. immediate bag-mask ventilation

   b. check the carotid pulse for signs of circulation

   c. stimulate the infant and check for responsiveness

   d. leave the infant to phone 911 or activate the emergency response system in your work setting

   The correct answer is c. Although the mother said that the infant had stopped breathing, a rapid cardiopulmonary assessment is appropriate. The infant had been crying, but you must evaluate the infant's responsiveness now. If the infant is unresponsive, assess the airway and effectiveness of breathing.

   Answer a is incorrect because you should not initiate bag-mask ventilation until you assess the infant's airway and breathing.

   Answer b is incorrect because you should not check for a pulse until you have assessed and supported the infant's airway and breathing. You check for a pulse and other signs of circulation after you deliver 2 rescue breaths. Note that in infants less than about 1 year of age, assessment of the brachial pulse is preferable to assessment of the carotid pulse.

   Answer d is incorrect because you should not leave an infant in distress to phone 911, particularly when others are present. The lone rescuer should perform initial assessment and approximately 1 minute of CPR (when needed) before leaving a child to activate the emergency response system (phone fast versus

   phone first for infants and children). The mother is present and may be able to phone 911 while you begin CPR for the infant.

2. **You are evaluating a 3-month-old infant with a history of apnea. On your initial assessment, you note that the infant is cyanotic and unresponsive to stimulation. You open the airway with a head tilt–chin lift and note that the infant is breathing (gasping) slowly and irregularly at a rate of approximately 6 breaths/min. Assuming that the full array of resuscitation equipment is available, what should your next action be?**

   a. provide rescue breathing with oxygen and a bag-mask device

   b. check for a brachial pulse and other signs of circulation to determine if chest compressions are needed

   c. administer oxygen but do not provide assisted ventilations

   d. perform an abdominal thrust (Heimlich maneuver) in case of an FBAO

   The correct answer is a. Although the infant has some respiratory effort (gasping at 6 breaths/min), this effort is *not* effective breathing. The infant with gasping breaths and cyanosis requires rescue breathing (assisted ventilation). Your rapid cardiopulmonary assessment reveals respiratory failure with impending respiratory arrest. After opening the airway, you should provide 2 effective breaths with supplementary oxygen. When resuscitation equipment is readily available, bag-mask ventilation with 100% FiO_2 is appropriate.

   Answer b is incorrect because you should not assess for signs of circulation until after you have delivered 2 effective breaths.

   Answer c is incorrect because supplementary oxygen will not be useful if the infant has inadequate respiratory effort.

   Answer d is incorrect because the infant has no signs of FBAO. If such signs were present, you would perform back blows and chest thrusts to attempt to relieve the obstruction. Abdominal thrusts are *not* recommended for relief of FBAO in infants less than approximately 1 year of age.

3. **You have provided 2 effective positive-pressure, bag-mask assisted breaths with oxygen for an unresponsive 4-year-old child with agonal respirations. You observe no effective breathing, coughing, or movement after the 2 breaths, but you do detect a carotid pulse rate of approximately 30 bpm (1 beat every 2 seconds). What should your next action be?**

   a. continue rescue breathing only at a rate of approximately 20 breaths/min

   b. administer 100% oxygen and place the child in a recovery position

   c. leave the child to phone 911 or other emergency response number

   d. begin chest compressions at a rate of approximately 100 compressions per minute

   The correct answer is d. Although the child has some initial agonal respiratory effort, this effort is *not* effective breathing. After opening the airway, you provided 2 effective breaths with extra oxygen, then assessed circulation. Your rapid cardiopulmonary assessment revealed respiratory failure with severe, symptomatic bradycardia and impending cardiorespiratory arrest. The child demonstrates severe bradycardia despite delivery of the initial rescue breaths. In this setting chest compressions should assist circulation.

   Answer a is incorrect because although the child does have a pulse, the rate is too slow to maintain effective circulation, so chest compressions should be provided in addition to effective rescue breathing.

Answer b is incorrect because this child has respiratory arrest with secondary hypoxic bradycardia and requires immediate ventilation and chest compressions. The child's chance of survival from respiratory arrest can be good if the child receives immediate CPR.

Answer c is incorrect. You should provide approximately 1 minute of CPR before leaving the child if necessary to activate the emergency response system. If you leave the child initially, the child may develop cardiopulmonary arrest.

4. **You are attempting to assess signs of circulation in a 3-month-old infant. The infant is unresponsive and is not breathing effectively, coughing, or moving after you provide 2 initial rescue breaths. Where should you feel for the pulse of an unresponsive infant victim?**

    a. the radial pulse (wrist)

    b. the carotid pulse (neck)

    c. the brachial pulse (upper arm)

    d. over the middle of the sternum (chest)

    The correct answer is c. It is difficult to palpate a pulse, so the healthcare provider may select the site with which he/she is most comfortable. The PALS guidelines, however, recommend palpation of the brachial pulse in infants because it is often easier to detect than a carotid pulse.

    Answer a is incorrect because the radial pulse is small and peripheral and may not be as easy to detect as a more central pulse in an emergency or when blood pressure is low.

    Answer b is incorrect because the carotid pulse is the preferred site for palpation of pulses in children 1 to 8 years of age and adults. The carotid pulse is centrally and reliably located with good surface landmarks. However, palpation of the carotid pulse in infants is *not* recommended because infants have short, chubby necks and there is a risk of stimulat-

ing the relatively hyperactive vagus nerve or compressing the infant's airway when trying to palpate the carotid pulse.

Answer d is incorrect because the sternum is a bone and will not allow sensitive palpation of a pulse.

5. **You are at a lake and have just helped pull a 10-month-old submersion victim from the water. The infant is limp and blue and does not respond to touch. What is the *first* thing that you should do?**

    a. send someone to phone 911 while you open the airway and prepare to provide rescue breathing

    b. attempt to eliminate water from the airway with a Heimlich abdominal thrust

    c. begin chest compressions as the first intervention

    d. get and attach an AED

    The correct answer is a. In situations in which compromise of airway and breathing are most likely (for infants and children and victims of all ages after submersion, trauma, or drug overdose), the lone rescuer should provide initial rescue breathing and any other steps of CPR needed before phoning 911. When other bystanders are present, the rescuer should send someone to phone 911 while the rescuer remains with the victim to begin CPR. When a primary cardiac cause of arrest is likely (eg, a child at risk for sudden cardiac arrest or arrhythmias), early access to defibrillators and ALS is most important, and the EMS system should be activated as soon as unresponsiveness is verified.

    Answer b is incorrect because delaying effective assessment and interventions such as rescue breathing and CPR to provide an abdominal thrust is *not* recommended. Maneuvers to relieve FBAO should be performed only when a foreign

body is suspected as the cause of inability to provide effective ventilation (ie, the chest does not rise with rescue breaths despite reopening of the airway).

Answer c is incorrect because chest compressions should not be provided until after you open the airway, check breathing, deliver 2 rescue breaths, and check for signs of circulation and find none (airway, breathing, circulation). Although chest compressions may be necessary, many infants and children will respond to initial rescue breathing alone.

Answer d is incorrect because submersion victims have compromise of airway, oxygenation and ventilation, so initial rescue breathing and CPR are the most important interventions needed. The AHA does not recommend for or against the use of AEDs in infants. However, for the submersion victim of any age, rescue breathing is the first priority.

6. **You are caring for a 7-year-old child who reportedly fell 20 feet from a rooftop and lost consciousness. She is now limp and unresponsive. Which of the following is the next step in the BLS sequence that you should take?**

    a. check for a pulse and signs of circulation

    b. open the airway with a head tilt–chin lift maneuver

    c. open the airway with a tongue–jaw lift maneuver and look for an FBAO

    d. open the airway with a jaw thrust without head tilt and maintain cervical spine stabilization

    The correct answer is d. This child has a history of significant trauma and may have a spinal injury. Although she needs a thorough evaluation, the ABCs should

(Continued on next page)

be first assessed and supported, starting with the airway. A jaw thrust without head tilt is the most appropriate initial maneuver in an unresponsive trauma victim. Simultaneous activation of EMS is appropriate if possible (other bystanders are present).

Answer a is incorrect because you should not check for signs of circulation until you have opened the airway and provided rescue breaths.

Answer b is incorrect because the airway should be opened without moving the head or neck, so the head tilt–chin lift is inappropriate.

Answer c is incorrect because the tongue-jaw lift should be used to open the airway only when an FBAO is suspected and is not recommended when trauma is the primary suspected injury.

7. **A 6-year-old child chokes on a piece of hard candy. The child tries to cough but is unable to cough, speak, or breathe effectively. Abdominal thrusts are not effective in dislodging the candy, and the child collapses to the ground without respiratory effort. After opening the airway with a tongue–jaw lift, which of the following actions should you perform next?**

   a. a blind finger sweep

   b. look for a foreign body and if you see it, use a finger sweep to remove it

   c. never attempt to remove a foreign body, even if it is seen

   d. perform back blows and chest thrusts

The correct answer is b. Healthcare providers should attempt to remove an object when a victim of FBAO becomes unresponsive. If no object is seen, the rescuer should open the airway and check breathing and if no adequate breathing is present, attempt rescue breaths and reattempt if necessary. If rescue breaths are not effective, perform abdominal thrusts and then repeat the sequence.

Answer a is incorrect because blind finger sweeps are *not* recommended in infants and children. They may injure the back of the throat or push a foreign body further back into the airway.

Answer c is incorrect because a foreign body should be removed if visible and accessible.

Answer d is incorrect because back blows may be an appropriate alternative maneuver for a responsive child with signs of airway obstruction, but they are not the primary recommended maneuver for relief of FBAO in the child. Abdominal thrusts (the Heimlich maneuver) are the recommended maneuver for relief of FBAO for healthcare providers to deliver to unresponsive children approximately 1 to 8 years of age.

References

1. Zaritsky A, Nadkarni V, Getson P, Kuehl K. CPR in children. *Ann Emerg Med.* 1987;16: 1107-1111.

2. Young KD, Seidel JS. Pediatric cardiopulmonary resuscitation: a collective review. *Ann Emerg Med.* 1999;33:195-205.

3. Hazinski MF. Is pediatric resuscitation unique? Relative merits of early CPR and ventilation versus early defibrillation for young victims of prehospital cardiac arrest. *Ann Emerg Med.* 1995;25:540-543.

4. Newacheck PW, Strickland B, Shonkoff JP, Perrin JM, McPherson M, McManus M, Lauver C, Fox H, Arango P. An epidemiologic profile of children with special health care needs. *Pediatrics.* 1998;102:117-123.

5. McPherson M, Arango P, Fox H, Lauver C, McManus M, Newacheck PW, Perrin JM, Shonkoff JP, Strickland B. A new definition of children with special health care needs. *Pediatrics.* 1998;102:137-140.

6. Committee on Pediatric Emergency Medicine, American Academy of Pediatrics. Emergency preparedness for children with special health care needs. *Pediatrics.* 1999;104:e53.

7. Spaite DW, Conroy C, Tibbitts M, Karriker KJ, Seng M, Battaglia N, Criss EA, Valenzuela TD, Meislin HW. Use of emergency medical services by children with special health care needs. *Prehosp Emerg Care.* 2000;4:19-23.

8. Schultz-Grant LD, Young-Cureton V, Kataoka-Yahiro M. Advance directives and do not resuscitate orders: nurses' knowledge and the level of practice in school settings. *J Sch Nurs.* 1998;14:4-10, 12-13.

9. Hoyert DL, Kochanek KD, Murphy SL. Deaths: final data for 1997. *Natl Vital Stat Rep.* 1999;47:1-104.

10. Clements F, McGowan J. Finger position for chest compressions in cardiac arrest in infants. *Resuscitation.* 2000;44:43-46.

11. Whitelaw CC, Slywka B, Goldsmith LJ. Comparison of a two-finger versus two-thumb method for chest compressions by healthcare providers in an infant mechanical model. *Resuscitation.* 2000;43:213-216.

12. Mejicano GC, Maki DG. Infections acquired during cardiopulmonary resuscitation: estimating the risk and defining strategies for prevention. *Ann Intern Med.* 1998;129:813-828.

13. Ruben HM, Elam JO, Ruben AM, Greene DG. Investigation of upper airway problems in resuscitation, 1: studies of pharyngeal x-rays and performance by laymen. *Anesthesiology.* 1961;22:271-279.

14. Safar P, Escarraga LA. Compliance in apneic anesthetized adults. *Anesthesiology.* 1959;20: 283-289.

15. Elam JO, Greene DG, Schneider MA, Ruben HM, Gordon AS, Hustead RF, Benson DW, Clements JA, Ruben A. Head-tilt method of oral resuscitation. *JAMA*. 1960;172:812-815.

16. Guildner CW. Resuscitation: opening the airway. A comparative study of techniques for opening an airway obstructed by the tongue. *JACEP*. 1976;5:588-590.

17. Roth B, Magnusson J, Johansson I, Holmberg S, Westrin P. Jaw lift—a simple and effective method to open the airway in children. *Resuscitation*. 1998;39:171-174.

18. Reber A, Wetzel SG, Schnabel K, Bongartz G, Frei FJ. Effect of combined mouth closure and chin lift on upper airway dimensions during routine magnetic resonance imaging in pediatric patients sedated with propofol. *Anesthesiology*. 1999;90:1617-1623.

19. Reber A, Paganoni R, Frei FJ. Effect of common airway manoeuvres on upper airway dimensions and clinical signs in anaesthetized, spontaneously breathing children. *Br J Anaesth*. 2001;86:217-222.

20. Reber A, Bobbia SA, Hammer J, Frei FJ. Effect of airway opening manoeuvres on thoraco-abdominal asynchrony in anaesthetized children. *Eur Respir J*. 2001;17:1239-1243.

21. Hammer J, Reber A, Trachsel D, Frei FJ. Effect of jaw thrust and continuous positive airway pressure on tidal breathing in deeply sedated infants. *J Pediatr*. 2001;138:826-830.

22. Herzenberg JE, Hensinger RN, Dedrick DK, Phillips WA. Emergency transport and positioning of young children who have an injury of the cervical spine: the standard backboard may be hazardous. *J Bone Joint Surg Am*. 1989;71:15-22.

23. Markenson D, Foltin G, Tunik M, Cooper A, Giordano L, Fitton A, Lanotte T. The Kendrick extrication device used for pediatric spinal immobilization. *Prehosp Emerg Care*. 1999;3:66-69.

24. Baskett P, Nolan J, Parr M. Tidal volumes which are perceived to be adequate for resuscitation. *Resuscitation*. 1996;31:231-234.

25. Ruppert M, Reith MW, Widmann JH, Lackner CK, Kerkmann R, Schweiberer L, Peter K. Checking for breathing: evaluation of the diagnostic capability of emergency medical services personnel, physicians, medical students, and medical laypersons. *Ann Emerg Med*. 1999;34:720-729.

26. Noc M, Weil MH, Sun S, Tang W, Bisera J. Spontaneous gasping during cardiopulmonary resuscitation without mechanical ventilation. *Am J Respir Crit Care Med*. 1994;150:861-864.

27. Poets CF, Meny RG, Chobanian MR, Bonofiglo RE. Gasping and other cardiorespiratory patterns during sudden infant deaths. *Pediatr Res*. 1999;45:350-354.

28. Handley AJ, Becker LB, Allen M, van Drenth A, Kramer EB, Montgomery WH. Single-rescuer adult basic life support: an advisory statement from the Basic Life Support Working Group of the International Liaison Committee on Resuscitation (ILCOR). *Resuscitation*. 1997;34:101-108.

29. Fulstow R, Smith GB. The new recovery position: a cautionary tale. *Resuscitation*. 1993;26:89-91.

30. Doxey J. Comparing 1997 Resuscitation Council (UK) recovery position with recovery position of 1992 European Resuscitation Council guidelines: a user's perspective. *Resuscitation*. 1998;39:161-169.

31. Turner S, Turner I, Chapman D, Howard P, Champion P, Hatfield J, James A, Marshall S, Barber S. A comparative study of the 1992 and 1997 recovery positions for use in the UK. *Resuscitation*. 1998;39:153-160.

32. Berg MD, Idris AH, Berg RA. Severe ventilatory compromise due to gastric distention during pediatric cardiopulmonary resuscitation. *Resuscitation*. 1998;36:71-73.

33. Zideman DA. Paediatric and neonatal life support. *Br J Anaesth*. 1997;79:178-187.

34. Nadkarni V, Hazinski MF, Zideman D, Kattwinkel J, Quan L, Bingham R, Zaritsky A, Bland J, Kramer E, Tiballs J. Pediatric resuscitation: an advisory statement from the Pediatric Working Group of the International Liaison Committee on Resuscitation. *Circulation*. 1997;95:2185-2195.

35. *Medical Treatment Effectiveness Research*. Rockville, Md: Agency for Health Care Policy and Research; 1990.

36. Tonkin SL, Davis SL, Gunn TR. Nasal route for infant resuscitation by mothers. *Lancet*. 1995;345:1353-1354.

37. Dembofsky CA, Gibson E, Nadkarni V, Rubin S, Greenspan JS. Assessment of infant cardiopulmonary resuscitation rescue breathing technique: relationship of infant and caregiver facial measurements. *Pediatrics*. 1999;103:E17.

38. Segedin E, Torrie J, Anderson B. Nasal airway versus oral route for infant resuscitation. *Lancet*. 1995;346:382.

39. Wilson-Davis SL, Tonkin SL, Gunn TR. Air entry in infant resuscitation: oral or nasal routes? *J Appl Physiol*. 1997;82:152-155.

40. Miller MJ, Martin RJ, Carlo WA, Fouke JM, Strohl KP, Fanaroff AA. Oral breathing in newborn infants. *J Pediatr*. 1985;107:465-469.

41. Moss ML. The veloepiglottic sphincter and obligate nose breathing in the neonate. *J Pediatr*. 1965;67:330-331.

42. Nowak AJ, Casamassimo PS. Oral opening and other selected facial dimensions of children 6 weeks to 36 months of age. *J Oral Maxillofac Surg*. 1994;52:845-847.

43. Stocks J, Godfrey S. Nasal resistance during infancy. *Respir Physiol*. 1978;34:233-246.

44. Rodenstein DO, Perlmutter N, Stanescu DC. Infants are not obligatory nasal breathers. *Am Rev Respir Dis*. 1985;131:343-347.

45. Terndrup TE, Kanter RK, Cherry RA. A comparison of infant ventilation methods performed by prehospital personnel. *Ann Emerg Med*. 1989;18:607-611.

46. Handley JA, Handley AJ. Four-step CPR: improving skill retention. *Resuscitation*. 1998;36:3-8.

47. Field D, Milner AD, Hopkin IE. Efficiency of manual resuscitators at birth. *Arch Dis Child*. 1986;61:300-302.

48. Hess D, Ness C, Oppel A, Rhoads K. Evaluation of mouth-to-mask ventilation devices. *Respir Care*. 1989;34:191-195.

49. Milner AD. Resuscitation at birth. *Eur J Pediatr*. 1998;157:524-527.

50. Terndrup TE, Warner DA. Infant ventilation and oxygenation by basic life support providers: comparison of methods. *Prehospital Disaster Med*. 1992;7:35-40.

51. Hirschman AM, Kravath RE. Venting vs ventilating: a danger of manual resuscitation bags. *Chest*. 1982;82:369-370.

52. Jesudian MC, Harrison RR, Keenan RL, Maull KI. Bag-valve-mask ventilation; two rescuers are better than one: preliminary report. *Crit Care Med*. 1985;13:122-123.

53. Wenzel V, Idris AH, Banner MJ, Fuerst RS, Tucker KJ. The composition of gas given by mouth-to-mouth ventilation during CPR. *Chest*. 1994;106:1806-1810.

54. Theophilopoulos DT, Burchfield DJ. Accuracy of different methods for heart rate determination during simulated neonatal resuscitations. *J Perinatol*. 1998;18:65-67.

55. Cavallaro DL, Melker RJ. Comparison of two techniques for detecting cardiac activity in infants. *Crit Care Med*. 1983;11:189-190.

56. Whitelaw CC, Goldsmith LJ. Comparison of two techniques for determining the presence of a pulse in an infant. *Acad Emerg Med*. 1997;4:153-154.

57. Lee CJ, Bullock LJ. Determining the pulse for infant CPR: time for a change? *Mil Med*. 1991;156:190-193.

58. Connick M, Berg RA. Femoral venous pulsations during open-chest cardiac massage. *Ann Emerg Med*. 1994;24:1176-1179.

59. Bush CM, Jones JS, Cohle SD, Johnson H. Pediatric injuries from cardiopulmonary resuscitation. *Ann Emerg Med*. 1996;28:40-44.

60. Spevak MR, Kleinman PK, Belanger PL, Primack C, Richmond JM. Cardiopulmonary resuscitation and rib fractures in infants: a postmortem radiologic-pathologic study. *JAMA*. 1994;272:617-618.

61. Kaplan JA, Fossum RM. Patterns of facial resuscitation injury in infancy. *Am J Forensic Med Pathol.* 1994;15:187-191.

62. Feldman KW, Brewer DK. Child abuse, cardiopulmonary resuscitation, and rib fractures. *Pediatrics.* 1984;73:339-342.

63. Nagel EL, Fine EG, Krischer JP, Davis JH. Complications of CPR. *Crit Care Med.* 1981;9:424.

64. Powner DJ, Holcombe PA, Mello LA. Cardiopulmonary resuscitation-related injuries. *Crit Care Med.* 1984;12:54-55.

65. Parke TR. Unexplained pneumoperitoneum in association with basic cardiopulmonary resuscitation efforts. *Resuscitation.* 1993;26:177-181.

66. Kramer K, Goldstein B. Retinal hemorrhages following cardiopulmonary resuscitation. *Clin Pediatr.* 1993;32:366-368.

67. Flesche CW, Neruda B, Breuer S, Tarnow J. Basic cardiopulmonary resuscitation skills: a comparison of ambulance staff and medical students in Germany. *Resuscitation.* 1994; 28:S25.

68. Eberle B, Dick WF, Schneider T, Wisser G, Doetsch S, Tzanova I. Checking the carotid pulse check: diagnostic accuracy of first responders in patients with and without a pulse. *Resuscitation.* 1996;33:107-116.

69. Flesche CW, Neruda B, Noetges T, Tarnow J. Do cardiopulmonary resuscitation skills among medical students meet current standards and patients' needs? *Resuscitation.* 1994;28:S25.

70. Bahr J, Klingler H, Panzer W, Rode H, Kettler D. Skills of lay people in checking the carotid pulse. *Resuscitation.* 1997;35:23-26.

71. Flesche CW, Breuer S, Mandel LP, Breivik H, Tarnow J. The ability of health professionals to check the carotid pulse. *Circulation.* 1994; 90(suppl 1):288.

72. Mather C, O'Kelly S. The palpation of pulses. *Anaesthesia.* 1996;51:189-191.

73. Cecchin F, Jorgenson DB, Berul CI, Perry JC, Zimmerman AA, Duncan BW, Lupinetti FM, Snyder D, Lyster TD, Rosenthal GL, Cross B, Atkins DL. Is arrhythmia detection by automatic external defibrillator accurate for children? Sensitivity and specificity of an automatic external defibrillator algorithm in 696 pediatric arrhythmias. *Circulation.* 2001;103:2483-2488.

74. Atkinson E, Mikysa B, Conway JA, Parker M, Christian K, Deshpande J, Knilans TK, Walker C, Stickney RE, Hamptom DR, Hazinski MF. Specificity and Sensitivity of Automated External Defibrillator Rhythm Analysis in Infants and Children. *Ann Emerg Med.* 2003. In Press.

75. Automated External Defibrillators for Children: an Update. An Advisory Statement by the Pediatric Advanced Life Support Task Force of the International Liaison Committee on Resuscitation (ILCOR). *Circulation* 2003. In press.

76. Maier GW, Tyson GS Jr, Olsen CO, Kernstein KH, Davis JW, Conn EH, Sabiston DC Jr, Rankin JS. The physiology of external cardiac massage: high-impulse cardiopulmonary resuscitation. *Circulation.* 1984;70:86-101.

77. Kouwenhoven WB, Jude JR, Knickerbocker GG. Closed-chest cardiac massage. *JAMA.* 1960;173:1064-1067.

78. Kern KB, Hilwig R, Ewy GA. Retrograde coronary blood flow during cardiopulmonary resuscitation in swine: intracoronary Doppler evaluation. *Am Heart J.* 1994;128:490-499.

79. Tucker KJ, Khan J, Idris A, Savitt MA. The biphasic mechanism of blood flow during cardiopulmonary resuscitation: a physiologic comparison of active compression-decompression and high-impulse manual external cardiac massage. *Ann Emerg Med.* 1994;24:895-906.

80. Forney J, Ornato JP. Blood flow with ventilation alone in a child with cardiac arrest. *Ann Emerg Med.* 1980;9:624-626.

81. Berg RA, Hilwig RW, Kern KB, Babar I, Ewy GA. Simulated mouth-to-mouth ventilation and chest compressions (bystander cardiopulmonary resuscitation) improves outcome in a swine model of prehospital pediatric asphyxial cardiac arrest. *Crit Care Med.* 1999;27:1893-1899.

82. Johnson JC. Quality assurance in EMS. Roush WR, Aranosian RD, Blair TMH, Handal KA, Kellow RC, Steward RD, eds. *Principles of EMS Systems: A Comprehensive Text for Physicians.* Dallas, Tex: American College of Emergency Physicians; 1989.

83. Dean JM, Koehler RC, Schleien CL, Berkowitz I, Michael JR, Atchison D, Rogers MC, Traystman RJ. Age-related effects of compression rate and duration in cardiopulmonary resuscitation. *J Appl Physiol.* 1990;68:554-560.

84. Nypaver M, Treloar D. Neutral cervical spine positioning in children. *Ann Emerg Med.* 1994;23:208-211.

85. Finholt DA, Kettrick RG, Wagner HR, Swedlow DB. The heart is under the lower third of the sternum: implications for external cardiac massage. *Am J Dis Child.* 1986;140:646-649.

86. Phillips GW, Zideman DA. Relation of infant heart to sternum: its significance in cardiopulmonary resuscitation. *Lancet.* 1986;1:1024-1025.

87. Orlowski JP. Optimum position for external cardiac compression in infants and young children. *Ann Emerg Med.* 1986;15:667-673.

88. Shah NM, Gaur HK. Position of heart in relation to sternum and nipple line at various ages. *Indian Pediatr.* 1992;29:49-53.

89. Burchfield D, Erenberg A, Mullett MD, Keenan WJ, Denson SE, Kattwinkel J, Bloom R. Why change the compression and ventilation rates during CPR in neonates? Neonatal Resuscitation Steering Committee, American Heart Association and American Academy of Pediatrics. *Pediatrics.* 1994;93:1026-1027.

90. Chandra N, Rudikoff M, Weisfeldt ML. Simultaneous chest compression and ventilation at high airway pressure during cardiopulmonary resuscitation. *Lancet.* 1980;1:175-178.

91. Babbs CF, Tacker WA, Paris RL, Murphy RJ, Davis RW. CPR with simultaneous compression and ventilation at high airway pressure in 4 animal models. *Crit Care Med.* 1982;10:501-504.

92. Hou SH, Lue HC, Chu SH. Comparison of conventional and simultaneous compression-ventilation cardiopulmonary resuscitation in piglets. *Jpn Circ J.* 1994;58:426-432.

93. Barranco F, Lesmes A, Irles JA, Blasco J, Leal J, Rodriguez J, Leon C. Cardiopulmonary resuscitation with simultaneous chest and abdominal compression: comparative study in humans. *Resuscitation.* 1990;20:67-77.

94. Kinney SB, Tibballs J. An analysis of the efficacy of bag-valve-mask ventilation and chest compression during different compression-ventilation ratios in manikin-simulated paediatric resuscitation. *Resuscitation.* 2000;43:115-120.

95. Wik L, Steen PA. The ventilation/compression ratio influences the effectiveness of two rescuer advanced cardiac life support on a manikin. *Resuscitation.* 1996;31:113-119.

96. Milander MM, Hiscok PS, Sanders AB, Kern KB, Berg RA, Ewy GA. Chest compression and ventilation rates during cardiopulmonary resuscitation: the effects of audible tone guidance. *Acad Emerg Med.* 1995;2:708-713.

97. Whyte SD, Wyllie JP. Paediatric basic life support: a practical assessment. *Resuscitation.* 1999;41:153-157.

98. Nadkarni V, Tice L, Randall D, Corddry D. Metabolic effects on rescuer of varying compression-ventilation ratios during infant, pediatric, and adult CPR. *Crit Care Med.* 1999;27:A43.

99. Nadkarni V, Goodie B, Tice L, Cox T, Rose MJ. Evaluation of a universal compression/ventilation ratio for one-rescuer CPR in infant, pediatric, and adult manikins. *Crit Care Med.* 1997;25:A61.

100. Assar D, Chamberlain D, Colquhoun M, Donnelly P, Handley AJ, Leaves S, Kern KB, Mayor S. A rationale for staged teaching of basic life support. *Resuscitation.* 1998;39:137-143.

101. Kern KB, Sanders AB, Raife J, Milander MM, Otto CW, Ewy GA. A study of chest compression rates during cardiopulmonary resuscitation in humans: the importance of rate-directed chest compressions. *Arch Intern Med.* 1992;152:145-149.

102. Kern KB, Hilwig RW, Berg RA, Ewy GA. Efficacy of chest compression-only BLS CPR in the presence of an occluded airway. *Resuscitation.* 1998;39:179-188.

103. Friesen RM, Duncan P, Tweed WA, Bristow G. Appraisal of pediatric cardiopulmonary resuscitation. *Can Med Assoc J.* 1982;126:1055-1058.

104. Kyriacou DN, Arcinue EL, Peek C, Kraus JF. Effect of immediate resuscitation on children with submersion injury. *Pediatrics.* 1994;94:137-142.

105. Hickey RW, Cohen DM, Strausbaugh S, Dietrich AM. Pediatric patients requiring CPR in the prehospital setting. *Ann Emerg Med.* 1995;25:495-501.

106. Sirbaugh PE, Pepe PE, Shook JE, Kimball KT, Goldman MJ, Ward MA, Mann DM. A prospective, population-based study of the demographics, epidemiology, management, and outcome of out-of-hospital pediatric cardiopulmonary arrest [published correction appears in Ann Emerg Med. 1999;33:358]. *Ann Emerg Med.* 1999;33:174-184.

107. Mogayzel C, Quan L, Graves JR, Tiedeman D, Fahrenbruch C, Herndon P. Out-of-hospital ventricular fibrillation in children and adolescents: causes and outcomes. *Ann Emerg Med.* 1995;25:484-491.

108. Biggart MJ, Bohn DJ. Effect of hypothermia and cardiac arrest on outcome of near-drowning accidents in children. *J Pediatr.* 1990;117:179-183.

109. Quan L, Gore EJ, Wentz K, Allen J, Novack AH. Ten-year study of pediatric drownings and near-drownings in King County, Washington: lessons in injury prevention. *Pediatrics.* 1989;83:1035-1040.

110. Fiser DH, Wrape V. Outcome of cardiopulmonary resuscitation in children. *Pediatr Emerg Care.* 1987;3:235-238.

111. Kemp AM, Sibert JR. Outcome in children who nearly drown: a British Isles study. *BMJ.* 1991;302:931-933.

112. Ornato JP, Hallagan LF, McMahan SB, Peeples EH, Rostafinski AG. Attitudes of BCLS instructors about mouth-to-mouth resuscitation during the AIDS epidemic. *Ann Emerg Med.* 1990;19:151-156.

113. Brenner BE, Van DC, Cheng D, Lazar EJ. Determinants of reluctance to perform CPR among residents and applicants: the impact of experience on helping behavior. *Resuscitation.* 1997;35:203-211.

114. Hew P, Brenner B, Kaufman J. Reluctance of paramedics and emergency medical technicians to perform mouth-to-mouth resuscitation. *J Emerg Med.* 1997;15:279-284.

115. Locke CJ, Berg RA, Sanders AB, Davis MF, Milander MM, Kern KB, Ewy GA. Bystander cardiopulmonary resuscitation: concerns about mouth-to-mouth contact. *Arch Intern Med.* 1995;155:938-943.

116. Van Hoeyweghen RJ, Bossaert LL, Mullie A, Calle P, Martens P, Buylaert WA, Delooz H. Quality and efficiency of bystander CPR. Belgian Cerebral Resuscitation Study Group. *Resuscitation.* 1993;26:47-52.

117. Berg RA, Kern KB, Sanders AB, Otto CW, Hilwig RW, Ewy GA. Bystander cardiopulmonary resuscitation: is ventilation necessary? *Circulation.* 1993;88:1907-1915.

118. Berg RA, Wilcoxson D, Hilwig RW, Kern KB, Sanders AB, Otto CW, Eklund DK, Ewy GA. The need for ventilatory support during bystander CPR. *Ann Emerg Med.* 1995;26:342-350.

119. Berg RA, Kern KB, Hilwig RW, Berg MD, Sanders AB, Otto CW, Ewy GA. Assisted ventilation does not improve outcome in a porcine model of single-rescuer bystander cardiopulmonary resuscitation. *Circulation.* 1997;95:1635-1641.

120. Berg RA, Kern KB, Hilwig RW, Ewy GA. Assisted ventilation during 'bystander' CPR in a swine acute myocardial infarction model does not improve outcome. *Circulation.* 1997;96:4364-4371.

121. Chandra NC, Gruben KG, Tsitlik JE, Brower R, Guerci AD, Halperin HH, Weisfeldt ML, Permutt S. Observations of ventilation during resuscitation in a canine model. *Circulation.* 1994;90:3070-3075.

122. Tang W, Weil MH, Sun S, Kette D, Kette F, Gazmuri RJ, O'Connell F, Bisera J. Cardiopulmonary resuscitation by precordial compression but without mechanical ventilation. *Am J Respir Crit Care Med.* 1994;150:1709-1713.

123. Noc M, Weil MH, Tang W, Turner T, Fukui M. Mechanical ventilation may not be essential for initial cardiopulmonary resuscitation. *Chest.* 1995;108:821-827.

124. Weil MH, Rackow EC, Trevino R, Grundler W, Falk JL, Griffel MI. Difference in acid-base state between venous and arterial blood during cardiopulmonary resuscitation. *N Engl J Med.* 1986;315:153-156.

125. Sanders AB, Otto CW, Kern KB, Rogers JN, Perrault P, Ewy GA. Acid-base balance in a canine model of cardiac arrest. *Ann Emerg Med.* 1988;17:667-671.

126. Lindner KH, Pfenninger EG, Lurie KG, Schurmann W, Lindner IM, Ahnefeld FW. Effects of active compression-decompression resuscitation on myocardial and cerebral blood flow in pigs. *Circulation.* 1993;88:1254-1263.

127. Chang MW, Coffeen P, Lurie KG, Shultz J, Bache RJ, White CW. Active compression-decompression CPR improves vital organ perfusion in a dog model of ventricular fibrillation. *Chest.* 1994;106:1250-1259.

128. Shultz JJ, Coffeen P, Sweeney M, Detloff B, Kehler C, Pineda E, Yakshe P, Adler SW, Chang M, Lurie KG. Evaluation of standard and active compression-decompression CPR in an acute human model of ventricular fibrillation. *Circulation.* 1994;89:684-693.

129. Baubin M, Haid C, Hamm P, Gilly H. Measuring forces and frequency during active compression decompression cardiopulmonary resuscitation: a device for training, research and real CPR. *Resuscitation.* 1999;43:17-24.

130. Cohen TJ, Tucker KJ, Lurie KG, Redberg RF, Dutton JP, Dwyer KA, Schwab TM, Chin MC, Gelb AM, Scheinman MM, et al. Active compression-decompression: a new method of cardiopulmonary resuscitation. Cardiopulmonary Resuscitation Working Group. *JAMA.* 1992;267:2916-2923.

131. Plaisance P, Adnet F, Vicaut E, Hennequin B, Magne P, Prudhomme C, Lambert Y, Cantineau JP, Leopold C, Ferracci C, Gizzi M, Payen D. Benefit of active compression-decompression cardiopulmonary resuscitation as a prehospital advanced cardiac life support: a randomized multicenter study. *Circulation.* 1997;95:955-961.

132. Mauer D, Schneider T, Dick W, Withelm A, Elich D, Mauer M. Active compression-decompression resuscitation: a prospective, randomized study in a two-tiered EMS system with physicians in the field. *Resuscitation.* 1996;33:125-134.

133. Mauer DK, Nolan J, Plaisance P, Sitter H, Benoit H, Stiell IG, Sofianos E, Keiding N, Lurie KG. Effect of active compression decompression resuscitation (ACD-CPR) on survival: a combined analysis using individual patient data. *Resuscitation.* 1999;41:249-256.

134. Stiell IG, Hebert PC, Wells GA, Laupacis A, Vandemheen K, Dreyer JF, Eisenhauer MA, Gibson J, Higginson LA, Kirby AS, Mahon JL, Maloney JP, Weitzman BN. The Ontario trial of active compression-decompression cardiopulmonary resuscitation for in-hospital and prehospital cardiac arrest. *JAMA.* 1996;275:1417-1423.

135. Skogvoll E, Wik L. Active compression-decompression cardiopulmonary resuscitation: a population-based, prospective randomised clinical trial in out-of-hospital cardiac arrest. *Resuscitation.* 1999;42:163-172.

136. Babbs CF. CPR techniques that combine chest and abdominal compression and decompression: hemodynamic insights from a spreadsheet model. *Circulation.* 1999;100:2146-2152.

137. Lurie KG. Recent advances in mechanical methods of cardiopulmonary resuscitation. *Acta Anaesthesiol Scand Suppl.* 1997;111: 49-52.

138. Tang W, Weil MH, Schock RB, Sato Y, Lucas J, Sun S, Bisera J. Phased chest and abdominal compression-decompression: a new option for cardiopulmonary resuscitation. *Circulation.* 1997;95:1335-1340.

139. Lindner KH, Wenzel V. New mechanical methods for cardiopulmonary resuscitation (CPR): literature study and analysis of effectiveness [in German]. *Anaesthesist.* 1997;46: 220-230.

140. Sack JB, Kesselbrenner MB. Hemodynamics, survival benefits, and complications of interposed abdominal compression during cardiopulmonary resuscitation. *Acad Emerg Med.* 1994;1:490-497.

141. Majumdar A, Sedman PC. Gastric rupture secondary to successful Heimlich manoeuvre. *Postgrad Med J.* 1998;74:609-610.

142. Reilly JS. Prevention of aspiration in infants and young children: federal regulations. *Ann Otol Rhinol Laryngol.* 1990;99:273-276.

143. Rimell FL, Thome A Jr, Stool S, Reilly JS, Rider G, Stool D, Wilson CL. Characteristics of objects that cause choking in children. *JAMA.* 1995;274:1763-1766.

144. *Data on Odds of Death Due to Choking.* National Center for Health Statistics and National Safety Council; 1998.

145. Rosen P, Stoto M, Harley J. The use of the Heimlich maneuver in near drowning: Institute of Medicine report. *J Emerg Med.* 1995; 13:397-405.

146. Fink JA, Klein RL. Complications of the Heimlich maneuver. *J Pediatr Surg.* 1989; 24:486-487.

147. Heimlich HJ. A life-saving maneuver to prevent food-choking. *JAMA.* 1975;234: 398-401.

148. Day RL, Crelin ES, DuBois AB. Choking: the Heimlich abdominal thrust vs back blows: an approach to measurement of inertial and aerodynamic forces. *Pediatrics.* 1982;70:113-119.

149. Fingerhut LA, Cox CS, Warner M. International comparative analysis of injury mortality: findings from the ICE on injury statistics. International Collaborative Effort on Injury Statistics. *Adv Data.* 1998;1-20.

150. Langhelle A, Sunde K, Wik L, Steen PA. Airway pressure with chest compressions versus Heimlich manoeuvre in recently dead adults with complete airway obstruction. *Resuscitation.* 2000;44:105-108.

151. Sternbach G, Kiskaddon RT. Henry Heimlich: a life-saving maneuver for food choking. *J Emerg Med.* 1985;3:143-148.

152. Redding JS. The choking controversy: critique of evidence on the Heimlich maneuver. *Crit Care Med.* 1979;7:475-479.

153. Gordon AS, Belton MK, Ridolpho PF. Emergency management of foreign body obstruction. Safar P, Elam JO, eds. *Advances in Cardiopulmonary Resuscitation.* New York, NY: Springer-Verlag, Inc; 1977.

154. Guildner CW, Williams D, Subitch T. Airway obstructed by foreign material: the Heimlich maneuver. *JACEP.* 1976;5: 675-677.

155. Bintz M, Cogbill TH. Gastric rupture after the Heimlich maneuver. *J Trauma.* 1996;40: 159-160.

156. Cowan M, Bardole J, Dlesk A. Perforated stomach following the Heimlich maneuver. *Am J Emerg Med.* 1987;5:121-122.

157. Kabbani M, Goodwin SR. Traumatic epiglottis following blind finger sweep to remove a pharyngeal foreign body. *Clin Pediatr.* 1995;34:495-497.

158. Hartrey R, Bingham RM. Pharyngeal trauma as a result of blind finger sweeps in the choking child. *J Accid Emerg Med.* 1995;12: 52-54.

159. Dykes EH, Spence LJ, Young JG, Bohn DJ, Filler RM, Wesson DE. Preventable pediatric trauma deaths in a metropolitan region. *J Pediatr Surg.* 1989;24:107-110.

160. Esposito TJ, Sanddal ND, Dean JM, Hansen JD, Reynolds SA, Battan K. Analysis of preventable pediatric trauma deaths and inappropriate trauma care in Montana. *J Trauma.* 1999;47:243-251.

161. Suominen P, Rasanen J, Kivioja A. Efficacy of cardiopulmonary resuscitation in pulseless paediatric trauma patients. *Resuscitation.* 1998;36:9-13.

162. Curran C, Dietrich AM, Bowman MJ, Ginn-Pease ME, King DR, Kosnik E. Pediatric cervical-spine immobilization: achieving neutral position? *J Trauma.* 1995;39: 729-732.

163. Huerta C, Griffith R, Joyce SM. Cervical spine stabilization in pediatric patients: evaluation of current techniques. *Ann Emerg Med.* 1987;16:1121-1126.

164. Treloar DJ, Nypaver M. Angulation of the pediatric cervical spine with and without cervical collar. *Pediatr Emerg Care.* 1997; 13:5-8.

165. Soud T, Pieper P, Hazinski MF. Pediatric trauma. In Hazinski MF, ed. *Nursing Care of the Critically Ill Child.* St. Louis, Mo: Mosby–Year Book; 1992:842-843.

166. Boyd R. Witnessed resuscitation by relatives. *Resuscitation.* 2000;43:171-176.

167. Doyle CJ, Post H, Burney RE, Maino J, Keefe M, Rhee KJ. Family participation during resuscitation: an option. *Ann Emerg Med.* 1987;16:673-675.

168. Hanson C, Strawser D. Family presence during cardiopulmonary resuscitation: Foote Hospital emergency department's nine-year perspective. *J Emerg Nurs.* 1992;18:104-106.

169. Barratt F, Wallis DN. Relatives in the resuscitation room: their point of view. *J Accid Emerg Med.* 1998;15:109-111.

170. Meyers TA, Eichhorn DJ, Guzzetta CE. Do families want to be present during CPR? A retrospective survey. *J Emerg Nurs.* 1998; 24:400-405.

171. Robinson SM, Mackenzie-Ross S, Campbell Hewson GL, Egleston CV, Prevost AT. Psychological effect of witnessed resuscitation on bereaved relatives. *Lancet.* 1998;352: 614-617.

172. Boie ET, Moore GP, Brummett C, Nelson DR. Do parents want to be present during invasive procedures performed on their children in the emergency department? A survey of 400 parents. *Ann Emerg Med.* 1999;34: 70-74.

173. Hampe SO. Needs of the grieving spouse in a hospital setting. *Nurs Res.* 1975;24: 113-120.

174. Offord RJ. Should relatives of patients with cardiac arrest be invited to be present during cardiopulmonary resuscitation? *Intensive Crit Care Nurs.* 1998;14:288-293.

175. Shaner K, Eckle N. Implementing a program to support the option of family presence during resuscitation. *The Association for the Care of Children's Health (ACCH) Advocate.* 1997;3:3-7.

176. Eichhorn DJ, Meyers TA, Mitchell TG, Guzzetta CE. Opening the doors: family presence during resuscitation. *J Cardiovasc Nurs.* 1996;10:59-70.

177. Todd KH, Braslow A, Brennan RT, Lowery DW, Cox RJ, Lipscomb LE, Kellermann AL. Randomized, controlled trial of video self-instruction versus traditional CPR training. *Ann Emerg Med.* 1998;31:364-369.

178. Doherty A, Damon S, Hein K, Cummins RO. Evaluation of CPR prompt and home learning system for teaching CPR to lay rescuers. *Circulation.* 1998;98(suppl I):I-410.

179. Starr LM. Electronic voice boosts CPR responses. *Occup Health Saf.* 1997;66: 30-37.

Airway, Ventilation, and Management of Respiratory Distress and Failure

Introductory Case Scenario

A 4-month-old infant is brought to the Emergency Department because he is "breathing funny." The mother says the infant's oral intake has decreased, he was fussy and irritable today, and he seemed unable to catch his breath when he tried to eat. The infant has had a cold for the past 2 days, and the breathing problems started today. The mother says that the infant felt warm but she did not take his temperature.

You see a tachypneic infant with labored breathing (nasal flaring and intercostal and subcostal retractions) and an anxious look on his face. The infant has a frequent wheezy-sounding cough, and he has noisy airway sounds during inspiration. His skin color appears somewhat mottled, but he is not overtly blue. He is attentive to his mother and watches you as you approach. His heart rate is 180 bpm, respiratory rate (counting for 30 seconds) is 60 per minute, temperature (rectal) is 37.8°C (99.9°F), and blood pressure is 88/60 mm Hg. His heart rhythm is regular without rubs or gallops, but you hear a short systolic ejection murmur. The infant has readily palpable pulses in his feet. Capillary refill is brisk, and his extremities are warm. Copious nasal secretions are present. During auscultation of the chest you hear bilateral moist crackles, scattered rhonchi, and expiratory wheezes. Air entry over the axillary lung fields seems diminished. The infant's anterior fontanelle is soft and flat.

- What is your rapid cardiopulmonary assessment for this infant?

- What are your initial treatment priorities?

- What type of airway or respiratory problem does this infant demonstrate?

- What would be signs of further deterioration in this infant?

- If respiratory failure develops in this infant, how would you manage it?

Learning Objectives

After completing this chapter the PALS provider should be able to

- Describe how the anatomy and physiology of the airway and respiratory system of infants and children differ from the anatomy and physiology of the airway and respiratory system of adults

- Explain what pulse oximetry measures and describe the limitations of this assessment tool

- Explain what exhaled CO_2 detectors measure and the limitations of these assessment devices

- Describe common oxygen delivery systems and their effectiveness in delivering different concentrations of oxygen to the infant or child

- Describe how to select and use oropharyngeal and nasopharyngeal airways

- Explain the differences between a self-inflating and a flow-inflating manual resuscitator and describe the advantages and disadvantages of each device

- Describe the techniques of bag-mask ventilation and tracheal intubation

- List the procedures that should be used to confirm proper position of the tracheal tube

- If appropriate for your training, describe the techniques of laryngeal mask airway (LMA) insertion, cricothyrotomy, and decompression of a pneumothorax

- Describe the signs of artificial airway obstruction and displacement

Introduction

Respiratory problems are common in infants and children, and these problems are an important cause of in-hospital and out-of-hospital cardiopulmonary arrest in the pediatric age group. Respiratory problems may result from upper airway obstruction, lower airway obstruction, alteration of the diffusion of gas from the alveolus to the capillaries, abnormal pulmonary blood flow, or alteration in the nerves and muscles that control breathing.

Respiratory status is frequently compromised by one or more of these factors. To prevent progression from respiratory compromise to respiratory failure and cardiopulmonary arrest, assessment and treatment decisions must be made quickly.

If respiratory failure or respiratory arrest is treated promptly, neurologically intact survival of the child is likely. Once *respiratory* arrest progresses to pulseless *cardiac* arrest, outcome is poor.[1,2] Therefore, early recognition and effective management of respiratory problems are fundamental to pediatric advanced life support.

This chapter describes the overall management of respiratory problems in children. The chapter reviews basic physiology and anatomy and describes the techniques and adjuncts used in airway management and treatment of respiratory failure. Timely and appropriate use of these techniques and adjuncts is critical for survival of the patient. The review questions and case scenarios at the end of this chapter highlight the priorities of assessment and treatment of the infant and child with respiratory insufficiency or failure.

Anatomic and Physiologic Considerations

The pediatric airway differs from the adult airway in several important anatomic and physiologic ways.[3] The pediatric upper airway has the following important developmental characteristics:

■ The airway of the infant or child is much smaller in diameter and shorter in length than the airway of the adult.

■ The infant's tongue is larger relative to the oropharynx than is the adult's tongue.

■ The larynx in infants and toddlers is relatively cephalad in position compared with the larynx in adults.

■ The epiglottis in infants and toddlers is long, floppy, narrow, and angled away from the long axis of the trachea.

■ The vocal cords have a lower attachment anteriorly in the infant and child than in the adult.

■ In children younger than 10 years, the narrowest portion of the airway is below the vocal cords at the level of the non-distensible cricoid cartilage, and the larynx is funnel shaped. In teenagers and adults the narrowest portion of the airway is at the glottic inlet (see Figure 1), and the larynx is cylinder shaped.

These anatomic differences have the following important clinical consequences:

■ A relatively small amount of airway edema or obstruction causes a relatively large reduction in the diameter of the pediatric airway. This reduction in diameter markedly increases resistance to airflow and therefore the work of breathing.

■ Posterior displacement of the tongue may cause severe airway obstruction. During tracheal intubation in a child, there often is less room to compress the tongue anteriorly, so that it may be difficult to control the position of the tongue with the laryngoscope blade.

■ The high position of the larynx makes the angle between the base of the tongue and glottic opening more acute. As a result, straight laryngoscope blades are often more useful than curved blades for creating a direct visual plane from the mouth to the glottis, particularly in infants.

■ Controlling the epiglottis with a laryngoscope blade is more difficult. You can overcome this difficulty by using a straight laryngoscope blade and by directly lifting the epiglottis, exposing the vocal cords.

■ Intubation of the child is more difficult than intubation of the adult. In the child the tracheal tube will easily enter the esophagus, or it may become caught at the anterior commissure of the vocal cords.

■ Tracheal tube size must be based on the size of the cricoid ring rather than the size of the glottic opening. Ideally if the tracheal tube size is appropriate, an air leak is detectable when a peak inspiratory pressure of 20 to 30 cm H_2O is created. Note that with a number of conditions (discussed below), the "ideal" tube size is inappropriate and a tighter airway seal may be desirable, particularly during initial stabilization of the patient.

In the infant and young child, the subglottic airway is smaller and more compliant and the supporting cartilage less developed than in the adult. The subglottic airway tends to collapse or narrow if there is upper airway obstruction (Figure 2C). Even a minor reduction in diameter of the infant's upper airway results in a clinically significant reduction in airway cross-sectional area, which results in an increase in airflow resistance and work of breathing (Figure 3).

FIGURE 1. Configuration of the adult **(A)** and the infant **(B)** larynx. Note the cylindrical shape of the adult larynx. The infant larynx is funnel shaped because of a narrow cricoid cartilage relative to the thyroid cartilage. A indicates anterior; P, posterior. Modified with permission from Coté and Todres.[6]

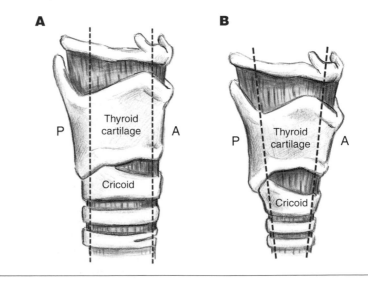

FIGURE 2. A, During *normal* expiration the chest wall muscles relax so that the elastic recoil of the lung becomes dominant, leading to subatmospheric pleural pressures. The elastic recoil also compresses the alveoli and airways, generating an intraluminal airway pressure greater than atmospheric, which leads to expiratory air flow. **B,** Respiratory dynamics during expiration with lower airway obstruction (eg, asthma or bronchiolitis). Increased effort is used to move air past narrowed or obstructed intrathoracic airways. Active chest wall muscle and abdominal muscle contraction narrow the chest and push the diaphragm up. These forces increase intrapleural and parenchymal pressure, compressing the small airways and worsening airway obstruction. **C,** During *normal* inspiration the muscles of the chest wall contract to maintain its configuration while the diaphragm actively contracts, pulling on the lung parenchyma. The net effect is to increase the elastic recoil of the lung parenchyma on the airways, which dilates the airways and lowers intraluminal airway pressure, resulting in gas flow into the lung. **D,** Extrathoracic airway obstruction during inspiration results in greater diaphragmatic muscle effort, producing greater subatmospheric intraluminal airway pressures. The larger pressure gradient between atmospheric and extrathoracic tracheal airway pressure leads to severe dynamic collapse of the extrathoracic trachea just beyond the level of obstruction. Adapted from Coté and Todres.[6]

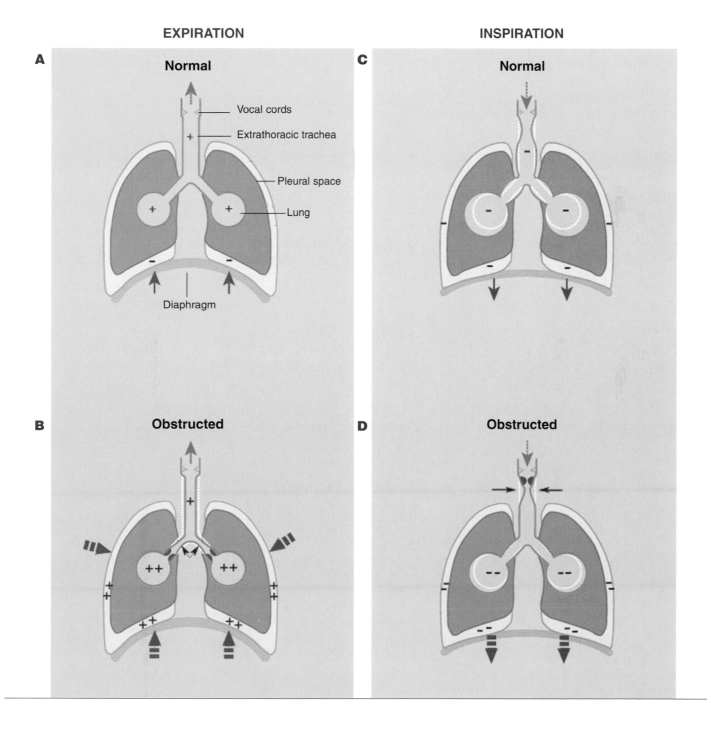

FIGURE 3. Effects of edema on airway resistance in the infant versus the adult. Normal airways are shown on the left; edematous airways (with 1 mm of circumferential edema) are on the right. Resistance to flow is inversely proportional to the *fourth* power of the radius of the airway lumen for laminar flow and to the *fifth* power for turbulent flow. The net result is a 75% decrease in cross-sectional area and a 16-fold increase in airway resistance in the infant versus a 44% decrease in cross-sectional area and a 3-fold increase in airway resistance in the adult during quiet breathing. Turbulent flow in the infant (eg, crying) increases airway resistance and thus the work of breathing from 16- to 32-fold. Modified with permission from Coté and Todres.[6]

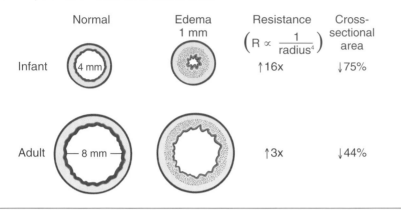

During quiet breathing, airflow is laminar and the resistance to airflow is inversely proportional to the fourth power of the airway radius. Thus, even during quiet breathing, *any* reduction in airway diameter results in an *exponential* increase in resistance to airflow and work of breathing. When airflow is *turbulent* (eg, during crying), resistance to airflow is inversely proportional to the *fifth* power of the radius. For these reasons the infant or child with airway obstruction should be kept as calm and quiet as possible to prevent generation of turbulent airflow, increased airway resistance (Figure 3), and markedly increased work of breathing.[6]

The pediatric airway is susceptible to dynamic collapse in the presence of airway obstruction.[7] Upper airway obstruction (eg, croup, presence of an extrathoracic foreign body, or epiglottitis) may cause tracheal collapse during inspiration because deeply negative intra-airway pressure causes the flexible supporting structures of the upper airway to collapse (Figure 2C). An intrathoracic foreign body or a disease that causes lower airway obstruction (eg, bronchiolitis or asthma) increases external pressure on the *intra-thoracic* airways during exhalation (Figure 2D). Application of positive end-expiratory pressure (PEEP) often improves gas exchange by opposing the forces causing dynamic airway collapse (Figure 4).

The pediatric patient has a high oxygen demand per kilogram of body weight because the child's metabolic rate is high. Oxygen consumption in infants is 6 to 8 mL/kg per minute compared with 3 to 4 mL/kg per minute in adults.[8,9] Consequently in the presence of apnea or inadequate alveolar ventilation, hypoxemia develops more rapidly in the child than in the adult.

An illness leading to respiratory distress or failure may cause hypoxemia by several mechanisms:

- The disease process directly interferes with exchange of oxygen and carbon dioxide, eg, pneumonia or acute respiratory distress syndrome (ARDS).

- Mismatch of ventilation and perfusion causes shunting of pulmonary blood through the lung so that hypoxemia and (to a lesser extent) hypercarbia occur, eg, asthma, bronchiolitis, or aspiration pneumonia.

- The disease process decreases lung compliance or increases airway resistance, resulting in increased work of breathing and increased oxygen consumption that exceeds delivery, eg, pneumonia, ARDS, or asthma.

- Infection of the central nervous system, trauma, drug overdose, and other conditions impair respiratory drive, resulting in hypoventilation or apnea.

FYI: The Mechanics of Breathing During Infancy and Childhood

During inspiration the intercostal muscles stiffen the chest as the diaphragm contracts, thereby increasing intrathoracic volume. When volume increases, intrathoracic pressure falls, causing air to flow into the lungs. If the lungs are abnormally stiff, the compliant chest wall of the infant or child may retract during inspiration, making ventilation less efficient. Because the chest wall of infants and young children is flexible,[4,5] the forceful contraction of the diaphragm can also pull the chest inward so that even maximum inspiratory efforts do not produce adequate tidal volume. Similarly, children with neuromuscular disorders have a weak chest wall and respiratory muscles that make breathing and coughing ineffective.

The normal diaphragm is dome shaped, and from this shape it contracts most forcefully. When the diaphragm is flattened, as occurs with lung hyperinflation (eg, as in acute asthma), diaphragm contraction is less forceful and ventilation is less efficient. If movement of the diaphragm is impeded by high intra-abdominal pressure (eg, gastric inflation) or by air trapping due to airway obstruction, respiration is compromised because the infant's intercostal muscles cannot effectively lift the chest wall to increase intrathoracic volume and compensate for the loss of diaphragm motion.

FIGURE 4. A, Upper airway obstruction caused by laryngospasm or mechanical obstruction (eg, croup) results in dynamic collapse of the extrathoracic trachea (green arrows) during inspiration. **B,** Application of approximately 10 cm H_2O positive end-expiratory pressure (PEEP) during spontaneous breathing often relieves obstruction (arrows) by keeping the airway patent. If this simple maneuver does not relieve obstruction, positive-pressure ventilation may be necessary. Reproduced with permission from Coté CJ. Pediatric anesthesia. In: Miller RD, ed. *Anesthesia*. 3rd ed. New York, NY: Churchill Livingstone; 1990:911.

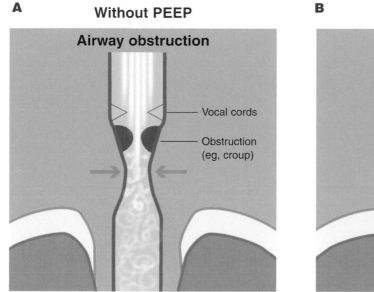
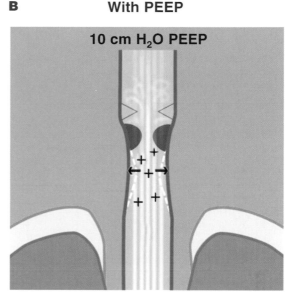

A Without PEEP
Airway obstruction

B With PEEP
10 cm H_2O PEEP

Vocal cords
Obstruction (eg, croup)

Foundation Facts: Symptoms of Airway Obstruction

- Obstruction of the *extrathoracic* airway (eg, nose, posterior pharynx, larynx, or subglottic space) results in symptoms predominantly during the *inspiratory* phase. Increased inspiratory effort often amplifies airway resistance by causing collapse of the compliant upper airway, producing stridor.

- Obstruction of the *intrathoracic* airway (eg, lower trachea, bronchi, or bronchioles) results in symptoms predominantly during the *expiratory* phase. Increased expiratory effort worsens airway obstruction by causing collapse of the intrathoracic airways, producing wheezing.

Devices to Monitor Respiratory Function
General Principles

The goal of emergency airway management is to support or restore respiratory function. To achieve that goal, the provider must anticipate and recognize respiratory problems and treat those problems as soon as possible. In an emergency it may be impossible to determine the cause of respiratory dysfunction before emergency airway management is initiated. But identification of the precise cause of respiratory dysfunction will enable targeted respiratory support.

Noninvasive Respiratory Monitoring
Pulse Oximetry

Pulse oximetry is an important noninvasive monitoring technique because it enables continuous evaluation of arterial oxygen saturation both out of hospital and in hospital.[10,11] Continuous monitoring of pulse oximetry will enable detection of hypoxemia[12] and response to therapy. Pulse oximetry is highly recommended during stabilization and transport because healthcare providers cannot reliably detect hypoxemia by clinical examination alone.[13] In children with cyanotic congenital heart disease, pulse oximeter readings correlate less well with measured oxygen saturation values than they do in other children, but pulse oximeters are still useful for assessing changes in oxygen saturation over time.[14] Pulse oximeters may be inaccurate in the presence of carboxyhemoglobinemia, which occurs with carbon monoxide poisoning, and methemoglobinemia, which may be congenital or may result from toxin or drug exposure (see FYI: "Accuracy of Pulse Oximetry in the Presence of Carboxyhemoglobin and Methemoglobinemia").

Pulse oximetry is a useful monitoring technique during attempts at tracheal intubation. Hyperoxygenation before intubation, however, can mask the decrease in arterial oxygen saturation that usually develops with incorrect (ie, esophageal) placement of the tube. In these patients the time required for a fall in oxyhemoglobin saturation will vary according to the patient's rate of oxygen consumption.[15,16]

Pulse oximeters evaluate *oxygenation;* they do not reflect the effectiveness of *ventilation* (ie, carbon dioxide elimination). Despite this limitation pulse oximetry is recommended throughout stabilization and transport. Outside the hospital intermittent pulse oximetry may be accomplished by use of finger probes. If available, pulse oximetry should be used before and during transport, on arrival, and whenever the patient is moved (eg, into the Emergency Department) because movement of the patient is most likely to result in tracheal tube displacement.[17]

The pulse oximeter requires pulsatile blood flow to determine oxygen saturation. Devices vary in accuracy and signal strength in the presence of shock and poor perfusion, and all are inaccurate unless they precisely track the heart rate. Low or absent pulse signals can occur if there is a problem with the skin-probe interface or if the photodiode sensor is not aligned across from the light-emitting diodes. In addition, if the child is actively moving, the pulse oximeter may have difficulty distinguishing between pulsatile changes and movement-induced changes in light absorption, although the introduction of filters and additional algorithms has reduced the problem of motion artifact in some models. Pulse oximeters are useless in the child in cardiac arrest (because of the absence of pulsatile blood flow).

If infant sensors are unavailable, an adult sensor may be placed around the hand or foot of an infant. If intense vasoconstriction is present and a pulsatile signal is not detected in the extremities, an infant pulse oximeter probe may be applied to the ear lobe. If the patient is unconscious, the probe may also be applied to the nares, the cheek at the corner of the mouth, and even to the tongue.[19] Do not use a sensor with a cracked surface because the light-emitting diodes may come in contact with the skin.[20,21]

Different brands of pulse oximeters vary greatly in their speed of response to the development of hypoxemia[22,23] and their accuracy in low-flow states. The validity of oximeter data must be confirmed by evaluating the patient's appearance and comparing the heart rate displayed by the oximeter with that displayed by the bedside cardiorespiratory monitor. If the displayed heart rate does not correlate with the patient's heart rate or if the patient's appearance does not correspond with the reported level of oxygenation, the accuracy of the oximeter must be questioned.

During pulse oximetry be sure to use compatible equipment as recommended by the manufacturer. Do not mix the probes of one manufacturer with the base unit of a different company. If perfusion is poor, rotate the sites of monitoring.[20,21]

Exhaled or End-Tidal CO₂ Monitoring

Evaluation of exhaled carbon dioxide can be used to estimate arterial carbon dioxide tension and to confirm tracheal tube placement. If there is a good match of ventilation and perfusion in the lungs and if there is no airway obstruction, exhaled CO_2 should correlate well with arterial P_{CO_2}. During acute stabilization, exhaled or end-tidal CO_2 monitoring is used to confirm tracheal tube placement. This technique is particularly accurate (both sensitive and specific) in confirming tracheal tube placement in children who weigh more than 2 kg and have a perfusing rhythm.

Exhaled CO_2 is typically monitored by attaching a CO_2 detector to a tracheal tube to capture and quantify the amount of carbon dioxide present in exhaled gas. Exhaled CO_2 is occasionally monitored by attaching a CO_2 detector to a nasal cannula.

FYI: Accuracy of Pulse Oximeters in the Presence of Carboxyhemoglobinemia and Methemoglobinemia

Most commercially available pulse oximeters use two light-emitting diodes and a photodetector in a sensor. The two diodes emit a red and an infrared light. These diodes should be placed across a pulsatile tissue bed (eg, a well-perfused finger) from the photodetector/sensor. Oxygenated hemoglobin in the pulsatile tissue bed primarily absorbs infrared light, but reduced (nonoxygenated) hemoglobin in the pulsatile tissue bed primarily absorbs red light. A microprocessor in the unit determines the relative absorption of red and infrared light to calculate the percentage of oxygenated versus reduced (nonoxygenated) hemoglobin present in the tissue bed.[18] Commercially available devices differ in the filters and algorithms used to reduce motion artifact and increase signal accuracy in low-flow states.

The light absorption of methemoglobin and carboxyhemoglobin is different from that of normal hemoglobin, so pulse oximeters will not accurately reflect total hemoglobin saturation in the presence of these two products.[18] With significant methemoglobinemia, pulse oximeters display an oxygen saturation of approximately 85%. With significant carboxyhemoglobinemia (such as occurs in carbon monoxide poisoning), the pulse oximeter will typically reflect the oxygen saturation of *normal* hemoglobin, not the percentage of hemoglobin bound to carbon monoxide. If these or other conditions affecting oxyhemoglobin saturation are present, arterial hemoglobin oxygen saturation must be determined by using co-oximetry.

FIGURE 5. A, Normal exhaled CO_2 capnograph waveform during mechanical ventilation through a tracheal tube in a patient with normal cardiac output. **B,** Exhaled CO_2 capnograph waveform through a tracheal tube during CPR with effective chest compressions (low cardiac output).

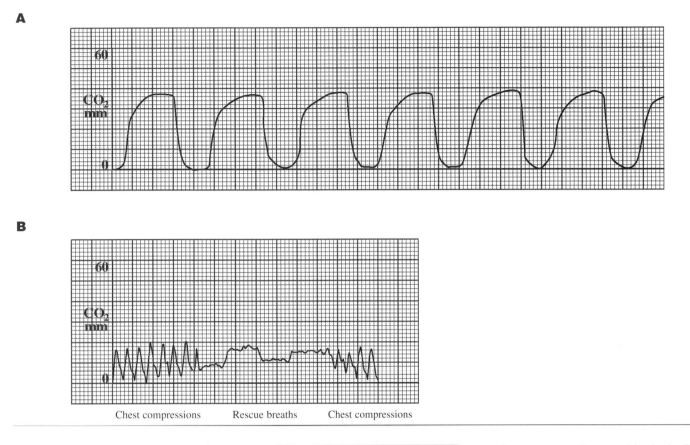

Several types of devices can be used to detect exhaled carbon dioxide. *Qualitative* monitors are based on a chemical reaction between exhaled CO_2 and a chemical detector impregnated in a strip of paper. When CO_2 is present, the color of the paper will change from purple to bright yellow (see Critical Concepts: "Memory Aid for Qualitative CO_2 Detectors").

Capnography devices are *quantitative* devices that measure the concentration of CO_2 using infrared absorption detectors. Carbon dioxide concentration is typically displayed by these devices as a continuous exhaled CO_2 concentration waveform with a digital display of end-tidal CO_2 (see Figure 5). For more information about exhaled CO_2 monitoring to confirm tracheal tube placement, see "Confirmation of Tracheal Tube Placement" later in this chapter.

Critical Concepts:
Memory Aid for Qualitative CO_2 Detectors

Qualitative CO_2 detectors change color from purple to bright yellow when carbon dioxide is present. To remember what the color changes indicate, use the following memory aid:

Purple = **P**roblem (no CO_2 detected)

Tan   = **T**hink (identify and rule out problems)

Yellow= **Y**es (CO_2 *is* present)

Arterial Blood Gas Analysis

Arterial blood gas analysis is the best way to determine the effectiveness of oxygenation and ventilation, to quantify respiratory or metabolic acidosis, and to monitor the response to therapy objectively. During CPR arterial PO_2 and pH may not accurately reflect tissue oxygenation and pH but instead indicate the effectiveness (or ineffectiveness) of ventilation.[24,25] The difference between arterial and central venous gas pH and PCO_2 may more accurately reflect the efficacy of perfusion.[25,26]

Discussion of arterial blood gas analysis in acute and chronic illness is beyond the scope of this text. In brief, the provider should not wait for the results of arterial blood gas analysis to identify respiratory distress and initiate therapy. When the patient has an acute illness, the provider generally *should* watch for the development of acidosis, hypoxemia, and hypercarbia. If the child has chronic lung disease, the development of significant acidosis or hypoxemia or hypercarbia exceeding the child's normal levels suggests deterioration in respiratory function.

If the child has asthma, initial hyperventilation and respiratory alkalosis may give way to normalization of pH and then to development of combined respiratory and metabolic acidosis as the child's condition deteriorates and hypoxemia and hypercarbia develop.

Oxygen Delivery Systems

Oxygen uptake and delivery are compromised during cardiac arrest and many other serious illnesses, so oxygen should be administered in high concentration to all seriously ill or injured patients with respiratory insufficiency, shock, or trauma, even if measured arterial oxygen tension is high. Add humidification as soon as practical to prevent obstruction of the small airways by dried secretions. Heated humidification systems are preferable to cool mist systems because cool mist systems may produce hypothermia in the small victim.

When you attempt to administer oxygen to an alert child, you must balance the desire to increase oxygen delivery against the potential adverse effects of increased agitation that may be produced by attaching a mask or cannula to the child. Anxiety increases oxygen consumption and possibly respiratory distress (see Figure 2). For this reason you should allow alert children in respiratory distress to remain with their parents, and you should introduce airway equipment, including oxygen, in a non-threatening manner.

If a child is upset by one method of oxygen support (eg, a mask), you should attempt to deliver the oxygen by an alternative technique (eg, a face tent or a "blow-by" stream of humidified oxygen held by a parent and directed toward the child's mouth and nose). To further prevent agitation, allow alert children with respiratory difficulty to remain in a position of comfort because they will usually assume a position that promotes optimal airway patency and minimizes respiratory effort.

If the child is somnolent or unconscious, the airway may become obstructed by a combination of neck flexion, relaxation of the jaw, posterior displacement of the tongue against the posterior wall of the pharynx, and collapse of the hypopharynx.[27,28] You should use noninvasive methods to open the airway (see Chapter 3, "Basic Life Support, Airway") before you use airway adjuncts.[29,30] If necessary, clear the airway by removing secretions, mucus, or blood from the oropharynx and nasopharynx with suction.

If spontaneous ventilation is *inadequate* despite a patent airway (as judged by insufficient chest movement and inadequate breath sounds), you must provide assisted ventilation. In most respiratory emergencies, infants and children can be successfully ventilated with a bag-mask device even in the presence of partial airway obstruction.[31] In spontaneously breathing patients, gentle positive-pressure breaths administered with a bag-mask device should be carefully timed to augment the child's inspiratory efforts. If the delivered breaths are not coordinated with the child's efforts, ventilation may be ineffective and may result in coughing, vomiting, laryngospasm, and gastric inflation, further impeding effective ventilation (see "Bag-Mask Ventilation," below).

If spontaneous ventilation is effective, you may administer oxygen by any of a number of devices. The choice of delivery system is determined by the child's clinical status and the desired concentration of oxygen. Oxygen delivery systems can be divided into low-flow and high-flow systems.[32] In a low-flow system, 100% oxygen mixes with entrained room air during inspiration because the oxygen flow is less than the patient's inspiratory flow. With a low-flow system, the delivered oxygen concentration is determined by the patient's minute ventilation rate and gas flow delivery rate (see FYI: "Effect of Patient Size and Minute Ventilation on Oxygen Delivery"). Low-flow systems theoretically can provide an oxygen concentration of 23% to 80%, although they do so unreliably.

In a *high-flow* system, the flow rate and reservoir capacity provide adequate gas flow to meet the total inspired flow requirements of the patient, so entrainment of room air does not occur. High-flow systems can reliably deliver either low or high inspired oxygen concentrations. They deliver a reliable inspired oxygen concentration by using a blender to adjust the final concentration of oxygen provided to the delivery system. High-flow systems should be used in emergency settings because they reliably deliver a high concentration of oxygen.

Oxygen Mask

Several types of oxygen masks may be used to administer humidified oxygen in a wide range of concentrations. The soft vinyl pediatric mask is often poorly tolerated by infants and toddlers, but it may be accepted by older children.

FYI: Effect of Patient Size and Minute Ventilation on Oxygen Delivery

A nasal cannula delivering 1 L of oxygen per minute provides approximately 16.67 mL of 100% oxygen per second. In a 2-kg infant with a normal tidal volume of approximately 12 mL (tidal volume ≈ 5 to 7 mL per kg), this flow rate exceeds the infant's tidal volume, so a high oxygen concentration is delivered even though the nasal cannula is a "low-flow" system. In comparison, in a 15-kg, 2-year-old child with a tidal volume of about 90 mL and an average inspiratory flow rate of approximately 180 mL/sec, the same 1 L/min flow rate will provide a much lower concentration of inspired oxygen.

FIGURE 6. Partial rebreathing mask.

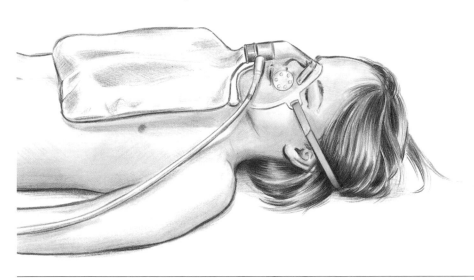

The simple oxygen mask is a low-flow device that delivers 35% to 60% oxygen with a flow rate of 6 to 10 L/min. The maximum inspired oxygen concentration is approximately 60% because inspiratory entrainment of room air occurs between the mask and the face and through exhalation ports in the side of the mask. Oxygen concentration delivered to the patient will be reduced if the patient's spontaneous inspiratory flow requirement is high, the mask is loose, or the oxygen flow into the mask is low. A minimum oxygen flow rate of 6 L/min must be used to maintain an increased inspired oxygen concentration and prevent rebreathing of exhaled carbon dioxide.

A *partial rebreathing mask* consists of a simple face mask with a reservoir bag (Figure 6). It reliably provides an inspired oxygen concentration of 50% to 60% (compared with 30% to 60% for standard masks). During exhalation some of the exhaled air flows into the reservoir bag and combines with fresh oxygen. Because this initial portion of the exhaled gas comes from the upper airway and was not involved in respiratory gas exchange during the prior breath, it remains oxygen rich. During inspiration the patient draws gas predominantly from the fresh oxygen inflow and from the reservoir bag, so entrainment of room air through the exhalation ports is minimized. Rebreathing of

exhaled carbon dioxide from the mask is prevented if the oxygen flow rate into the bag is consistently maintained above the patient's minute ventilation. If the oxygen flow rate is sufficient and the mask fits securely, the reservoir bag will not empty completely during inspiration. An oxygen flow rate of 10 to 12 L/min generally is required.

A *nonrebreathing mask* consists of a face mask and reservoir bag with the following additions: (1) a valve incorporated into one or both exhalation ports to prevent entrainment of room air during inspiration and (2) a valve placed between the reservoir bag and the mask to prevent flow of exhaled gas into the reservoir. On inspiration the patient draws 100% oxygen from the reservoir bag and the oxygen inflow. Oxygen flow into the mask is adjusted to prevent collapse of the bag. An inspired oxygen concentration of 95% can be achieved with an oxygen flow rate of 10 to 15 L/min and the use of a well-sealed face mask.

A Venturi-type mask is a high-flow system designed to reliably and predictably provide controlled, low to moderate (25% to 60%) inspired oxygen concentrations. This system uses a special oxygen outlet at the mask that creates a subatmospheric pressure designed to entrain a specific quantity of room air with the oxygen flow.

Face Tent

A face tent or face shield is a high-flow, soft plastic "bucket" that is often better tolerated by children than a face mask. Even with a high oxygen flow rate (10 to 15 L/min), stable inspired oxygen concentrations greater than 40% cannot be reliably provided. An advantage of the face tent is that it permits access to the face (eg, for suctioning) without interrupting oxygen flow.

Oxygen Hood

An oxygen hood is a clear plastic shell that encompasses the patient's head. It is well tolerated by infants; allows easy access to the chest, trunk, and extremities; and permits control of inspired oxygen concentration, gas temperature, and humidity. A gas inflow rate ≥10 to 15 L/min maintains approximately the same oxygen concentration within the hood as at the gas source. An inspired oxygen concentration of 80% to 90% may be achieved. As a rule, a hood is too small to use with children older than approximately 1 year.

Oxygen Tent

The oxygen tent is a clear plastic shell that encloses the child's upper body. It can deliver more than 50% oxygen with high flow rates, but it cannot reliably provide a stable inspired oxygen concentration. Room air may enter the tent whenever the tent is opened. The tent also limits access to the patient. If humidified oxygen is used, the resulting mist may impede observation of the patient. In practice a tent does not provide satisfactory supplementation of inspired oxygen if more than 30% inspired oxygen is required.

Nasal Cannula

A nasal cannula is a low-flow oxygen delivery device suitable for infants and children who require only low levels of supplemental oxygen; the net FiO_2 depends on the child's respiratory rate, respiratory effort, and size.[33] High oxygen concentrations may be delivered by nasal cannula to small infants (see FYI: "Effect of Patient Size and Minute Ventilation on Oxygen Delivery"). The inspired oxygen concentration cannot be reliably determined from the nasal oxygen flow rate because inspired oxygen concentration is influenced by other factors, such as nasal resistance, oropharyngeal resistance, inspiratory flow rate, tidal volume, and nasopharyngeal and oropharyngeal volume. A high oxygen flow rate (>4 L/min) irritates the nasopharynx and may not appreciably improve oxygenation. A nasal cannula typically does not provide humidified oxygen and may not deliver sufficient oxygen if the nares are obstructed.

Oropharyngeal and Nasopharyngeal Airways

Oropharyngeal Airway

An oropharyngeal airway consists of a flange, a short bite-block segment, and a curved body usually made of plastic and shaped to provide an air channel and suction conduit through the mouth. The curved body of the oropharyngeal airway is designed to fit over the back of the tongue to hold it and the soft hypopha-

ryngeal structures away from the posterior wall of the pharynx. An oropharyngeal airway may be used in the *unconscious* infant or child if procedures to open the airway (eg, head tilt–chin lift or jaw thrust) fail to provide and maintain a clear, unobstructed airway. An oropharyngeal airway should *not* be used in a *conscious* or *semiconscious* patient because it may stimulate gagging and vomiting. The key assessment is to check whether the patient has an intact cough and gag reflex; if so, do not use the oropharyngeal airway.

FIGURE 7. Selection of an oral airway. An airway of the proper size will relieve obstruction caused by the tongue without damaging laryngeal structures. The appropriate size can be estimated by holding the airway next to the child's face (**A**). The tip of the airway should end just cephalad to the angle of the mandible (dashed line), resulting in proper alignment with the glottic opening (**B**). If the oral airway is too large, the tip will align posterior to the angle of the mandible (**C**) and obstruct the glottic opening by pushing the epiglottis down (**C**, arrow). If the oral airway is too small, the tip will align well above the angle of the mandible (**D**) and exacerbate airway obstruction by pushing the tongue into the hypopharynx (**D**, arrows). Adapted with permission from Coté and Todres.[6]

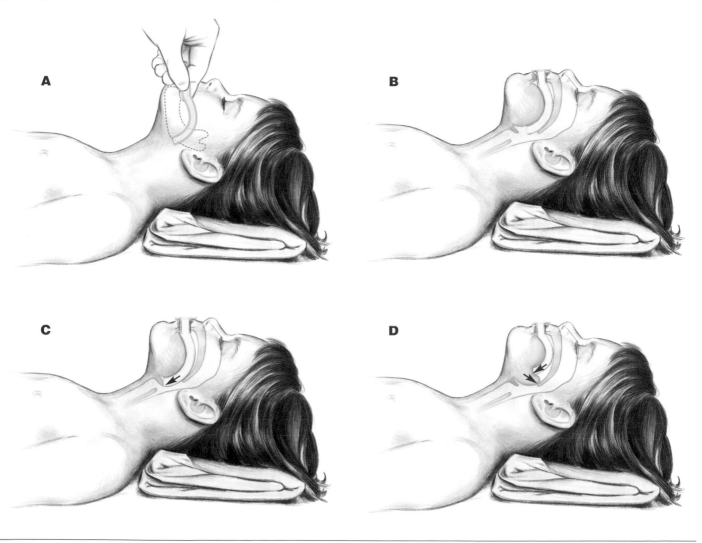

Airway sizes range from 4 to 10 cm in length (Guedel sizes 000 to 4), which should fit children of all ages. The proper size may be estimated by placing the oropharyngeal airway against the side of the face (Figure 7A). With the flange at the corner of the child's mouth, the tip of the airway should reach the angle of the jaw (Figure 7B). If the oropharyngeal airway is too large, it may obstruct the larynx, make a tight mask fit difficult, and traumatize laryngeal structures (Figure 7C). If the oropharyngeal airway is too small or is inserted improperly, it pushes the tongue posteriorly, obstructing the airway (Figure 7D). The oropharyngeal airway should be inserted while a tongue depressor holds the tongue on the floor of the mouth. The head and jaw must be positioned properly to maintain a patent airway even after insertion of an oropharyngeal airway.

Nasopharyngeal Airway

A nasopharyngeal airway is a soft rubber or plastic tube that provides a conduit for airflow between the nares and the pharynx (Figure 8A). Unlike oral airways, nasopharyngeal airways may be used in conscious patients (patients with an intact cough and gag reflex). They also may be useful in children with impaired consciousness or neurologically impaired children with poor pharyngeal tone or coordination leading to upper airway obstruction.

A shortened tracheal tube may be used as a nasopharyngeal airway. A shortened tracheal tube has the advantage of being more rigid; therefore, it maintains the patency of the airway when large adenoids are present. Its rigidity may also be a disadvantage because it is more likely to injure the soft tissues during passage. Nasopharyngeal airways are available in sizes 12F to 36F. A 12F nasopharyngeal airway (approximately the size of a 3-mm tracheal tube) will generally fit the nasopharynx of a full-term infant.

When selecting a nasopharyngeal airway, carefully check the outer diameter. The airway should not be so large that it causes

FIGURE 8. A, Nasopharyngeal airways. A shortened tracheal tube may be substituted (to reduce resistance). **B,** Placement of a nasopharyngeal airway. **C,** Shortened (cut) tracheal tube used as a nasopharyngeal airway. Note that the standard 15-mm adapter must be firmly reinserted into the tracheal tube.

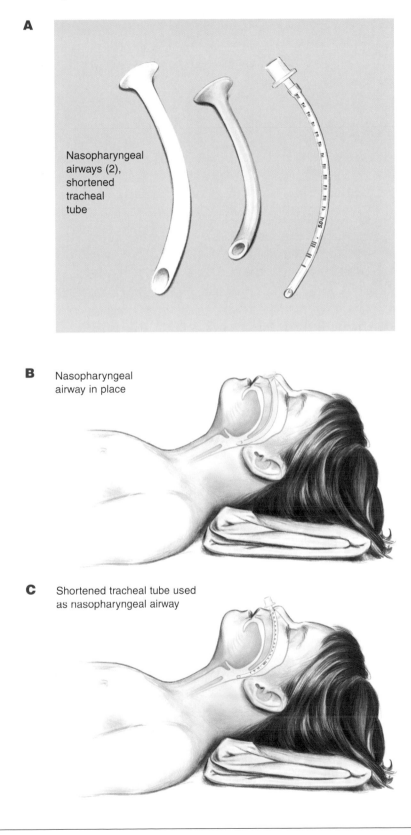

A

Nasopharyngeal airways (2), shortened tracheal tube

B Nasopharyngeal airway in place

C Shortened tracheal tube used as nasopharyngeal airway

sustained blanching of the alae nasi. The proper airway length is approximated by the distance from the tip of the nose to the tragus of the ear. The airway is lubricated and inserted through a nostril in a posterior direction perpendicular to the plane of the face and passed gently along the floor of the nasopharynx (Figure 8B). If passage does not occur readily, attempt passage through the other nostril because patients may have differently sized nasal passages. Insert the airway gently because it can irritate the mucosa or lacerate adenoidal tissue and cause bleeding, which may aggravate airway obstruction and complicate airway management.

Mucus, blood, vomitus, or the soft tissues of the pharynx can obstruct the nasopharyngeal airway, which has a small internal diameter. Frequent evaluation and suctioning of the airway may be necessary to ensure patency. A shortened tracheal tube is unlikely to become obstructed by external compression (Figure 8A). If a shortened tracheal tube is used, a 15-mm adapter must be firmly attached to prevent accidental advancement of the shortened tracheal tube beyond the nares.

If the nasopharyngeal airway is too long, it may cause bradycardia through vagal stimulation, or it may injure the epiglottis or vocal cords. Physical irritation of the larynx or lower pharynx may stimulate coughing, vomiting, or laryngospasm.

Suction Devices

Suctioning of secretions, blood, vomitus, or meconium (in newly born infants) from the oropharynx, nasopharynx, or trachea may be necessary to achieve or maintain a patent airway. Portable suction devices are easy to transport but may not provide adequate suction power. A suction force of −80 to −120 mm Hg is generally necessary. A wall-mounted suction unit should provide a vacuum of more than 300 mm Hg when the tube is clamped at full suction.[34] To avoid airway trauma, the suction device should have an adjustable suction regulator when used in children and intubated patients. Large-bore, non-collapsible suction tubing should always be joined to the suction unit, and semi-rigid pharyngeal tips (tonsil suction tips) and appropriately sized catheters should be available.

Flexible plastic suction catheters are useful for aspiration of thin secretions from the tracheal tube, trachea, nasopharynx, or mouth. Rigid wide-bore suction cannulas (tonsil tips) provide more effective suctioning of the pharynx and are useful for removing thick secretions and particulate matter.

During suctioning monitor the child's heart rate and clinical appearance (see FYI: "Tracheal Tube Suction Technique"). Vagal stimulation with resultant bradycardia may occur from stimulation of the posterior pharynx, larynx, or trachea.

Bag-Mask Ventilation
Ventilation Face Mask

A ventilation face mask allows the rescuer to ventilate and oxygenate a patient. It is used for patients with an oropharyngeal or nasopharyngeal airway or during spontaneous, assisted, or controlled ventilation.

A ventilation mask consists of a rubber or plastic body, a standardized 15-mm/22-mm connecting port, and a rim or face seal. Most disposable masks used for infants and children have a soft, inflatable cuff with a relatively large under-mask volume. In infants and toddlers the under-mask volume should be as low as possible to decrease dead space and minimize rebreathing of exhaled gases. Ideally the mask should be transparent, permitting the rescuer to observe the color of the child's lips and condensation on the mask (indicating exhalation) and to detect regurgitation.

Face masks are available in a variety of sizes. The mask should extend from the

---

FYI: Tracheal Tube Suction Technique

Healthcare providers should use sterile technique during tracheal suctioning to reduce the likelihood of airway contamination. A side opening at the proximal end of the suction catheter is used to control negative pressure. Gently insert the catheter into the tracheal tube just to or slightly (1 to 2 cm) beyond the end of the tube. Insertion of the catheter beyond the tip of the tracheal tube is not recommended because it may injure the tracheal mucosa. Apply suction by occluding the side opening while withdrawing the catheter with a rotating *or* twisting motion.

Suction attempts should not exceed 10 seconds, and they should be preceded and followed by a short period of ventilation with 100% oxygen to avoid hypoxemia. To help remove thick mucus or other material from the airway, 1 or 2 mL of sterile saline may be instilled into the airway before suctioning.

Monitor the child's heart rate and clinical appearance during suctioning. If bradycardia develops or clinical appearance deteriorates, interrupt suctioning and provide ventilation with a high oxygen concentration until the heart rate returns to normal.

FIGURE 9. Proper area of the face for face mask application. Note that no pressure is applied to the eyes.

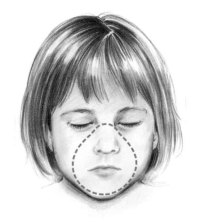

Critical Concepts:
Role of Bag-Mask Ventilation

In most emergency situations where assisted ventilation is required, bag-mask ventilation is the initial treatment of choice. All healthcare providers responsible for providing assisted ventilation should master this technique.

During bag-mask ventilation you must first open the airway and then deliver sufficient volume to make the chest rise visibly. If airway resistance or lung compliance reduces the effectiveness of bag-mask ventilation, use a 2-person procedure if possible. In the 2-person technique, one rescuer uses both hands to open the airway and hold the mask to the face, and the other rescuer squeezes the bag. Both rescuers look for bilateral chest rise (see Chapter 3).

Gastric inflation may complicate bag-mask ventilation. Cricoid pressure (the Sellick maneuver) may be used to limit gastric inflation in *unconscious* patients.

Tracheal intubation should be performed only by properly trained providers.

FIGURE 10. One-handed E-C clamp face mask application technique. **A,** Note that the fingers form an 'E' and lift the jaw (**B**) while avoiding pressure on the soft tissues of the neck that could cause laryngeal/tracheal compression. The mask is held to the face with the thumb and the forefinger forming a 'C.' Modified from Foltin GL, Tunik MG, Cooper A, Markenson D, Treiber M, Phillips R, Karpeles T. *Teaching Resource for Instructors in Prehospital Pediatrics.* New York, NY: Center for Pediatric Emergency Medicine, 1998. Maternal Child Health Bureau, Emergency Medical Services for Children grant.

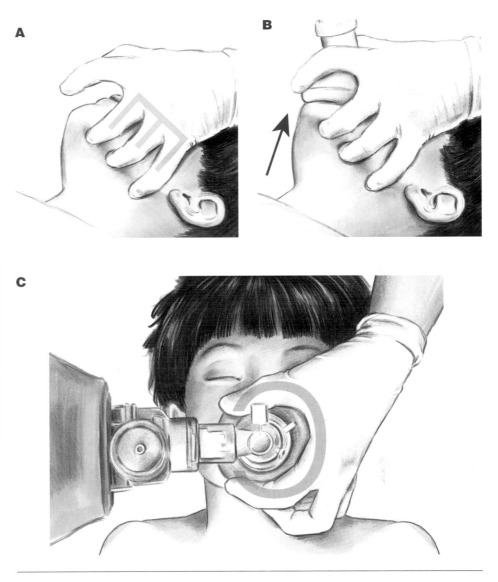

bridge of the nose to the cleft of the chin, enveloping the nose and mouth but avoiding compression of the eyes (Figure 9). The mask should provide an airtight seal. If an airtight seal is not maintained, the inspired oxygen concentration is lowered during spontaneous respiration, and assisted or controlled ventilation cannot be effectively provided.

Bag-Mask Ventilation Technique

Ventilation through a properly placed tracheal tube is the most effective and reliable method of assisted ventilation. This "gold standard" method requires technical skill to successfully and safely place and maintain a tube in the airway.

Intubation may not always be appropriate outside the hospital, depending on factors such as the experience and training of the healthcare providers and the transport time interval. In some EMS systems the success rate for pediatric intubation is relatively low and the complication rate is high.[35] These findings probably reflect the infrequent use of intubation skills by paramedics in a single-tiered system (see Chapter 1). In multitiered EMS systems,

second-tier prehospital providers may have sufficient training and experience to perform intubation safely and effectively.[2] Dedicated critical care or interhospital transport personnel (including helicopter transport personnel) also have a high success rate for tracheal intubation.[36,37]

Anyone providing prehospital BLS care for infants and children should be trained to deliver effective oxygenation and ventilation using the bag-mask technique as the primary method of ventilatory support, particularly if transport time is short. Similarly, in-hospital healthcare providers should master bag-mask ventilation.

To provide bag-mask ventilation, open the airway, seal the mask to the face, and deliver a tidal volume that makes the chest rise. To open the airway and seal the mask to the face in the absence of suspected cervical spine injury, tilt the head back while using 2 or 3 fingers positioned under the angle of the mandible to lift the mandible up and forward, moving the tongue off the posterior pharynx. This technique of opening the airway and sealing the mask to the face is called the E-C clamp technique (Figure 10). The third, fourth, and fifth fingers of one hand (forming an E) are positioned along the jaw to lift it forward; then the thumb and index finger of the same hand (forming a C) hold the mask on the child's face. Avoid pressure underneath the chin (in the submental area) because it can cause airway compression and obstruction.

More effective ventilation can be achieved with 2 persons than with 1 person, and 2-rescuer ventilation may be necessary when there is significant airway obstruction or poor lung compliance.[38] One rescuer uses both hands to open the airway and maintain a tight mask-to-face seal while the other rescuer compresses the ventilation bag (Figure 11). Both rescuers should observe the chest to ensure that the chest rises with each breath.

During bag-mask ventilation it may be necessary to move the head and neck gently through a range of positions to determine the optimum position for airway patency and effectiveness of ventilation. A neutral "sniffing" position without hyperextension of the neck is usually appropriate for infants and toddlers. The sniffing position is achieved by flexing the neck forward while extending the head on the neck. It is achieved by positioning the opening of the external ear canal even with or in front of the shoulder while the head is extended (see Figure 12). Avoid

extreme hyperextension in infants because it may produce airway obstruction. Children older than 2 years may require padding under the occiput to obtain optimal airway patency. In younger children and infants, padding may need to be placed under the torso to prevent excessive flexion of the neck.

If effective ventilation is not achieved (ie, the chest does not rise), reposition the head, ensure that the mask is sealed snugly against the face, lift the jaw, and consider suctioning the airway. Also ensure that the bag and gas source are functioning properly.

In the child with spontaneous ventilatory effort and partial airway obstruction, application of 5 to 10 cm H_2O continuous positive airway pressure (CPAP) by face mask may maintain adequate airway patency and oxygenation without the need for assisted ventilation. This technique requires a tight mask fit and a breathing circuit capable of delivering CPAP.

Inflation of the stomach frequently occurs during assisted or controlled ventilation with a face mask. Gastric inflation is especially likely when assisted or controlled ventilation is provided in the presence of partial airway obstruction or poor lung compliance. It may also occur if an excessive inspiratory flow rate or ventilation pressure is used. Gastric inflation after prolonged bag-mask ventilation can limit effective ventilation,[39] but the inflation can be relieved by placing a nasogastric tube.

Gastric inflation in unconscious or obtunded patients can be minimized by increasing inspiratory time to 1 to 1½ seconds and by delivering just enough tidal volume to make the chest rise. The rescuer must properly pace the rate of ventilation and ensure adequate time for exhalation.[35] To reduce gastric inflation, a second rescuer can apply cricoid pressure (Figure 13) in an *unconscious* victim (ie, a victim without a cough or gag reflex).[40] Cricoid pressure also may prevent regurgitation and aspiration of gastric contents.[41,42]

Cricoid pressure occludes the proximal esophagus by displacing the cricoid

FIGURE 11. Two-rescuer bag-mask ventilation technique may provide more effective ventilation than one-rescuer ventilation when there is significant airway obstruction or poor lung compliance. One rescuer uses both hands to open the airway and maintain a tight mask-to-face seal while the other rescuer compresses the ventilation bag.

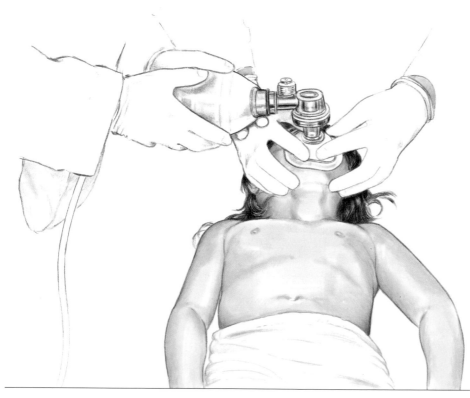

FIGURE 12. Correct positioning of the child more than 2 years of age for ventilation and tracheal intubation. **A,** With the patient on a flat surface (eg, bed or table), the oral (O), pharyngeal (P), and tracheal (T) axes pass through three divergent planes. **B,** A folded sheet or towel placed under the occiput aligns the pharyngeal and tracheal axes. **C,** Extension of the atlanto-occipital joint results in alignment of the oral, pharyngeal, and tracheal axes. Note that proper positioning places the external ear canal anterior to the shoulder. **D,** Incorrect position with neck flexion. **E,** Correct position for infant. Note that the external ear canal is anterior to the shoulder. Reproduced with permission from Coté and Todres.[6]

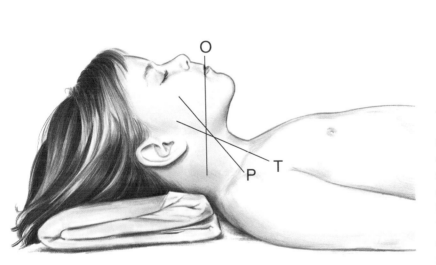

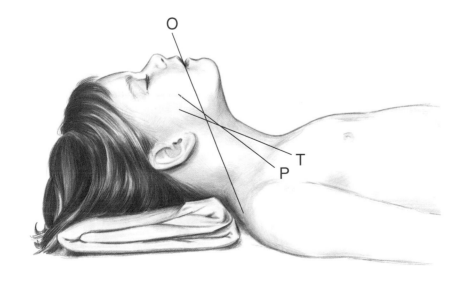

cartilage posteriorly; the esophagus is compressed between the rigid cricoid ring and the cervical spine. The cricoid cartilage is the first tracheal ring, located by palpating the prominent horizontal band inferior to the thyroid cartilage and cricothyroid membrane. Cricoid pressure is applied by a second rescuer using one fingertip in infants and the thumb and index finger in children. Avoid excessive cricoid pressure because it may produce tracheal compression and obstruction or distortion of the upper airway anatomy.[43]

Types of Ventilation Bags (Manual Resuscitators)

There are 2 basic types of manual resuscitators: self-inflating and flow-inflating. Ventilation bags used for resuscitation should be self-inflating and should be available in sizes suitable for the entire pediatric age range, ie, child and adult sizes.

Neonatal (250 mL) ventilation bags may be inadequate to support effective tidal volume and the longer inspiratory times

FIGURE 13. Cricoid pressure (the Sellick maneuver).

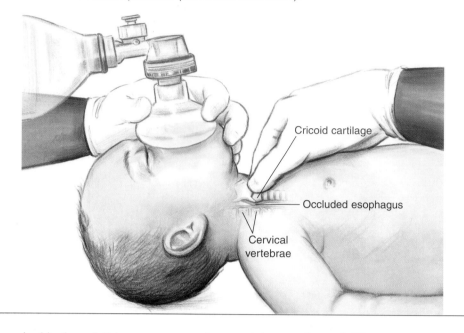

Cricoid cartilage

Occluded esophagus

Cervical vertebrae

bags.[45] *Regardless of the size of the manual resuscitator, you should use only the force and tidal volume necessary to make the chest just visibly rise.*

Excessive ventilation volume and airway pressure may reduce cardiac output by raising the intrathoracic pressure and distending alveoli, increasing afterload of the right heart. In patients with small-airway obstruction (eg, in asthma and bronchiolitis), excessive tidal volume and rate can result in air trapping, barotrauma, air leak, and reduced cardiac output. In head-injured and postarrest patients, excessive ventilation volume and rate may result in hyperventilation and decreased cerebral blood flow and perfusion with adverse effects on neurologic outcome. The routine target of ventilation in postarrest and head-injured patients should be physiologic oxygenation and ventilation (see Chapter 9, "Postarrest Stabilization and Transport").

required by large full-term neonates and infants.[44] For this reason resuscitation bags used for ventilation of full-term newly borns, infants, and children *should have a minimum volume of 450 to 500 mL.* Studies using infant manikins showed that effective infant ventilation can be accomplished using pediatric (and larger) resuscitation

FIGURE 14. Self-inflating manual resuscitator bag with face mask, with (**A** and **B**) and without (**C** and **D**) oxygen reservoir. **A,** Reexpansion of bag *with* oxygen reservoir. When the rescuer's hand releases the bag, oxygen flows into the bag from the oxygen source and from the reservoir, so the concentration of oxygen in the bag remains 100%. **B,** Compression of bag *with* oxygen reservoir delivers 100% oxygen to the patient (purple arrow). Oxygen continuously flows into the reservoir. **C,** Reexpansion of the bag *without* an oxygen reservoir. When the rescuer's hand releases the bag, oxygen flows into the bag from the oxygen source, but ambient air is also entrained into the bag, so the bag becomes filled with a *mixture* of oxygen and ambient air. **D,** Compression of the bag *without* oxygen reservoir delivers oxygen *mixed* with room air (aqua arrow). Note that with both setups exhaled patient air flows into the atmosphere between the mask and the bag (see gray arrows from mask in **A** and **C**).

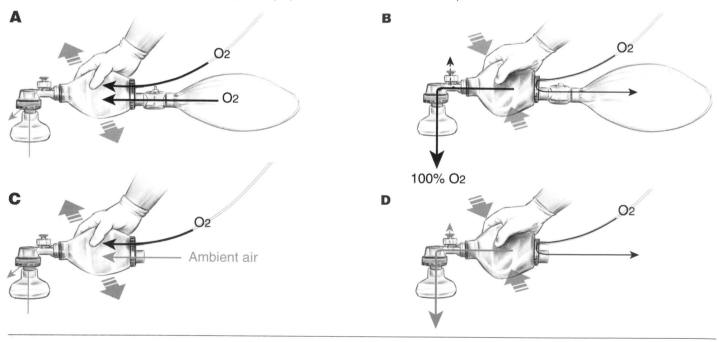

A

O₂

O₂

B

O₂

100% O₂

C

O₂

Ambient air

D

O₂

Self-Inflating Manual Resuscitator Devices

A self-inflating bag-valve device with a face mask provides a rapid means of ventilating a patient in an emergency and does not require an oxygen source.[32] The bag recoil mechanism fills the self inflating bag from a gas source (if available) or from room air. During bag reinflation the gas intake valve opens, and supplemental oxygen, if available (Figure 14A), or room air (Figure 14B) is drawn into the bag. During bag compression the gas intake valve closes, and a second valve opens to permit gas flow to the patient. During patient exhalation the bag outlet valve (nonrebreathing valve) closes, and the patient's exhaled gases are vented to the atmosphere to prevent rebreathing of carbon dioxide. If secretions or vomitus occlude the nonrebreathing valve and interfere with its function, inability to ventilate or rebreathing of carbon dioxide may occur.

As noted, a self-inflating bag-mask device delivers room air (21% oxygen) unless supplemental oxygen is provided. At an oxygen inflow rate of 10 L/min, pediatric self-inflating bag-mask devices without oxygen reservoirs deliver 30% to 80% oxygen to the patient, depending on patient size and minute ventilation.[33] An oxygen reservoir is used to deliver a consistently high oxygen concentration (60% to 95%). A minimum oxygen inflow rate of 10 to 15 L/min is required to maintain adequate oxygen volume in the reservoir.[33] Adult self-inflating bag-mask devices, which have larger reinflating bags, require an oxygen inflow rate of 15 L/min or greater to reliably deliver high oxygen concentrations. High oxygen flow rates may cause some spring-loaded ball or disk outlet valves to chatter or stick. If this occurs, the flow rate should be reduced just until the chattering or sticking is eliminated.

Before you initiate ventilation, confirm that oxygen is flowing into the bag. Listen over the tail of the bag for the sound of oxygen flow, and ensure that the oxygen tubing is correctly attached to an oxygen outlet. If an oxygen tank is used, verify adequate tank pressure. If no flow is heard, confirm that the oxygen flow regulator is turned on. Oxygen flow should also be verified whenever the patient's condition deteriorates.

Many self-inflating bags are equipped with a pressure-limited pop-off valve set at 35 to 45 cm H_2O to prevent barotrauma. Ventilation during CPR may require pressures exceeding these limits. When lung compliance is poor or airway resistance is high, an automatic pop-off valve may result in insufficient tidal volume being delivered, as indicated by inadequate chest expansion.[46] Bags used for resuscitation should have *no pop-off valve* or one that is easily occluded. To occlude the pop-off valve, depress the valve with a finger during ventilation or twist the valve into the closed position. Peak ventilation pressure can be monitored with a manometer placed in line with the bag-mask device.

The bag-mask device must be appropriate for the patient's size and condition so that the operator has a "feel" for the patient's lung compliance. Sudden decreases in lung compliance (ie, increased stiffness during ventilation) may indicate intubation of a main bronchus (usually the right one), an obstructed tracheal tube (caused by secretions, blood, or a kink), or a pneumothorax. Lung overdistension, from excessive inflating pressures, PEEP or high assisted respiratory rates, and short exhalation time, may also cause "stiff lungs" during ventilation.

Self-inflating manual resuscitator devices with a fish-mouth or leaf-flap–operated outlet (nonrebreathing) valve should *not* be used to provide supplemental oxygen during spontaneous ventilation. This valve opens *only* if the bag is squeezed *or* the child's inspiratory effort is significant. Although these valves can open during inspiration, many infants cannot generate the increased inspiratory effort required to open the outlet valve, so they will not inspire the oxygen-enriched gas mixture contained in the bag.

PEEP may be provided during controlled or assisted ventilation by adding a compatible spring-loaded ball or disk or *a magnetic-disk PEEP valve* to the bag-mask outlet. Self-inflating manual resuscitators equipped with PEEP valves should *not* be used to provide CPAP *during spontaneous breathing* because the outlet valve in the bag requires high negative inspiratory pressure to open.

Flow-Inflating (Anesthesia) Ventilation Systems

Flow-inflating ventilation systems[47] consist of a reservoir bag, an overflow port, a fresh gas inflow port, and a standard 15-mm/22-mm connector for mask or tracheal tube connection (Figure 15). The overflow port usually includes an adjustable clamp or valve. The volume of the reservoir bag for infants is 500 mL; for children, 600 to 1000 mL; and for adults, 1500 to 2000 mL.

FIGURE 15. Flow-inflating manual resuscitator.

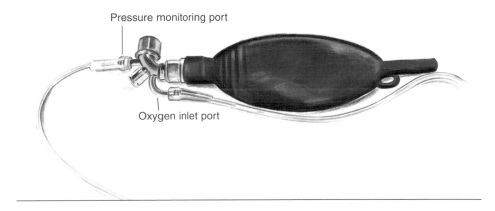

Pressure monitoring port

Oxygen inlet port

Safe and effective ventilation with these devices requires more experience than is needed to use self-inflating manual resuscitators. To achieve ventilation the rescuer must be able to adjust the flow of fresh gas, adjust the outlet control valve, and ensure proper fit of the face mask. For these reasons only trained and experienced persons should use flow-inflating manual resuscitators.[48]

Flow-inflating bags do not contain a non-rebreathing valve, so the composition of inspired gas is determined by fresh gas flow. The only valve in the system is the expiratory or pressure-relief valve, which must be adjusted to maintain gas volume in the reservoir bag yet permit a sufficient oxygen inflow rate to wash out exhaled gases. If the pressure-relief valve offers too much resistance to flow, the bag will become distended, producing high airway pressure and the potential for barotrauma and its complications. If the gas flow is reduced while the pressure-relief valve is too tight, insufficient washout of exhaled gases may result in rebreathing of exhaled air and resultant hypercapnia. In addition, the bag may refill slowly, limiting the rate of ventilation.

If the pressure-relief valve is opened too much, gases will escape from the bag too quickly, and the reservoir bag will collapse when compressed. If the bag collapses, effective ventilation will be impossible until the reservoir refills.

During ventilation with a flow-inflating bag, fresh gas inflow should be adjusted to at least 250 mL/kg per minute. An increase in the fresh gas inflow rate decreases the rebreathing of carbon dioxide and is therefore an effective method of preventing hypercarbia. Use of an inline pressure manometer is recommended as a guide to prevent barotrauma and as a way to monitor breath-by-breath inflation consistency. Effective ventilation, however, is determined by observing the patient for adequate chest movement rather than by reading a pressure manometer.

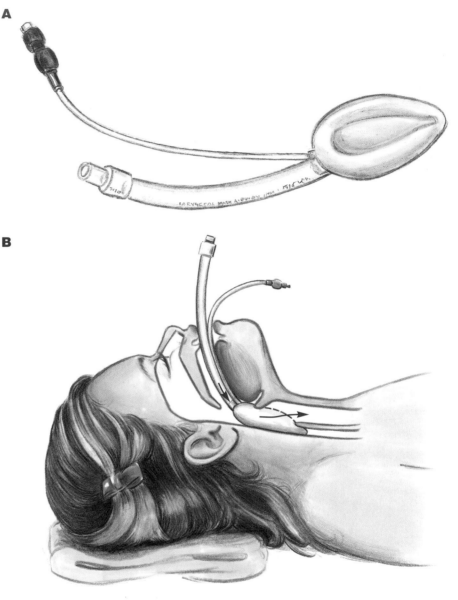

FIGURE 16. Laryngeal mask airway (LMA). The LMA consists of a soft cuff that is deflated before insertion (**A**). After correct insertion, the tip of the LMA is positioned in the esophagus (**B**). The LMA opening is positioned at the glottis. Inflation of the cuff helps secure the tube in the proper position so that air passes through the tube into the trachea.

A

B

Flow-inflating ventilation systems *can* be used to provide supplemental oxygen during spontaneous respiration, even in small infants, because there are no flow valves to be opened during inspiration. In this situation the fresh gas flow rate must be at least three times the patient's minute ventilation, or removal of exhaled CO_2 may be inefficient. In addition, PEEP or CPAP may be provided through this bag by partially closing the adjustable pressure-relief valve until the desired level of PEEP (5 to 10 cm H_2O) is achieved. PEEP or CPAP may be delivered only by using a tight-fitting mask or a tracheal or tracheostomy tube.

Laryngeal Mask Airway

The LMA is a device used to secure the airway in an unconscious patient. It is available in a range of sizes. It consists of a tube with a cuffed, masklike projection at the distal end (Figure 16). The LMA is introduced into the pharynx and advanced until resistance is felt as the tube enters the hypopharynx. The balloon cuff is then inflated, which seals the hypopharynx, leaving the distal opening of the tube just above the glottic opening and providing a clear, secure airway.

LMAs are widely used in the operating room, and they provide an effective means of ventilation and oxygenation. But use of an LMA is contraindicated in an infant or child with an intact gag reflex. LMAs may be useful in patients with facial trauma or abnormal upper airway anatomy, and they have been used successfully for emergency airway control in adults both in and out of hospital.[49,50] They can be placed safely and reliably in infants and children,[51] although proper training and supervision are needed to master the technique.[52,53] Data also suggests that mastering LMA insertion may be easier than mastering tracheal intubation.[54] In one study, for example, nurses were successfully trained to insert an LMA in adults in cardiac arrest.[55] In another study paramedics trained to insert an LMA had a higher success rate for LMA insertion than for tracheal intubation.[56]

Although LMAs do not protect the airway from aspiration of refluxed gastric contents, recent data suggests that aspiration is uncommon when LMAs are used in the operating room[57] and is less common with LMAs than with bag-mask ventilation in adults undergoing in-hospital CPR.[58] In the setting of cardiac or respiratory arrest, LMAs may be an effective alternative for establishing the airway when inserted by *properly trained* healthcare providers. Data comparing LMAs with bag-mask ventilation or tracheal intubation in emergency resuscitation of pediatric patients is limited. Thus, individual provider systems must determine if and when LMAs should be used. Training for healthcare providers in the use of the LMA should not replace training in the use of bag-mask ventilation.

An LMA may be more difficult to maintain during patient movement than a tracheal tube, making it problematic to use during transport. Careful attention is needed to ensure that the position of the LMA is maintained. LMAs are relatively expensive, although they can be reused, and a number of sizes are needed to provide airway support for children of all sizes.

Tracheal Airway

In the past a tracheal tube was called an "endotracheal tube," but the terminology was changed to be consistent with international usage. A tracheostomy tube is also placed in the trachea, but it is inserted through the neck into the trachea. Tracheal tube ventilation is the most effective and reliable method of assisted ventilation for the following reasons:

- The airway is isolated, permitting adequate ventilation and oxygen delivery without inflating the stomach.
- Pulmonary aspiration of gastric contents is reduced.
- Secretions and other debris can be suctioned from the airways.
- Interposition of ventilations with chest compressions can be accomplished efficiently.
- Inspiratory time and peak inspiratory pressures can be controlled.
- PEEP can be delivered if needed.

Indications for tracheal intubation include

- Inadequate control of ventilation by the central nervous system
- Functional or anatomical airway obstruction
- Loss of protective airway reflexes (cough, gag)
- Excessive work of breathing, which may lead to fatigue and respiratory failure
- Need for high peak inspiratory pressure (PIP) to maintain effective alveolar gas exchange
- Need for airway protection and control of ventilation during deep sedation for diagnostic studies
- Potential occurrence of any of the above if patient transport is needed

The Tracheal Tube

The tracheal tube should be sterile, disposable, and constructed of translucent polyvinyl chloride with a radiopaque marker. A tracheal tube of uniform internal diameter is preferable to a tapered tube. A standard 15-mm adapter is firmly affixed to the proximal end for attachment to a ventilating device. The distal end of the tracheal tube may provide an opening in the side wall (Murphy eye) to reduce the risk of atelectasis of the right upper lobe. The Murphy eye also reduces the likelihood of complete tracheal tube obstruction if the end opening is occluded. The tracheal tube should have calibrated marks (in centimeters) to use as reference points during placement and to facilitate detection of unintentional movement of the tube. The tube may also have a vocal cord mark. When this mark is placed at the level of the glottic opening, the tip of the tube should be in the midtrachea (Figure 17).

A *cuffed* tracheal tube should have a low-pressure, high-volume cuff. This tracheal tube is generally indicated for children

FIGURE 17. Tracheal tube with distance markers.

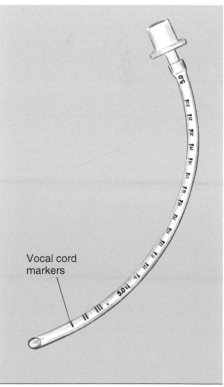

Vocal cord markers

aged 8 to 10 years or older. In children younger than 8 to 10 years, the normal anatomic narrowing at the level of the cricoid cartilage provides a functional "cuff," eliminating the need for a cuffed tracheal tube under most conditions. Small cuffed tracheal tubes are available for younger children who need high inspiratory pressure. For example, a child in respiratory failure due to status asthmaticus or ARDS might benefit from use of a cuffed tracheal tube because the tube would permit use of high ventilatory pressures. Data suggests that use of cuffed tracheal tubes in critically ill children results in complication rates that are no different from those for uncuffed tubes provided cuff pressure is closely monitored.[59,60]

Whether an uncuffed or a cuffed tube is used, if the child has normal airway resistance and lung compliance, an audible air leak should develop when ventilation is delivered to a pressure of 20 to 30 cm H_2O. The absence of an air leak may indicate the following problems:

- The tracheal tube is too large
- The cuff (if present) is inflated excessively
- Laryngospasm is occurring around the tracheal tube

These conditions may lead to excessive pressure on the inner surface of the trachea. Nonetheless, if successful intubation has been difficult to achieve, even a "tight" tracheal tube should be left in place until the patient is stabilized. Moreover, high cuff pressures may be needed to eliminate an air leak when high inflation pressures are required to ensure effective ventilation. As soon as possible, if the patient is improved or stable, replace a tube that is too large or reduce cuff pressure to minimize the risk of airway injury.

If a patient is intubated with an uncuffed tracheal tube that is too small, a large air leak around the tube may prevent adequate ventilation, particularly if the patient has high airway resistance or stiff lungs (poor lung compliance). If a large air leak occurs,

the tracheal tube should be replaced with a larger tube when possible. If the patient is unstable, the rescuer often can provide adequate ventilation by applying cricoid pressure (essentially a Sellick maneuver) to seal the larynx around the tube and by increasing the inspiratory volume to help compensate for the air lost around the tube. Once the patient is adequately oxygenated and ventilated, the tube can be electively replaced.

Although the internal diameter of the tracheal tube may appear to be roughly equivalent to the size of the victim's little finger, estimation of tube size by this method may be difficult and unreliable.[61,62] An alternate method of estimating tube size is based on the child's *body length*, which provides a more accurate estimation of appropriate tracheal tube size than does the child's age.[63] Length-based resuscitation tapes may be helpful in identifying the correct tracheal tube size for children who weigh up to approximately 35 kg

Critical Concepts:
Selection of a Tracheal Tube

Selection and placement of a tracheal tube require assessment of the patient's size and anticipated need for high airway pressures.

- Uncuffed tracheal tubes are generally recommended for children <8 years old.

- Correct tracheal tube size may be estimated by using age-based formulas or body length.

- An appropriately sized tube will permit an audible air leak around the tube when the peak inflation pressure exceeds 20 to 30 cm H_2O.

- Cuffed tracheal tubes may be needed in children with high airway resistance (eg, status asthmaticus) or stiff lungs (eg, pneumonia or ARDS).

(see Critical Concepts: "Selection of a Tracheal Tube").[63]

Several other formulas can be used to estimate the correct tracheal tube size. For example, in children older than 2 years, tracheal tube size (internal diameter [ID] in millimeters) may be estimated as follows:

Uncuffed Tracheal Tube Size (mm ID) =
$$\frac{\text{Age (years)}}{4} + 4$$

If a cuffed tracheal tube is used, the correct size may be approximated using a modification of the previous formula:[60]

Cuffed Tracheal Tube Size (mm ID) =
$$\frac{\text{Age (years)}}{4} + 3$$

All of these strategies only *estimate* proper tube size. Tracheal tubes 0.5 mm smaller and larger than the estimated size should be readily available. After intubation verify the adequacy of tube size and tube position. Recommended tracheal tube sizes are listed in the Table at the end of this chapter.

Most tracheal tubes are inscribed with a vocal cord mark. When this mark is placed at the vocal cords, the tube should be inserted to the proper depth when the child's head is in the neutral position. Formulas may also be used to estimate the proper depth of tube insertion. The proper distance (depth) of insertion in centimeters (from the distal end of the tube to the alveolar ridge of the teeth) for children older than 2 years can be approximated by adding one-half the patient's age to 12:

Depth of Insertion (cm) =
$$\frac{\text{Age (years)}}{2} + 12$$

Use of this formula will generally result in placement of the tip of the tracheal tube above the carina. Alternatively, the distance of insertion (in centimeters) from the distal end of the tube to the lip can be estimated by multiplying the internal diameter of a properly selected tube by 3:

ID = 3.5 mm
Depth of Insertion = 3.5 × 3 = 10.5 cm

The Laryngoscope

The laryngoscope consists of a handle with a battery and a blade with a light source. The blade is used to expose the glottis by moving the tongue laterally, placing the tip of the blade in the vallecula, and lifting the base of the tongue toward the floor of the mouth. If the glottic opening is not exposed by this maneuver, the blade is advanced so that it lifts the epiglottis directly. Adult and pediatric laryngoscope handles fit all blades interchangeably and differ only in diameter and length. The laryngoscope blade may be curved or straight (Figure 18A and 18B). Several sizes are available. A straight blade is preferred for infants and toddlers because it provides better visualization of the relatively cephalad and anterior glottis, but a curved blade is often preferred for older children because its broader base and flange facilitate displacement of the tongue and improve visualization of the glottis.

When combined with proper positioning of the head and neck, laryngoscopy permits a straight visual path through the mouth and pharynx to the larynx. When this path has been established, you can pass a tracheal tube for tracheal intubation, a suction catheter for suctioning, or Magill forceps for extraction of foreign material.

Preparation for Intubation

Elective or planned intubation is preferable to urgent intubation. Before elective intubation, assemble the appropriate intubation and monitoring equipment and personnel (see Critical Concepts: "Intubation Equipment").

If the child has a perfusing rhythm, administer supplementary oxygen before tracheal intubation. Assist ventilation only if the patient's effort is inadequate. If rapid sequence intubation (RSI) is planned (see Chapter 14, "Rapid Sequence Intubation"), avoid assisted (bag-mask) ventilation if possible because it may inflate the stomach and increase the risk of vomiting and aspiration. If trauma to the head and neck or multiple trauma is present, immobilize the cervical spine during intubation.

If the child is in cardiac arrest, perform intubation immediately without stopping to apply physiologic monitors. In virtually all other circumstances, continuously monitor the heart rate and (if possible) oxygen saturation by pulse oximetry during the procedure (see Critical Concepts: "Preparation for Intubation").

The laryngoscope and suction equipment should be checked *before* laryngoscopy to ensure that they are in working order. To attach the blade to the handle, insert its U-shaped indentation onto the small bar at the end of the handle. After the indentation is aligned with the bar, press the blade forward, clip it onto the bar, and elevate it until it snaps into position perpendicular to the handle (Figure 18C). If the light on the flange of the blade is dim, flickers, or does not illuminate, the blade may be improperly seated on the handle or the bulb or batteries (encased in the handle) may be faulty.

During intubation of patients with a perfusing rhythm, monitoring with a pulse oximeter whenever possible is highly recommended. Continuous evaluation of oxygen saturation is especially important if the bradycardic response to hypoxemia has been blunted by atropine.

FIGURE 18. Laryngoscope blades. **A,** Curved blade. **B,** Straight blade. **C,** Attachment of laryngoscope blade to handle.

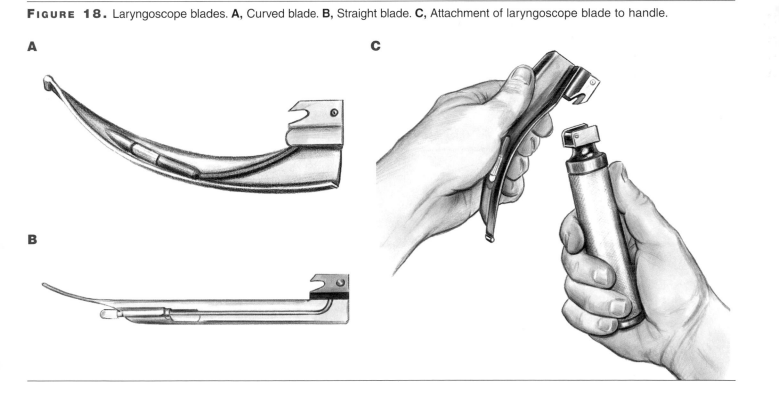

Before attempting intubation, assemble the following equipment:

- A cardiorespiratory monitor and pulse oximeter. These devices should be applied before intubation to patients with a perfusing rhythm.

- A tonsil-tipped suction device or a large-bore suction catheter attached to a suction machine.

- A suction catheter of appropriate size that will fit into the tracheal tube.

- A properly functioning manual resuscitator and oxygen source and an appropriately sized face mask.

- A stylet to provide rigidity to the tracheal tube and to help guide it through and beyond the vocal cords. If a stylet is used, place the tip 1 to 2 cm proximal to the distal end of the tracheal tube to prevent trauma to the trachea. A sterile, water-soluble lubricant may be helpful to moisten the stylet and aid its removal from the tracheal tube after successful placement.

- Three tracheal tubes: 1 tube of the estimated required size and tubes 0.5 mm smaller and 0.5 mm larger.

- A laryngoscope blade and handle with a functioning bright light.

- Tape to secure the tube and gauze to dry the face. Consider using an adhesive solution to secure the tube to the face if using tape, or use a tracheal tube holder.

- An exhaled CO_2 detector (capnography or colorimetric device) or, in older children and adolescents, an esophageal tube detector.

Atropine can minimize the unfavorable responses (bradycardia and asystole) to vagal stimulation resulting from laryngoscopy, hypoxia, or succinylcholine administration. Anticholinergics decrease oral secretions, making it easier to visualize landmarks during intubation. Anticholinergics are indicated for infants less than 1 year of age, children from 1 to 5 years of age receiving succinylcholine, and the unusual older child or adolescent who receives a second dose of succinylcholine because of inability to successfully intubate after the initial dose.[64]

Anticholinergics should be considered for any child who is bradycardic at the time of intubation. Anticholinergics also should be considered when ketamine is used to prevent increased oral secretions associated with administration of this agent. The atropine dose is 0.01 to 0.02 mg/kg IV (maximum single dose: 1 mg; minimum single dose: 0.1 mg) given 1 to 2 minutes before intubation. When given IM, a dose of 0.04 mg/kg is used. For more information see Chapter 14, "Rapid Sequence Intubation."

The most common side effect of anticholinergics is tachycardia. Anticholinergics block the bradycardic response to hypoxia, so continuous pulse oximetry is strongly recommended.[64] If the patient is apneic or in cardiac arrest, intubation should proceed without atropine if its administration would delay intubation.

The Intubation Technique

To directly visualize the glottis, the axes of the mouth, pharynx, and trachea must be aligned (see Figure 12). Use manual cervical stabilization to maintain a neutral position if cervical spine injury is suspected.

In children older than 2 years without suspected cervical spine trauma, anterior displacement of the neck or cervical spine and simultaneous extension of the neck (ie, lifting the chin into the sniffing position) can be facilitated by placing the child's head on a small pillow.[65]

Before intubation open the child's airway and provide oxygen if the child is spontaneously breathing. If the child is not breathing, provide bag-mask ventilation before you attempt intubation.

- Monitor the heart rate and oxygen saturation (pulse oximetry) before you attempt intubation *unless* the patient is in cardiac arrest. In cardiac arrest and cardiopulmonary failure there is no pulse, so monitoring with pulse oximetry is impossible.

- Check the intubation equipment (ie, laryngoscope, cuff on tracheal tube, suction device, bag-mask device) before you begin intubation.

- Follow universal precautions to reduce the risk of infection.

Infants and toddlers younger than 2 years should be placed on a flat surface with the chin lifted into the sniffing position for intubation.[65] These young patients do not require anterior displacement of the neck because such displacement occurs naturally when the relatively prominent occiput is placed on a flat surface with the child supine. Because the prominent occiput of the infant or toddler may cause neck flexion, you may need to place a small pillow or blanket under the patient's torso to achieve proper alignment of the mouth, pharynx, and trachea. For all patients appropriate alignment of the head and neck is typically achieved when the opening of the ear canal is above or just even with the top of the shoulder when you look at the patient from the side (Figure 12). When the head and neck are in correct alignment, the child looks as if he is putting his head forward to sniff a flower.

Intubation attempts should be brief. Attempts lasting longer than 30 seconds may produce profound hypoxemia, especially in infants, whose small lung volumes and increased oxygen requirements rapidly consume oxygen reserves. An intubation attempt is generally interrupted if significant hypoxemia, cyanosis, pallor, or a decreased heart rate develops. But if the patient is unstable and difficult to oxygenate or ventilate by bag-mask, the clinician may judge that the need to achieve airway control supersedes the need to correct a transient fall in oxygenation or heart rate during the intubation. In this situation intubation is probably best performed or closely supervised by the most skilled provider. If intubation is interrupted, immediately ventilate the patient with 100% oxygen using a mask and manual resuscitator to improve heart rate and oxygenation before you reattempt intubation.

Orotracheal intubation is preferred during resuscitation because it can be performed more rapidly than nasotracheal intubation. Hold the laryngoscope handle in your left hand, and insert the blade into the mouth in the midline, following the natural contour of the pharynx to the base of the tongue (Figures 19 and 20). Once the

FIGURE 20. A, Introduction of the laryngoscope. **B,** Operator's view of the anatomy with landmarks.

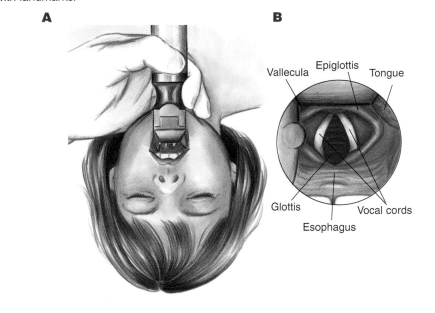

tip of the blade is at the base of the tongue (in the vallecula: the space between the epiglottis and the base of the tongue) and the epiglottis is seen, move the proximal end of the blade to the right side of the mouth and then sweep the tongue toward the middle to achieve control of the tongue.

An alternative way to achieve control of the tongue is to insert the blade along the right side of the mouth to the base of the tongue. Once you see the epiglottis, sweep the proximal end of the blade and the handle to the midline. This movement toward the midline provides a channel in

FIGURE 19. Position of laryngoscope blade when using (**A**) a straight blade and (**B**) a curved blade. Note that a straight blade may often be used in the same manner as a curved blade (ie, the tip of the blade can be placed in the vallecula).

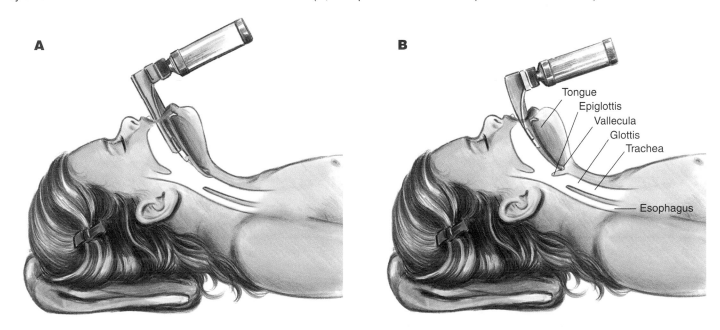

the right third of the mouth to pass the tracheal tube while maintaining direct visualization of the laryngeal structures.

The risk of laryngeal trauma is increased if the blade is initially inserted into the esophagus and then slowly withdrawn to visualize the glottis. Avoid this practice.

Either a straight or a curved blade may be used for intubation of children. Ideally with a straight blade the tip of the blade is used to lift the epiglottis and visualize the glottic opening (Figure 19A). The tip of a curved blade is inserted into the vallecula to displace the tongue anteriorly (Figure 19B). After the blade is properly positioned, traction is exerted *upward* in the direction of the long axis of the handle to displace the base of the tongue and the epiglottis anteriorly, exposing the glottis. The handle and blade *must not* be used for prying or levering, nor should the upper gums or teeth be used as a fulcrum. These practices may damage the teeth and reduce the ability to visualize the larynx.

To avoid visual obstruction of the glottic opening by the tracheal tube, insert the tracheal tube from the right corner of the mouth, not down the barrel of the laryngoscope blade. The rescuer should see the tracheal tube pass through the glottic opening. Having an assistant displace the right corner of the mouth often improves visualization of passage of the tube. In addition, application of cricoid pressure by an assistant may facilitate visualization of the glottic opening. The black glottic marker of the tube is placed at the level of the vocal cords; this position places the tip of the tracheal tube in the midtrachea. Cuffed tracheal tubes are inserted until the cuff is positioned just below the vocal cords.

Confirmation of Tracheal Tube Placement

Once the tube is inserted, confirm its position using both primary and secondary confirmation techniques (see Critical Concepts: "Primary and Secondary Confirmation of Tracheal Tube Placement"). Although no

Critical Concepts:
Primary and Secondary Confirmation of Tracheal Tube Placement

During intubation the provider should see the tube passing through the cords and should place the vocal cord (glottic) mark on the tube at the level of the vocal cords. After the tube is inserted, provide positive-pressure ventilation and perform a clinical evaluation (primary assessment) to confirm proper tube position. This *primary confirmation* includes the following steps:

- Look for chest rise (symmetric* bilateral chest rise during positive-pressure ventilation).

- Look for water vapor in the tracheal tube during exhalation. The presence of water vapor is encouraging, but it does *not* definitively confirm tracheal tube position.[66]

- Listen for breath sounds over the peripheral lung fields (equal* bilateral breath sounds confirmed by listening over axillae).

- Listen for breath sounds over the upper abdomen (if the tube is in the trachea, breath sounds should be virtually absent over the upper abdomen).[67]

Symmetry and equality of breath sounds after tracheal intubation may be affected by the patient's underlying disease or injury. If breath sounds are asymmetric before intubation (eg, as the result of a pleural effusion or pneumothorax), the findings of the preintubation examination should serve as the baseline for comparison after intubation.

Secondary confirmation of tracheal tube position involves evaluation of exhaled CO_2 and oxygenation.

- Look for evidence of exhaled CO_2. If the tube is in the *trachea* of a child who weighs more than 2 kg and has a perfusing cardiac rhythm, exhaled CO_2 should be detected within 6 manual breaths (see "Exhaled or End-Tidal CO_2 Monitoring" later in this chapter).

- *Note:* If a child is in cardiac arrest, exhaled CO_2 may not be detected despite correct placement of the tracheal tube. In cardiac arrest, cardiac output is so low that little CO_2 is delivered to the lungs and exhaled. Observation of a consistent color change, however, confirms tracheal tube placement.

- If the tube is in the *esophagus*, exhaled CO_2 will not be detected after 6 positive-pressure breaths. These 6 breaths eliminate any exhaled gas that might have been forced into the stomach during bag-mask ventilation before intubation.

- Look for improvement in or sustained excellent oxygen saturation. In a patient monitored by continuous pulse oximetry, oxygen saturation typically increases or remains excellent after successful tracheal intubation and ventilation with 100% oxygen (unless the child has a severe compromise in oxygen diffusion or a severe ventilation-perfusion mismatch).

If there is any doubt about tracheal position of the tube, use the laryngoscope to verify tube position by visualizing the tube passing through the glottic opening.

confirmation method is 100% reliable, the use of primary and secondary confirmation techniques reduces the risk of undetected tube misplacement or displacement. Providers should confirm tracheal tube placement immediately after tube insertion, during patient transport, after the patient is moved (eg, from a gurney to a hospital bed), and whenever the patient's condition deteriorates.

Several points about the use of supplemental respiratory monitoring devices to confirm tracheal tube position after intubation deserve emphasis[68]:

■ No single confirmation technique is 100% reliable under all circumstances.

■ Always use a device to confirm tracheal tube placement in the patient with a perfusing rhythm. Confirmation is highly recommended in the patient in cardiac arrest because physical examination alone is unreliable.

■ If the infant or child has a perfusing rhythm, exhaled CO_2 detection is the best method (most sensitive and specific) for verification of tube placement (see "Exhaled or End-Tidal CO_2 Monitoring to Confirm Tracheal Tube Placement," in the next section).

■ Once tracheal placement is confirmed, secure the tube and record the tube position at the level of the lip or teeth.

■ Repeated confirmation of tracheal tube position or continuous monitoring of exhaled CO_2 is highly recommended during stabilization and transport out-of-hospital or in-hospital.

Exhaled or End-Tidal CO_2 Monitoring to Confirm Tracheal Tube Placement

Because *clinical* confirmation of tracheal tube placement may be unreliable, use of exhaled CO_2 (either with a colorimetric device or continuous capnography) is recommended to confirm tube placement in all patients who weigh >2 kg and have a perfusing rhythm. *These devices are very sensitive and specific for confirming tracheal tube placement if the patient has a perfusing rhythm.* If no CO_2 is detected, the tube is not in the trachea. If CO_2 *is* detected, the tube *is* in the trachea (see Critical Concepts: "Primary and Secondary Confirmation of Tracheal Tube Placement"). In patients with a perfusing cardiac rhythm, a positive color change or the presence of a capnography waveform showing exhaled CO_2 after 6 ventilations confirms tube position in the trachea.[69,70] Six ventilations are recommended to wash out CO_2 that may be present in the stomach and esophagus after bag-mask ventilation. After 6 ventilations, any detected CO_2 can be assumed to come from the trachea because there is negligible CO_2 in the air or in the stomach.

Note that although detection of exhaled CO_2 indicates the tube is in the trachea, it does *not* confirm that the tube is in the *ideal position* in the trachea. For example, exhaled CO_2 may be detected with intubation of the right main bronchus. For this reason use of exhaled CO_2 does *not* replace the need to document proper tube position in the trachea by clinical examination and a postintubation chest x-ray.

An adult-sized colorimetric end-tidal CO_2 detector will add a large amount of dead space to a child's ventilator circuit. If child-sized colorimetric devices are unavailable, an adult-sized device should be used intermittently to confirm tracheal tube placement, but the device should probably not remain attached to the circuit.

Although detection of exhaled CO_2 in patients *with a perfusing rhythm* is both specific and sensitive for tube placement in the trachea, exhaled CO_2 detection is not as reliable for confirmation of tube placement in patients *in cardiac arrest*. In patients with cardiac arrest, a positive color change or exhaled CO_2 waveform will reliably confirm tracheal tube placement. *But the absence of detectable CO_2 does not confirm esophageal tube placement* (ie, it will not rule out tracheal tube placement). This failure to detect CO_2 despite tracheal tube placement occurs because patients in cardiac arrest often have limited pulmonary blood flow and therefore undetectable exhaled CO_2 (see Figure 5).[69,71] In cardiac arrest the absence of detectable exhaled CO_2 may indicate either esophageal or tracheal tube placement (see FYI: "Use of Exhaled CO_2 in Cardiac Arrest").[71-73] If placement is uncertain, tube position must be confirmed by clinical examination and direct laryngeal examination.

In addition to cardiac arrest, other conditions causing very low exhaled CO_2 also may produce misleading exhaled CO_2 results. Clinical experience in adults, for example, suggests that severe airway obstruction (eg, status asthmaticus) and pulmonary edema may impair CO_2 elimination sufficiently to cause a false-negative test result.[72,74] If the colorimetric detector is contaminated with acidic gastric contents or acidic drugs, such as tracheally administered epinephrine, the *results* may be unreliable. You should suspect contamination of the detector if it remains yellow during the entire respiratory cycle. Finally, administration of an IV bolus of epinephrine in cardiac arrest patients may transiently reduce pulmonary blood flow and thus reduce exhaled CO_2 below the limits of detection.[75]

Monitoring of exhaled CO_2 may be useful in children with a right-to-left pulmonary shunt because any therapeutic maneuver that increases effective pulmonary blood flow in this setting (eg, use of inhaled nitric oxide in children with reactive pulmonary vascular beds) increases exhaled CO_2 concentration. In other conditions exhaled CO_2 is affected by respiratory function rather than pulmonary blood flow. For example, patients with severe small-airway obstruction (eg, status asthmaticus) or pulmonary edema interfering with gas exchange at the alveolus (eg, ARDS) may have exhaled CO_2 concentrations below the limits of detection.

Esophageal Detector Devices

The use of esophageal detector devices to confirm tracheal tube placement is based on the assumption that you can readily aspirate air from the cartilage-supported trachea by drawing from gas in the lower airways. In contrast, if the tracheal tube is placed in the esophagus, the walls of the esophagus collapse when aspiration is attempted with an esophageal detector device, preventing filling of the syringe or self-inflating rubber bulb.[73] In adults the esophageal detector device is very sensitive in identifying esophageal tube placement when used in emergency intubations in patients with or without a perfusing rhythm.[86-88] In adults with cardiac arrest, the esophageal detector device can be used to supplement the potentially misleading information provided by the exhaled CO_2 detector to confirm tracheal tube placement.[88]

Although an esophageal detector device has been used successfully in a small number of normal children,[89] it appears to be unreliable in infants <1 year of age.[90] It is also unreliable in morbidly obese patients[91] and patients in the late stages of pregnancy.[92] In summary, there is insufficient data in infants and children to recommend routine use of an esophageal detector device. The device may be used reliably in adolescents, especially adolescents *in cardiac arrest*, because exhaled CO_2 detection is less reliable for confirming tracheal tube position in cardiac arrest.

Confirming Tracheal Tube Placement When Findings Are Equivocal

As noted above, in low-cardiac-output states and cardiac arrest, tracheal (exhaled)

CO_2 levels may be minimal, especially in infants.[72,93] If exhaled CO_2 is not detected and other clinical findings are equivocal, or if epigastric distention occurs during positive-pressure ventilation via the tube, esophageal intubation should be suspected. When esophageal placement is strongly suspected, remove the tracheal tube and maintain ventilation with a bag-mask device. If tube placement is uncertain, direct visualization of the tube's position using a laryngoscope is recommended.

If chest movement or breath sounds are asymmetrical, particularly if breath sounds are heard only over the right lung, intubation of the right or left main bronchus should be suspected (see Foundation Facts: "Trouble Shooting When Lung Expansion Is Inadequate"). The tracheal tube should be withdrawn until equal breath sounds are heard bilaterally and chest expansion is symmetric. Confirm proper position of the tracheal tube by chest x-ray as soon as possible.

Securing the Tracheal Tube

Once the tracheal tube is placed and secured, maintain the patient's head in a neutral position. Excessive head movement may displace the tube. Flexion of the head or neck moves the tube farther into the airway, and extension of the head displaces the tube farther out of the airway.[94,95] In a responsive patient, placement of an oral airway adjacent to the tracheal tube, but not deeply enough into the oropharynx to stimulate a gag reflex, prevents the child from biting down on the tube and obstructing the airway.

After intubation secure the tracheal tube to the patient's face with adhesive (eg, tincture of benzoin) and tape to prevent unintentional extubation. During active CPR it is difficult to tape the tube in place; therefore, the tube must be held securely and its position reconfirmed at regular intervals. If spontaneous circulation is restored, listen for equal breath sounds before you tape the tracheal tube in place. Exhaled CO_2 detection is also useful to confirm tracheal tube position

FYI: Use of Exhaled CO_2 in Cardiac Arrest

Although the absence of detected exhaled CO_2 may not confirm esophageal tube placement in cardiac arrest, the absence of exhaled CO_2 *may* provide prognostic information in this setting. Experience in animals[76] and adults[77-79] shows that absent or low detectable exhaled CO_2 during cardiac arrest correlates with poor outcome. In addition, efforts that improve closed-chest compressions increase exhaled CO_2.[80,81] This finding is consistent with data correlating cardiac output with exhaled CO_2 concentration.[82,83]

Data relating exhaled CO_2 to outcome in pediatric cardiac arrest is limited,[71] and animal data emphasizes the need to evaluate the concentration of exhaled CO_2 after providing several minutes of adequate ventilation in asphyxial arrests because the initial values will be elevated.[84,85] Because the data is limited, no recommendation can be made about the use of exhaled CO_2 to *predict outcome* in children with cardiac arrest.

The mechanisms producing low exhaled CO_2 are summarized in Figure 5. During

cardiac arrest global and pulmonary blood flow are greatly reduced. Carbon dioxide accumulates in venous blood during low-flow states, particularly in cardiac arrest.[25] At the same time, during resuscitation alveolar ventilation is high relative to alveolar capillary blood flow, resulting in low alveolar carbon dioxide concentrations as alveolar CO_2 is washed out and not replaced by CO_2 brought by pulmonary blood flow into the lungs. Pulmonary venous and systemic arterial blood contain low concentrations of CO_2 because ventilation is often excessive during resuscitation.

If more effective chest compressions or a return of spontaneous circulation increases pulmonary (and thus alveolar capillary) blood flow, high concentrations of CO_2 will be delivered to the alveolus and will be detected in the exhaled gas. Conversely, if anything compromises cardiac output, delivery of CO_2 to the alveolus will fall and exhaled CO_2 may fall below the limits of detection.

TABLE. Guidelines for Laryngoscope, Tracheal Tube, and Suction Catheter Sizes

Age of Patient	Laryngoscope	Internal Diameter of Tracheal Tube (mm)*	Distance From Midtrachea to Lips or Gums (cm)*	Suction Catheter (F)*
		$\dfrac{\text{Age (years)}}{4} + 4$	<44 weeks gestational age: 6 + Weight (kg) >44 weeks gestational age: 3 × TT size	2 × TT size
Preterm infant	Miller 0†	2.5, 3.0 uncuffed	8	5-6
Term infant	Miller 0-1† Wis-Hipple 1 Robertshaw 0	3.0, 3.5 uncuffed	9-10	6-8
6 months		3.5, 4.0 uncuffed	10.5-12	8
1 year	Miller 1 Wis-Hipple 1½ Robertshaw 1	4.0, 4.5 uncuffed	12-13.5	8
2 years	Miller 2 Macintosh 2 Flagg 2	4.5 uncuffed 4.0 cuffed	13.5	8
4 years		5.0, 5.5 uncuffed 4.5 cuffed	15	10
6 years		5.5 uncuffed 5.0 cuffed	16.5	10
8 years	Miller 2 Macintosh 2	6.0 cuffed	18	12
10 years		6.5 cuffed	19.5	12
12 years	Macintosh 3	7.0 cuffed	21	12
Adolescent	Macintosh 3 Miller 3	7.0, 8.0 cuffed	21	12

*Formulas provide estimates of appropriate tracheal tube size, the tracheal tube distance marker that is aligned with the lip when the tube is at the proper depth, and appropriate suction catheter size. A tracheal tube 0.5 mm larger and one 0.5 mm smaller than the estimated size should be readily available. TT indicates tracheal tube size (in mm).

†Oxyscope modifications are available for Miller 0 and 1 blades. These devices may reduce the likelihood of hypoxemia during laryngoscopy in infants.

before taping. The distance marker at the lips should be noted in the medical record to allow detection of unintentional tracheal tube displacement (see the Table for distance from midtrachea to teeth).

Managing Airway and Ventilation Emergencies

Causes of Acute Deterioration in Intubated Patients

Intubated patients are at risk for a variety of problems that may result in life-threatening loss of artificial airway function, including loss of oxygen supply, occlusion or kinking of the airway, and displacement of the airway. Precautions must be taken to reduce the probability of such events, and patients must be monitored carefully to enable early detection and prompt correction of these events.

When respiratory distress develops in the patient with an artificial airway, the first priority is rapid assessment of the patient's status. Evaluate the adequacy of air exchange and oxygenation by observation of chest expansion, use of noninvasive monitoring devices (eg, pulse oximeter or exhaled CO_2 monitor), and auscultation over both axillae of the chest and over the stomach. Heart rate should be appropriate for age and clinical condition. This assessment will determine the urgency of the required response. If tracheal tube position remains uncertain, direct visualization of the tube passing through the glottis is advised.

If the condition of an intubated patient deteriorates, consider the possible causes, which can be recalled by the mnemonic "**DOPE**": **D**isplacement of the tube from the trachea, **O**bstruction of the tube, **P**neumothorax, and **E**quipment failure (see Critical Concepts: "Causes of Inadequate Improvement or Acute Deterioration in the Intubated Patient"). Evaluate tracheal tube position by visual inspection and auscultation. If the patient is mechanically ventilated, temporarily disconnect the patient from the ventilator circuit and provide *manual ventilation* with a resuscitation bag. Carefully auscultate the lung fields during manual ventilation and try to determine a "feeling" for increased resistance while squeezing the resuscitation bag. These assessments will aid in the assessment of airway patency and tube position. If breath sounds are poor and there is no movement of the chest with manual inflation, the tracheal tube may be displaced from the trachea or obstructed (in which case there will be high resistance to manual inflation). A tension pneumothorax may also be present (see "Tension Pneumothorax," below).

If the tracheal tube is obstructed, attempt to clear the obstruction by instilling saline into the trachea and suctioning the tube with a catheter. Pass the suction catheter just beyond the distal end of the tube. After suctioning, resume manual ventilation and reassess breath sounds, airway resistance, and adequacy of chest movement. If the tracheal tube appears to be properly positioned and adequate ventilation is achieved with manual inflation, the problem may be located in the ventilator or the ventilator circuit. Manually ventilate the patient until the problem is identified and corrected.

If the tracheal tube is occluded and suctioning does not restore patency, you *must* remove and replace the tracheal tube. Reintubation should be a semielective procedure except in rare situations in which

---

Foundation Facts:
Troubleshooting When Lung Expansion Is Inadequate

If the tube is properly placed within the trachea but lung expansion is inadequate, or if inadequate oxygenation or ventilation is documented by pulse oximetry, end-tidal CO_2 monitoring, or arterial blood gas analysis, consider one of the following problems:

- The tracheal tube is too small, producing a large air leak. Replacement of the tube with a larger one may be necessary. In circumstances where high airway pressures are needed, a cuffed tracheal tube may be used safely in young children.[59] When a cuffed tracheal tube is used, the cuff should be inflated just until the air leak disappears.

- The pop-off valve on the resuscitation bag is open and ventilations are escaping into the atmosphere. This problem is most likely to occur when the child's lung compliance is poor (eg, submersion or pulmonary edema[46]) or when airway resistance is high (eg, bronchiolitis or asthma). An increase in inflation and cuff pressures may be required to achieve effective ventilation in these patients.

- A leak is present at any of several connections in the bag-mask device. Leaks may be detected by separating the bag-mask device from the patient and occluding the tracheal connection while compressing the bag. No air should leak from the bag during compression.

- The operator is providing inadequate tidal volume. This problem is easily confirmed by delivering a larger volume breath while observing the chest wall for movement and listening for breath sounds.

- Miscellaneous causes of inadequate lung expansion or lung collapse (pneumothorax, hemothorax, obstruction of tracheal tube, etc).

After you tape the tube, confirm its position within the trachea by chest x-ray because transmitted breath sounds may be heard over the left hemithorax despite intubation of the right main bronchus. In addition, if the tube is located high in the trachea, the tube may become dislodged.

ventilation cannot be achieved with a bag and mask.

If tracheal tube position and patency are confirmed and mechanical ventilation failure and pneumothorax are ruled out, it is possible that the patient's agitation, excessive movement, or pain is interfering with adequate ventilation. If so, the patient may require analgesia for pain control (eg, fentanyl or morphine) or sedation to treat confusion, anxiety, or agitation (eg, lorazepam, midazolam, or ketamine). Occasionally neuromuscular blocking agents combined with analgesia or sedation are needed to optimize ventilation and minimize the risk of barotrauma or accidental tube dislodgment. In the hospital continuous capnography is helpful in mechanically ventilated patients to avoid hypoventilation or hyperventilation, which may occur inadvertently during intrahospital transport and diagnostic procedures.[96]

The management of obstructed tracheostomy tubes is similar to that used for obstructed tracheal tubes. If the tube is completely occluded and ventilation cannot be accomplished, the tube should be immediately removed and replaced with a new tube. If replacement is impossible, the patient must be ventilated by bag and mask or intubated orally (see Chapter 11, "Care of the Child With Special Healthcare Needs").

Tension Pneumothorax

Tension pneumothorax may complicate trauma or positive-pressure ventilation. The presence of a pneumothorax should be suspected in the victim of blunt chest trauma or in any intubated patient who deteriorates suddenly during positive-pressure ventilation (including overzealous ventilation by bag and mask). Because the tracheal tube tends to enter the *right* main bronchus if displaced too far into the airway, a tension pneumothorax most frequently occurs on the *right* side. As pressure increases within the chest, it directly impedes venous return to the heart. Venous return is further impaired by a shift of the mediastinum, resulting in mechanical obstruction in venous return by distortion of the great veins.

Tension pneumothorax is indicated by signs of low cardiac output and the following clinical signs: severe respiratory distress, hyperresonance to chest percussion, diminished breath sounds on the affected side, and deviation of the trachea and mediastinal structures away from the affected side. Keep in mind that only some of these signs may be present in a patient with a tension pneumothorax.

Treatment of a tension pneumothorax consists of immediate needle decompression without a confirmatory chest x-ray because delay can be fatal. An 18- to 20-gauge over-the-needle catheter is inserted through the second intercostal space, over the top of the third rib, in the midclavicular line. A gush of air will be heard after successful needle decompression. A chest tube should be placed as soon as feasible.

Critical Concepts:
Causes of Inadequate Improvement or Acute Deterioration in the Intubated Patient

Causes of inadequate improvement following intubation:

- Inadequate tidal volume
- Excessive leak around the tracheal tube
- Air trapping and impaired cardiac output due to excessive tidal volume or respiratory rate
- Failure to compress the pop-off valve on the manual resuscitator
- Leak or disconnection in the manual resuscitator or ventilator system
- "DOPE" (see below)
- Inadequate PEEP
- Inadequate O_2 flow from gas source

Sudden deterioration in an intubated patient may be caused by one of the following complications, which can be recalled using the mnemonic **DOPE**:

- **D**isplacement of the tracheal tube. The tube may be displaced out of the trachea or beyond the carina into a bronchus.
- **O**bstruction of the tracheal tube. Obstruction may be caused by secretions, blood, pus, a foreign body, or kinking of the tube.
- **P**neumothorax. A simple pneumothorax usually results in sudden deterioration of oxygenation or a sudden increase in ventilating pressure and P_{CO_2}. A tension pneumothorax is more likely to result in hypotension or reduced cardiac output (see below). Pneumothorax is more likely in patients with lower airway or parenchymal lung disease.
- **E**quipment failure. Equipment may fail for a number of reasons, such as disconnection of the oxygen supply from the tracheal tube, leak in the ventilator or ventilator circuit, or failure of the power supply to the ventilator.

Carefully observe the patient, looking for chest rise and symmetry of chest movement. Check pulse oximetry and, if available, capnography. If the patient is mechanically ventilated, disconnect the ventilator and provide manual ventilation while listening carefully over the lateral lung fields for asymmetry in breath sounds or evidence of airway obstruction (rhonchi or wheezes). Use sedatives, analgesics, or neuromuscular blockers if needed to reduce the patient's agitation, but administer these agents only *after* you rule out a correctable cause of the acute distress.

Cricothyrotomy to Treat Airway Obstruction

Standard methods to open the airway, including repositioning of the head and jaw, use of an oropharyngeal or nasopharyngeal airway, and tracheal intubation or reintubation, will permit adequate oxygenation and ventilation in most circumstances. When these methods fail, cricothyrotomy can be used. Cricothyrotomy is the percutaneous or surgical insertion of a needle or catheter into the trachea to enable oxygenation, and in some circumstances ventilation, through the needle or catheter. Cricothyrotomy is rarely required, but it may enable oxygen administration to children with complete upper airway obstruction caused by a foreign body, severe orofacial injuries, upper airway infection, or laryngeal fracture.

Oxygen administration through the cricothyrotomy is often successful, but ventilation may be limited. If the patient with total airway obstruction is breathing spontaneously through the catheter or cricothyroid tube, delivery of 100% oxygen through the catheter may be all that is required to sustain life. Suboptimal ventilation may be tolerated because short periods of hypercarbia, in the absence of hypoxemia, may be well tolerated by seriously ill infants and children.[97] Oxygen flow rates should be relatively low (average of approximately 100 mL/kg per minute; total, 1 to 5 L/min) to minimize the risk of barotrauma. Exhalation of gas will generally occur through the upper airway and out the oropharynx. If upper airway obstruction is complete, it may be necessary to pause between insufflations to allow passive exhalation.

Percutaneous needle cricothyrotomy with a large-bore (14- to 16-gauge) intravenous catheter results in high resistance to air flow because of the small diameter of the catheter. This high resistance frequently prohibits effective ventilation by a bag-mask device coupled to the intravenous catheter with a 3-mm-ID tracheal tube connector. Nonetheless, oxygenation with moderate hypercarbia may be possible.[98]

The pop-off valve of the bag-mask ventilating device must be disabled to achieve the high peak inflation pressures needed.

To achieve effective ventilation or oxygenation with cricothyrotomy, a transtracheal cannula of adequate size and an appropriate ventilating device are necessary. If effective ventilation *and* oxygenation are required, a transtracheal cannula with an ID of 3 mm or larger and a bag-mask device can be used in children and small adults.[99]

Percutaneous needle cricothyrotomy may be used to provide effective ventilation and oxygenation in children during anesthesia if a jet ventilator is used,[100,101] although there is a risk of barotrauma.[100] There are only anecdotal reports of emergency oxygenation and ventilation using a transtracheal catheter in children,[102] so further evaluation is required. Effective ventilation (ie, maintenance of a normal $Paco_2$) through a 14- to 16-gauge intravenous catheter can also be accomplished in patients with a patent upper airway using specialized high-flow jet oxygen ventilation devices, but these devices are not widely available.[101,103]

There is very little published information about percutaneous catheter cricothyrotomy in infants and small children for emergency airway management. Optimal sizes of intravenous catheters for this purpose have not been determined. Significant and life-threatening barotrauma (eg, pneumothorax, pneumomediastinum, or subcutaneous emphysema) may result from attempts at jet ventilation if the tip of the catheter is not in the lumen of the trachea.[100,104]

Theoretically cricothyrotomy should facilitate effective delivery of oxygen to most patients with upper airway obstruction because the most common site of pediatric airway obstruction is at or above the glottis. If a foreign body is located *below* the level of the cricoid cartilage (inferior to the cricothyroid membrane), cricothyrotomy probably will be ineffective. But a rescuer typically cannot predict the precise site of obstruction, so cricothyrotomy should be considered if all other methods have failed to establish a patent airway (see FYI: "Technique of Cricothyrotomy").

Summary Points

Management of respiratory emergencies is a key element of effective pediatric advanced life support. This chapter reviews the anatomic and physiologic differences in the airway and lungs of infants and children versus adults. These differences emphasize the importance of proper positioning of the infant and child to best open the airway and support ventilation. Because of their large occiput, infants often require padding under the trunk; older children often need padding under the occiput to place the head in a sniffing position.

Effective bag-mask ventilation will usually provide adequate oxygenation and ventilation until definitive control of the airway can be achieved. In the out-of-hospital environment, bag-mask ventilation is often sufficient for patient transport if the transport interval is short. It may be the optimal method to use if the provider is inexperienced in pediatric intubation. Properly trained providers may intubate the trachea or insert an LMA.

In the Emergency Department and hospital, tracheal intubation is the preferred method of airway control. Tracheal intubation should be attempted by only properly trained providers. Before intubation is attempted, patients should be placed on a cardiorespiratory monitor and pulse oximeter if a perfusing rhythm is present. In patients with cardiac arrest, intubation may be attempted immediately without delay to institute monitoring. After tracheal intubation the position of the tracheal tube must be confirmed using clinical findings and a confirmatory test, such as exhaled CO_2 detection, particularly in children with a perfusing rhythm. For children in cardiac arrest, exhaled CO_2 detection is a less sensitive indicator of tracheal tube position, but it remains highly specific, ie, if exhaled CO_2 is detected, the tube is in the trachea.

FYI: Technique of Cricothyrotomy

Safe performance of cricothyrotomy requires specialized training. Cricothyrotomy may be performed either by surgical incision or by needle puncture. In the pediatric patient, particularly the infant and toddler, surgical cricothyrotomy is associated with significant risk of injury to vital structures such as the carotid arteries or jugular veins. This procedure should be performed only by persons with surgical training. The technique of needle cricothyrotomy is presented here for highly skilled medical providers who encounter complete upper airway obstruction that is unresponsive to standard treatment techniques.

Place a roll of sheets or towels under the child's shoulders to hyperextend the neck and position the larynx as far anterior as possible. Locate the cricothyroid membrane. This membrane extends from the cricoid to the thyroid cartilage (Figure 21), and it can be palpated with a fingernail. Locate the anterior and midline transverse indentation between the two cartilages (Figure 21 and 22A). The cricothyroid membrane is relatively avascular, so you should puncture it and enter the underlying trachea percutaneously. Initially insert a small-bore (20-gauge) needle attached to a syringe, and aspirate to verify proper position (only air should appear in the syringe) for subsequent puncture. Then insert a large-bore catheter-over-needle cannula (14 to 16 gauge) through the cricothyroid membrane (Figure 22C and 22D). Direct the cannula toward the midline caudally and posteriorly at a 45° angle. Aspirate a second time. Aspiration of air signifies entry into the trachea (Figure 22E).

Advance the catheter into the trachea, remove the needle, and again aspirate air to confirm intraluminal position. Then connect the cannula to an oxygen source and manual resuscitator bag or to a high-pressure oxygen source.[105] Intravenous catheters may be attached to most 3-mm-ID tracheal tube adapters (15 mm) to provide a connection for ventilating devices (22 mm) (Figure 22F). The size of 15-mm/3-mm adapters varies from manufacturer to manufacturer, so you should assemble cricothyrotomy equipment before it is needed.

An alternative method of cricothyrotomy uses a modified Seldinger technique. A small-bore needle is inserted through the cricothyroid membrane, and a wire is passed through the needle. A dilator is advanced over the wire to enable ultimate insertion of a 3-mm-ID tube. Experience with percutaneous dilational cricothyrotomy has been limited primarily to adult patients.[106]

FIGURE 21. Cricothyroid membrane anatomy. Note that the cricothyroid membrane is between the thyroid and cricoid cartilages.

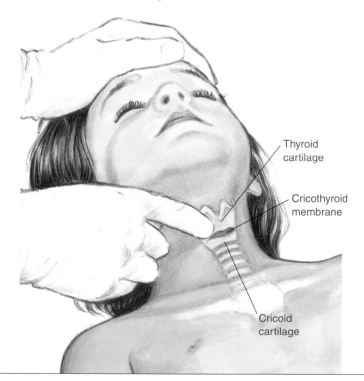

Thyroid cartilage

Cricothyroid membrane

Cricoid cartilage

The case scenarios below illustrate the major types of conditions that cause respiratory distress or failure in infants and children. Although children may have combinations of these causes, rapid and thorough cardiopulmonary assessment and physical examination will often identify the site and type of problem (see Foundation Facts: "Causes and Presentation of Respiratory Failure or Arrest").

Additional key points are summarized below.

Definitions

- Respiratory distress and respiratory failure are prearrest conditions that can progress to respiratory or cardiac arrest.
- *Respiratory failure* is a clinical state of inadequate oxygenation, inadequate ventilation, or both.
  — Often accompanied by r*espiratory distress* (ie, increased respiratory effort, rate, and work of breathing)

FIGURE 22. Percutaneous cricothyrotomy. Extend the head in the midline by placing a rolled towel or folded sheet beneath the shoulders. Stand to the left of the patient, and stabilize the trachea with the right hand. Locate the cricothyroid membrane with the tip of the left index finger. This membrane is between the thyroid and cricoid cartilages (**A**). This space is very narrow (1 mm) in an infant, and only a fingernail can discern it. Stabilize the trachea between the middle finger and thumb of the left hand while using the fingernail of the left index finger to mark the crico-thyroid membrane. Introduce a catheter-over-needle cannula (14 to 16 gauge) that is attached to a syringe (**B**) through the membrane. If air is aspirated (**C**), advance the catheter through the cricothy-roid membrane in the trachea (**D**), and remove the needle (**E**). Aspirate air with a 3-mL syringe to confirm intraluminal position. Most 3-mm adapters from a pediatric tracheal tube can be attached to the intravenous catheter. To provide ventilation, connect the catheter to a breathing circuit with a standard 22-mm connector (**F**). Alternatively, leave the barrel of the 3-mL syringe attached to the intravenous catheter, insert an 8-mm tracheal tube adapter into the barrel of the syringe, and attach the adapter to a venti-lating system with a standard 22-mm adapter. Reproduced with permission from Coté et al.[6]

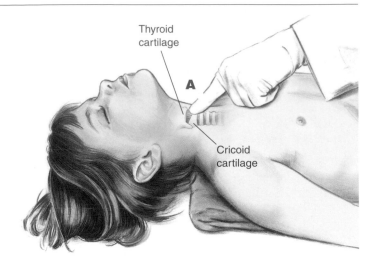

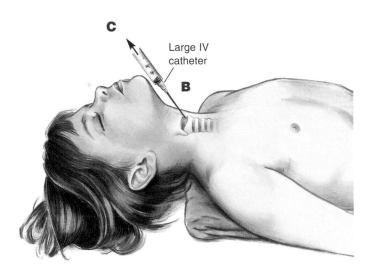

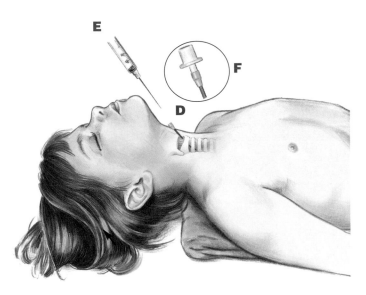

— May also result from inadequate respiratory effort with no signs of distress

— Abnormalities in oxygenation or ventilation should be evaluated in the context of the child's baseline respiratory function

■ *Respiratory arrest* is the absence of breathing (ie, apnea). Note that agonal respirations or gasping respirations are treated as respiratory arrest.

Initial Management of Respiratory Distress

■ Allow the child to assume a position of comfort.

■ Administer oxygen as tolerated.

■ Consider pulse oximetry and ECG moni-toring. Cardiorespiratory monitoring of oxyhemoglobin saturation is indicated for children with respiratory distress and a perfusing rhythm when advanced airway support is provided.

■ Upper airway obstruction: consider steroids and aerosolized epinephrine.

■ Lower airway obstruction: consider steroids and nebulized β_2-agonists.

Management of Suspected Respiratory Failure

■ Control or secure the airway. Be sure the airway is patent.

■ Administer 1 Fio$_2$ (100% oxygen).

■ Assist or provide ventilation.

Foundation Facts:
Causes and Presentation of Respiratory Failure or Arrest

Four general types of respiratory problems lead to respiratory failure or arrest. These problems are indicated by the following signs and symptoms:

- **Upper airway obstruction:** The major clinical signs occur during the *inspiratory* phase of the respiratory cycle. The child may have stridor, a frightened appearance, drooling, hoarseness, or a change in voice or cry. Inspiratory retractions, use of accessory muscles, and nasal flaring are present. The respiratory rate is often only mildly elevated.

- **Lower airway obstruction:** The major clinical signs occur during the *expiratory* phase of the respiratory cycle. The child often has wheezing, retractions, and a prolonged expiratory phase requiring increased effort. The respiratory rate is usually elevated, particularly in infants.

- **Parenchymal lung disease:** The child's lungs become stiff, requiring increased respiratory effort during both inspiration and exhalation. Retractions are common, and hypoxemia is often marked because of alveolar collapse or reduced oxygen diffusion caused by pulmonary edema fluid and inflammatory debris in alveoli. Tachypnea is common. The patient frequently attempts to counteract alveolar and small-airway collapse by increasing efforts to maintain an elevated end-expiratory pressure; this effort is usually manifested by grunting respirations.

- **Abnormal control of ventilation:** The breathing pattern is irregular; often the parent will say the child is "breathing funny." There may be periods of increased rate or effort followed by decreased rate or effort, or the child's respiratory rate or effort may be continuously inadequate. The net effect is hypoventilation. This condition results from a host of conditions, such as injury to the brain or brainstem or drug overdose.

— A leak anywhere in the manual resuscitator or ventilator system.

— Disconnection of oxygen tubing from the manual self-inflating resuscitator system (or other failure of the oxygen delivery system).

— Presence of a pneumothorax.

— The need to provide increased end-expiratory pressure secondary to parenchymal lung disease and alveolar collapse.

— Stomach distention caused by accumulation of air in the stomach during bag-mask ventilation before tracheal intubation.

- Causes of sudden deterioration in an intubated patient are recalled by the **DOPE** mnemonic:

— **D**isplacement of the tracheal tube out of the airway or into a main bronchus

— **O**bstruction of the tracheal tube

— **P**neumothorax

— **E**quipment failure

Case Scenarios
Case Scenario 1

A 2-year-old is brought to the Emergency Department. For the past 2 days he has had labored breathing that has progressively worsened. Initially he had a runny nose, but yesterday he began to have a barky cough, and today he started making a high-pitched sound on inspiration. Earlier today he was playful and took fluids well, but now the parents are concerned because he seems very anxious.

Initial Assessment

You see an anxious toddler who is sitting on his mom's lap and working hard to breathe. He has obvious nasal flaring and intercostal and suprasternal retractions. You hear a high-pitched inspiratory sound with each breath, and he has an occasional harsh, barky cough. His mucus membranes and skin look pale. The child's heart rate is 165 bpm, respiratory rate is 35 per

- Monitor pulse oximetry and ECG.

- Establish vascular access.

- Provide nothing by mouth in case intubation is required.

- *Anticipate further patient deterioration.* Advance preparation includes ensuring that a correctly sized laryngoscope blade, tracheal tubes, suction equipment, and bag-mask devices are ready. Selection of equipment and medication dosing may be aided by use of a length-based estimation system.

- *Confirm tracheal tube placement* after intubation by auscultation and detection of exhaled CO_2. Confirmation of midtracheal tube position requires a chest x-ray.

- *If the patient does not improve* after tracheal intubation and appropriate

confirmation of tracheal tube placement, consider the following potential causes:

— Inadequate tidal volume. Adequate tidal volume should produce bilateral chest rise, adequate bilateral breath sounds, and clinical improvement in the patient.

— An excessive leak around the tracheal tube. An excessive air leak usually results from use of a tube that is too small (or from high inspiratory pressures).

— Failure to compress the pop-off valve on the manual resuscitator. This problem can result in inadequate lung expansion in a patient with increased lower airway resistance or poor lung compliance.

minute, blood pressure is 115/75 mm Hg, and temperature (axillary) is 99.2°F (37.4°C). When you examine his lungs, you hear transmitted upper airway sounds centrally and diminished air entry over the axillary regions bilaterally. No rales or wheezes are noted. Heart sounds are normal, and capillary refill in his fingers is <2 seconds.

Acceptable Actions and Rationale

The following actions are generally *acceptable* for assessment and management of this child with respiratory distress:

■ *Perform a rapid cardiopulmonary assessment:* This child clearly demonstrates respiratory distress with potential respiratory failure. Note the phase of the respiratory cycle associated with the most significant symptoms (eg, ask yourself, Are the noise and increased effort noted on inspiration, expiration, or both?)

— If the airway obstruction is located *at or above the thoracic inlet,* symptoms are most notable during *inspiration.* Typical inspiratory symptoms include stridor and retractions, as noted in this child. Typically the child with *upper airway* obstruction breathes at a relatively slow rate because higher rates increase airflow turbulence and thus increase airway resistance and the work of breathing. Therefore, a respiratory rate >60 per minute in an infant and >50 per minute in a child is unlikely to occur with obstruction restricted to the upper airway.

— If the airway obstruction is at the *level of the glottis* (vocal cords) or just below, the child's cough often sounds like the *bark of a seal*; hoarseness is more common in older children. When the *obstruction is higher*, the voice may sound muffled. A muffled voice is often noted with a retropharyngeal abscess or markedly enlarged tonsils (eg, due to infectious mononucleosis), and

the patient often sounds as if he/she is talking while holding something hot in the mouth (like a mouthful of hot potato). With more severe upper airway obstruction, audible sounds associated with increased respiratory distress may be heard during inspiration and expiration.

■ *Obtain a targeted history:* In this child the symptoms of upper respiratory tract infection, nontoxic appearance, and low-grade fever suggest croup (ie, laryngotracheobronchitis).

— A history of high fever and rapid onset of respiratory distress suggests supraglottitis or bacterial tracheitis, whereas a history of sudden onset of respiratory distress and upper airway obstruction in a previously well child suggests foreign-body aspiration.

— Other important questions to ask are if the child was premature, was mechanically ventilated (which increases the risk of upper airway injury, predisposing to upper airway obstruction with subsequent infections), or has had episodes of croup in the past. Previous episodes of croup suggest an underlying airway problem such as subglottic stenosis, constricting vascular ring, airway hemangioma, or laryngeal papillomatosis.

■ *Allow the child to assume a position of comfort:* Because this child is alert and interactive, avoid causing additional agitation while providing therapy and continuing your evaluation. Increased agitation causes faster breathing, turbulent airflow, and greater airway resistance, resulting in increased work of breathing. As upper airway resistance increases, the pressure drop across the airway obstruction increases, which tends to collapse that portion of the airway. The subsequent narrowing further increases resistance to airflow and causes the child to work harder to move air (eg, causing intercostal and suprasternal retractions and nasal flaring).

■ *Provide oxygen by a method that does not cause agitation:* For the same reasons as noted above, avoid additional agitation. Administration of humidified oxygen is desirable but not essential for short-term therapy. Humidification reduces drying of airway secretions and irritation of the airway.

■ *Monitor the child:* Cardiorespiratory monitoring provides continuous information about the child's heart rate and respiratory rate.

— If the child struggles to breathe and becomes more anxious secondary to increasing airway obstruction, the heart rate increases. If the child's respiratory distress *decreases* in response to therapy, the heart rate will likely decrease.

— A rapid *fall* in heart rate associated with grunting, gasping, or other ominous signs of respiratory distress strongly suggests the development of respiratory failure and imminent respiratory or cardiac arrest (need for urgent intervention).

— *Pulse oximetry* provides continuous assessment of the child's oxyhemoglobin saturation. If the patient's distal perfusion is adequate and the displayed heart rate correlates closely with the heart rate on the cardiac monitor, the pulse oximeter oxygen saturation correlates well with the patient's measured arterial oxygen saturation.

— A *significant fall* in oxyhemoglobin saturation is a sign of respiratory failure. Improvement in oxygen saturation in response to therapy is reassuring, but it does *not* exclude the possibility of respiratory failure because respiratory failure is defined as inadequate oxygenation or ventilation. Inadequate ventilation and resulting hypercarbia are *not* detected by pulse oximetry.

■ *Provide specific therapy:* Begin therapy while completing the initial cardiopulmonary assessment and instituting monitoring. Do not wait to complete an assessment when the patient demonstrates significant respiratory distress. For this patient with upper airway obstruction, you should strongly consider the use of nebulized epinephrine (either racemic or L-epinephrine). Oral, intramuscular, or intravenous dexamethasone is also typically used if croup is the most likely diagnosis.

■ *Reassess frequently:* The condition of patients with acute respiratory distress is dynamic and requires frequent, careful examination to detect changes in status requiring more urgent therapy.

Unacceptable Actions and Rationale

The following actions would be inappropriate in this clinical situation:

■ *Failure* to identify the prearrest condition of respiratory distress with the potential for development of respiratory failure.

■ *Immediate tracheal intubation.* This child does not have signs or symptoms of respiratory failure *at this time* and thus docs not require immediate invasive airway intervention. Signs of respiratory failure include a declining level of consciousness, marked respiratory effort with poor air movement on examination, *or* a decline in respiratory effort often associated with a decline in consciousness.

■ *Attempting to lay the child on a stretcher or bed to obtain vascular access.* The initial cardiopulmonary assessment documented that the child was alert and responsive, so it is most appropriate to carefully monitor the child and allow him/her to assume a *position of comfort* while implementing specific therapy as appropriate. Vascular access is very stressful and is not a high priority in the acute management of this patient.

Case Scenario 1 Progression and Summary

After helping his mother administer oxygen by a high-flow device and 3 mL of nebulized L-epinephrine, you reassess the patient. The child appears less distressed and is more interactive with his parents. His retractions have diminished, and there is better air entry in the distal lung fields and minimal inspiratory stridor. His oxygen saturation rises from 92% to 99%, and his heart rate decreases to 130 bpm.

The child has clearly improved, but he still requires careful observation because his symptoms may recur as the therapeutic effects of the epinephrine subside. A dose of dexamethasone is appropriate in this setting.

In summary, upper airway obstruction causes respiratory distress that is more apparent during *inspiration*. If tracheal intubation is needed in a patient with upper airway obstruction secondary to respiratory failure, a tracheal tube smaller than normally estimated is appropriate secondary to anticipated narrowing of the airway.

Case Scenario 2

You are an advanced EMS provider called to the home of a 7-year-old girl with acute breathing difficulty. Her mother says the girl has asthma and has used her home nebulizer every hour for the past 3 hours because of increasing breathing difficulty.

Initial Assessment

On initial rapid cardiopulmonary assessment you see an awake, anxious child sitting upright and using her accessory muscles. She is unable to say more than one word at a time. She has marked intercostal and suprasternal retractions during inspiration, a forced, prolonged expiratory phase, and occasional grunting. On auscultation you note that air entry is markedly decreased over her distal lung fields, and you hear high-pitched wheezing centrally throughout exhalation. Her

heart rate is 144 bpm, and respiratory rate is 24 per minute. Heart sounds are normal, although they sound somewhat distant, and distal pulses are weak. You note that her radial pulse disappears and reappears in a somewhat rhythmic manner every few heart beats.

Acceptable Actions and Rationale

The following actions are generally acceptable for assessment and management of this child with respiratory distress:

■ *Perform a rapid cardiopulmonary assessment:* Treatment of the child with respiratory distress is determined by the degree of physiologic impairment revealed during both the rapid cardiopulmonary assessment and a more complete physical examination.

■ *Provide cardiorespiratory monitoring and pulse oximetry:* Any patient with acute respiratory distress needs careful monitoring while treatment is initiated. Continuous evaluation of pulse oximetry provides useful information, but you must ensure that the oximeter is working properly. The variability in this child's palpable pulse volume may result in inaccurate pulse oximetry readings. The fluctuations in pulse are a sign of *pulsus paradoxus.* Severe air trapping in the lower airways is causing hyperinflation; with each inspiratory effort the heart is squeezed by the overinflated lungs and by the pericardium (see Figure 23). Squeezing by the pericardium occurs because the pericardium is attached to the diaphragm, and the diaphragm is flattened in patients with severe asthma. Each time the patient breathes in, the diaphragm moves downward, adding additional tension to the pericardium and impairing filling of the heart.

■ *Provide oxygen:* Oxygen administration is always appropriate for an infant or child with respiratory distress, and it rarely impairs ventilatory drive in children with chronic respiratory disease. Deliver oxygen using a high flow system, preferably a nonrebreathing mask with an oxygen reservoir.

- *Begin specific therapy:* This child has asthma; nebulized albuterol is the appropriate treatment. Audible wheezing during exhalation suggests that the intrathoracic airways are the most likely site of air turbulence and obstruction. Although the child received albuterol at home, it is appropriate to give another dose in this setting. The home nebulizer may generate large particles, or its operational efficiency may be impaired, particularly if it has not been well maintained. Patients using meter dose inhalers (MDIs) at home may fail to recognize that the canister is empty. Finally, EMS systems and Emergency Departments use oxygen to drive nebulization, so they may produce better drug delivery since oxygen administration may result in some degree of airway relaxation.

- *Allow the child to assume a position of comfort:* A child with respiratory distress will generally assume the position that best maintains ventilation. The healthcare provider should not inter-

fere with that position unless doing so is required to provide definitive care.

- *Anticipate the need for advanced airway intervention:* Advance preparation is appropriate for this child. Children with status asthmaticus may rapidly deteriorate. Rapid deterioration would require emergent bag-mask ventilation and possible invasive airway support.

- *Rapidly transport the patient to the Emergency Department:* Rapid transport to the Emergency Department with continuous monitoring and nebulizer therapy is important.

Unacceptable Actions and Rationale

The following actions would be unacceptable in this case scenario:

- Failing to identify respiratory distress with potential for respiratory failure.

- Attempting to establish vascular access before treating the respiratory distress. Vascular access may be appropriate to establish during transport, but it generally should not be attempted if it causes

increased agitation and respiratory distress.

- Giving oxygen by nasal cannula only.

- Forcing the patient to lie down.

- Immediately placing a chest tube or performing needle thoracostomy. (Although this patient is at risk for pneumothorax, she does not show symptoms of tension pneumothorax.)

Case Scenario 2 Progression and Summary

The patient initially appears to improve somewhat during albuterol nebulizer therapy in the transport vehicle because her respiratory effort decreases. But as therapy continues, she suddenly falls back against the stretcher and does not respond to verbal stimulation. Her heart rate and pulse oximetry saturation quickly fall, and she has no spontaneous respiratory effort.

One provider opens her airway with a 2-handed jaw thrust maneuver and seals the face mask to her face while the second provider compresses the manual resuscitator. Two initial breaths are provided as signs of circulation are assessed. Distal pulses are palpable, although they continue to come and go in association with the manual ventilation cycle: they disappear during the inspiratory phase and reappear during the expiratory phase. Because pulses are palpable, chest compression is not indicated. Manual ventilation is provided at a rate of 10 to 12 breaths per minute to provide adequate time for exhalation. (Note that this is a slower rate than one might expect for an apneic patient who is likely to be hypercarbic). Sufficient pressure is used to make the chest rise, but large breaths are avoided (see Critical Concepts: "Complications of Air Trapping").

Note: There have been anecdotal reports of successful bag-mask ventilation in a patient with severe asthma and overinflated lungs by provision of lateral chest wall compressions during exhalation. This technique may improve ventilation and reduce the magnitude of hyperinflation.

FIGURE 23. Chest x-ray of a child with asthma illustrates the relationship between the lungs and heart. As lung volume increases, the heart is compressed. In addition, the parietal pericardium is attached to the diaphragm. As the child inhales, the diaphragm flattens more and pulls the pericardium more tightly around the heart. Both of these actions impede venous return and thus impair stroke volume during inspiration, leading to *pulsus paradoxus.*

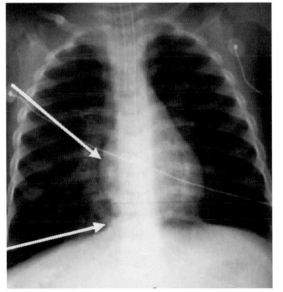

Hyperinflated lungs compress the heart

Pericardium is attached to the diaphragm. When diaphragm descends, it squeezes the heart

The possibility of a tension pneumothorax should now be considered. If the findings of examination suggest a tension pneumothorax, a needle thoracostomy may be appropriate. The patient arrives in the Emergency Department (see Case Scenario 3).

Case Scenario 3

You are working in the Emergency Department and receive a call from the EMS team about the child from Case Scenario 2. Bag-mask ventilation is continued on arrival in the Emergency Department. The child is pale, unresponsive, and apneic on arrival. The cardiac monitor shows a heart rate of 110 bpm. The pulse oximeter shows that oxygen saturation is fluctuating between 84% and 90%, but the oximeter displays a numeric value only intermittently and seems unreliable.

Acceptable Actions and Rationale

The following actions are generally *acceptable* for assessment and management of this child with respiratory distress:

- *Treat respiratory arrest:* Airway support, oxygenation, and ventilation must be adequate to prevent progression to cardiopulmonary arrest.

- *Prepare equipment for tracheal intubation:* Advance preparation is important. A manual resuscitator, face mask, tracheal tubes, laryngoscope and blades, working suction system, and suction catheters are necessary. A length-based resuscitation tape is useful to help select the correct equipment sizes. Personnel should be organized so that each person knows exactly what to do when the patient arrives.

- *Perform a rapid cardiopulmonary assessment:* The rapid cardiopulmonary assessment directs subsequent treatment: establishment of an airway and support of ventilation are urgently required in this child with respiratory failure.

- *Obtain a targeted history:* A rapid, targeted history may identify important

information that affects subsequent therapy. In addition to asking about the history of asthma, ask if the child has required hospitalization, an ICU stay, and intubation. A history of previous episodes of respiratory decompensation requiring ICU admission or mechanical ventilation are associated with a higher risk of respiratory failure and death with this episode.

- *Continue bag-mask ventilation:* While preparing for tracheal intubation, continue assisted manual ventilation. Because the patient has high airway resistance, a 2-person technique may be needed to provide adequate ventilation. If the patient remains unresponsive, a third person should provide *cricoid pressure* to limit inflation of the stomach. Cricoid pressure should be maintained during tracheal intubation to reduce the risk of regurgitation and aspiration.

- *Obtain vascular access:* Vascular access enables both drug and fluid administration. If the patient remains unresponsive, drugs will not be needed for sedation. But neuromuscular blockade and sedation may be required after tracheal intubation if the patient becomes responsive and resists ventilation. Fluid administration is often required to counteract the adverse effects of positive-pressure ventilation (ie, decreased preload and cardiac output).

- *Intubate the trachea with a properly selected tracheal tube:* Although *cuffed* tracheal tubes are generally reserved for children 8 years or older, use of a cuffed tracheal tube is appropriate to prevent an air leak, which may compromise effective ventilation in this child. High airway pressures likely will be required to support effective ventilation despite high airway resistance. Once the patient is stabilized, be sure to check the cuff pressure and attempt to reduce it to the minimum inflation pressure that permits adequate chest expansion with minimal

air leak. As noted previously, do *not* attempt to correct this patient's hypercarbia by ventilating at high rates or using large tidal volumes.

- *Confirm proper tracheal tube position:* After tracheal intubation carefully listen over both lateral lung fields. Chest expansion, humidification (vapor) in the tube, and auscultation of adequate bilateral breath sounds are not completely reliable indicators of correct tracheal tube position, so confirm tracheal tube position by exhaled CO_2 detection. Detection of exhaled CO_2 does *not* confirm that the tube is properly positioned *in* the trachea; it may be in a main bronchus. Therefore, confirmation of tracheal tube position by chest x-ray is appropriate once the patient is adequately stabilized.

- *Secure the tracheal tube:* You must secure the tracheal tube, and you should

Critical Concepts: Complications of Air Trapping

In patients with severe lower airway disease characterized by air trapping, rapid respiratory rates result in further air trapping. This trapped air increases the risk of pneumothorax and often further compromises cardiac output.

Patients with severe air trapping may die or experience severe neurologic morbidity due to hypoxia or ischemia (ischemia results from the adverse effects of air trapping on cardiac output). Patients typically tolerate severe hypercarbia without adverse effects. Therefore, the initial goal in this setting is to ensure adequate *oxygenation* and cardiac output rather than rapid correction of hypercarbia. To support oxygenation and cardiac output, use a slow respiratory rate and allow adequate time for exhalation. Administration of fluid to increase cardiac preload and output is also appropriate.

record the position of the tube at the teeth, gum line, or lips to serve as a landmark for subsequent confirmation of tube position (eg, after transport).

■ *Decompress the stomach with a nasogastric or orogastric tube:* This patient required bag-mask ventilation using high pressure; it is likely that this procedure caused stomach inflation. Decompression of the stomach may improve ventilation and reduce the likelihood of vomiting and subsequent aspiration.

■ *Continue therapy for acute asthma:* Asthma-specific therapy includes nebulized albuterol and ipratropium bromide and intravenous corticosteroid therapy. You may consider treatment with intravenous magnesium sulfate and terbutaline.

Unacceptable Actions and Rationale

The following actions would be unacceptable for the assessment and treatment of this child:

■ Failure to recognize the severity of the child's condition or failure to recognize respiratory arrest and the need to support the airway, oxygenation, and ventilation.

■ Delaying tracheal intubation or advanced airway management to obtain vascular access.

■ Providing assisted ventilation at a rapid rate or using very large tidal volumes.

■ Beginning chest compressions.

■ Failure to perform secondary confirmation of tracheal tube placement.

Case Scenario 3 Progression and Summary

The child's trachea is successfully intubated with a 5.5-mm cuffed tracheal tube. Clinical examination and colorimetric exhaled CO_2 detection confirm tracheal location. A chest x-ray confirms that the tube is in the midtrachea. Sufficient air is added to the cuff to cause visible chest expansion during inspiration and an audible air leak when airway pressure exceeds 25 cm H_2O. A healthcare provider

ventilates the child at a rate of 10 breaths per minute. Oxygenation improves with these interventions (92% oxygen saturation). The child's heart rate is 124 bpm, and pulses are now more readily and consistently palpable. Vascular access is obtained, and 2 mg/kg methylprednisolone is given intravenously along with 10 mL/kg normal saline and 2 g of magnesium sulfate. The patient is transferred to the intensive care unit for subsequent therapy.

Reactive airway disease with wheezing (asthma) is the most common cause of lower airway obstruction in children requiring hospitalization. In infants viral bronchiolitis (eg, respiratory syncytial virus) is a common cause of wheezing. The treatment principles outlined above can also be applied to the infant with bronchiolitis, although the clinical condition of infants is often complicated by symptoms of pneumonia.

Lower airway obstructive disease is characterized by a prolonged expiratory phase and the presence of wheezes or other sounds during forced exhalation. Severe lower airway obstruction results in air trapping, which often impairs cardiac output by interfering with venous return. If cardiac output is compromised, fluid administration may help to restore perfusion, but fluids should be given cautiously to avoid creating pulmonary edema. Thus, in this case a 10 mL/kg bolus rather than the more typical 20 mL/kg bolus was infused. Additional fluid can be administered as needed after reevaluation of the patient's condition.

Case Scenario 4

You are examining a 2-year-old patient with increasing respiratory distress in the Emergency Department. The child was previously well, and his past medical history is unremarkable. He was found at home with a bottle of lamp oil that he apparently opened. The mother called EMS immediately when she noted he was "breathing funny." EMS personnel administered oxygen by high-flow face mask, and this therapy was continued

during transport and on arrival at the ED. The child's pulse oximetry reading during transport and on arrival was in the mid to high 90s.

Initial Assessment

Your rapid cardiopulmonary assessment reveals a tachypneic, anxious toddler with grunting respirations, nasal flaring, and increased respiratory effort indicated by intercostal and suprasternal retractions. Heart rate is 145 bpm, respirations are 50 per minute, blood pressure is 115/ 75 mm Hg, and temperature (axillary) is 97.8°F (36.6°C). His oxygen saturation during administration of high-flow oxygen is 85%. On auscultation you hear moist crackles (rales) throughout his lung fields and decreased air entry over his axillary lung fields; there are coarse breath sounds centrally. He has good distal perfusion with readily palpable pulses and brisk capillary refill.

Acceptable Actions and Rationale

The following actions would be appropriate during the initial assessment and management of this patient:

■ *Perform a rapid cardiopulmonary assessment:* This child is in respiratory distress with respiratory failure; rapid intervention is needed to prevent further deterioration.

■ *Place the patient on a cardiorespiratory monitor and pulse oximeter:* Continuous monitoring of heart rate, heart rhythm, and oxygen saturation provides helpful insight into the patient's response to interventions and progression of the disease process.

■ *Provide oxygen and specific therapy:* High-flow oxygen is clearly indicated because of the initial oxygen saturation. In this case a nonrebreathing mask should be used to maximize oxygen administration. In some centers a tight-fitting face mask may be used to deliver CPAP. In infants and children with parenchymal lung disease, CPAP may recruit alveoli, improving oxygenation.

■ *Anticipate the need for tracheal intubation:* This child has serious impairment of oxygenation and is at high risk for respiratory failure. Advance preparation for tracheal intubation is indicated.

■ *Obtain an arterial blood gas analysis:* Arterial blood gas analysis provides objective information about the adequacy of ventilation and confirms the impairment of oxygenation revealed by pulse oximetry.

■ *Obtain a portable chest x-ray:* This child is too ill to go to the radiology suite for an x-ray. A portable chest X-ray can help sort out the possible diagnoses.

■ *Obtain vascular access if possible,* especially if rapid sequence intubation or resuscitation is expected. Note that vascular access should *not* take priority over appropriate airway management. If vascular access is attempted, the child's condition must be carefully monitored during the attempt. The attempt should be interrupted if deterioration occurs. If the need for vascular access is thought to justify the risk of further deterioration (eg, to enable immediate provision of rapid sequence intubation medications), then access should be achieved by an experienced provider.

Unacceptable Actions and Rationale

The following actions would be unacceptable for the care of this toddler:

■ Failure to identify the presence of respiratory failure.

■ Obtaining vascular access before providing additional therapy to improve oxygenation.

■ Giving a fluid bolus instead of providing appropriate airway management.

■ Treating this child as for upper airway obstruction. It is unlikely such treatment would be helpful because there is no upper airway obstruction by examination. Albuterol may be considered, but there

is no evidence of wheezing, and this toddler's major problem appears to be oxygenation rather than ventilation.

■ Failure to provide oxygen therapy or airway support until results of arterial blood gas analysis are available.

■ Sending the patient for an x-ray without appropriate monitoring and support.

Case Scenario 4 Progression and Summary

The child's condition continues to deteriorate over the next 30 minutes. He receives 100% oxygen by nonrebreathing, tight-fitting mask and albuterol aerosol, but his oxygen saturation declines to 78%. His respiratory rate is close to 60 breaths per minute, and his heart rate is up to 160 bpm. His pulses are still readily palpable, but he is lethargic and barely cries or withdraws in response to needle sticks. Vascular access was successfully obtained, and his chest x-ray shows diffuse infiltrates, opacification of both lung fields, and a normal-sized heart. While you await the results of blood gas analysis, the patient becomes unresponsive, and his respiratory effort and heart rate rapidly decline.

Using universal precautions, ED personnel provide 2-person bag-mask ventilation while the previously selected equipment is assembled to perform tracheal intubation. The pulse is readily palpable. Cricoid pressure is maintained during bag-mask ventilation in this unresponsive patient. A 4.5-mm uncuffed tracheal tube is placed, and tracheal position is confirmed by auscultation and by detection of exhaled CO_2 using a colorimetric detector. After intubation the toddler's oxygen saturation increases to a maximum of 86% with an FiO_2 of 1, so ventilation is continued with a PEEP of 10 cm H_2O. A chest x-ray is ordered to confirm the position of the tube in the midtrachea.

The toddler's arterial blood gas (ABG) values before intubation were pH 7.24, PO_2 38 mm Hg, PCO_2 55 mm Hg, and Base Deficit –5.

The toddler's preintubation ABG values confirm respiratory failure with significant impairment of both oxygenation and ventilation, consistent with the diffuse parenchymal lung disease seen on his chest x-ray. Aspiration of certain hydrocarbon products (like lamp oil) may cause diffuse injury to the alveoli and small airways. The priority of treatment is to maintain adequate oxygenation and organ perfusion; attempts to normalize arterial carbon dioxide tension are not advisable because such attempts would require high tidal volume and high inspiratory pressure, which can produce airway and parenchymal lung trauma and impaired cardiac output. Recent data shows that "permissive hypercapnia" is preferable to production of normocarbia in patients with ARDS.[107]

In patients with parenchymal lung disease and alveolar collapse, oxygenation may be improved by increasing PEEP. Prolonging inspiratory time increases mean airway pressure, which also can improve oxygenation. A detailed discussion of ventilator management is beyond the scope of this chapter.

Case Scenario 4 Further Case Progression

The patient improves with application of 10 cm H_2O of PEEP; his oxygen saturation increases to 92%, and his heart rate declines to 140 bpm. He is transferred uneventfully to the ICU. A repeated chest x-ray is obtained on admission to the ICU. Immediately after the child is removed from the x-ray plate, his oxygen saturation and heart rate fall and he deteriorates.

In this setting consider causes of sudden deterioration in an intubated child. These causes can be recalled by the DOPE mnemonic (see "Managing Airway and Ventilation Emergencies" in this chapter). Examination shows that the tracheal tube was displaced from the trachea, so 2-person bag-mask ventilation is provided using a flow-inflating manual resuscitator with a pressure manometer. The trachea is then successfully reintubated, and correct tube position is confirmed by exhaled CO_2 detection. Oxygenation and ventilation improve immediately.

Case Scenario 5

An 11-year-old boy is in the intermediate care unit pending surgical resection of a newly diagnosed brain tumor, which is scheduled for tomorrow morning. He presented to the Emergency Department earlier today with vomiting and double vision, and a CT scan revealed the diagnosis. He was treated with steroids and admitted to the hospital, and his condition was clinically improved several hours later. You are called to his room the night before surgery because his mother says he is "breathing funny." On your initial cardiopulmonary assessment and examination, he is unresponsive to you and his mother. His breathing is characterized by periods of several slow, deep breaths followed by pauses. His color is pale. Heart rate is irregular and averages 60 bpm, and respiratory rate is around 12 per minute and irregular as noted. His radial pulse is readily palpable, and he has brisk capillary refill. You firmly pinch his finger, which results in grimacing and rigid extension of his arms and legs. Blood pressure is 135/90 mm Hg. His pupils are 4 to 5 mm and appear to be sluggishly reactive to light. No seizure activity was reported.

Acceptable Actions and Rationale

The following actions are acceptable during the initial assessment and management of this patient:

- *Shout for help and activate the EMS response system* per local protocol: The patient shows signs of increased intracranial pressure and impending brain herniation. If emergent interventions are not provided, this patient will likely progress rapidly to brainstem herniation and cardiopulmonary arrest.

- *Open the airway and provide ventilation:* This child has erratic ventilatory effort and does not demonstrate adequate

ventilation. Hypoventilation is present and is likely causing hypercarbia and hypoxia. In this patient the major concern is that he has increased intracranial pressure and impending brain herniation. Noxious stimulation caused decerebrate (ie, extensor) posturing. Because either hypercapnia or hypoxemia can contribute to increased intracranial pressure, you should attempt to correct both. If a bag-mask manual resuscitator is not readily available, mouth-to-barrier device ventilation is appropriate.

- *Provide cricoid pressure:* The child may have recently eaten and is unresponsive. For these reasons application of cricoid pressure is appropriate to reduce the risk of gastric inflation with resultant regurgitation and the risk of aspiration. Cricoid pressure is a noxious stimulus; if the pressure causes the patient to cough, gag, or become agitated, discontinue cricoid pressure until medications for rapid sequence intubation are administered.

- *Prepare for tracheal intubation and attempt vascular access:* Vascular access may be attempted while the equipment for tracheal intubation is assembled. If vascular access is established, many healthcare providers will use a sequence of medications (typically sedatives and neuromuscular blockers or muscle relaxants) to minimize the development of increased intracranial pressure during intubation. (For more information, see Chapter 14, "Rapid Sequence Intubation," in the *PALS Provider Manual*). Because this child is scheduled for surgery in the morning, vascular access may already be established, allowing rapid administration of dexamethasone.

- *Apply a cardiorespiratory monitor and pulse oximeter* to continuously monitor the heart rate and oxyhemoglobin saturation during attempted tracheal intubation. If oxyhemoglobin saturation or heart rate falls during the intubation attempt, interrupt the attempt to provide oxygenation and ventilation.

- *Administer specific therapies:* Intravenous mannitol may be useful to reduce intracranial pressure, but it will not work as rapidly as effective hyperventilation. Thus, provide ventilation while mannitol is being prepared for administration and definitive treatment is being planned.

Unacceptable Actions and Rationale

The following actions would be unacceptable during the assessment and treatment of this child:

- Failure to recognize a prearrest condition and the need for immediate support of oxygenation and ventilation

- Failure to rapidly initiate ventilation in this child with signs of brain or brainstem herniation

- Delaying ventilation to obtain vascular access

- Giving mannitol alone without providing ventilation

- Transporting the child for a CT scan without first ensuring that the airway is secure and ventilation is adequate

Case Scenario 5 Progression and Summary

The child receives mask ventilation, and his oxyhemoglobin saturation is 100% by pulse oximetry. The most experienced healthcare provider successfully intubates the child's trachea with a 6.5-mm cuffed tracheal tube using a rapid sequence technique. Clinical assessment and exhaled CO_2 detection confirm tracheal tube placement. His heart rate is 88 bpm and blood pressure is 110/65 mm Hg after tracheal intubation and mild hyperventilation. A chest x-ray is ordered to confirm midtracheal tube position. He is ventilated at 20 breaths per minute, and postintubation arterial blood gas analysis shows pH 7.48, P_{O_2} 589 mm Hg, P_{CO_2} 30 mm Hg, and Base Excess −0.2. End-tidal CO_2 by capnography is 28 mm Hg.

The child is transported to the CT scanner with continuous ECG, exhaled CO_2, and pulse oximetry monitoring. His CT *scan shows new bleeding in his tumor with increased edema surrounding the tumor. He is rapidly transported to the operating room for tumor resection. Two weeks after the tumor is removed, a neurologic examination is performed, and the findings are normal.*

Note that hyperventilation for *routine* ventilation of patients with cardiopulmonary failure or *brain injury* is discouraged. But hyperventilation *is* appropriate when there are signs of impending cerebral (brain or brainstem) herniation, as in this patient. Inadequate or abnormal central nervous system control of respiratory drive is an additional cause of respiratory failure, but symptoms of respiratory distress may not be present. Nonetheless, this condition can still result in respiratory failure.

Review Questions

1. You are examining a 6-week-old infant with a 2-day history of increasing coughing and breathing difficulty. The infant appears alert. The infant has mild to moderate intercostal and sternal retractions and nasal flaring during inspiration. You hear no abnormal noises during inspiration, but on chest auscultation you hear bilateral wheezes and an occasional grunt during exhalation. The infant's skin color is pink. Which *one* of the following statements is *true*?

   a. the infant has respiratory distress and likely has upper airway obstruction

   b. the infant has respiratory distress and likely has lower airway obstruction

   c. the infant has no respiratory distress and likely has foreign-body airway obstruction

   d. the infant has no respiratory distress and likely has disordered control of ventilation

The correct answer is b. Retractions, nasal flaring, and grunting are symptoms of respiratory distress in an infant. Normal inspiratory noises and *expiratory* wheezes are most consistent with *lower* airway obstruction.

Answer a is incorrect because upper airway obstruction would likely cause abnormal *inspiratory* noises.

Answer c is also incorrect. Although a foreign body can cause symptoms of either upper or lower airway obstruction, this infant's age and the duration of symptoms make foreign-body airway obstruction unlikely. The infant's history is also inconsistent with foreign-body airway obstruction. The infant has no acute distress; the onset of symptoms was gradual rather than abrupt.

Answer d is incorrect because disordered control of ventilation is characterized by inadequate or absent ventilatory effort.

2. For the infant described in question 1, which of the following options is the *most* appropriate *initial* management?

   a. immediate vascular access

   b. immediate tracheal intubation

   c. immediate administration of oxygen

   d. no immediate therapy, but order a stat chest x-ray

The correct answer is c. This infant has respiratory distress, so immediate oxygen administration is appropriate. Oxyhemoglobin saturation should be monitored using a pulse oximeter.

Answer a is incorrect because there is no indication for immediate vascular access. The infant is alert, interactive, and well perfused.

Answer b is incorrect because there are no indications for immediate tracheal intubation based on your rapid cardiopulmonary assessment. The infant is alert and has no signs of severe airway compromise or need for immediate mechanical ventilation.

Answer d is incorrect because obtaining a chest x-ray is not the best immediate course of action. Although a chest X-ray may be appropriate, it will not immediately help this child in distress.

3. A 5-year-old with a history of sickle cell anemia presents with fever and rapid breathing. You are asked to see the child because the mother is concerned that his distress is getting worse. On initial examination you see an anxious child with labored, rapid respirations, nasal flaring, and grunting. The child is receiving 3 L/min oxygen by nasal cannula, and pulse oximetry indicates an oxygen saturation of 85% to 88%. He has rapid, bounding peripheral pulses, a heart rate of 135 bpm, and blood pressure is 92/45 mm Hg. On auscultation of the chest, you hear adequate bilateral breath sounds and bilateral moist crackles. The child has a rapid but regular cardiac rhythm and a loud systolic ejection murmur. Which *one* of the following most accurately describes the child's respiratory distress?

   a. the child likely has upper airway obstruction

   b. the child likely has lower airway obstruction

   c. the child likely has a tension pneumothorax

   d. the child likely has parenchymal lung disease (eg, pneumonia)

The correct answer is d. This child has respiratory distress with increased work of breathing (retractions, nasal flaring, grunting), hypoxemia despite oxygen therapy, and moist crackles on auscultation, all of which are symptoms of parenchymal lung disease. Children with sickle cell disease are at increased risk for development of respiratory failure due to "acute chest syndrome." This syndrome is often triggered by pneumonia, and it causes diffuse parenchymal lung disease. The symptoms correlate with obstruction of the capillaries in the lung by sickled red blood cells. Ventilation and perfusion are often not well matched.

Answers a and **b** are incorrect because the absence of turbulent noises during inspiration (consistent with upper airway obstruction) or expiration (consistent with lower airway obstruction) suggests that airway obstruction is less likely.

Answer c is incorrect because there is no reason to suspect a tension pneumothorax in this patient. Although his distress has come on somewhat suddenly, there is no hemodynamic compromise, and equal bilateral breath sounds are present.

4. **For the child described in question 3, which of the following is *not* a treatment priority *at this time*?**

   a. immediate tracheal intubation

   b. cardiorespiratory monitoring

   c. provision of oxygen using a high-flow device such as a partial non-rebreathing face mask

   d. consultation and support in a monitored ICU environment

   The correct answer is a. This child is in acute respiratory distress with hypoxemia, but he is still alert and does not require immediate tracheal intubation. Instead the child requires careful monitoring of his response to treatment. To improve oxygenation, a high-flow oxygen delivery system is preferable to a nasal cannula. If available, CPAP with ventilatory assistance may be provided using a tight-fitting face mask (BiPAP).

   Answer b is incorrect because this child is in distress with respiratory symptoms. Cardiorespiratory monitoring *is* appropriate.

   Answer c is incorrect because high-flow oxygen administration *is* indicated for this hypoxemic child.

   Answer d is incorrect because this child is clearly at risk for respiratory failure. Preparation for tracheal intubation and early consultation and transfer to an ICU *are* appropriate.

5. **Despite efforts to support and improve oxygenation, the child in questions 3 and 4 deteriorates, and gasping respirations, bradycardia, and cyanosis develop. After tracheal intubation, which one of the following would provide the most *reliable* indicator that the tracheal tube is in the trachea for *this* patient?**

   a. presence of equal breath sounds over the lungs on auscultation

   b. presence of water vapor in the tracheal tube

   c. absence of breath sounds over the abdomen

   d. presence of exhaled CO_2 after 6 breaths as determined by a colorimetric detector device

   The correct answer is d. This patient has a *perfusing cardiac rhythm*, so under these conditions the presence of exhaled CO_2 is a sensitive and specific indicator of placement of the tube in the trachea. To avoid error due to detection of CO_2 from the stomach (resulting from bag-mask ventilation), the result should be interpreted after 6 breaths are delivered.

   Answers a, b, and **c** are incorrect. Although all are important clinical signs of proper tube placement, extensive experience in the operating room confirms that they are not always sensitive and specific indicators of tube placement in the trachea or displacement from the trachea. Pulse oximetry provides a useful monitor of tube placement after tracheal intubation. But if the patient has severe lung disease, oxygen saturation may remain low even when the tracheal tube is properly placed.

6. **After tracheal intubation and mechanical ventilation, the child described in questions 3, 4, and 5 improves (oxygen saturation increases to 94%). Approximately 4 hours later he suddenly deteriorates. Rapid cardiopulmonary assessment reveals weak pulses and poor color. Breath sounds are absent over the right chest. Oxygen saturation is 80% and falling. The end-tidal CO_2 (capnography) reading falls from 40 mm Hg to 30 mm Hg. You remove the patient from mechanical ventilation and provide hand ventilation, but his condition does not change. A suction catheter is rapidly and easily passed beyond the tracheal tube and does not meet resistance. Which one of the following causes of acute deterioration of the intubated patient is *most* likely to be present *in this child*?**

   a. displacement of the tracheal tube out of the airway

   b. obstruction of the tracheal tube

   c. pneumothorax

   d. equipment failure (ie, ventilator failure)

   The correct answer is c. Causes of acute deterioration of the intubated child are recalled by the DOPE mnemonic. **P**neumothorax, especially tension pneumothorax, is the most likely possibility. Pneumothorax occurs more commonly on the right than the left side because the tracheal tube often enters the right main bronchus, resulting in overdistention of that lung. Tension pneumothorax is characterized by sudden hemodynamic deterioration secondary to a sudden rise in intrathoracic pressure, which impairs venous return and cardiac output.

   Answer a is incorrect because exhaled CO_2 is detected, so the tube is still located in the airway. **D**isplacement of the tracheal tube often occurs during movement of the patient or during procedures, so it should be suspected if deterioration develops immediately after the patient is moved or procedures are completed. Displacement out of the trachea should be suspected if the exhaled CO_2 level falls rapidly in the patient with a perfusing rhythm.

   Answer b is incorrect because **O**bstruction of the tube is unlikely. Breath sounds are present unilaterally, and a suction catheter passes easily through the tube.

   Answer d, Equipment failure, is incorrect because when you removed the patient from the ventilator circuit and provided ventilation using a manual resuscitator, there was no improvement in his clinical condition.

References

1. Young KD, Seidel JS. Pediatric cardiopulmonary resuscitation: a collective review. *Ann Emerg Med.* 1999;33:195-205.

2. Sirbaugh PE, Pepe PE, Shook JE, Kimball KT, Goldman MJ, Ward MA, Mann DM. A prospective, population-based study of the demographics, epidemiology, management, and outcome of out-of-hospital pediatric cardiopulmonary arrest. *Ann Emerg Med.* 1999; 33:174-184.

3. Eckenhoff J. Some anatomic considerations of the infant larynx influencing endotracheal anesthesia. *Anesthesiology.* 1951;12:401-410.

4. Mansell A, Bryan C, Levison H. Airway closure in children. *J Appl Physiol.* 1972;33: 711-714.

5. Anthonisen NR, Danson J, Robertson PC, Ross WR. Airway closure as a function of age. *Respir Physiol.* 1969;8:58-65.

6. Coté CJ, Ryan JF, Todres ID, Groudsouzian NG, eds. *A Practice of Anesthesia for Infants and Children.* 2nd ed. Philadelphia, Pa: WB Saunders; 1993.

7. Wittenborg MH. Development-radiologic reevaluation: an overview. *Am J Roentgenol Radium Ther Nucl Med.* 1967;100:228-231.

8. Cross KW, Tizard JP, Trythall DA. The gaseous metabolism of the newborn infant. *Acta Paediatr.* 1957;46:265-285.

9. Epstein RA, Hyman AI. Ventilatory requirements of critically ill neonates. *Anesthesiology.* 1980;53:379-384.

10. Bota GW, Rowe BH. Continuous monitoring of oxygen saturation in prehospital patients with severe illness: the problem of unrecognized hypoxemia. *J Emerg Med.* 1995;13: 305-311.

11. Aughey K, Hess D, Eitel D, Bleecher K, Cooley M, Ogden C, Sabulsky N. An evaluation of pulse oximetry in prehospital care. *Ann Emerg Med.* 1991;20:887-891.

12. Anderson AB, Zwerdling RG, Dewitt TG. The clinical utility of pulse oximetry in the pediatric emergency department setting. *Pediatr Emerg Care.* 1991;7:263-266.

13. Brown LH, Manring EA, Kornegay HB, Prasad NH. Can prehospital personnel detect hypoxemia without the aid of pulse oximeters? *Am J Emerg Med.* 1996;14:43-44.

14. Schmitt HJ, Schuetz WH, Proeschel PA, Jaklin C. Accuracy of pulse oximetry in children with cyanotic congenital heart disease. *J Cardiothorac Vasc Anesth.* 1993;7:61-65.

15. Poirier MP, Gonzalez Del-Rey JA, McAneney CM, DiGiulio GA. Utility of monitoring capnography, pulse oximetry, and vital signs in the detection of airway mishaps: a hyperoxemic animal model. *Am J Emerg Med.* 1998; 6:350-352.

16. Birmingham PK, Cheney FW, Ward RJ. Esophageal intubation: a review of detection techniques. *Anesth Analg.* 1986;65:886-891.

17. Beyer AJ, III, Land G, Zaritsky A. Nonphysician transport of intubated pediatric patients: A system evaluation. *Crit Care Med.* 1992; 20:961-966.

18. Wahr JA, Tremper KK, Diab M. Pulse oximetry. *Respir Care Clin N Am.* 1995;1:77-105.

19. Coté CJ, Daniels AL, Connolly M, Szyfelbein SK, Wickens CD. Tongue oximetry in children with extensive thermal injury: comparison with peripheral oximetry. *Can J Anaesth.* 1992;39:454-457.

20. Murphy KG, Secunda JA, Rockoff MA. Severe burns from a pulse oximeter. *Anesthesiology.* 1990;73:350-352.

21. Sobel DB. Burning of a neonate due to a pulse oximeter: arterial saturation monitoring. *Pediatrics.* 1992;89:154-155.

22. Reynolds LM, Nicolson SC, Steven JM, Escobar A, McGonigle ME, Jobes DR. Influence of sensor site location on pulse oximetry kinetics in children. *Anesth Analg.* 1993;76:751-754.

23. Severinghaus JW, Naifeh KH, Koh SO. Errors in 14 pulse oximeters during profound hypoxia. *J Clin Monit.* 1989;5:72-81.

24. Steedman DJ, Robertson CE. Acid-base changes in arterial and central venous blood during cardiopulmonary resuscitation. *Arch Emerg Med.* 1992;9:169-176.

25. Weil M, Rackow E, Trevino R, Grundler W, Falk J, Griffel M. Difference in acid-base state between venous and arterial blood during cardiopulmonary resuscitation. *N Engl J Med.* 1986;315:153-156.

26. Johnson BA, Weil MH. Redefining ischemia due to circulatory failure as dual defects of oxygen deficits and of carbon dioxide excesses. *Crit Care Med.* 1991;19:1432-1438.

27. Hudgel DW, Hendricks C. Palate and hypopharynx—sites of inspiratory narrowing of the upper airway during sleep. *Am Rev Respir Dis.* 1988;138:1542-1547.

28. Abernethy LJ, Allan PL, Drummond GB. Ultrasound assessment of the position of the tongue during induction of anaesthesia. *Br J Anaesth.* 1990;65:744-748.

29. Galloway DW. Upper airway obstruction by the soft palate: influence of position of head, jaw, and neck. *Br J Anaesth.* 1990;64:383-384.

30. Morikawa S, Safar P, DeCarlo J. Influence of the head-jaw position upon upper airway patency. *Anesthesiology.* 1961;22:265-270.

31. Davis HW, Gartner JC, Galvis AG, Michaels RH, Mestad PH. Acute upper airway obstruction: croup and epiglottitis. *Pediatr Clin North Am.* 1981;28:859-880.

32. McPherson SP. *Respiratory Therapy Equipment.* 3rd ed. St. Louis, MO: CV Mosby Co; 1985.

33. Finer NN, Barrington KJ, Al-Fadley F, Peters KL. Limitations of self-inflating resuscitators. *Pediatrics.* 1986;77:417-420.

34. Zander J, Hazinski MF. Pulmonary disorders: airway obstruction. In: Hazinski MF, ed. *Nursing Care of the Critically Ill Child.* St Louis, MO: Mosby—Year Book; 1992.

35. Gausche M, Lewis RJ, Stratton SJ, Haynes BE, Gunter CS, Goodrich SM, Poore PD, McCollough MD, Henderson DP, Pratt FD, Seidel JS. Effect of out-of-hospital pediatric endotracheal intubation on survival and neurological outcome: a controlled clinical trial. *JAMA.* 2000;283:783-790.

36. Thomas SH, Harrison T, Wedel SK. Flight crew airway management in four settings: a six-year review. *Prehosp Emerg Care.* 1999; 3:310-315.

37. Sing RF, Rotondo MF, Zonies DH, Schwab CW, Kauder DR, Ross SE, Brathwaite CC. Rapid sequence induction for intubation by an aeromedical transport team: a critical analysis. *Am J Emerg Med.* 1998;16:598-602.

38. Jesudian MC, Harrison RR, Keenan RL, Maull KI. Bag-valve-mask ventilation: two rescuers are better than one: preliminary report. *Crit Care Med.* 1985;13.

39. Berg MD, Idris AH, Berg RA. Severe ventilatory compromise due to gastric distention during pediatric cardiopulmonary resuscitation. *Resuscitation.* 1998;36:71-73.

40. Moynihan RJ, Brock-Utne JG, Archer JH, Feld LH, Kreitzman TR. The effect of cricoid pressure on preventing gastric insufflation in infants and children. *Anesthesiology.* 1993;78: 652-656.

41. Salem MR, Wong AY, Mani M, Sellick BA. Efficacy of cricoid pressure in preventing gastric inflation during bag-mask ventilation in pediatric patients. *Anesthesiology.* 1974;40: 96-98.

42. Sellick BA. Cricoid pressure to control regurgitation of stomach contents during induction of anesthesia. *Lancet.* 1961;2:404-406.

43. Hartsilver EL, Vanner RG. Airway obstruction with cricoid pressure. *Anaesthesia.* 2000; 55:208-211.

44. Field D, Milner AD, Hopkin IE. Efficiency of manual resuscitators at birth. *Arch Dis Child.* 1986;61:300-302.

45. Terndrup TE, Kanter RK, Cherry RA. A comparison of infant ventilation methods performed by prehospital personnel. *Ann Emerg Med.* 1989;18:607-611.

46. Hirschman AM, Kravath RE. Venting vs ventilating. A danger of manual resuscitation bags. *Chest.* 1982;82:369-370.

47. Dorsch JA, Dorsch SE. *Understanding Anesthesia Equipment: Construction, Care, and Complications*. 2nd ed. Baltimore, MD: Williams & Wilkins Co; 1984.

48. Mondolfi AA, Grenier BM, Thompson JE, Bachur RG. Comparison of self-inflating bags with anesthesia bags for bag-mask ventilation in the pediatric emergency department. *Pediatr Emerg Care*. 1997;13:312-316.

49. Rumball CJ, MacDonald D. The PTL, Combitube, laryngeal mask, and oral airway: a randomized prehospital comparative study of ventilatory device effectiveness and cost-effectiveness in 470 cases of cardiorespiratory arrest. *Prehosp Emerg Care*. 1997;1:1-10.

50. Martin SE, Ochsner MG, Jarman RH, Agudelo WE, Davis FE. Use of the laryngeal mask airway in air transport when intubation fails. *J Trauma*. 1999;47:352-357.

51. Berry AM, Brimacombe JR, Verghese C. The laryngeal mask airway in emergency medicine, neonatal resuscitation, and intensive care medicine. *Int Anesthesiol Clin*. 1998;36:91-109.

52. Lopez-Gil M, Brimacombe J, Alvarez M. Safety and efficacy of the laryngeal mask airway. A prospective survey of 1400 children. *Anaesthesia*. 1996;51:969-972.

53. Lopez-Gil M, Brimacombe J, Cebrian J, Arranz J. Laryngeal mask airway in pediatric practice: a prospective study of skill acquisition by anesthesia residents. *Anesthesiology*. 1996;84:807-811.

54. Brimacombe J. The advantages of the LMA over the tracheal tube or facemask: a meta-analysis. *Can J Anaesth*. 1995;42:1017-1023.

55. Leach A. The use of the laryngeal mask airway by nurses during cardiopulmonary resuscitation. Results of a multicentre trial. *Anaesthesia*. 1994;49:3-7.

56. Pennant JH, Walker MB. Comparison of the endotracheal tube and laryngeal mask in airway management by paramedical personnel. *Anesth Analg*. 1992;74:531-534.

57. Brimacombe JR, Berry A. The incidence of aspiration associated with the laryngeal mask airway: a meta-analysis of published literature. *J Clin Anesth*. 1995;7:297-305.

58. Stone BJ, Chantler PJ, Baskett PJ. The incidence of regurgitation during cardiopulmonary resuscitation: a comparison between the bag valve mask and laryngeal mask airway. *Resuscitation*. 1998;38:3-6.

59. Deakers TW, Reynolds G, Stretton M, Newth CJ. Cuffed endotracheal tubes in pediatric intensive care. *J Pediatr*. 1994;125:57-62.

60. Khine HH, Corddry DH, Kettrick RG, Martin TM, McCloskey JJ, Rose JB, Theroux MC, Zagnoev M. Comparison of cuffed and uncuffed endotracheal tubes in young children during general anesthesia. *Anesthesiology*. 1997;86:627-631.

61. King BR, Baker MD, Braitman LE, Seidl-Friedman J, Schreiner MS. Endotracheal tube selection in children: a comparison of four methods. *Ann Emerg Med*. 1993;22:530-534.

62. van den Berg AA, Mphanza T. Choice of tracheal tube size for children: finger size or age-related formula? *Anaesthesia*. 1997;52:701-703.

63. Luten RC, Wears RL, Broselow J, Zaritsky A, Barnett TM, Lee T, Bailey A, Valley R, Brown R, Rosenthal B. Length-based endotracheal tube and emergency equipment in pediatrics. *Ann Emerg Med*. 1992;21:900-904.

64. Gerardi MJ, Sacchetti AD, Cantor RM, Santamaria JP, Gausche M, Lucid W, Foltin GL. Rapid-sequence intubation of the pediatric patient. Pediatric Emergency Medicine Committee of the American College of Emergency Physicians. *Ann Emerg Med*. 1996;28:55-74.

65. Westhorpe RN. The position of the larynx in children and its relationship to the ease of intubation. *Anaesth Intensive Care*. 1987;15:384-388.

66. Kelly JJ, Eynon CA, Kaplan JL, de Garavilla L, Dalsey WC. Use of tube condensation as an indicator of endotracheal tube placement. *Ann Emerg Med*. 1998;31:575-578.

67. Andersen KH, Schultz-Lebahn T. Oesophageal intubation can be undetected by auscultation of the chest. *Acta Anaesthesiol Scand*. 1994;38:580-582.

68. O'Connor R, Swor RA. National Association of EMS Physicians Position Paper: Verification of endotracheal tube placement following intubation. *Prehosp Emerg Care*. 1999;3:248-250.

69. Bhende MS, Thompson AE, Orr RA. Utility of an end-tidal carbon dioxide detector during stabilization and transport of critically ill children. *Pediatrics*. 1992;89:1042-1044.

70. Bhende MS, Thompson AE, Cook DR, Saville AL. Validity of a disposable end-tidal CO_2 detector in verifying endotracheal tube placement in infants and children. *Ann Emerg Med*. 1992;21:142-145.

71. Bhende MS, Thompson AE. Evaluation of an end-tidal CO2 detector during pediatric cardiopulmonary resuscitation. *Pediatrics*. 1995;95:395-399.

72. Ornato JP, Shipley JB, Racht EM, Slovis CM, Wrenn KD, Pepe PE, Almeida SL, Ginger VF, Fotre TV. Multicenter study of a portable, hand-size, colorimetric end-tidal carbon dioxide detection device. *Ann Emerg Med*. 1992;21:518-523.

73. Cardoso MM, Banner MJ, Melker RJ, Bjoraker DG. Portable devices used to detect endotracheal intubation during emergency situations: a review. *Crit Care Med*. 1998;26:957-964.

74. Ward KR, Yealy DM. End-tidal carbon dioxide monitoring in emergency medicine, Part 1: Basic principles. *Acad Emerg Med*. 1998;5:628-638.

75. Cantineau JP, Merckx P, Lambert Y, Sorkine M, Bertrand C, Duvaldestin P. Effect of epinephrine on end-tidal carbon dioxide pressure during prehospital cardiopulmonary resuscitation. *Am J Emerg Med*. 1994;12:267-270.

76. Kern KB, Sanders AB, Voorhees WD, F BC, Tacker WA, Ewy GA. Changes in expired end-tidal carbon dioxide during cardiopulmonary resuscitation in dogs: A prognostic guide for resuscitation efforts. *JACC*. 1989;13:1184-1189.

77. Callaham M, Barton C. Prediction of outcome of cardiopulmonary resuscitation from end-tidal carbon dioxide concentration. *Crit Care Med*. 1990;18:358-362.

78. Levine RL, Wayne MA, Miller CC. End-tidal carbon dioxide and outcome of out-of-hospital cardiac arrest. *N Engl J Med*. 1997;337:301-306.

79. Varon AJ, Morrina J, Civetta JM. Clinical utility of a colorimetric end-tidal CO_2 detector in cardiopulmonary resuscitation and emergency intubation. *J Clin Monit*. 1991;7:289-293.

80. Ward K, Sullivan JR, Zelenak RR, Summer WR. A comparison of interposed abdominal compression CPR and standard CPR by monitoring end-tidal P_{CO_2}. *Ann Emerg Med*. 1989;18:831-837.

81. Ward KR, Menegazzi JJ, Zelenak RR, Sullivan RJ, McSwain N, Jr. A comparison of chest compressions between mechanical and manual CPR by monitoring end-tidal P_{CO_2} during human cardiac arrest. *Ann Emerg Med*. 1993;22:669-674.

82. Weil MH, Bisera J, Trevino RP, Rackow EC. Cardiac output and end-tidal carbon dioxide. *Crit Care Med*. 1985;13:907-909.

83. Ornato JP, Garnett AR, Glauser FL. Relationship between cardiac output and the end-tidal carbon dioxide tension. *Ann Emerg Med*. 1990;19:1104-1106.

84. Bhende MS, Karasic DG, Karasic RB. End-tidal carbon dioxide changes during cardiopulmonary resuscitation after experimental asphyxial cardiac arrest. *Am J Emerg Med.* 1996;14:349-350.

85. Berg RA, Henry C, Otto CW, Sanders AB, Kern KB, Hilwig RW, Ewy GA. Initial end-tidal CO_2 is markedly elevated during cardiopulmonary resuscitation after asphyxial cardiac arrest. *Pediatr Emerg Care.* 1996;12:245-248.

86. Kasper CL, Deem S. The self-inflating bulb to detect esophageal intubation during emergency airway management. *Anesthesiology.* 1998;88:898-902.

87. Zaleski L, Abello D, Gold MI. The esophageal detector device. Does it work? *Anesthesiology.* 1993;79:244-247.

88. Bozeman WP, Hexter D, Liang HK, Kelen GD. Esophageal detector device versus detection of end-tidal carbon dioxide level in emergency intubation. *Ann Emerg Med.* 1996;27:595-599.

89. Wee MY, Walker AK. The oesophageal detector device. An assessment with uncuffed tubes in children. *Anaesthesia.* 1991;46:869-871.

90. Haynes SR, Morton NS. Use of the oesophageal detector device in children under one year of age. *Anaesthesia.* 1990;45:1067-1069.

91. Lang DJ, Wafai Y, Salem MR, Czinn EA, Halim AA, Baraka A. Efficacy of the self-inflating bulb in confirming tracheal intubation in the morbidly obese. *Anesthesiology.* 1996;85:246-253.

92. Baraka A, Khoury PJ, Siddik SS, Salem MR, Joseph NJ. Efficacy of the self-inflating bulb in differentiating esophageal from tracheal intubation in the parturient undergoing cesarean section. *Anesth Analg.* 1997;84:533-537.

93. Bhende MS, Karasic DG, Menegazzi JJ. Evaluation of an end-tidal CO_2 detector during cardiopulmonary resuscitation in a canine model for pediatric cardiac arrest. *Pediatr Emerg Care.* 1995;11:365-368.

94. Donn SM, Kuhns LR. Mechanism of endotracheal tube movement with change of head position in the neonate. *Pediatr Radiol.* 1980;9:37-40.

95. Hartrey R, Kestin IG. Movement of oral and nasal tracheal tubes as a result of changes in head and neck position. *Anaesthesia.* 1995;50:682-687.

96. Tobias JD, Lynch A, Garrett J. Alterations of end-tidal carbon dioxide during the intrahospital transport of children. *Pediatr Emerg Care.* 1996;12:249-251.

97. Goldstein B, Shanon DC, Todres ID. Supercarbia in children: clinical course and outcome. *Crit Care Med.* 1990;18:166-168.

98. Coté CJ, Eavey RD, Todres ID, Jones DE. Cricothyroid membrane puncture: oxygenation and ventilation in a dog model using an intravenous catheter. *Crit Care Med.* 1988;16:615-619.

99. Neff CC, Pfister RC, Van Sonnenberg E. Percutaneous transtracheal ventilation: experimental and practical aspects. *J Trauma.* 1983;23:84-90.

100. Depierraz B, Ravussin P, Brossard E, Monnier P. Percutaneous transtracheal jet ventilation for paediatric endoscopic laser treatment of laryngeal and subglottic lesions. *Can J Anaesth.* 1994;41:1200-1207.

101. Ravussin P, Bayer-Berger M, Monnier P, Savary M, Freeman J. Percutaneous transtracheal ventilation for laser endoscopic procedures in infants and small children with laryngeal obstruction: report of two cases. *Can J Anaesth.* 1987;34:83-86.

102. Smith RB, Schaer WB, Pfaeffle H. Percutaneous transtracheal ventilation for anaesthesia and resuscitation: a review and report of complications. *Can Anaesth Soc J.* 1975;22:607-612.

103. Stothert JC, Jr., Stout MJ, Lewis LM, Keltner RM, Jr. High pressure percutaneous transtracheal ventilation: the use of large gauge intravenous-type catheters in the totally obstructed airway. *Am J Emerg Med.* 1990;8:184-189.

104. Benumof JL, Scheller MS. The importance of transtracheal jet ventilation in the management of the difficult airway. *Anesthesiology.* 1989;71:769-778.

105. Peak DA, Roy S. Needle cricothyroidotomy revisited. *Pediatr Emerg Care.* 1999;15:224-226.

106. Barrachina F, Guardiola JJ, Ano T, Ochagavia A, Marine J. Percutaneous dilatational cricothyroidotomy: outcome with 44 consecutive patients. *Intensive Care Med.* 1996;22:937-940.

107. The Acute Respiratory Distress Syndrome Network. Ventilation with lower tidal volumes as compared with traditional tidal volumes for acute lung injury and the acute respiratory distress syndrome. *N Engl J Med.* 2000;342:1301-1308.

Chapter 5

Fluid Therapy and Medications for Shock and Cardiac Arrest

Introductory Case Scenario

A 4-year-old girl is brought to her pediatrician's office with a complaint of increasing lethargy, fever, and dizziness when she tries to stand. She has had chickenpox for 5 days, and her mother notes that several of the lesions on her abdomen have become red, tender, and swollen over the last 18 hours.

On physical examination the child is lying supine and listless and appears very ill. She does not answer questions appropriately but withdraws appropriately from painful stimulation. Her heart rate is 175 bpm; respiratory rate, 60 breaths/min with deep breaths that are not labored; oral temperature, 39.4°C (103°F); and blood pressure, 70/29 mm Hg. Her extremities are cool and mottled below the elbows and knees, and peripheral pulses are barely palpable. Capillary refill time is 6 to 8 seconds.

- What is your initial cardiopulmonary assessment?

- What initial treatment should you provide?

- What type of fluid resuscitation should you provide? How much? How fast?

- What medications should you administer to improve blood pressure and cardiac output?

Learning Objectives

After completing this chapter the PALS provider should be able to

- Discuss the principles of acute fluid resuscitation for circulatory shock and select appropriate resuscitation fluids for a child in shock

- Discuss the pharmacology of medications for cardiac arrest and their indications and which medications to administer for treatment of a child in cardiac arrest

- Describe the indications, doses, and precautions for medications to (1) prevent progression from shock to cardiac arrest and (2) treat postresuscitation myocardial dysfunction

Acute Fluid Resuscitation for Circulatory Shock

The objectives of fluid administration during resuscitation for circulatory shock are to

- Rapidly restore effective circulating volume in shock states such as hypovolemic and distributive shock

- Restore oxygen-carrying capacity in hemorrhagic shock states

- Correct metabolic imbalances secondary to volume depletion

Expansion of circulating blood volume is a critical component of treatment for circulatory shock (see Critical Concepts: "Hypovolemia and Shock"). Early restitution of circulating blood volume is important to prevent progression to refractory shock or cardiac arrest[1] and to reduce the risk of postshock organ dysfunction.

Critical Concepts:
Hypovolemia and Shock

Hypovolemia is the most common cause of shock in children worldwide. For all forms of shock you should determine the need for initial volume resuscitation.

Hypovolemia is the most common cause of shock in children worldwide. It frequently results from diarrhea, vomiting, diabetic ketoacidosis, or sudden large volume losses associated with burns or trauma. The volume loss is often complicated by inadequate fluid intake. Although septic, anaphylactic, neurogenic, and other so-called distributive forms of shock are not typically classified as hypovolemic shock, all are characterized in large part by *relative* hypovolemia that results from vasodilation, increased capillary permeability, and plasma loss into the interstitium. You should consider the need for volume administration during initial resuscitation of *all* forms of shock, although cardiogenic shock may require alternative therapies. Therefore, quickly establish vascular access in all patients showing signs of shock, preferably with 1 or 2 large-bore, short-length vascular catheters (see Chapter 6: "Vascular Access").

The ideal fluid for volume expansion in children with hypovolemic shock is controversial. Volume expansion is probably best achieved with isotonic crystalloid solutions such as normal saline or Ringer's lactate.[2,3] Isotonic crystalloid solutions are inexpensive and readily available and do not produce sensitivity reactions. They effectively expand the interstitial water space and correct sodium deficits. But they do not efficiently expand the intravascular (circulating) volume because only approximately one fourth of administered isotonic crystalloid solution remains in the intravascular compartment.[4] As a result a large quantity of crystalloid solution (potentially 4 or 5 times the deficit) must be administered to restore intravascular volume to the hypovolemic patient. Rapid infusion of this quantity is well tolerated by a healthy young patient but may cause pulmonary edema in the critically ill child with underlying cardiac or pulmonary disease.

Colloid solutions remain in the intravascular compartment hours longer than crystalloid solutions.[4] As a result blood and colloid solutions, such as 5% albumin, fresh frozen plasma, and synthetic colloid solutions (eg, hetastarch, dextran 40, dextran 60), are more efficient volume expanders than crystalloid solutions. But colloid solutions may cause sensitivity reactions and other complications. As with crystalloids, excessive administration of colloids may lead to pulmonary edema, particularly in patients with cardiac or pulmonary disease.

One meta-analysis of studies comparing crystalloid with colloid administration in various types of shock suggests that colloid administration may be associated with an increased mortality rate.[2,3] But a recent second meta-analysis called these results into question.[5] Few children were included in the studies analyzed, and no firm recommendation can be made against the use of colloid solutions for circulatory shock in infants and children. Indeed, in a large case series of children with meningococcemia, septic shock was treated effectively with colloid solution and outcomes were better than previously reported

when patients are stratified by severity of illness on presentation.[6] More information is needed about the use of colloid solutions in treatment of shock.

Blood products should be administered only when specifically indicated for replacement of blood loss or correction of coagulopathies (see Critical Concepts: "Isotonic Crystalloid vs Blood for Volume Resuscitation"). Blood and blood products may be useful in the treatment of non-traumatic hypovolemic shock but are not the first choice for volume expansion because the risk of blood-borne infection cannot be eliminated.[7]

Blood is recommended for fluid replacement of volume loss in pediatric trauma victims with inadequate perfusion despite administration of 2 to 3 boluses of crystalloid solution (ie, approximately 40 to 60 mL/kg). Under these circumstances administer blood (10 to 15 mL/kg of packed red blood cells or 20 mL/kg of whole blood) as soon as it is available. With a physician order type O blood may be administered before crossmatch (O-negative blood may be reserved for girls and women of childbearing age to avoid Rh isoimmunization). Blood component therapy may

Critical Concepts:
Isotonic Crystalloid vs Blood for Volume Resuscitation

Initial volume resuscitation for hypovolemic shock should usually be 20 mL/kg of isotonic crystalloid; smaller volumes may be administered if myocardial dysfunction is present or suspected. Red blood cell transfusion (typically 10 to 15 mL/kg of packed red blood cells) is recommended for pediatric trauma victims when signs of shock or hemodynamic instability persist despite administration of approximately 40 to 60 mL/kg (2 to 3 boluses) of isotonic crystalloid solution.

also be valuable in correction of coagulopathies, although such treatment may be palliative until the cause of the coagulopathy is identified and treated.

Rapid infusion of blood or blood products, particularly in large volumes, may produce several complications.[7] Rapid administration of cold blood products can produce hypothermia, which can complicate the management of the trauma or submersion victim who may already be hypothermic from exposure to the environment. Hypothermia may adversely affect cardiovascular function and compromise several metabolic functions, including the metabolism of citrate, which is present in stored blood. Inadequate citrate clearance in turn causes ionized hypocalcemia. The combined effects of hypothermia and ionized hypocalcemia can result in significant myocardial dysfunction. To minimize these problems, blood and blood products should be warmed before or during rapid IV administration if possible.

Hypovolemic shock results from depletion of intravascular and extravascular volume. If the hypovolemia is severe or sustained, vascular tone may decrease and capillary permeability may increase, resulting in extravascular fluid shift and greater depletion of intravascular volume. Thus adequate fluid resuscitation often requires IV infusions that exceed the estimated volume losses in order to replace transcapillary fluid loss and fill the expanded vascular compartment.

Volume therapy is indicated when a child demonstrates signs of shock (eg, tachycardia, mottled or pale color, cool skin, diminished peripheral pulses, change in mental status, oliguria, and delayed capillary refill despite normal ambient temperature). Shock may be present despite a "normal" blood pressure. Blood pressure measurements are used to distinguish *compensated* from *decompensated* shock in children. In decompensated shock systolic blood pressure is less than the 5th percentile for age (for children 1 to 10 years of age, this 5th percentile systolic blood pressure is estimated to be 70 mm Hg plus twice the child's age in years). Prompt and effective treatment of early signs of compensated shock may prevent the development of decompensated shock and the high rates of morbidity and mortality associated with it.

When signs of hypovolemic shock are detected, rapidly administer a fluid bolus and assess the child's response. Provide additional fluid boluses until systemic perfusion improves and signs of shock are corrected. Be prepared to modify your approach to shock resuscitation for specific conditions (see FYI: "Advanced Provider Information—Fluid Therapy for Diabetic Ketoacidosis, Burns, and Poisonings").

In bolus fluid resuscitation therapy, 20 mL/kg of isotonic crystalloid solution is administered very rapidly (generally in a range of 5 to 20 minutes) immediately after obtaining intravascular or intraosseous (IO) access. If severe myocardial dysfunction is present, administer a smaller (5 to 10 mL/kg) fluid bolus. If the fluid deficit is mild or you suspect that myocardial function is not optimal, you may administer a bolus of 10 to 20 mL/kg. Normal saline or Ringer's lactate solution is appropriate for initial crystalloid infusion. Do not infuse large volumes of dextrose-containing solutions during resuscitation because the resultant hyperglycemia may induce osmotic diuresis and produce or aggravate hypokalemia.

For shock resuscitation the PALS guidelines recommend administration of fluid boluses over 5 to 20 minutes (see Critical Concepts: "Rapidity of Fluid Bolus Administration"). If the child has a severe volume deficit (eg, the trauma victim with significant hemorrhage), this interval should be at the shorter end of the range (5 to 10 minutes or less). If the child has a less severe fluid deficit or significant myocardial dysfunction (eg, the child with calcium channel blocker poisoning), you would likely administer the fluid bolus more slowly (over 10 to 20 minutes). Monitor cardiovascular function and assess for pul-

FYI: Advanced Provider Information—Fluid Therapy for Diabetic Ketoacidosis, Burns, and Poisonings

Diabetic Ketoacidosis

Although patients in diabetic ketoacidosis are typically dehydrated and may be in shock, the recommended fluid therapy is less aggressive than for other causes of shock. Clinically significant cerebral edema is an infrequent but often deadly complication of diabetic ketoacidosis and its therapy.[8] The pathophysiology of this cerebral edema is poorly understood. Several risk factors for cerebral edema have been proposed, including a higher initial BUN, severity of acidosis and hypocapnia at presentation,[8,9] sodium bicarbonate therapy, rapid volume administration,[10] and rapid decreases in serum osmolality during therapy.[11-13] In several studies smaller increases in serum sodium concentration during reduction in hyperglycemia have been linked to development of cerebral edema.[8,11-13]

In one study a less aggressive fluid management strategy (bolus of 10 mL/kg isotonic saline plus continuous infusion of replacement and maintenance fluid therapy over 48 hours) was administered to children with diabetic ketoacidosis.[11] With this regimen fewer patients developed neurologic complications or died. The authors suggest that rehydration should generally not exceed 2500, 3200, or 4000 mL/m^2 per day for 5%, 7.5%, and 10% dehydration, respectively.[11]

During therapy monitor serum sodium concentration and ensure that it rises appropriately as serum glucose falls. Serum sodium should rise approximately 1.6 mEq/L for every 100 mg/dL fall in glucose.[8,11-13]

Burns

Thermal injury results in loss of fluid through the burn wound and into adjacent tissue (third space loss), particularly during the first 12 to 36 hours after the burn injury. There is also loss of fluid into tissues distant from the burn when the burn injury is significant.

Fluid resuscitation is critical to replace fluid losses and prevent dehydration and hypovolemia. A variety of formulas can be used to guide fluid resuscitation; all are based on the size of the burn and the child's size. Most formulas, including those endorsed by the American College of Surgeons and the American Burn Association, recommend administration of a balanced salt solution at a rate of approximately 2 to 4 mL/kg per percent of body surface area burned per 24 hours.[14] This therapy is reevaluated and modified after the first 24 to 48 hours.

Poisonings

Poisonings with drugs such as calcium channel blockers, and β-adrenergic blockers can cause hypotension associated with poor myocardial contractility and acute congestive heart failure. If hypotension results from known or suspected calcium channel blocker or β-blocker overdose, provide smaller initial fluid boluses of 5 to 10 mL/kg and monitor the child closely for development of pulmonary edema. Repeat small boluses as needed.

For further information see Chapter 12: "Toxicology."

Critical Concepts: Rapidity of Fluid Bolus Administration

The current PALS guidelines allow the provider some discretion in determining the size and speed of administration of fluid boluses because children with shock are not all alike. The guidelines generally recommend a bolus volume of 20 mL/kg with the following caveats:

■ If the child demonstrates severe signs of hypovolemic shock (eg, after trauma and hemorrhage or with severe dehydration), a 20 mL/kg bolus is indicated, delivered rapidly (over 5 to 10 minutes).

■ If the child demonstrates less severe signs of shock or the provider is concerned that there is some impairment in myocardial function, a bolus of 10 mL/kg may be appropriate.

■ If the child has calcium channel blocker or β-adrenergic blocker poisoning, hypotension is treated with smaller fluid boluses (5 to 10 mL/kg) delivered more slowly (over 10 to 20 minutes) because severe myocardial dysfunction is often present.

The PALS guidelines recommend that the fluid bolus for shock be delivered over 5 to 20 minutes, based on the child's clinical condition:

■ If the child has severe hemorrhage after trauma, severe dehydration, hypovolemia, or decompensated shock, administer the fluid bolus as quickly as possible (in less than 5 to 10 minutes).

■ If the shock is less severe or you think the child may have associated myocardial dysfunction (eg, with calcium channel blocker or β-adrenergic blocker poisoning), you should probably administer the fluid bolus over approximately 10 to 20 minutes.

These ranges are not absolute, and clinical judgment is needed. The provider should assess the child's response to therapy and repeat the boluses if needed.

monary edema during and after administration of fluid boluses.

The minidrip IV systems used for routine pediatric fluid therapy may not allow rapid administration of fluid boluses. Placement of a 3-way stopcock in-line in the IV tubing system can facilitate rapid fluid delivery. A 35- to 60-mL syringe can be used to push fluids through the stopcock.

Reassess the child during and immediately after each bolus infusion. A child with hypovolemic shock may require administration of 40 to 60 mL/kg of fluid during the first hour of resuscitation and as much as 200 mL/kg during the first few hours of therapy. When septic shock is present, 60 to 80 mL/kg of fluid is often required

during the first hour of therapy[1,6] (for management of septic shock, see "Medications to Maintain Adequate Cardiac Output" later in this chapter). Persistent shock despite volume administration in a seriously injured child is an indication that surgical intervention may be required.

The efficacy of IV fluid administration during cardiac arrest is controversial. In normovolemic adult animal models, volume administration has been shown to *decrease* myocardial perfusion by elevating right atrial pressure and decreasing coronary perfusion pressure.[15,16] The results of these studies, however, may not be applicable to pediatric patients with hypovolemic cardiac arrest.

Consider administration of a crystalloid bolus (20 mL/kg) during resuscitation of the child with prehospital cardiac arrest of unknown cause if the child fails to respond to provision of adequate oxygenation, ventilation, chest compressions, and epinephrine (especially if child abuse is suspected). Unsuspected child abuse and internal hemorrhage may be responsible for hypovolemic shock, which may respond to volume administration plus standard resuscitation therapy. However, avoid excessive fluid administration because it may compromise vital organ blood flow and lead to pulmonary edema.[15]

Medications Administered During Cardiac Arrest

The objectives of administration of medications during cardiac arrest are

■ To increase coronary and cerebral (vital organ) perfusion pressure and therefore blood flow

■ To stimulate spontaneous or more forceful myocardial contractility

■ To accelerate heart rate

■ To correct metabolic acidosis

■ To suppress or treat arrhythmias (see Chapter 8: "Rhythm Disturbances")

General Issues in Cardiac Arrest Medications

Children in cardiac arrest are unresponsive with no effective breathing and no signs of circulation, including a pulse. Some of these children demonstrate VF or pulseless VT, but most have terminal bradycardia or asystolic arrest secondary to progressive hypoxic or ischemic events or both.[17-20] A small number may have organized electrical activity but such profound hypotension that the central pulses cannot be palpated, although they may be appreciated with intra-arterial monitoring or Doppler echocardiography; this phenomenon has been called "pseudo-pulseless electrical activity."[21,22]

Clearly, different interventions are appropriate for each cardiac arrest rhythm. The pharmacology of drugs used for resuscitation from cardiac arrest and in ALS is presented below with therapeutic considerations, indications, doses, routes of administration, and precautions. Also refer to Chapter 8: "Rhythm Disturbances," particularly for information about management of VF, pulseless VT, and pulseless electrical activity.

The venous system is the preferred route for administration of drugs in emergencies, but this system may be difficult to access.[23-31] Resuscitation medications, including catecholamines, adenosine, fluids, and blood products, have been safely and effectively administered via the bone marrow, a noncollapsible venous plexus.[25,29-32] (See Chapter 6: "Vascular Access.") During cardiac arrest in children, IO access may be the initial access site of choice for delivery of medications and fluids, because it can be established quickly, safely, and reliably.[25-27] In addition, the IO route is preferable to the tracheal route because drug absorption from the tracheobronchial tree is unpredictable.[33-36]

Critical Concepts:
Establishment of Vascular Access During Resuscitation

The intravascular route is preferred for administration of medications during emergencies. IO access may be the initial vascular access site of choice for medications and fluid during cardiac arrest. Providers should use the technique in which they are most proficient and the one that will provide the most rapid vascular access under these conditions. All medications should be followed by a saline flush of at least 5 mL.

During external chest compressions, central venous administration of medications theoretically provides a more rapid onset and higher peak concentration than peripheral venous injection.[37,38] In a single study of adult animals, drug injection into the central supradiaphragmatic venous system achieved better drug delivery into the circulation than IV injection below the diaphragm.[39] These differences, however, have not been demonstrated in pediatric resuscitation models and may not be important during pediatric CPR.[40]

In a pediatric animal model, drug infusion into a peripheral vein provided drug distribution comparable to that achieved by central venous administration.[40]

During resuscitation of the infant or small child, either peripheral or central venous drug administration is acceptable. If both access sites are present, central venous administration is preferred. All medications should be followed by a saline flush of at least 5 mL to move the drug from the peripheral to the central circulation.

Direct intracardiac injections are not recommended because they are associated with significant complications, including coronary artery laceration, pneumothorax, cardiac tamponade, and intractable arrhythmias.[41-44] In addition, intracardiac injections require interruption of cardiac compressions.

Cardiac output often remains depressed in patients following return of spontaneous circulation after cardiac arrest. These patients may benefit from administration of agents that increase cardiac contractility (eg, catecholamines). Occasionally they may require an agent that increases peripheral vascular resistance to maintain adequate perfusion pressure.

For continuous infusion, catecholamines (epinephrine, dopamine, dobutamine, and norepinephrine) may be diluted in a number of IV solutions, including 5% dextrose and water, normal saline, or Ringer's lac-

tate. When starting a drug infusion, flush the IV tubing with the catecholamine solution to the point where the IV tubing joins the vascular catheter. Initially infuse the drug at a rapid rate (eg, up to 20 mL/h) until the heart rate increases, indicating a response to the entry of catecholamine in the circulation. You can then reduce the infusion rate and titrate the infusion dose to produce the desired effects. The initial rapid infusion rate will prevent any delay in the delivery of medication to the patient through the tubing. All catecholamines are rapidly metabolized, so titration of the infusion rate to the patient's cardiovascular response (including heart rate), will reduce the likelihood of undesirable side effects.

Drug tables, charts, or tapes should be readily available to expedite the preparation of drug infusions. The use of length-based resuscitation tapes facilitates rapid estimation of the appropriate drug dose.[45]

Tracheal Administration of Medications

Until vascular access is obtained, the tracheal route may be used for administration of the lipid-soluble drugs lidocaine, epinephrine, atropine, and naloxone (these medications can be recalled with the mnemonic "LEAN").[46] Drugs that are not lipid soluble (eg, sodium bicarbonate and calcium) should *not* be administered by this route because they will injure tracheal tissue.

Optimal dosages for the tracheal administration of medications are unknown because drug absorption across the alveolar and bronchiolar epithelium during cardiac arrest may vary widely. Data from animal models,[34] including a neonatal piglet model[35] and one adult human study,[33] however, suggests that tracheal administration of a standard IV dose of epinephrine results in a serum concentration that is one tenth of that achieved by intravenous administration. For this reason the recommended tracheal dose of epinephrine given during pediatric resuscitation is 10 times the dose given via an intravascular route. Doses of other resuscitation drugs administered tracheally probably should also be increased compared with the IV dose.

Animal data suggests that when drugs administered by the tracheal route are diluted in up to 5 mL of normal saline and are followed by 5 manual ventilations, absorption and pharmacologic effects are equivalent to those observed after drug administration through a catheter or feeding tube inserted into the tracheal tube.[36] Direct tracheal administration is preferred because the use of catheters or feeding tubes is cumbersome and requires additional equipment, which may delay drug administration. Tracheal tubes with drug administration ports are now available.

Antiarrhythmic Medications

Antiarrhythmic medications may be indicated for treatment of (1) atrial and ventricular arrhythmias in order to prevent cardiogenic shock and cardiac arrest, (2) shock-resistant VF/pulseless VT, and (3) control of atrial or ventricular arrhythmias in symptomatic patients. Indications for these medications and their pharmacologic properties are discussed in Chapter 8: "Rhythm Disturbances."

Medications Used to Treat Cardiac Arrest

Epinephrine

Therapeutic Considerations

Epinephrine (adrenaline) is an endogenous catecholamine with potent α- and β-adrenergic stimulating properties. The α-adrenergic action (vasoconstriction) increases systemic vascular resistance and elevates systolic and diastolic blood pressure. α-Adrenergic vasoconstriction reduces blood flow to the splanchnic, renal, muscular, and dermal vascular beds. The β-adrenergic receptor action increases myocardial contractility and heart rate and relaxes smooth muscle in the skeletal muscle vascular bed and bronchi.

In cardiac arrest, α-adrenergic–mediated vasoconstriction is the most important pharmacologic action of epinephrine. Vasoconstriction increases aortic diastolic pressure and coronary perfusion pressure, a critical determinant of the success or failure of resuscitation.[47,48] Epinephrine-induced elevation of coronary perfusion pressure during chest compression enhances delivery of oxygen to the heart. Epinephrine also enhances the contractile state of the heart, stimulates spontaneous contractions, and increases the vigor and intensity of VF, increasing the success of defibrillation.[49] During CPR intense epinephrine-induced peripheral vasoconstriction in nonessential vascular beds directs limited cardiac output to the brain.[50,51]

The following cardiovascular effects have been observed after administration of epinephrine in the doses used during resuscitation:

■ Increased cardiac automaticity

■ Increased heart rate

■ Increased myocardial contractility

■ Increased systemic vascular resistance

■ Increased blood pressure (due to increased myocardial contractility and increased systemic vascular resistance)

■ Increased myocardial oxygen requirements (due to increased heart rate, increased myocardial contractility, and increased systemic vascular resistance)

Indications

Indications for administration of epinephrine during PALS are

■ Cardiac arrest

■ Symptomatic bradycardia unresponsive to ventilation and administration of oxygen

■ Hypotension unrelated to volume depletion

The elevation of coronary perfusion pressure associated with administration of epinephrine makes this drug useful in the treatment of all forms of cardiac arrest.[47-49] Asystole and bradyarrhythmias are the

most common presenting rhythms in pediatric patients with cardiac arrest.[17-20] In these settings epinephrine can successfully stimulate electrical and mechanical activity of the heart. VF is less common in children than in adult victims of cardiac arrest. Although rapid defibrillation is the treatment of choice for VF, epinephrine is recommended for VF unresponsive to defibrillation attempts or during CPR until a defibrillator is available.[47,48]

The presence of acidosis may depress the action of catecholamines.[52,53] Although sodium bicarbonate was previously recommended for treatment of severe metabolic acidosis, its value in this setting is not clear (see "Sodium Bicarbonate"). Treatment of metabolic acidosis in cardiac arrest includes administration of oxygen, support of adequate ventilation, and restoration of effective systemic perfusion.

Dose

The recommended initial resuscitation dose of epinephrine for cardiac arrest is 0.01 mg/kg (0.1 mL/kg of 1:10 000 solution) by the IV or IO route or 0.1 mg/kg (0.1 mL/kg of 1:1000 solution) by the tracheal route. For persistent arrest, the ECC guidelines recommend repeating doses every 3 to 5 minutes. For second and subsequent doses for unresponsive asystolic and pulseless arrest, the same dose of epinephrine is recommended, but higher doses (0.1 to 0.2 mg/kg [0.1 to 0.2 mL/kg of 1:1000 solution], so-called "high-dose" epinephrine) by any intravascular route may be considered (see Critical Concepts: "Epinephrine Doses During Resuscitation"). These recommendations use 2 different dilutions of epinephrine. *It is critical to select the correct concentration and dose.*

If intra-arterial pressure monitoring is available during CPR (eg, for resuscitation in the ICU), epinephrine doses can be titrated to effect. For example, standard epinephrine doses are appropriate if aortic diastolic pressure is greater than approximately 20 to 30 mm Hg, whereas higher epinephrine doses may be considered if diastolic pressure is substantially lower.

Critical Concepts:
Epinephrine Doses During Resuscitation

The key medication for resuscitation from cardiac arrest is intravascular epinephrine. The following doses of epinephrine are recommended during PALS:

- 0.01 mg/kg (0.1 mL/kg of 1:10 000 solution) IV or IO

- 0.1 mg/kg (0.1 mL/kg of 1:1000 solution [high dose]) by tracheal route

- The PALS provider may consider a higher IV or IO dose on second or subsequent doses: 0.1 mg/kg (0.1 mL/kg of 1:1000 solution).

Epinephrine is absorbed when administered by the tracheal route, although absorption and resulting plasma levels are unpredictable.[33-36,54] For children the recommended tracheal dose is 0.1 mg/kg (0.1 mL/kg of a 1:1000 solution). Once vascular access is obtained, administer intravascular epinephrine immediately if the victim remains in cardiac arrest, beginning with a standard initial dose of 0.01 mg/kg (0.1 mL/kg of 1:10 000 solution). You are assuming that the tracheal dose has not been adequately absorbed.

If perfusion remains inadequate, a continuous infusion of epinephrine may be useful once spontaneous circulation is restored. The hemodynamic effects of infused epinephrine are dose related: low-dose infusions (less than 0.3 µg/kg per minute) generally produce prominent β-adrenergic action, and higher-dose infusions (greater than 0.3 µg/kg per minute) result in both β-adrenergic actions and α-adrenergic–mediated vasoconstriction.[55] Because there is great interpatient variability in catecholamine pharmacology,[56-64] the infused dose should be titrated to the desired effect.

High-Dose Epinephrine

High-dose epinephrine (0.05 to 0.2 mg/kg) improves myocardial and cerebral blood flow during CPR, and it may improve rates of *initial* return of spontaneous circulation, particularly in animals with prolonged cardiac arrest.[65-74] Administration of high-dose epinephrine, however, can lead to a toxic postresuscitation hyperadrenergic state with atrial tachycardia or VT, severe hypertension, and worse postresuscitation cardiac dysfunction.[74-78] Retrospective adult and pediatric studies suggest that higher cumulative epinephrine doses are associated with worse neurologic outcome.[17,79-84] In contrast, a single poorly controlled pediatric study suggests that rescue therapy with high-dose epinephrine after failure of standard-dose epinephrine may improve outcome of *witnessed* cardiac arrest due to asystole or pulseless electrical activity.[85]

Many randomized, controlled studies in adults or animals and a few less rigorous pediatric investigations have demonstrated that initial high-dose epinephrine does not improve outcome.[65-75,81-84] Therefore, high-dose epinephrine is not recommended for the *initial* dose. Because of the scant dosage data on rescue therapy with high-dose epinephrine in patients who fail to respond to a standard dose, recommendations for its use are less firm. For second and subsequent doses in refractory pediatric cardiac arrest, high-dose epinephrine (0.1 mg/kg [0.1 mL/kg of 1:1000 solution]) is not recommended as the treatment of choice but is considered an acceptable alternative to standard-dose epinephrine. There is great interpatient variability in catecholamine pharmacokinetics and response[56-64]; a dangerous dose for one person may be a lifesaving dose for another.

For neonatal resuscitation the recommended tracheal dose is 0.01 to 0.03 mg/kg (0.1 to 0.3 mL/kg of 1:10 000 solution) repeated every 3 to 5 minutes. The evidence concerning the safety and efficacy of higher-dose epinephrine in neonates is inadequate. Prolonged hypertension after administration of high-dose tracheal epinephrine is especially worrisome in neonates because of the potential for intraventricular hemorrhage. See Chapter 13.

Precautions

It is important to note that the *volume* of epinephrine administered is 0.1 mL/kg whether standard or high-dose epinephrine is provided. The *dose* of epinephrine is determined by the *concentration of the drug: the standard dose is 0.1 mL/kg of 1:10 000 solution, and the high dose is 0.1 mL/kg of 1:1000 solution.* The recommended tracheal dose of epinephrine for children is 0.1 mL/kg of 1:1000 concentration or 0.1 mg/kg.

Epinephrine should be administered through a secure vascular catheter, preferably into the central circulation. If the drug infiltrates tissues, it may cause local ischemia, leading to tissue injury and ulceration. Epinephrine (and other catecholamines) are inactivated in alkaline solutions and therefore should not be mixed with sodium bicarbonate. In patients with a perfusing rhythm, epinephrine infusions cause tachycardia and often a wide pulse pressure and may produce ventricular ectopy. Continuous infusions of high-dose epinephrine may produce excessive vasoconstriction, compromising extremity, mesenteric, and renal blood flow and resulting in severe hypertension and tachyarrhythmias.

Supraventricular tachycardia, VT, and severe hypertension occur more frequently after administration of high-dose epinephrine, and postresuscitation myocardial dysfunction tends to be worse.[67,74-78] The benefits of high-dose epinephrine in relation to improved myocardial perfusion during CPR and perhaps an improved initial resuscitation rate must be weighed against the potential dangers of a postresuscitation hyperadrenergic state, excessive vasoconstriction, and adverse neurologic effects.[67,74-78,86]

Vasopressin

Therapeutic Considerations

Vasopressin is an endogenous hormone that acts at specific receptors to mediate systemic vasoconstriction (V_1 receptor) and reabsorption of water in the renal tubule (V_2 receptor). Marked secretion of vasopressin occurs in circulatory shock states and causes relatively selective vasoconstriction of blood vessels in the skin, skeletal muscle, intestine, and fat with relatively less vasoconstriction of the coronary, cerebral, and renal vascular beds. In experimental models of cardiac arrest the hemodynamic actions of vasopressin increase blood flow to the heart and brain and improve long-term survival rates when compared with epinephrine.[87-89] In swine models, however, this potent, long-acting vasoconstrictive effect decreases splanchnic blood flow during CPR and the early postresuscitation period.[90-92]

Vasopressin can be used as an alternative to epinephrine for treatment of shock-refractory VF in adults. In the prehospital setting vasopressin produced a higher return of spontaneous circulation than epinephrine.[92a] In the hospital setting vasopressin produced a survival-to-hospital-discharge rate equivalent to that of epinephrine in adult victims of cardiac arrest.[93] In a piglet model of prolonged asphyxial (pediatric) cardiac arrest, vasopressin was less effective than epinephrine.[94] Promising animal studies and limited clinical data[95,96] suggest that vasopressin may have an emerging role in treatment of shock-refractory VF in children. It has also been reported to be successful in the treatment of vasodilatory shock in limited pediatric reports.[97] The data is inadequate, however, to evaluate its efficacy and safety. Thus vasopressin is not presently recommended for treatment of cardiac arrest in children.

Glucose

Therapeutic Considerations

Small infants and chronically ill children have limited stores of glycogen that may be rapidly depleted during episodes of cardiopulmonary distress, resulting in hypoglycemia. Clinical signs of hypoglycemia may mimic those of hypoxemia, ischemia, or cardiac arrest (ie, poor perfusion, diaphoresis, tachycardia, hypothermia, irritability or lethargy, and hypotension). For this

reason you should monitor the serum glucose concentration in all infants and children with coma, shock, or respiratory failure.

Because glucose is the major metabolic substrate for the neonatal myocardium, hypoglycemia may depress neonatal myocardial function. Although fatty acids normally function as the major metabolic substrate for the myocardium of older infants and children, glucose provides a significant energy source during episodes of ischemia.

Data from newborn animals suggests that the ischemic neonatal brain may benefit from administration of glucose.[98] Data from adult animals, however, suggests that the mature brain may be harmed by glucose administration, particularly if glucose is administered immediately before or during cardiac arrest and resuscitation.[99-102] Clinical studies in children with severe head injury, submersion, and shock have demonstrated an association between hyperglycemia and poor neurologic outcome.[103-105] This association does not prove a cause-and-effect relationship; hyperglycemia may simply be a marker of a severe ischemic insult with diffuse cellular injury.

In the absence of convincing data showing benefit or harm of hyperglycemia *after* arrest, the current recommendation is to ensure that the serum glucose concentration is at least normal during resuscitation and to avoid hypoglycemia after resuscitation. Administer glucose if blood glucose or clinical signs suggest hypoglycemia.

> ## Critical Concepts:
> ### Glucose Administration During Resuscitation
>
> Ensure that serum glucose is not low (hypoglycemia) during and after resuscitation. Administer glucose to treat hypoglycemia.

Indications

The indications for administration of glucose during PALS are

■ Documented hypoglycemia

■ Suspected hypoglycemia:

— A rapid bedside glucose screen suggests hypoglycemia

— If a bedside glucose screen is unavailable and the clinical situation suggests hypoglycemia, consider empiric treatment with glucose (0.5 to 1 g/kg)

Dose

Glucose boluses of 0.5 to 1 g/kg IV or IO will generally correct profound hypoglycemia. A dose of 2 to 4 mL/kg of 25% glucose (25 g/100 mL = 250 mg/mL) will provide 0.5 to 1 g/kg; 5 to 10 mL/kg of 10% glucose (100 mg/mL) may be infused to deliver a similar quantity of glucose. To avoid local vascular and tissue injury, concentrations of 25% dextrose or less via a peripheral vein are recommended. $D_{50}W$ can be diluted 1:1 with sterile water to prepare $D_{25}W$ or 1:4 with sterile water to produce $D_{10}W$. Further dilutions are possible if volume administration is required (0.5 g/kg = 1 mL/kg of $D_{50}W$ = 2 mL/kg of $D_{25}W$ = 5 mL/kg of $D_{10}W$ = 10 mL/kg of D_5NS or D_5LR). Bolus glucose therapy for treatment of documented hypoglycemia should generally be followed by continuous glucose infusion.

Precautions

Hypertonic glucose (eg, $D_{25}W$ or $D_{50}W$) is very hyperosmolar and may cause sclerosis of the peripheral veins. Repeated administration of hypertonic glucose may result in hyperglycemia and an increase in serum osmolality. These changes have been associated with poor outcome in children with severe head injury, submersion, and shock.[103,105]

In general the concentration of intravenous glucose administered to neonates should not exceed 12.5%.

Calcium Chloride

Therapeutic Considerations

Calcium is essential in myocardial excitation-contraction coupling. Routine administration of calcium, however, does not improve outcome of cardiac arrest.[106] In addition, several studies have implicated cytoplasmic calcium accumulation in the final common pathway of cell death.[107] Calcium accumulation results from calcium entering cells after ischemia and during reperfusion of ischemic organs. Increased cytoplasmic calcium concentration activates intracellular enzyme systems, resulting in cellular necrosis.

Although calcium has been recommended in the treatment of pulseless electrical activity, including electromechanical dissociation, experimental evidence for its efficacy in either setting is lacking.[106,108,109] Therefore, routine administration of calcium during resuscitation of asystolic patients cannot be recommended. Calcium is indicated for treatment of documented hypocalcemia and hyperkalemia,[110] particularly in patients with hemodynamic compromise. Ionized hypocalcemia is relatively common in critically ill children, particularly those with sepsis.[111,112] Calcium should also be considered for treatment of hypermagnesemia[113] and calcium channel blocker overdose.[114]

There is little information about the optimal emergency dose of calcium. The currently recommended dose of 5 to 7 mg/kg of elemental calcium is based on extrapolation from adult data and limited pediatric data.[115] Calcium chloride 10% (100 mg/mL) is the calcium preparation of choice in critically ill children because it provides greater bioavailability of calcium than calcium gluconate.[115] A dose of 0.2 mL/kg of 10% calcium chloride will provide 20 mg/kg of the salt and 5.4 mg/kg of elemental calcium. The dose should be infused by slow IV push over 10 to 20 seconds during cardiac arrest or over 5 to 10 minutes in perfusing patients. In cardiac arrest the dose may be repeated after 10 minutes if required. Further doses should be based on measured deficits of ionized calcium.

Indications

Calcium administration is appropriate for the following documented or suspected conditions:

- Hypocalcemia (preferably documented as ionized hypocalcemia)

- Hyperkalemia

- Hypermagnesemia

- Calcium channel blocker overdose

Dose

A dose of 20 mg/kg of calcium chloride 10% (0.2 mL/kg) IV or IO is equivalent to 5.4 mg/kg of elemental calcium. Calcium chloride 10% contains approximately 27.2 mg/mL of elemental calcium, whereas calcium gluconate 10% contains approximately 9 mg/mL of elemental calcium. Therefore, the dose and volume of calcium gluconate must be 3 times the dose and volume of calcium chloride to provide an equivalent dose of elemental calcium.

Precautions

Rapid administration of calcium may induce significant bradycardia and even asystole; this response is more likely if the patient is receiving digoxin. Calcium forms an insoluble precipitate in the presence of sodium bicarbonate. When infusing calcium or sodium bicarbonate emergently, irrigate the tubing with normal saline before and after the infusion to avoid formation of an insoluble precipitate in the catheter lumen. Calcium can cause sclerosis of the peripheral veins and produce a severe chemical burn if it infiltrates the surrounding tissue.

Sodium Bicarbonate

Therapeutic Considerations

Although sodium bicarbonate was previously recommended for treatment of severe metabolic acidosis in cardiac arrest, routine administration of sodium bicarbonate does not consistently improve outcome of cardiac arrest.[116,117] Respiratory failure is the major cause of cardiac arrest in children. Because sodium bicarbonate transiently elevates CO_2 tension, administration of this drug to the pediatric patient during resuscitation may worsen existing respiratory acidosis. For these reasons the treatment priorities for metabolic acidosis in the infant or child in cardiac arrest should be to assist ventilation, support oxygenation, and restore effective systemic perfusion (to correct tissue hypoxia and ischemia). Once effective ventilation is established and epinephrine plus chest compressions are provided to maximize circulation, use of sodium bicarbonate may be considered for the patient with prolonged cardiac arrest.

The PALS provider may also consider administering sodium bicarbonate when shock is associated with documented severe metabolic acidosis, although clinical trials in critically ill adults with acidosis failed to show a beneficial effect of sodium bicarbonate on hemodynamics despite correction of metabolic acidosis.[118,119] The decision to administer sodium bicarbonate is determined by the acuity and severity of the acidosis and the child's circulatory state, among other factors. For example, a child with shock and marked metabolic acidosis from dehydration due to diabetic ketoacidosis does not require sodium bicarbonate in most circumstances and will respond well to fluid resuscitation and insulin administration alone.

Sodium bicarbonate is the treatment of choice for tricyclic antidepressant overdose and other sodium channel blocker poisonings. For these patients administer sodium bicarbonate in bolus infusions of 1 to 2 mEq/kg until the serum pH is above 7.45 (and 7.50 to 7.55 for severe poisoning), and then provide infusions of a solution of 150 mEq $NaHCO_3$ per liter to maintain the alkalosis. For further information see Chapter 12.

Indications

Potential indications for sodium bicarbonate therapy in PALS are[120,121]

- Severe metabolic acidosis with effective ventilatory support

- Hyperkalemia

- Hypermagnesemia
- Tricyclic antidepressant poisoning
- Sodium channel blocker poisoning

Dose

The initial dose of sodium bicarbonate is 1 mEq/kg (1 mL/kg of 8.4% solution) IV or IO (higher doses may be needed for tricyclic antidepressant poisoning). A dilute solution (0.5 mEq/mL of 4.2% solution) should be used in neonates to limit the osmotic load (see "Precautions," below), but there is no evidence that the dilute solution is beneficial in older infants or children. Subsequent doses of sodium bicarbonate may be based on blood gas analyses, or if such measurements are unavailable, subsequent doses of 0.5 to 1 mEq/kg may be considered after every 10 minutes of continued arrest. Even if available, arterial blood gas analysis may not accurately reflect tissue and venous pH during cardiac arrest or severe shock.[122,123] The role of sodium bicarbonate remains unclear in children who have documented metabolic acidosis immediately after resuscitation.

Precautions

Excessive administration of sodium bicarbonate may result in metabolic alkalosis and other detrimental effects:

- Displacement of the oxyhemoglobin dissociation curve to the left with impaired release of oxygen to tissues
- Acute intracellular shift of potassium with lowering of serum potassium concentration
- Decreased plasma ionized calcium concentration caused by greater binding of calcium to serum proteins
- Decreased VF threshold
- Sodium and water overload (1 mEq of sodium is delivered with each milliequivalent of bicarbonate)

The standard 8.4% solution of sodium bicarbonate is very hyperosmolar (2000 mOsm/L) compared with plasma (280 mOsm/L), and repeated doses can produce symptomatic hypernatremia and hyperosmolarity as well as transient vasodilation and hypotension.[118,119] In premature infants this hyperosmolarity correlates with an increased risk for periventricular-intraventricular hemorrhage.[124] For this reason the 4.2% solution (0.5 mEq/mL) should be used in premature infants (see Table 1).

Production of CO_2 is transiently increased after administration of sodium bicarbonate. This newly formed CO_2 can cross the blood-brain barrier and cell membranes much more rapidly than HCO_3^-, causing paradoxical cerebrospinal fluid and intracellular acidosis.[125,126] This is particularly problematic when metabolic acidosis is prolonged (eg, diabetic ketoacidosis).

Irrigate IV and IO tubing with normal saline before and after infusions of sodium bicarbonate. Catecholamines may be inactivated by bicarbonate solutions. In addition, calcium salts plus bicarbonate can precipitate into insoluble calcium carbonate crystals that may obstruct the IV catheter or tubing. Because sodium bicarbonate is hyperosmolar, it may cause sclerosis of small veins and produce a chemical burn if extravasated into the subcutaneous tissues. Sodium bicarbonate should not be administered into the tracheobronchial tree for treatment of metabolic acidosis.

Medications to Maintain Adequate Cardiac Output

Medications to maintain adequate cardiac output may help prevent cardiac arrest and treat postresuscitation myocardial dysfunction. The pharmacokinetics (ie, the relationship between dose and plasma concentration) and pharmacodynamics (ie, the relationship between plasma concentration and drug effects) of these vasoactive and inotropic agents vary from patient to patient and even from hour to hour in the same patient. The effects of these agents are influenced by the child's age and maturity, underlying disease process (which influences receptor density and response), metabolic state, acid-base balance, autonomic and endocrine responses, and hepatic and renal function. The recommended infusion doses are starting points; you must titrate the infusion to achieve the desired therapeutic effect (eg, increased heart rate, systemic perfusion, or blood pressure or correction of acidosis) while minimizing side or toxic effects.

During treatment of shock or following resuscitation from cardiac arrest the patient may demonstrate hemodynamic compromise associated with poor myocardial function or inappropriate systemic or pulmonary vascular resistance.[127-131] Most children with septic shock have decreased systemic vascular resistance, although clinical data suggests that children with *fluid-refractory* septic shock have high rather than low systemic vascular resistance and poor myocardial function.[128,132] Management of these patients will involve both fluid resuscitation and pharmacologic support of cardiovascular function. Children with cardiogenic shock typically have poor myocardial function and a compensatory increase in systemic and pulmonary vascular resistance as the body attempts to maintain adequate blood pressure.

The agents used to support circulatory function are classified as inotropes, vasopressors, vasodilators, and inodilators. Inotropes increase cardiac function and often increase heart rate as well. Vasopressors increase systemic and pulmonary vascular resistance and are most commonly used in children with inappropriately low systemic vascular resistance. If myocardial function is adequate, vasopressors will typically increase systemic and pulmonary artery pressures. Vasodilators are designed to reduce systemic and pulmonary vascular resistance. Although vasodilators do not directly increase myocardial contractility, they reduce ventricular afterload, which often improves stroke volume and cardiac output. Vasodilators are the only class of agents that can increase cardiac output and simultaneously reduce myocardial oxygen demand.

TABLE 1. Drugs Used in Pediatric Advanced Life Support (see Table 3, page 237)

Drug	Dosage (Pediatric)	Remarks
Calcium chloride (27.2 mg/mL elemental calcium)	20 mg/kg (0.2 mL/kg of 10% solution)	Give slowly
Dobutamine hydrochloride	2 to 20 µg/kg per minute	Titrate to desired effect
Dopamine hydrochloride	2 to 20 µg/kg per minute	α-Adrenergic action predominates at higher infusion rates
Epinephrine for symptomatic bradycardia*	IV/IO: 0.01 mg/kg (0.1 mL/kg 1:10 000) Tracheal: 0.1 mg/kg (0.1 mL/kg 1:1000)	
Epinephrine for asystolic or pulseless arrest*	**First dose:** IV/IO: 0.01 mg/kg (0.1 mL/kg of 1:10 000 concentration) Tracheal: 0.1 mg/kg (0.1 mL/kg of 1:1000 concentration) **Subsequent doses:** • Repeat same dose as above every 3 to 5 minutes during CPR: 0.01 mg/kg (0.1 mL/kg of 1:10 000 concentration) • Consider higher dose: 0.1 to 0.2 mg/kg (0.1 to 0.2 mL/kg of 1:1000 concentration) for special conditions	
Epinephrine infusion	0.1 to 1 µg/kg per minute Use higher infusion dose if asystole is present	Titrate to desired effect
Glucose	1 to 2 mL/kg $D_{50}W$ (0.5 to 1 g/kg) or 2 to 4 mL/kg $D_{25}W$ or 5 to 10 mL/kg $D_{10}W$ or 10 to 20 mL/kg D_5NS	
Milrinone	Loading: 50 to 75 µg/kg Infusion: 0.5 to 0.75 µg/kg per minute	Monitor for hypotension during loading dose; consider infusion without loading dose
Naloxone*	Patient <5 years old or ≤20 kg: 0.1 mg/kg Patient ≥5 years old or >20 kg: 2 mg	Titrate to desired effect
Norepinephrine	0.1 to 2 µg/kg per minute IV/IO infusion	Titrate to desired effect
Prostaglandin E₁	0.05 to 0.1 µg/kg per minute IV/IO infusion†	Monitor for apnea, hypotension, hypoglycemia
Sodium bicarbonate	1 mEq/kg per dose IV/IO	Infuse slowly and only if ventilation is adequate
Sodium nitroprusside	1 to 8 µg/kg per minute IV/IO infusion Do not mix with normal saline	Monitor blood pressure closely Titrate to desired effect

*For tracheal administration, the IV dose is the minimum to be administered by tracheal route and higher doses are often required. Dilute drug with normal saline to a volume of 3 to 5 mL and follow with several positive-pressure ventilations.

†Doses as low as 0.01 µg/kg per minute may be effective.

Inodilators improve cardiac contractility and reduce afterload.

The optimal use of vasoactive agents requires knowledge of the patient's cardiovascular physiology, which is not always clearly discerned from the clinical examination. Invasive hemodynamic monitoring, including measurement of central venous pressure, pulmonary capillary wedge pressure, and cardiac output, may be needed.[128] Optimal use also requires knowledge of the drugs because a number of vasoactive agents have different hemodynamic effects at different infusion rates. For example, at low infusion rates epinephrine is a potent inotrope and lowers systemic vascular resistance through a prominent action on vascular β-adrenergic receptors. At higher infusion rates, epinephrine remains a potent inotrope and increases systemic vascular resistance by activating vascular α-adrenergic receptors.

The infusion rate and therapeutic effects achieved may be limited by drug side effects. For example, higher infusion rates of epinephrine may substantially

Critical Concepts: Classification of Drugs to Support Cardiac Output

Four major classes of medications are used to support cardiac output in PALS:

- Inotropes: increase cardiac contractility and often heart rate
- Vasopressors: increase vascular resistance and blood pressure
- Vasodilators: decrease vascular resistance and cardiac afterload and promote peripheral perfusion
- Inodilators: increase cardiac contractility and reduce afterload

Titrate these drugs to achieve the desired effect and minimize side effects.

improve blood pressure but may reduce renal blood flow and urine output and produce tachyarrhythmias. Because the pharmacokinetic and pharmacodynamic responses will vary, you must carefully monitor the patient's response to each vasoactive agent.

There is no single ideal drug regimen for cardiovascular support; drug selection should be individualized and titrated to patient response (Figure 1). The management of most forms of shock combines support of intravascular volume with titration of fluid therapy plus possible vasoactive support. An algorithm for treatment of septic shock illustrates this combination therapy (Figure 2). The goals of PALS are restoration of adequate blood pressure and effective perfusion and correction of hypoxia and acidosis.

Dopamine

Therapeutic Considerations

Dopamine is an endogenous catecholamine with complex cardiovascular effects. Low doses of dopamine stimulate dopaminergic receptors that relax vascular tone in selected vascular beds and thereby increase renal, splanchnic, coronary, and cerebral blood flow.[55,63] At higher infusion rates dopamine produces both direct stimulation of cardiac β-adrenergic receptors and indirect stimulation through the release of norepinephrine stored in cardiac sympathetic nerves.[55,63] If norepinephrine stores are depleted, as in chronic congestive heart failure, the inotropic effects of dopamine are diminished.[55,133]

In the peripheral vascular bed, dopamine also has both direct and indirect actions at α- and β-adrenergic receptors. In low doses vasodilatory effects predominate; at higher doses α-adrenergic vasoconstriction occurs.[55]

Wide interpatient variability in plasma clearance is well documented.[58,61-63] An infusion of 5 μg/kg per minute in one patient may produce a plasma dopamine concentration that is the same as that produced by an infusion of 25 μg/kg per minute in

another patient. There is also wide variability in pharmacodynamics, meaning that the same plasma concentration will result in different hemodynamic effects in different patients.[58] Not surprisingly, increases in cardiac output and blood pressure have been noted with infusion rates as low as 0.5 to 1 μg/kg per minute.[58]

Indications

Potential indications for dopamine infusion are

- Inadequate cardiac output
- Hypotension
- Need for enhanced splanchnic blood flow and urine output

Dopamine may be used for treatment of hypotension or poor peripheral perfusion in the pediatric patient with adequate intravascular volume and a stable rhythm. Low doses (0.5 to 5 μg/kg per minute) may enhance renal and splanchnic blood flow and urine output, although this is not a consistent effect. In one study doses of 7 to 12 μg/kg per minute improved renal function more than a dose of 3 μg/kg per minute.[134]

Dose

As with all catecholamines, there is wide interpatient variability in the pharmacokinetics of dopamine and hemodynamic responses to it. Therefore, the PALS provider should titrate the infusion rate to the desired clinical response. The typical infusion rate of dopamine is 2 to 20 μg/kg per minute, but the optimal infusion rate may be substantially lower or higher.

Dopamine has a short plasma half-life and should be delivered by constant infusion controlled by an infusion pump. The infusion can be prepared by adding 6 mg of dopamine multiplied by the child's body weight in kilograms to sufficient diluent to create a solution totaling 100 mL. Infusions of 1 mL/h of this mixture deliver 1 μg/kg per minute (see Table 2). An infusion of 10 mL/h or 10 μg/kg per minute is a reasonable starting dose for the child with shock. The infusion can then be

FIGURE 1. Approach to selection of vasoactive medications for postresuscitation hemodynamic stabilization.

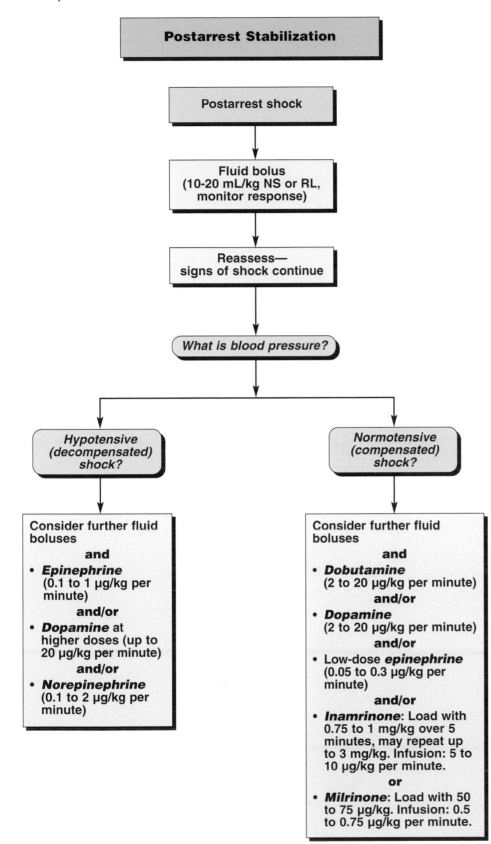

adjusted after evaluating the patient's hemodynamic status, including urine output, systemic perfusion, and blood pressure.

Dopamine infusion rates greater than 20 µg/kg per minute may produce predominantly vasoconstrictive effects without further inotropic effect. If additional *inotropic* effect is needed, epinephrine or dobutamine may be preferable to dopamine infusions that exceed 20 µg/kg per minute. If further *vasopressor* support is needed to maintain blood pressure, epinephrine or norepinephrine is generally preferred.

Precautions

Dopamine may produce tachycardia (which increases myocardial oxygen demand), arrhythmias, and hypertension. Reported dopamine-induced arrhythmias include premature ventricular contractions, supraventricular tachycardia, and VT.[55,135] High infusion rates of dopamine (greater than 20 µg/kg per minute) may produce severe peripheral vasoconstriction and ischemia in the child with shock.

Dopamine infusions should be delivered through a secure, large-bore peripheral venous catheter. High concentrations and large-volume infusions should be administered via a central venous catheter. Extravasation of the infusion can result in local ischemia and tissue necrosis. Dopamine and other catecholamines should not be mixed with sodium bicarbonate because they are inactivated by alkaline pH.

If dopamine infusions are continued for several days, thyroid function may be affected because of inhibition of thyrotropin-stimulating hormone (TSH) release from the pituitary gland.[136]

Dobutamine

Therapeutic Considerations

Dobutamine is a synthetic catecholamine possessing a relatively selective action at β_1-adrenergic receptors. Dobutamine increases cardiac contractility and heart rate, often with mild dilation of the peripheral vascular bed.[55] Unlike dopamine, dobutamine acts directly on β_1 receptors and does not depend on the presence of adequate stores of norepinephrine to produce these effects. Dobutamine has no dopaminergic effects, so it does not affect renal or splanchnic blood flow directly. In children with cardiogenic shock, dobutamine increases cardiac output and decreases pulmonary capillary pressure and systemic vascular resistance.[57,64,137,138] Dobutamine may be less effective than epinephrine in septic shock, particularly if hypotension is present, because it may increase existing systemic vasodilation.[138]

Indications

Potential indications for dobutamine infusion are

- Myocardial dysfunction

- Inadequate cardiac output, particularly in patients with elevated systemic or pulmonary vascular resistance

Dobutamine is an effective agent for treatment of poor perfusion despite adequate intravascular volume. It is particularly useful for treatment of low cardiac output secondary to poor myocardial function.[55,139] Clinical data and the results of animal studies indicate that dobutamine can be effective in treating postresuscitation myocardial dysfunction.[127,129-131] A theoretical advantage of dobutamine is its ability to decrease peripheral vascular resistance in this setting, but this can be a disadvantage if the patient is hypotensive.

In one study dobutamine infusions were superior to dopamine infusions for improving renal function in critically ill patients[140]; a more recent study drew the opposite conclusion.[134] Perhaps improved cardiac output has a greater effect on splanchnic perfusion than dopaminergic effects for some critically ill patients.

Dose

Like other catecholamines, dobutamine has a short plasma half-life and should be administered by constant infusion via a large-bore venous catheter regulated by an infusion pump. High doses should generally be administered by a central venous catheter. Prepare the infusion by adding 6 mg of dobutamine multiplied by the child's body weight in kilograms to sufficient diluent to create a solution totaling 100 mL (see Table 2). Infusions of this solution are often started at 5 to 10 mL/h, which delivers 5 to 10 µg/kg per minute.

A typical infusion dose ranges from 2 to 20 µg/kg per minute.

The pharmacokinetics of dobutamine and the therapeutic response to it vary greatly among children.[57,59-61,64,141] In 2 studies infusion rates of 0.5 µg/kg per minute improved cardiac output by more than 10% in most children, although some children needed much higher infusion rates for demonstrable inotropic effects.[57,64] As with other catecholamines, plasma clearance varies by at least 3-fold to 5-fold among patients.[57,59-61,64,141] That is, plasma concentrations may be the same in one patient receiving 3 µg/kg per minute and another receiving 15 µg/kg per minute. The infusion rate should be adjusted as needed for optimal hemodynamic effect.

Precautions

Dobutamine may produce tachycardia, tachyarrhythmias, or ectopic beats. Nausea, vomiting, hypertension, and hypotension are less frequent side effects. Extravasation of dobutamine may produce tissue ischemia and necrosis, although the limited α-adrenergic effects of dobutamine make this much less of a problem with dobutamine infusions than with other

---

TABLE 2. Preparation of Vasoactive Drug Infusions in Infants and Children

Medication	Dilution*	Delivery Rate
Epinephrine Norepinephrine	0.6 × body weight (kg) equals milligrams to add to sufficient diluent† to create a total volume of 100 mL	1 mL/h delivers 0.1 µg/kg per minute
Prostaglandin E$_1$	0.3 × body weight (kg) equals milligrams to add to sufficient diluent† to create a total volume of 50 mL	0.5 mL/h infusion delivers 0.05 µg/kg per minute
Dopamine Dobutamine Sodium nitroprusside	6 × body weight (kg) equals milligrams to add to sufficient diluent† to create a total volume of 100 mL	1 mL/h delivers 1.0 µg/kg per minute
Infusion rate (mL/h) =	$$\dfrac{\text{Weight (kg)} \times \text{desired dose (µg/kg per minute)} \times 60 \text{ min/h}}{\text{Concentration (µg/mL)}}$$	

*This provides an initial concentration only. Drug concentration can be adjusted based on the patient's fluid requirements or limitations.

In large patients the amount of drug used to create 100 mL of infusion may deplete the available supply of the drug. To reduce the volume of drug needed to prepare the infusion, decrease the drug concentration by a factor of 10 and increase the hourly infusion rate by a factor of 10.

If high doses of the drug are required (eg, ≥10 µg/kg per minute), the resulting amount of fluid delivered may be excessive for small infants or children. Under these conditions, the concentration of the drug may be *increased* by a factor of 3, 5, or 10 and the rate of infusion *decreased* by the same factor.

†Diluent may be D$_5$W, 5% dextrose in half-normal saline, normal saline, or Ringer's lactate. Mix sodium nitroprusside in D$_5$W only.

FIGURE 2. Proposed algorithm for treatment of septic shock. Modified with permission from Carcillo JA, et al.[132]

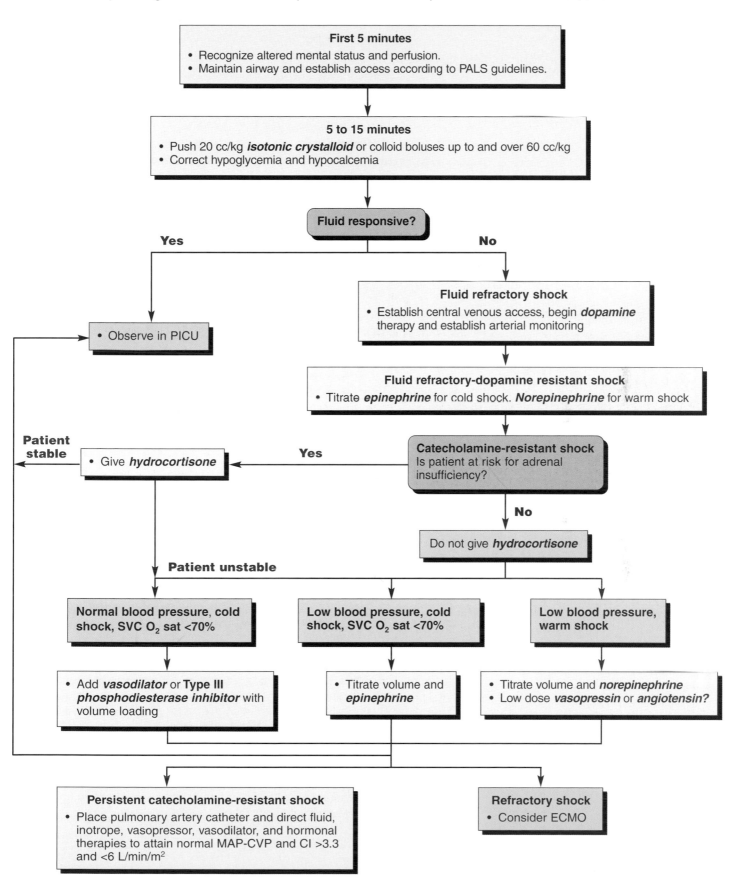

catecholamine infusions. Like other catecholamines, dobutamine is inactivated in alkaline solutions.

Epinephrine

Therapeutic Considerations

The actions of epinephrine were summarized earlier in this chapter. Epinephrine is a potent catecholamine that acts directly on the adrenergic receptors rather than through a release of stored norepinephrine. Epinephrine infusion has dose-related actions. Lower-dose infusions are primarily associated with β-adrenergic effects, including an increase in myocardial contractility, heart rate, pulse pressure (due to reduced systemic vascular resistance), and systolic blood pressure. As the infusion dose is increased, α-adrenergic effects predominate and are likely to produce an increase in systolic and diastolic blood pressures and a narrowing of pulse pressure.[55,56]

Indications

Potential indications for epinephrine infusion in PALS are

- Inadequate cardiac output
- Hypotension
- Symptomatic bradycardia
- Pulseless cardiac arrest
- Septic shock

Indications for epinephrine infusion are signs of poor systemic perfusion or hypotension in the patient with adequate intravascular volume and a stable rhythm.[142,143] Epinephrine infusion may also be indicated for hemodynamically significant bradycardia. An infusion of epinephrine may be initiated during resuscitation of a patient with asystolic or pulseless arrest if intermittent bolus therapy fails to restore a perfusing cardiac rhythm. Epinephrine is preferable to dopamine for the patient who may have depleted myocardial norepinephrine stores, such as the infant or child with chronic congestive heart failure.[55,133] Epinephrine can be effective for septic and cardiogenic shock.[142-145]

Dose

Epinephrine has a short half-life (2 to 4 minutes), and plasma epinephrine concentrations reach a steady state within 20 minutes of each change in the infusion rate. When epinephrine is needed emergently, it is generally advisable to begin with an infusion of approximately 20 mL/h until a clinical response in the form of tachycardia is detected. This indicates that the drug has passed from the intravenous tubing and entered the patient's circulation, producing a response. The infusion is then reduced to the desired rate (generally 0.1 to 1 µg/kg per minute).

For treatment of acute life-threatening cardiovascular dysfunction, the infusion rate is often adjusted every 5 minutes (or more frequently) until the desired clinical effect (eg, increased heart rate or blood pressure or improved systemic perfusion) is achieved.

As with other catecholamines, there is wide interpatient variability in pharmacokinetics and hemodynamic response.[56,144] Doses as low as 0.01 µg/kg per minute may produce an adequate clinical response. However, side effects including tachyarrhythmias, may develop with doses as low as 0.1 µg/kg per minute. Doses as high as 5 µg/kg per minute may occasionally be necessary for adequate effect, although the patient must be monitored closely for evidence of tachyarrhythmias and other side effects.

Epinephrine infusions should be delivered through a well-secured peripheral venous catheter or, preferably, a central venous catheter to ensure a reliable route of administration and minimize the risk of extravasation. Prepare the infusion by multiplying 0.6 by the patient's weight in kilograms. The result is the number of milligrams of epinephrine to add to an appropriate diluent to yield a total volume of 100 mL. Infusion of the solution at a rate of 1 mL/h will deliver 0.1 µg/kg per minute of epinephrine (see Table 2).

Precautions

Epinephrine can produce significant supraventricular tachycardia or VT and ventricular ectopy. Higher-dose infusions (generally more than 0.5 µg/kg per minute) may produce profound vasoconstriction that compromises perfusion of the extremities and the skin. Even in lower doses epinephrine may decrease renal and hepatic blood flow, but renal function as assessed by urine output will usually improve if shock is treated successfully.[145] Infiltration of tissue by an epinephrine infusion can cause local ischemia and tissue necrosis. Sodium bicarbonate should not be infused with epinephrine because the alkaline pH inactivates epinephrine.

Norepinephrine

Therapeutic Considerations

Norepinephrine is the catecholamine neurotransmitter released from sympathetic nerves. It is a potent inotropic agent that also activates peripheral α- and β-adrenergic receptors. At the infusion rates used clinically, α-adrenergic effects predominate, producing both beneficial and adverse effects. Because norepinephrine is a potent vasoconstricting agent, it is generally reserved for children with low systemic vascular resistance that is unresponsive to fluid resuscitation. This is most commonly seen in children with septic shock but also may be seen with spinal shock, anaphylaxis, and certain drug overdoses.

Although intuitive reasoning suggests that norepinephrine would worsen renal and splanchnic perfusion secondary to its vasoconstrictive actions, clinical data in adults shows that it improves splanchnic perfusion and renal function in hypotensive patients with septic shock,[146,147] particularly if combined with dobutamine.[148] Furthermore, infusing low doses of dopamine with norepinephrine appears to increase splanchnic blood flow and urine output, providing some degree of protection from excessive vasoconstriction.[149,150] Certainly urine output and the magnitude of metabolic acidosis should be monitored carefully during a norepinephrine infusion.

Indications

Potential indications for the use of norepinephrine in PALS are

- Hypotension (especially due to vasodilation)
- Inadequate cardiac output
- Spinal shock
- α-Adrenergic blockade

Norepinephrine is generally used in patients with low systemic vascular resistance, such as septic shock, spinal shock, anaphylaxis, and certain drug overdoses (eg, tricyclic antidepressant and neuroleptic drugs that have prominent α-adrenergic blocking effects).[151,152]

Dose

Prepare a norepinephrine infusion as noted in Table 2. Begin the infusion at 0.1 μg/kg per minute and titrate to patient response. Doses of 0.1 to 2 μg/kg per minute are generally used. The distribution, metabolism, and excretion of norepinephrine is similar to that of other catecholamines (see epinephrine, dopamine, and dobutamine). The half-life of norepinephrine is approximately 2 to 4 minutes, and there is wide interpatient variability in pharmacokinetics and hemodynamic response. Therefore, the infusion rate must be titrated to the desired clinical effect (eg, improved blood pressure, perfusion, cardiac output). Infusion doses as low as 0.1 μg/kg per minute may result in excessive vasoconstriction and tachycardia; however, infusion rates greater than 1 μg/kg per minute may be required for adequate vasopressor effect in some patients, especially for α-adrenergic blockade.

Precautions

The most common side effects of norepinephrine are hypertension, organ ischemia (including distal extremity ischemia and renal failure), and arrhythmias. Norepinephrine should be infused through a secure vascular line, preferably one placed centrally. Because of the prominent vasoconstrictive effects of norepinephrine, extravasation can result in severe tissue ischemia and necrosis. Like other catecholamines,

norepinephrine is inactivated in alkaline solutions.

Sodium Nitroprusside

Therapeutic Considerations

Sodium nitroprusside is a vasodilator that reduces tone in all vascular beds by stimulating local nitric oxide production. It has no direct effect on the myocardium when infused at therapeutic doses, but cardiac output often increases after administration of nitroprusside because it improves effective myocardial function by reducing systemic and pulmonary vascular resistance (ie, ventricular afterload). Sodium nitroprusside is indicated for treatment of shock or low cardiac output states characterized by high vascular resistance.[153-155] It is also the treatment of choice for severe life-threatening hypertension.[154]

Sodium nitroprusside also has venodilating effects, thereby increasing venous capacitance and decreasing preload.[156] Thus, if the patient has volume depletion, sodium nitroprusside is relatively contraindicated because hypotension is likely to develop.

Indications

Potential indications for sodium nitroprusside infusion in PALS are

- Hypertensive emergencies
- Inadequate cardiac output with high systemic or pulmonary vascular resistance
- Cardiogenic shock

Sodium nitroprusside is the agent of choice for acute vasodilator therapy in the critical care setting because it is a powerful vasodilator and it has a short half-life. Thus its useful effects can be rapidly attained and adverse effects rapidly resolved. Small changes in the cross-sectional diameter of the arterial tree can have profound effects on vascular resistance and thereby blood pressure. Severe hypotension is an important side effect of sodium nitroprusside, particularly when treating cardiogenic shock. Longer-acting vasodilators are even more dangerous in this setting because the vasodilatory effects do not abate rapidly.

Dose

Sodium nitroprusside is rapidly metabolized and therefore must be infused continuously. The drug must be prepared with a dextrose-containing solution and cannot be infused with saline; this often creates the need for a separate vascular infusion site. The solution should be wrapped promptly in aluminum foil or another opaque material or specialized administration set to protect it from deterioration on exposure to light. Once prepared, the solution should be used immediately. The freshly prepared solution may have a very faint brownish tint without any change in drug potency. In aqueous solution nitroprusside will react with a variety of substances to form highly colored reaction products. If this occurs, the infusion should be replaced. Infusions are typically started at approximately 0.1 to 1 μg/kg per minute and adjusted as needed up to 8 μg/kg per minute.

Precautions

Systemic arterial pressure must be closely monitored during infusions of nitroprusside. Hypotension is the most common adverse reaction; it can be profound and life-threatening. Rapid reduction in blood pressure in patients with severe hypertension can lead to renal failure or stroke because the cerebral and renal vascular beds may need high perfusion pressures to maintain adequate organ blood flow.

Nitroprusside undergoes metabolism by endothelial cells and red blood cells, releasing nitric oxide and cyanide. Cyanide is rapidly metabolized in the liver to thiocyanate if hepatic function is adequate. High infusion rates or diminished hepatic function may exceed the ability of the liver to metabolize cyanide, resulting in clinical cyanide toxicity.[157] Furthermore, the hepatic metabolite thiocyanate must be renally excreted. In patients with poor renal function, thiocyanate may accumulate, leading to central nervous system dysfunction that ranges from irritability to seizures, tinnitus, visual blurring, hyperreflexia, abdominal pain, nausea, and vomiting.

Thiocyanate levels should be measured in patients receiving prolonged sodium nitroprusside infusions (more than 2 to 3 days), particularly if the infusion rate exceeds 2 µg/kg per minute. Although sodium nitroprusside is generally the acute vasodilator of choice for critically ill patients in a well-monitored setting, these metabolism issues make it a poor choice for more prolonged usage.

Milrinone

Therapeutic Considerations

Milrinone is an inodilator, a class of agents that combines inotropic stimulation of the heart with vasodilation of the systemic and pulmonary vascular beds. Unlike catecholamines, inodilators do not depend on activation of receptors. Instead, these agents inhibit phosphodiesterase type III. This inhibition increases the intracellular concentration of cAMP. In the myocardium cAMP acts as a second messenger, increasing cardiac contractility. Heart rate is increased to a lesser extent because phosphodiesterase type III is more predominant in myocytes and vascular smooth muscle than in the pacemaker cells of the heart.[158-161] Indeed the action of inodilators is most notable in vascular smooth muscle, so this class of agents acts much like a combination of sodium nitroprusside and a selective inotrope such as dobutamine.

Inodilators are used to treat children with myocardial dysfunction and increased systemic or pulmonary vascular resistance. Milrinone is particularly well suited for conditions such as congestive heart failure in postoperative cardiac surgical patients and dilated cardiomyopathy and even in selected children with septic shock and myocardial dysfunction with high systemic vascular resistance.[158-161] Like vasodilators, inodilators have the ability to augment cardiac output with little effect on myocardial oxygen demand and produce little change in heart rate. Blood pressure is generally well maintained, provided that the patient has adequate intravascular volume. In the presence of hypovolemia,

the potent vasodilating action will result in hypotension.

Indications

Potential indications for milrinone infusion during PALS are

- Inadequate cardiac output with high systemic or pulmonary vascular resistance
- Cardiogenic shock
- Septic shock

Milrinone can be effective in the treatment of children with myocardial dysfunction and increased systemic or pulmonary vascular resistance, including selected children with septic shock.[148-151]

Dose

Because of its relatively long half-life (more than 1 hour), a loading dose (commonly a bolus of 50 to 75 µg/kg) is necessary for rapid attainment of a therapeutic steady-state plasma concentration.[158-161] Alternatively milrinone can be infused without a loading dose, reaching a steady-state plasma concentration in approximately 4½ hours. The gradual achievement of steady-state concentration avoids the severe acute hypotension that may occur with a loading dose. Typical continuous infusion rates are 0.5 to 0.75 µg/kg per minute.[158-161]

Precautions

As with all vasodilator therapy for hemodynamically unstable patients, the most important life-threatening side effect is hypotension, particularly when the patient is relatively volume depleted before infusion of milrinone. If hypotension develops during the loading dose, provide a rapid infusion bolus of 5 to 10 mL/kg of normal saline or other appropriate fluid. Place the patient in the Trendelenburg position (head tilted in a dependent fashion). If the patient remains hypotensive despite fluid loading, administer a vasopressor.

The major disadvantage of these agents is their relatively long elimination half-life. Milrinone is often administered with a loading dose followed by a continuous infusion. The infusion may lead to a false

sense that a change in the infusion rate results in a rapid change in hemodynamic effect. Hemodynamic changes occur as a result of significant changes in the plasma concentration. *A new steady-state concentration will be achieved approximately 4½ hours after changing a milrinone infusion rate* because 3 half-lives are needed to reach about 90% of the steady-state concentration at a given infusion rate, assuming a 1½-hour half-life.[160] Hemodynamic changes will occur in less than the full 4½ hours but not in seconds to minutes as with catecholamine infusions. Similarly, if toxicity occurs, the adverse effects will continue as the drug is metabolized over hours.

Milrinone is cleared by the kidney. In infants less than 4 weeks of age and in patients with renal dysfunction, milrinone clearance will be decreased, leading to a greater risk of toxicity.[160] Thrombocytopenia can develop with milrinone therapy but is less frequent and less severe than with inamrinone.[160,161] Routinely monitor platelet counts during milrinone infusions.

Miscellaneous PALS Medications

Prostaglandin E₁

Therapeutic Considerations

Various endogenous prostaglandins mediate constriction or dilation of the ductus arteriosus during the perinatal period. IV infusions of prostaglandin E₁ can maintain the patency of the ductus arteriosus in infants with cyanotic congenital heart diseases and other complex congenital heart diseases, such as interrupted aortic arch.[162-166] These infants depend on ductal patency for adequate pulmonary or systemic blood flow. Ductal-dependent cardiac lesions can include transposition of the great vessels, aortic coarctation, and tricuspid atresia. Neonates with ductal-dependent systemic blood flow may present in profound shock when the ductus closes, sometimes days after birth. Immediate treatment with a continuous infusion of prostaglandin E₁ may be lifesaving.

Maximum therapeutic effect is usually noted within 30 minutes in infants with cyanotic lesions but may take several hours for those with acyanotic lesions.

Indications

Prostaglandin E_1 is indicated to maintain or reopen the ductus arteriosus in neonates with congenital cardiovascular disease when adequate systemic or pulmonary blood flow depends on ductal patency. Neonates with such diseases may present with cyanosis or shock. A neonatologist, pediatric cardiologist, or pediatric intensivist should be involved in the care of these patients as soon as possible.

Dose

Prostaglandin E_1 has a very short half-life; 90% is metabolized in one passage through a normal lung.[167] Administration as a continuous intravascular infusion is therefore indicated. Clinical efficacy is usually initially achieved at doses ranging from 0.05 to 0.1 µg/kg per minute. Maintenance infusion rates should be titrated to clinical effect; lower infusion rates (0.01 to 0.05 µg/kg per minute) are often adequate.

Prepare an infusion by multiplying 0.3 by the infant's weight in kilograms. The result is the number of milligrams of prostaglandin to add to sufficient diluent (D_5W or NS) to create a solution totaling 50 mL. An infusion rate of 0.5 mL/h controlled by an infusion pump will deliver 0.05 µg/kg per minute.

Precautions

Side effects from prostaglandin E_1 infusions are common and potentially life-threatening.[168,169] The prominent vasodilator effects can result in cutaneous flushing, hypotension, and peripheral edema. Because systemic vasodilation is more common and more severe after intra-aortic infusion, an IV route is preferred. Apnea, hyperpyrexia, and jitteriness are relatively common central nervous system effects; convulsions are much less common. Prepare for tracheal intubation before infusing prostaglandin E_1. Diarrhea, rhythm distur-

bances, hypoglycemia, hypocalcemia, renal failure, and coagulopathies may occur. Prostaglandin E_1 should be refrigerated until administered.

Naloxone

Therapeutic Considerations

Naloxone hydrochloride, a pure narcotic (opiate) antagonist, reverses the effects of narcotic poisoning.[170-178] Naloxone acts rapidly (less than 2 minutes to onset of drug action) with a 45-minute average duration of action. Although naloxone administration is generally well tolerated,[172,173] both animal and clinical data document adverse effects, including ventricular arrhythmias, acute pulmonary edema, asystole, and seizures.[174-176]

The opioid system and adrenergic systems are interrelated; opioid antagonists stimulate sympathetic nervous system activity.[177] Moreover, hypercapnia stimulates the sympathetic nervous system. Animal data suggests that when ventilation is provided to normalize the partial pressure of arterial CO_2 *before* administration of naloxone, the sudden rise in epinephrine concentration and its attendant toxic effects are blunted.[174] Thus ventilation is recommended before administration of naloxone. Initial doses may be repeated at 2-minute intervals until the desired degree of narcotic reversal is achieved. A continuous IV infusion of naloxone may be desirable if the narcotic involved has a longer duration of action than naloxone.[178]

Indications

Naloxone may be used to reverse the effects of narcotic poisoning, including respiratory depression, sedation, hypotension, and hypoperfusion. Naloxone may also be used to reverse the effects of therapeutic doses of narcotics when excessive sedation and hypoventilation occur.

Dose

The recommended dose of naloxone is 0.1 mg/kg for infants and children from birth to less than 5 years of age or up to

20 kg of body weight. Children 5 years of age or older or weighing more than 20 kg may be given 2 mg. Naloxone doses ranging from 0.001 to 0.4 mg/kg have been reported in the literature. Very low doses of naloxone (1 to 10 µg/kg or 0.001 to 0.01 mg/kg) may be appropriate for reversal of adverse effects of narcotics when complete reversal of the analgesic effect is not desirable (see Chapter 15: "Sedation"), whereas higher doses (0.1 mg/kg) are administered for opioid poisoning (see Chapter 12: "Toxicology").

Therapy should be titrated to produce the desired effect. Continuous IV infusions of 0.04 to 0.16 mg/kg per hour have been well tolerated. This dose will generally achieve total reversal of narcotic effects. If total reversal is not required, smaller doses may be used. This is often the case when reversal of excessive sedation is desired after a therapeutic dose of a narcotic, but full reversal with return of pain is not desirable.

The IV route of naloxone administration is recommended when a narcotic (opiate) or unknown toxic ingestion is suspected. No well-controlled studies in infants and children directly compare the efficacy of various routes of administration (IV and intratracheal versus intramuscular or subcutaneous). Absorption of intramuscular or subcutaneous medications may be erratic in patients with hypotension or hypoperfusion.

Precautions

Even at high doses naloxone is quite safe. Side effects of naloxone are rare and are generally related to abrupt reversal of narcotic depression. These side effects include nausea and vomiting, tachycardia, hypertension, tremulousness, seizures, ventricular arrhythmias, asystole, and acute pulmonary edema.[170-178] Adequate ventilation should be established before naloxone administration to minimize many of the adrenergic side effects (see above).

The relatively short duration of action of naloxone (40 to 60 minutes) may result in a recurrence of symptoms of narcotic intoxication. In infants of addicted mothers, administer naloxone with caution immediately after birth because it may precipitate abrupt narcotic withdrawal and seizures.

Summary Points

Selection of fluid therapy, drugs, and doses for PALS must be individualized, based on the patient's clinical condition, age, and target cardiovascular effects. The PALS provider must be familiar with drug indications, recommended dose ranges, compatibilities, and side effects.

- Volume resuscitation usually begins with a fluid bolus of 20 mL/kg of isotonic crystalloid administered over 5 to 20 minutes

- Blood transfusion is indicated to replace volume losses in pediatric trauma victims with continued hypovolemic shock despite administration of 2 to 3 boluses of isotonic crystalloid solution.

- Modification of fluid resuscitation is appropriate for the child with shock associated with diabetic ketoacidosis, burns, and some poisonings (particularly calcium channel blocker and β-adrenergic blocker overdoses).

- The goals of medication administration during cardiac arrest are to
  — Increase coronary and cerebral perfusion pressure and blood flow
  — Stimulate spontaneous or more forceful myocardial contractility
  — Accelerate heart rate
  — Correct metabolic acidosis
  — Suppress or treat arrhythmias

- The 4 major classifications of medications used to support circulation in the prearrest period are
  — Inotropes: increase cardiac contractility and often heart rate
  — Vasopressors: increase vascular resistance and blood pressure
  — Vasodilators: decrease vascular resistance and afterload on the heart and promote peripheral perfusion
  — Inodilators: increase cardiac contractility and reduce afterload

- Catecholamines administered by continuous infusion should be titrated to maximize the desired therapeutic effects while minimizing side or toxic effects. These drugs have a short half-life.

- Inodilators may be administered to augment cardiac output and reduce systemic vascular resistance. These drugs have a long half-life, so a longer time is needed to reach a steady-state plasma concentration when the infusion is started (unless a loading dose is administered) or increased (unless a bolus is administered). If side or toxic effects develop, it will take a longer time for drug levels to fall.

Case Scenario

Note: Additional case scenarios involving the management of shock are presented in Chapter 7: "Case Scenarios in Shock." Refer to this chapter for additional case scenarios, including one similar to the scenario below.

Introductory Case Scenario

A 4-year-old girl is brought to her pediatrician's office with a complaint of increasing lethargy, fever, and dizziness when she tries to stand. She has had chickenpox for 5 days, and her mother notes that several of the lesions on her abdomen have become red, tender, and swollen over the last 18 hours.

On physical examination the child is lying supine and listless and appears very ill. She does not answer questions appropriately but withdraws appropriately from painful stimulation. Her heart rate is 175 bpm; respiratory rate is 60 breaths/min with deep breaths that are not labored; oral temperature is 39.4°C (103°F); and blood pressure is 70/29 mm Hg. Her extremities are cool and mottled distal to the elbows and knees, and peripheral pulses are barely palpable. Capillary refill time is 6 to 8 seconds.

Introductory Case Scenario Review Questions and Answers

1. *What is your initial cardiopulmonary assessment?*

This child demonstrates decompensated shock. She has signs of altered level of consciousness (complaint of increasing lethargy, does not answer questions appropriately) and dizziness when she tries to stand. She is hypotensive for her age (the minimum systolic blood pressure for a 4-year-old should be 70 mm Hg plus twice her age in years: 78 mm Hg), and her peripheral pulses are barely palpable. She is tachypneic without labored respirations, and her extremities are cool and mottled.

2. *What initial treatment should you provide?*

Administer 100% oxygen, ensure that the airway is patent, and monitor the effectiveness of ventilation (chest expansion, breath sounds). Establish continuous ECG monitoring and monitoring of pulse oximetry. Establish IV access and prepare to give a fluid bolus.

3. *What type of fluid resuscitation should you provide? How much? How fast?*

This child may have septic shock. She has a history of viral infection (varicella) and may have a secondary bacterial infection with possible infection of the varicella lesions. Provide an immediate isotonic crystalloid fluid bolus of 20 mL/kg and reassess systemic perfusion. Attempt to palpate the liver to determine if there is any evidence of congestive heart failure (myocardial dysfunction). Administer repeat fluid boluses as needed to improve systemic perfusion and blood pressure. Watch for signs of increased respiratory distress that may signal the development of pulmonary edema.

4. *What medications should you administer to improve blood pressure and cardiac output and prevent progression to cardiac arrest?*

A variety of medications could be provided to improve blood pressure and systemic perfusion. If the child's blood pressure improves with volume administration, dobutamine can increase cardiac output while lowering systemic vascular resistance. Administration of dopamine in moderate doses may also be useful. If the child remains hypotensive despite fluid therapy consider epinephrine. If a catecholamine infusion is used, monitor the child's heart rate. It should decrease with fluid resuscitation and improved cardiac output.

Review Questions

1. **Which of the following statements about the effects of epinephrine during attempted resuscitation is *true*?**

   a. epinephrine decreases peripheral vascular resistance and reduces myocardial afterload, so ventricular contractions are more effective

   b. epinephrine can improve coronary artery perfusion pressure and can stimulate spontaneous contractions when asystole is present

   c. epinephrine is not useful in VF because it will increase myocardial irritability

   d. epinephrine decreases myocardial oxygen consumption

   The correct answer is b. Epinephrine improves coronary artery perfusion pressure and myocardial oxygen delivery during CPR by increasing peripheral vascular resistance and aortic diastolic pressure. Epinephrine may also stimulate spontaneous cardiac contractions, so it may restore cardiac activity when asystole is present.

   Answer a is incorrect because epinephrine *increases* peripheral vascular resistance, ventricular afterload, and oxygen demand.

   Answer c is incorrect because epinephrine *is* useful in the treatment of VF, increasing the coarseness of VF and enhancing the potential for defibrillation.

   Answer d is incorrect because epinephrine *increases* myocardial oxygen consumption. Although epinephrine-induced elevation of coronary artery perfusion pressure during chest compressions enhances oxygen delivery to the heart, oxygen consumption is increased.

2. **A pale and obtunded 3-year-old child with a history of diarrhea is brought to the hospital. The child's** respirations are 45 breaths/min with no distress and good breath sounds bilaterally. The heart rate is 150 bpm, and blood pressure is 88/64 mm Hg. Capillary refill time is 5 seconds, and peripheral pulses are weak. After placing the child on a 10 L/min flow of 100% oxygen and obtaining vascular access, which of the following is the *most appropriate* immediate treatment for this child?

   a. obtain a chest x-ray

   b. administer a maintenance crystalloid infusion

   c. administer a 20 mL/kg bolus of IV or IO isotonic fluids

   d. administer a dopamine infusion at a rate of 2 to 5 µg/kg per minute

   The correct answer is c. This child has signs of compensated shock, including prolonged capillary refill, weak peripheral pulses, and tachycardia with a blood pressure that is above the 5th percentile systolic blood pressure for her age (70 mm Hg plus twice the child's age in years = 76 mm Hg) although it is lower than the median systolic blood pressure for a 3-year-old (90 mm Hg plus twice the age in years = 96 mm Hg). The shock is probably caused by hypovolemia secondary to diarrhea, so administration of an isotonic crystalloid fluid bolus is needed.

   Answer a is incorrect because a chest x-ray is not indicated during initial stabilization of the child. The child's respiratory rate is 45 breaths/min with clear breath sounds and no distress.

   Answer b is incorrect because fluid boluses (20 mL/kg) must be given to correct hypovolemic shock. Maintenance fluids are inadequate to correct the shock that is present.

   Answer d is incorrect because fluid resuscitation is needed. Vasopressors like dopamine may be unnecessary if fluid resuscitation is adequate.

For the advanced provider:

3. **You are caring for a 3-year-old child who presents with ventricular arrhythmias and profound hypotension after ingesting his grandmother's blood pressure medication (a calcium channel blocker). After establishing IV access, you prepare to administer a fluid bolus. Which of the following would be the most appropriate fluid bolus to give this child?**

   a. 20 mL/kg isotonic crystalloid as quickly as possible (5 to 10 minutes)

   b. 5 to 10 mL/kg isotonic crystalloid over 10 to 20 minutes

   c. 10 mL/kg of packed red blood cells over 5 to 10 minutes

   d. 5 to 10 mL/kg infusions of sodium bicarbonate over 10 to 20 minutes

   The correct answer is b. Patients with calcium channel blocker or β-blocker overdose may present with severe hypotension and myocardial dysfunction. You should administer fluid cautiously in small amounts and monitor the patient for pulmonary edema. Repeat the fluid bolus as needed and consider adding a vasopressor.

   Answer a is incorrect because administration of a 20 mL/kg fluid bolus may worsen myocardial dysfunction, cause pulmonary edema, and fail to improve systemic perfusion.

   Answer c is incorrect because this child has no history of blood loss and no need for transfusion.

   Answer d is incorrect because administration of sodium bicarbonate in doses of 1 to 2 mEq/kg is appropriate for tricyclic antidepressant overdose but not for calcium channel blocker overdose.

References

1. Carcillo JA, Davis AL, Zaritsky A. Role of early fluid resuscitation in pediatric septic shock. *JAMA*. 1991;266:1242-1245.

2. Schierhout G, Roberts I. Fluid resuscitation with colloid or crystalloid solutions in critically ill patients: a systematic review of randomised trials. *BMJ*. 1998;316:961-964.

3. Human albumin administration in critically ill patients: systematic review of randomised controlled trials. Cochrane Injuries Group Albumin Reviewers. *BMJ*. 1998;317:235-240.

4. Griffel MI, Kaufman BS. Pharmacology of colloids and crystalloids. *Crit Care Clin*. 1992;8:235-253.

5. Wilkes MM, Navickis RJ. Patient survival after human albumin administration. A meta-analysis of randomized, controlled trials. *Ann Intern Med*. 2001;135:149-164.

6. Pollard AJ, Britto J, Nadel S, DeMunter C, Habibi P, Levin M. Emergency management of meningococcal disease. *Arch Dis Child*. 1999;80:290-296.

7. Nacht A. The use of blood products in shock. *Crit Care Clin*. 1992;8:255-291.

8. Glaser N, Barnett P, McCaslin I, Nelson D, Trainor J, Louie J, Kaufman F, Quayle K, Roback M, Malley R, Kuppermann N. Risk factors for cerebral edema in children with diabetic ketoacidosis. The Pediatric Emergency Medicine Collaborative Research Committee of the American Academy of Pediatrics. *N Engl J Med*. 2001;344:264-269.

9. Mahoney CP, Vlcek BW, DelAguila M. Risk factors for developing brain herniation during diabetic ketoacidosis. *Pediatr Neurol*. 1999;21:721-727.

10. Adrogue HJ, Barrero J, Eknoyan G. Salutary effects of modest fluid replacement in the treatment of adults with diabetic ketoacidosis. Use in patients without extreme volume deficit. *JAMA*. 1989;262:2108-2113.

11. Harris GD, Fiordalisi I. Physiologic management of diabetic ketoacidemia: a 5-year prospective pediatric experience in 231 episodes. *Arch Pediatr Adolesc Med*. 1994;148:1046-1052.

12. Harris GD, Fiordalisi I, Harris WL, Mosovich LL, Finberg L. Minimizing the risk of brain herniation during treatment of diabetic ketoacidemia: a retrospective and prospective study [published correction appears in *J Pediatr*. 1991;118:166-167]. *J Pediatr*. 1990;117(pt 1):22-31.

13. Duck SC, Wyatt DT. Factors associated with brain herniation in the treatment of diabetic ketoacidosis. *J Pediatr*. 1988;113(pt 1):10-14.

14. Pietsch J, Pietsch J. Care of the child with burns. In: Hazinski MF, ed. *Manual of Pediatric Critical Care*. St. Louis, MO: Mosby; 1999.

15. Ditchey RV, Lindenfeld J. Potential adverse effects of volume loading on perfusion of vital organs during closed-chest resuscitation. *Circulation*. 1984;69:181-189.

16. Voorhees WD, Ralston SH, Kougias C, Schmitz PM. Fluid loading with whole blood or Ringer's lactate solution during CPR in dogs. *Resuscitation*. 1987;15:113-123.

17. Young KD, Seidel JS. Pediatric cardiopulmonary resuscitation: a collective review. *Ann Emerg Med*. 1999;33:195-205.

18. Mogayzel C, Quan L, Graves JR, Tiedeman D, Fahrenbruch C, Herndon P. Out-of-hospital ventricular fibrillation in children and adolescents: causes and outcomes. *Ann Emerg Med*. 1995;25:484-491.

19. Hickey RW, Cohen DM, Strausbaugh S, Dietrich AM. Pediatric patients requiring CPR in the prehospital setting. *Ann Emerg Med*. 1995;25:495-501.

20. Sirbaugh PE, Pepe PE, Shook JE, Kimball KT, Goldman MJ, Ward MA, Mann DM. A prospective, population-based study of the demographics, epidemiology, management, and outcome of out-of-hospital pediatric cardiopulmonary arrest [published correction appears in *Ann Emerg Med*. 1999;33:358]. *Ann Emerg Med*. 1999;33:174-184.

21. Paradis NA, Martin GB, Goetting MG, Rivers EP, Feingold M, Nowak RM. Aortic pressure during human cardiac arrest: identification of pseudo-electromechanical dissociation. *Chest*. 1992;101:123-128.

22. Berg RA, Hilwig RW, Kern KB, Ewy GA. "Bystander" chest compressions and assisted ventilation independently improve outcome from piglet asphyxial pulseless "cardiac arrest". *Circulation*. 2000;101:1743-1748.

23. Rosetti VA, Thompson BM, Aprahamian C, Darin JC, Mateer JR. Difficulty and delay in intravascular access in pediatric arrests [abstract]. *Ann Emerg Med*. 1984;13:406.

24. Lillis KA, Jaffe DM. Prehospital intravenous access in children. *Ann Emerg Med*. 1992;21:1430-1434.

25. Fiser DH. Intraosseous infusion. *N Engl J Med*. 1990;322:1579-1581.

26. Banerjee S, Singhi SC, Singh S, Singh M. The intraosseous route is a suitable alternative to intravenous route for fluid resuscitation in severely dehydrated children. *Indian Pediatr*. 1994;31:1511-1520.

27. Glaeser PW, Losek JD, Nelson DB, Bonadio WA, Smith DS, Walsh-Kelly C, Hennes H. Pediatric intraosseous infusions: impact on vascular access time. *Am J Emerg Med*. 1988;6:330-332.

28. Daga SR, Gosavi DV, Verma B. Intraosseous access using butterfly needle. *Trop Doct*. 1999;29:142-144.

29. Glaeser PW, Hellmich TR, Szewczuga D, Losek JD, Smith DS. Five-year experience in prehospital intraosseous infusions in children and adults. *Ann Emerg Med*. 1993;22:1119-1124.

30. Guy J, Haley K, Zuspan SJ. Use of intraosseous infusion in the pediatric trauma patient. *J Pediatr Surg*. 1993;28:158-161.

31. Berg RA. Emergency infusion of catecholamines into bone marrow. *Am J Dis Child*. 1984;138:810-811.

32. Andropoulos DB, Soifer SJ, Schreiber MD. Plasma epinephrine concentrations after intraosseous and central venous injection during cardiopulmonary resuscitation in the lamb. *J Pediatr*. 1990;116:312-315.

33. Quinton DN, O'Byrne G, Aitkenhead AR. Comparison of endotracheal and peripheral intravenous adrenaline in cardiac arrest: is the endotracheal route reliable? *Lancet*. 1987;1:828-829.

34. Ralston SH, Voorhees WD, Babbs CF. Intrapulmonary epinephrine during prolonged cardiopulmonary resuscitation: improved regional blood flow and resuscitation in dogs. *Ann Emerg Med*. 1984;13:79-86.

35. Kleinman ME, Oh W, Stonestreet BS. Comparison of intravenous and endotracheal epinephrine during cardiopulmonary resuscitation in newborn piglets. *Crit Care Med*. 1999;27:2748-2754.

36. Jasani MS, Nadkarni VM, Finkelstein MS, Mandell GA, Salzman SK, Norman ME. Effects of different techniques of endotracheal epinephrine administration in pediatric porcine hypoxic-hypercarbic cardiopulmonary arrest. *Crit Care Med*. 1994;22:1174-1180.

37. Hedges JR, Barsan WB, Doan LA, Joyce SM, Lukes SJ, Dalsey WC, Nishiyama H. Central versus peripheral intravenous routes in cardiopulmonary resuscitation. *Am J Emerg Med*. 1984;2:385-390.

38. Kuhn GJ, White BC, Swetnam RE, Mumey JF, Rydesky MF, Tintinalli JE, Krome RL, Hoehner PJ. Peripheral vs central circulation times during CPR: a pilot study. *Ann Emerg Med*. 1981;10:417-419.

39. Dalsey WC, Barsan WG, Joyce SM, Hedges JR, Lukes SJ, Doan LA. Comparison of superior vena caval and inferior vena caval access using a radioisotope technique during normal perfusion and cardiopulmonary resuscitation. *Ann Emerg Med*. 1984;13:881-884.

40. Fleisher G, Caputo G, Baskin M. Comparison of external jugular and peripheral venous administration of sodium bicarbonate in puppies. *Crit Care Med*. 1989;17:251-254.

41. Davison R, Barresi V, Parker M, Meyers SN, Talano JV. Intracardiac injections during cardiopulmonary resuscitation: a low-risk procedure. *JAMA*. 1980;244:1110-1111.

42. Harrison EE. Intracardiac injections [letter]. *JAMA.* 1981;245:1315.

43. Pun KK. Cardiac tamponade after intracardiac injection. *Anaesth Intensive Care.* 1984;12:66-67.

44. Vijay NK, Schoonmaker FW. Cardiopulmonary arrest and resuscitation. *Am Fam Physician.* 1975;12:85-90.

45. Lubitz DS, Seidel JS, Chameides L, Luten RC, Zaritsky AL, Campbell FW. A rapid method for estimating weight and resuscitation drug dosages from length in the pediatric age group. *Ann Emerg Med.* 1988;17:576-581.

46. Johnston C. Endotracheal drug delivery. *Pediatr Emerg Care.* 1992;8:94-97.

47. Niemann JT, Criley JM, Rosborough JP, Niskanen RA, Alferness C. Predictive indices of successful cardiac resuscitation after prolonged arrest and experimental cardiopulmonary resuscitation. *Ann Emerg Med.* 1985;14:521-528.

48. Sanders AB, Ewy GA, Taft TV. Prognostic and therapeutic importance of the aortic diastolic pressure in resuscitation from cardiac arrest. *Crit Care Med.* 1984;12:871-873.

49. Otto CW, Yakaitis RW, Blitt CD. Mechanism of action of epinephrine in resuscitation from asphyxial arrest. *Crit Care Med.* 1981;9:364-365.

50. Schleien CL, Dean JM, Koehler RC, Michael JR, Chantarojanasiri T, Traystman R, Rogers MC. Effect of epinephrine on cerebral and myocardial perfusion in an infant animal preparation of cardiopulmonary resuscitation. *Circulation.* 1986;73:809-817.

51. Michael JR, Guerci AD, Koehler RC, Shi AY, Tsitlik J, Chandra N, Niedermeyer E, Rogers MC, Traystman RJ, Weisfeldt ML. Mechanisms by which epinephrine augments cerebral and myocardial perfusion during cardiopulmonary resuscitation in dogs. *Circulation.* 1984;69:822-835.

52. Huang YG, Wong KC, Yip WH, McJames SW, Pace NL. Cardiovascular responses to graded doses of three catecholamines during lactic and hydrochloric acidosis in dogs. *Br J Anaesth.* 1995;74:583-590.

53. Preziosi MP, Roig JC, Hargrove N, Burchfield DJ. Metabolic acidemia with hypoxia attenuates the hemodynamic responses to epinephrine during resuscitation in lambs. *Crit Care Med.* 1993;21:1901-1907.

54. Chernow B, Holbrook P, D'Angona DSJ, Zaritsky A, Casey LC, Fletcher JR, Lake CR. Epinephrine absorption after intratracheal administration. *Anesth Analg.* 1984;63:829-832.

55. Zaritsky AL. Catecholamines, inotropic medications, and vasopressor agents. In: Chernow B, ed. *The Pharmacologic Approach to the Critically Ill Patient.* 3rd ed. Baltimore, MD: Williams & Wilkins; 1994:387-404.

56. Fisher DG, Schwartz PH, Davis AL. Pharmacokinetics of exogenous epinephrine in critically ill children. *Crit Care Med.* 1993;21:111-117.

57. Berg RA, Donnerstein RL, Padbury JF. Dobutamine infusions in stable, critically ill children: pharmacokinetics and hemodynamic actions. *Crit Care Med.* 1993;21:678-686.

58. Padbury JF, Agata Y, Baylen BG, Ludlow JK, Polk DH, Goldblatt E, Pescetti J. Dopamine pharmacokinetics in critically ill newborn infants. *J Pediatr.* 1987;110:293-298.

59. Habib DM, Padbury JF, Anas NG, Perkin RM, Minegar C. Dobutamine pharmacokinetics and pharmacodynamics in pediatric intensive care patients. *Crit Care Med.* 1992;20:601-608.

60. Martinez AM, Padbury JF, Thio S. Dobutamine pharmacokinetics and cardiovascular responses in critically ill neonates. *Pediatrics.* 1992;89:47-51.

61. Berg RA, Padbury JF. Sulfoconjugation and renal excretion contribute to the interpatient variation of exogenous catecholamine clearance in critically ill children. *Crit Care Med.* 1997;25:1247-1251.

62. Zaritsky A, Lotze A, Stull R, Goldstein DS. Steady-state dopamine clearance in critically ill infants and children. *Crit Care Med.* 1988;16:217-220.

63. Notterman DA, Greenwald BM, Moran F, DiMaio-Hunter A, Metakis L, Reidenberg MM. Dopamine clearance in critically ill infants and children: effect of age and organ system dysfunction. *Clin Pharmacol Ther.* 1990;48:138-147.

64. Berg RA, Padbury JF, Donnerstein RL, Klewer SE, Hutter JJJ. Dobutamine pharmacokinetics and pharmacodynamics in normal children and adolescents. *J Pharmacol Exp Ther.* 1993;265:1232-1238.

65. Stiell IG, Hebert PC, Weitzman BN, Wells GA, Raman S, Stark RM, Higginson LA, Ahuja J, Dickinson GE. High-dose epinephrine in adult cardiac arrest. *N Engl J Med.* 1992;327:1045-1050.

66. Brown CG, Martin DR, Pepe PE, Stueven H, Cummins RO, Gonzalez E, Jastremski M. A comparison of standard-dose and high-dose epinephrine in cardiac arrest outside the hospital. The Multicenter High-Dose Epinephrine Study Group. *N Engl J Med.* 1992;327:1051-1055.

67. Callaham M, Madsen CD, Barton CW, Saunders CE, Pointer J. A randomized clinical trial of high-dose epinephrine and norepinephrine vs standard-dose epinephrine in prehospital cardiac arrest. *JAMA.* 1992;268:2667-2672.

68. Lipman J, Wilson W, Kobilski S, Scribante J, Lee C, Kraus P, Cooper J, Barr J, Moyes D. High-dose adrenaline in adult in-hospital asystolic cardiopulmonary resuscitation: a double-blind randomised trial. *Anaesth Intensive Care.* 1993;21:192-196.

69. Lindner KH, Ahnefeld FW, Prengel AW. Comparison of standard and high-dose adrenaline in the resuscitation of asystole and electromechanical dissociation. *Acta Anaesthesiol Scand.* 1991;35:253-256.

70. Sherman BW, Munger MA, Foulke GE, Rutherford WF, Panacek EA. High-dose versus standard-dose epinephrine treatment of cardiac arrest after failure of standard therapy. *Pharmacotherapy.* 1997;17:242-247.

71. Choux C, Gueugniaud PY, Barbieux A, Pham E, Lae C, Dubien PY, Petit P. Standard doses versus repeated high doses of epinephrine in cardiac arrest outside the hospital. *Resuscitation.* 1995;29:3-9.

72. Woodhouse SP, Cox S, Boyd P, Case C, Weber M. High dose and standard dose adrenaline do not alter survival, compared with placebo, in cardiac arrest. *Resuscitation.* 1995;30:243-249.

73. Gueugniaud PY, Mols P, Goldstein P, Pham E, Dubien PY, Deweerdt C, Vergnion M, Petit P, Carli P. A comparison of repeated high doses and repeated standard doses of epinephrine for cardiac arrest outside the hospital. European Epinephrine Study Group. *N Engl J Med.* 1998;339:1595-1601.

74. Berg RA, Otto CW, Kern KB, Hilwig RW, Sanders AB, Henry CP, Ewy GA. A randomized, blinded trial of high-dose epinephrine versus standard-dose epinephrine in a swine model of pediatric asphyxial cardiac arrest. *Crit Care Med.* 1996;24:1695-1700.

75. Berg RA, Otto CW, Kern KB, Sanders AB, Hilwig RW, Hansen KK, Ewy GA. High-dose epinephrine results in greater early mortality after resuscitation from prolonged cardiac arrest in pigs: a prospective, randomized study. *Crit Care Med.* 1994;22:282-290.

76. Hornchen U, Lussi C, Schuttler J. Potential risks of high-dose epinephrine for resuscitation from ventricular fibrillation in a porcine model. *J Cardiothorac Vasc Anesth.* 1993;7:184-187.

77. Tang W, Weil MH, Sun S, Noc M, Yang L, Gazmuri RJ. Epinephrine increases the severity of postresuscitation myocardial dysfunction. *Circulation.* 1995;92:3089-3093.

78. Rivers EP, Wortsman J, Rady MY, Blake HC, McGeorge FT, Buderer NM. The effect of the total cumulative epinephrine dose administered during human CPR on hemodynamic, oxygen transport, and utilization variables in the postresuscitation period. *Chest.* 1994;106:1499-1507.

79. Behringer W, Kittler H, Sterz F, Domanovits H, Schoerkhuber W, Holzer M, Mullner M, Laggner AN. Cumulative epinephrine dose during cardiopulmonary resuscitation and neurologic outcome. *Ann Intern Med.* 1998;129:450-456.

80. Gedeborg R, Silander HC, Ronne-Engstrom E, Rubertsson S, Wiklund L. Adverse effects of high-dose epinephrine on cerebral blood flow during experimental cardiopulmonary resuscitation. *Crit Care Med.* 2000;28:1423-1430.

81. Dieckmann RA, Vardis R. High-dose epinephrine in pediatric out-of-hospital cardiopulmonary arrest. *Pediatrics.* 1995;95:901-913.

82. Ronco R, King W, Donley DK, Tilden SJ. Outcome and cost at a children's hospital following resuscitation for out-of-hospital cardiopulmonary arrest. *Arch Pediatr Adolesc Med.* 1995;149:210-214.

83. Kuisma M, Suominen P, Korpela R. Paediatric out-of-hospital cardiac arrests: epidemiology and outcome. *Resuscitation.* 1995;30:141-150.

84. Carpenter TC, Stenmark KR. High-dose epinephrine is not superior to standard-dose epinephrine in pediatric in-hospital cardiopulmonary arrest. *Pediatrics.* 1997;99:403-408.

85. Goetting MG, Paradis NA. High-dose epinephrine improves outcome from pediatric cardiac arrest. *Ann Emerg Med.* 1991;20:22-26.

86. Hilwig RW, Berg RA, Kern KB, Ewy GA. Endothelin-1 vasoconstriction during swine cardiopulmonary resuscitation improves coronary perfusion pressures but worsens postresuscitation outcome. *Circulation.* 2000;101:2097-2102.

87. Lindner KH, Prengel AW, Pfenninger EG, Lindner IM, Strohmenger HU, Georgieff M, Lurie KG. Vasopressin improves vital organ blood flow during closed-chest cardiopulmonary resuscitation in pigs. *Circulation.* 1995;91:215-221.

88. Prengel AW, Lindner KH, Keller A. Cerebral oxygenation during cardiopulmonary resuscitation with epinephrine and vasopressin in pigs. *Stroke.* 1996;27:1241-1248.

89. Wenzel V, Lindner KH, Krismer AC, Voelckel WG, Schocke MF, Hund W, Witkiewicz M, Miller EA, Klima G, Wissel J, Lingnau W, Aichner FT. Survival with full neurologic recovery and no cerebral pathology after prolonged cardiopulmonary resuscitation with vasopressin in pigs. *J Am Coll Cardiol.* 2000;35:527-533.

90. Prengel AW, Lindner KH, Wenzel V, Tugtekin I, Anhaupl T. Splanchnic and renal blood flow after cardiopulmonary resuscitation with epinephrine and vasopressin in pigs. *Resuscitation.* 1998;38:19-24.

91. Wenzel V, Lindner KH, Krismer AC, Miller EA, Voelckel WG, Lingnau W. Repeated administration of vasopressin but not epinephrine maintains coronary perfusion pressure after early and late administration during prolonged cardiopulmonary resuscitation in pigs. *Circulation.* 1999;99:1379-1384.

92. Voelckel WG, Lindner KH, Wenzel V, Bonatti J, Hangler H, Frimmel C, Kunszberg E, Lingnau W. Effects of vasopressin and epinephrine on splanchnic blood flow and renal function during and after cardiopulmonary resuscitation in pigs. *Crit Care Med.* 2000;28:1083-1088.

92a. Lindner KH, Dirks B, Strohmenger HU, Prengel AW, Lindner IM, Lurie KG. Randomised comparison of epinephrine and vasopressin in patients with out-of-hospital ventricular fibrillation. *Lancet.* 1997;349:535-537.

93. Stiell IG, Hebert PC, Wells GA, Vandemheen KL, Tang AS, Higginson LA, Dreyer JF, Clement C, Battram E, Watpool I, Mason S, Klassen T, Weitzman BN. Vasopressin versus epinephrine for inhospital cardiac arrest: a randomised controlled trial. *Lancet.* 2001;358:105-109.

94. Voelckel WG, Lurie KG, Lindner KH, McKnite S, Zielinski T, Lindstrom P, Wenzel V. Comparison of epinephrine and vasopressin in a pediatric porcine model of asphyxial cardiac arrest. *Circulation.* 1999;36:1115-1118.

95. Katz K, Lawler J, Wax J, O'Connor R, Nadkarni V. Vasopressin pressor effects in critically ill children during evaluation for brain death and organ recovery. *Resuscitation.* 2000;47:33-40.

96. Mann K, Berg RA, Nadkarni V. Vasopressin for shock refractory VF in children: a case series. *Resuscitation.* In press.

97. Liedal JL, Meadow W, Nachman J, Koogler T, Kahana MD. Use of vasopressin in refractory hypotension in children with vasodilatory shock; five cases of review of the literature. *Pediatr Crit Care Med.* 2002;3:15-18.

98. Voorhies TM, Rawlinson D, Vannucci RC. Glucose and perinatal hypoxic-ischemic brain damage in the rat. *Neurology.* 1986;36:1115-1118.

99. Sieber FE, Traystman RJ. Special issues: glucose and the brain. *Crit Care Med.* 1992;20:104-114.

100. Pulsinelli WA, Waldman S, Rawlinson D, Plum F. Moderate hyperglycemia augments ischemic brain damage: a neuropathologic study in the rat. *Neurology.* 1982;32:1239-1246.

101. Nakakimura K, Fleischer JE, Drummond JC, Scheller MS, Zornow MH, Grafe MR, Shapiro HM. Glucose administration before cardiac arrest worsens neurologic outcome in cats. *Anesthesiology.* 1990;72:1005-1011.

102. D'Alecy LG, Lundy EF, Barton KJ, Zelenock GB. Dextrose containing intravenous fluid impairs outcome and increases death after eight minutes of cardiac arrest and resuscitation in dogs. *Surgery.* 1986;100:505-511.

103. Michaud LJ, Rivara FP, Longstreth WTJ, Grady MS. Elevated initial blood glucose levels and poor outcome following severe brain injuries in children. *J Trauma.* 1991;31:1356-1362.

104. Cherian L, Goodman JC, Robertson CS. Hyperglycemia increases brain injury caused by secondary ischemia after cortical impact injury in rats. *Crit Care Med.* 1997;25:1378-1383.

105. Ashwal S, Schneider S, Tomasi L, Thompson J. Prognostic implications of hyperglycemia and reduced cerebral blood flow in childhood near-drowning. *Neurology.* 1990;40:820-823.

106. Stueven HA, Thompson B, Aprahamian C, Tonsfeldt DJ, Kastenson EH. The effectiveness of calcium chloride in refractory electromechanical dissociation. *Ann Emerg Med.* 1985;14:626-629.

107. Katz AM, Reuter H. Cellular calcium and cardiac cell death [editorial]. *Am J Cardiol.* 1979;44:188-190.

108. Stueven HA, Thompson B, Aprahamian C, Tonsfeldt DJ, Kastenson EH. Lack of effectiveness of calcium chloride in refractory asystole. *Ann Emerg Med.* 1985;14:630-632.

109. Redding JS, Haynes RR, Thomas JD. Drug therapy in resuscitation from electromechanical dissociation. *Crit Care Med.* 1983;11:681-684.

110. Bisogno JL, Langley A, Von Dreele MM. Effect of calcium to reverse the electrocardiographic effects of hyperkalemia in the isolated rat heart: a prospective, dose-response study. *Crit Care Med.* 1994;22:697-704.

111. Cardenas-Rivero N, Chernow B, Stoiko MA, Nussbaum SR, Todres ID. Hypocalcemia in critically ill children. *J Pediatr.* 1989;114:946-951.

112. Zaritsky A, Nadkarni V, Getson P, Kuehl K. CPR in children. *Ann Emerg Med.* 1987;16:1107-1111.

113. Bohman VR, Cotton DB. Supralethal magnesemia with patient survival. *Obstet Gynecol.* 1990;76(pt 2):984-986.

114. Ramoska EA, Spiller HA, Winter M, Borys D. A one-year evaluation of calcium channel blocker overdoses: toxicity and treatment. *Ann Emerg Med.* 1993;22:196-200.

115. Broner CW, Stidham GL, Westenkirchner DF, Watson DC. A prospective, randomized, double-blind comparison of calcium chloride and calcium gluconate therapies for hypocalcemia in critically ill children. *J Pediatr.* 1990;117:986-989.

116. Vukmir RB, Bircher NG, Radovsky A, Safar P. Sodium bicarbonate may improve outcome in dogs with brief or prolonged cardiac arrest. *Crit Care Med.* 1995;23:515-522.

117. Levy MM. An evidence-based evaluation of the use of sodium bicarbonate during cardio-pulmonary resuscitation. *Crit Care Clin.* 1998;14:457-483.

118. Cooper DJ, Walley KR, Wiggs BR, Russell JA. Bicarbonate does not improve hemodynamics in critically ill patients who have lactic acidosis: a prospective, controlled clinical study. *Ann Intern Med.* 1990;112:492-498.

119. Mathieu D, Neviere R, Billard V, Fleyfel M, Wattel F. Effects of bicarbonate therapy on hemodynamics and tissue oxygenation in patients with lactic acidosis: a prospective, controlled clinical study. *Crit Care Med.* 1991;19:1352-1356.

120. Ettinger PO, Regan TJ, Oldewurtel HA. Hyperkalemia, cardiac conduction, and the electrocardiogram: a review. *Am Heart J.* 1974;88:360-371.

121. Hoffman JR, Votey SR, Bayer M, Silver L. Effect of hypertonic sodium bicarbonate in the treatment of moderate-to-severe cyclic antidepressant overdose. *Am J Emerg Med.* 1993;11:336-341.

122. Weil MH, Rackow EC, Trevino R, Grundler W, Falk JL, Griffel MI. Difference in acid-base state between venous and arterial blood during cardiopulmonary resuscitation. *N Engl J Med.* 1986;315:153-156.

123. Steedman DJ, Robertson CE. Acid-base changes in arterial and central venous blood during cardiopulmonary resuscitation. *Arch Emerg Med.* 1992;9:169-176.

124. Howell JH. Sodium bicarbonate in the perinatal setting—revisited. *Clin Perinatol.* 1987;14:807-816.

125. Berenyi KJ, Wolk M, Killip T. Cerebrospinal fluid acidosis complicating therapy of experimental cardiopulmonary arrest. *Circulation.* 1975;52:319-324.

126. Arieff AI, Leach W, Park R, Lazarowitz VC. Systemic effects of NaHCO3 in experimental lactic acidosis in dogs. *Am J Physiol.* 1982;242:F586-F591.

127. Lucking SE, Pollack MM, Fields AI. Shock following generalized hypoxic-ischemic injury in previously healthy infants and children. *J Pediatr.* 1986;108:359-364.

128. Ceneviva G, Paschall JA, Maffei F, Carcillo JA. Hemodynamic support in fluid-refractory pediatric septic shock. *Pediatrics.* 1998;102:e19.

129. Kyriacou DN, Arcinue EL, Peek C, Kraus JF. Effect of immediate resuscitation on children with submersion injury. *Pediatrics.* 1994;94(pt 1):137-142.

130. Kern KB, Hilwig RW, Rhee KH, Berg RA. Myocardial dysfunction after resuscitation from cardiac arrest: an example of global myocardial stunning. *J Am Coll Cardiol.* 1996;28:232-240.

131. Kern KB, Hilwig RW, Berg RA, Rhee KH, Sanders AB, Otto CW, Ewy GA. Postresuscitation left ventricular systolic and diastolic dysfunction: treatment with dobutamine. *Circulation.* 1997;95:2610-2613.

132. Carcillo JA, et al. Revised ACCM/SCCM clinical practice parameters for hemodynamic support of pediatric and neonatal septic shock. *Crit Care Med.* In press.

133. Leier CV, Heban PT, Huss P, Bush CA, Lewis RP. Comparative systemic and regional hemodynamic effects of dopamine and dobutamine in patients with cardiomyopathic heart failure. *Circulation.* 1978;58:466-475.

134. Ichai C, Soubielle J, Carles M, Giunti C, Grimaud D. Comparison of the renal effects of low to high doses of dopamine and dobutamine in critically ill patients: a single-blind randomized study. *Crit Care Med.* 2000;28:921-928.

135. Guller B, Fields AI, Coleman MG, Holbrook PR. Changes in cardiac rhythm in children treated with dopamine. *Crit Care Med.* 1978;6:151-154.

136. Van den Berghe G, de Zegher F, Lauwers P. Dopamine suppresses pituitary function in infants and children. *Crit Care Med.* 1994;22:1747-1753.

137. Schranz D, Stopfkuchen H, Jungst BK, Clemens R, Emmrich P. Hemodynamic effects of dobutamine in children with cardiovascular failure. *Eur J Pediatr.* 1982;139:4-7.

138. Perkin RM, Levin DL, Webb R, Aquino A, Reedy J. Dobutamine: a hemodynamic evaluation in children with shock. *J Pediatr.* 1982;100:977-983.

139. Liang CS, Sherman LG, Doherty JU, Wellington K, Lee VW, Hood WBJ. Sustained improvement of cardiac function in patients with congestive heart failure after short-term infusion of dobutamine. *Circulation.* 1984;69:113-119.

140. Duke GJ, Briedis JH, Weaver RA. Renal support in critically ill patients: low-dose dopamine or low-dose dobutamine? *Crit Care Med.* 1994;22:1919-1925.

141. Banner WJ, Vernon DD, Minton SD, Dean JM. Nonlinear dobutamine pharmacokinetics in a pediatric population. *Crit Care Med.* 1991;19:871-873.

142. Bollaert PE, Bauer P, Audibert G, Lambert H, Larcan A. Effects of epinephrine on hemodynamics and oxygen metabolism in dopamine-resistant septic shock. *Chest.* 1990;98:949-953.

143. Benzing Gd, Helmsworth JA, Schreiber JT, Kaplan S. Nitroprusside and epinephrine for treatment of low output in children after open-heart surgery. *Ann Thorac Surg.* 1979;27:523-528.

144. Clutter WE, Bier DM, Shah SD, Cryer PE. Epinephrine plasma metabolic clearance rates and physiologic thresholds for metabolic and hemodynamic actions in man. *J Clin Invest.* 1980;66:94-101.

145. Coffin LHJ, Ankeney JL, Beheler EM. Experimental study and clinical use of epinephrine for treatment of low cardiac output syndrome. *Circulation.* 1966;33(suppl):I78-I85.

146. Martin C, Papazian L, Perrin G, Saux P, Gouin F. Norepinephrine or dopamine for the treatment of hyperdynamic septic shock? *Chest.* 1993;103:1826-1831.

147. Redl-Wenzl EM, Armbruster C, Edelmann G, Fischl E, Kolacny M, Wechsler-Fordos A, Sporn P. The effects of norepinephrine on hemodynamics and renal function in severe septic shock states. *Intensive Care Med.* 1993;19:151-154.

148. Levy B, Bollaert PE, Charpentier C, Nace L, Audibert G, Bauer P, Nabet P, Larcan A. Comparison of norepinephrine and dobutamine to epinephrine for hemodynamics, lactate metabolism, and gastric tonometric variables in septic shock: a prospective, randomized study. *Intensive Care Med.* 1997;23:282-287.

149. Hoogenberg K, Smit AJ, Girbes AR. Effects of low-dose dopamine on renal and systemic hemodynamics during incremental norepinephrine infusion in healthy volunteers. *Crit Care Med.* 1998;26:260-265.

150. Juste RN, Panikkar K, Soni N. The effects of low-dose dopamine infusions on haemodynamic and renal parameters in patients with septic shock requiring treatment with noradrenaline. *Intensive Care Med.* 1998;24:564-568.

151. Teba L, Schiebel F, Dedhia HV, Lazzell VA. Beneficial effect of norepinephrine in the treatment of circulatory shock caused by tricyclic antidepressant overdose. *Am J Emerg Med.* 1988;6:566-568.

152. Tran TP, Panacek EA, Rhee KJ, Foulke GE. Response to dopamine vs norepinephrine in tricyclic antidepressant-induced hypotension. *Acad Emerg Med.* 1997;4:864-868.

153. Cohn JN, Burke LP. Nitroprusside. *Ann Intern Med.* 1979;91:752-757.

154. Palmer RF, Lasseter KC. Drug therapy: sodium nitroprusside. *N Engl J Med.* 1975;292:294-297.

155. Guiha NH, Cohn JN, Mikulic E, Franciosa JA, Limas CJ. Treatment of refractory heart failure with infusion of nitroprusside. *N Engl J Med.* 1974;291:587-592.

156. Miller RR, Fennell WH, Young JB, Palomo AR, Quinones MA. Differential systemic arterial and venous actions and consequent cardiac effects of vasodilator drugs. *Prog Cardiovasc Dis.* 1982;24:353-374.

157. Rindone JP, Sloane EP. Cyanide toxicity from sodium nitroprusside: risks and management [published correction appears in Ann Pharmacother. 1992;26:1160]. *Ann Pharmacother.* 1992;26:515-519.

158. Barton P, Garcia J, Kouatli A, Kitchen L, Zorka A, Lindsay C, Lawless S, Giroir B. Hemodynamic effects of i.v. milrinone lactate in pediatric patients with septic shock: a prospective, double-blinded, randomized, placebo-controlled, interventional study. *Chest.* 1996;109:1302-1312.

159. Bailey JM, Miller BE, Lu W, Tosone SR, Kanter KR, Tam VK. The pharmacokinetics of milrinone in pediatric patients after cardiac surgery. *Anesthesiology.* 1999;90:1012-1018.

160. Lindsay CA, Barton P, Lawless S, Kitchen L, Zorka A, Garcia J, Kouatli A, Giroir B. Pharmacokinetics and pharmacodynamics of milrinone lactate in pediatric patients with septic shock. *J Pediatr.* 1998;132:329-334.

161. Ramamoorthy C, Anderson GD, Williams GD, Lynn AM. Pharmacokinetics and side effects of milrinone in infants and children after open heart surgery. *Anesth Analg.* 1998; 86:283-289.

162. Coceani F, Olley PM. The response of the ductus arteriosus to prostaglandins. *Can J Physiol Pharmacol.* 1973;51:220-225.

163. Heymann MA, Berman WJ, Rudolph AM, Whitman V. Dilatation of the ductus arteriosus by prostaglandin E1 in aortic arch abnormalities. *Circulation.* 1979;59:169-173.

164. Lewis AB, Takahashi M, Lurie PR. Administration of prostaglandin E1 in neonates with critical congenital cardiac defects. *J Pediatr.* 1978;93:481-485.

165. Freed MD, Heymann MA, Lewis AB, Roehl SL, Kensey RC. Prostaglandin E1 infants with ductus arteriosus-dependent congenital heart disease. *Circulation.* 1981;64:899-905.

166. Heymann MA. Pharmacologic use of prostaglandin E_1 in infant with congenital heart disease. *Am Heart J.* 1981;101:837-843.

167. Ferreira SH, Vane JR. Prostaglandins: their disappearance from and release into the circulation. *Nature.* 1967;216:868-873.

168. Hallidie-Smith KA. Prostaglandin E_1 in suspected ductus dependent cardiac malformation. *Arch Dis Child.* 1984;59:1020-1026.

169. Lewis AB, Freed MD, Heymann MA, Roehl SL, Kensey RC. Side effects of therapy with prostaglandin E1 in infants with critical congenital heart disease. *Circulation.* 1981;64: 893-898.

170. American Academy of Pediatrics. Emergency drug doses for infants and children and naloxone use in newborns: clarification. *Pediatrics.* 1989;83:803.

171. American Academy of Pediatrics Committee on Drugs. Naloxone dosage and route of administration for infants and children: addendum to emergency drug doses for infants and children. *Pediatrics.* 1990;86:484-485.

172. Sporer KA, Firestone J, Isaacs SM. Out-of-hospital treatment of opioid overdoses in an urban setting. *Acad Emerg Med.* 1996;3: 660-667.

173. Yealy DM, Paris PM, Kaplan RM, Heller MB, Marini SE. The safety of prehospital naloxone administration by paramedics. *Ann Emerg Med.* 1990;19:902-905.

174. Mills CA, Flacke JW, Flacke WE, Bloor BC, Liu MD. Narcotic reversal in hypercapnic dogs: comparison of naloxone and nalbuphine. *Can J Anaesth.* 1990;37:238-244.

175. Prough DS, Roy R, Bumgarner J, Shannon G. Acute pulmonary edema in healthy teenagers following conservative doses of intravenous naloxone. *Anesthesiology.* 1984;60: 485-486.

176. Osterwalder JJ. Naloxone—for intoxications with intravenous heroin and heroin mixtures—harmless or hazardous? A prospective clinical study. *J Toxicol Clin Toxicol.* 1996;34:409-416.

177. Kienbaum P, Thurauf N, Michel MC, Scherbaum N, Gastpar M, Peters J. Profound increase in epinephrine concentration in plasma and cardiovascular stimulation after mu-opioid receptor blockade in opioid-addicted patients during barbiturate-induced anesthesia for acute detoxification. *Anesthesiology.* 1998;88:1154-1161.

178. Tenenbein M. Continuous naloxone infusion for opiate poisoning in infancy. *J Pediatr.* 1984;105:645-648.

Vascular Access

Introductory Case Scenario

Note: Indications for an approach to vascular access are included in Chapter 7.

A 2-month-old girl arrives at the Emergency Department in cardiac arrest. Other providers promptly begin ventilation and perform chest compressions. You need to establish vascular access to administer fluids and medications.

- What is the optimal site for immediate vascular access for this infant?
- If resuscitative efforts are successful, what is the optimal site for vascular access during the *postresuscitation* period?

Learning Objectives

After completing this chapter the PALS provider should be able to

- Prioritize sites of vascular access for different clinical circumstances
- Describe the risks and benefits of peripheral venous, central venous, and intraosseous (IO) vascular access
- Describe the IO access technique

Some students may require detailed information about techniques of vascular access. "Vascular Access Techniques" (later in this chapter) describes peripheral venous, central venous, and arterial catheterization.

Selection of Site and Priorities of Vascular Access

Vascular access is vital for drug and fluid administration during advanced life support, but it may be difficult to achieve in the pediatric patient.[1-5] For CPR and treatment of *decompensated* shock, the preferred access site is the one that is most readily accessible. During CPR you should attempt to establish vascular access at a site that will not require interruption of compressions or ventilation.[6] For treatment of *compensated* shock, ideally you should use a large-bore peripheral catheter to enable rapid delivery of a large volume of fluid. During the postresuscitation phase, a central venous catheter provides secure access and enables monitoring of central venous pressure.

Intracardiac administration of drugs during closed-chest CPR is not recommended. Intracardiac injections increase the risk of coronary artery laceration, cardiac tamponade, pneumothorax, and intramyocardial injection with resultant acute myocardial necrosis.[7-9]

Arterial cannulation provides a direct means to measure blood pressure continuously and to sample blood for evaluation of arterial oxygenation, carbon dioxide tension, and acid-base balance.

Emergency Vascular Access During CPR and Treatment of Decompensated Shock

Priorities of Vascular Access

During pediatric CPR or treatment of severe shock, you should establish *IO* access if you cannot rapidly achieve venous access.[5,10-13]

A practical approach is to pursue IO and peripheral or central venous access simultaneously. The experience and expertise of the providers should determine the sites and techniques attempted. The safest central venous access site during CPR or decompensated shock is the femoral vein. Establishing access through the femoral vein does not require interruption of CPR, and airway management is less likely to be jeopardized if this site is used (see Critical Concepts: "Priorities of Vascular Access During CPR and Treatment of Decompensated Shock").

During attempted resuscitation, if a tracheal tube is in place but vascular access is not yet available, you may administer lipid-soluble resuscitation drugs such as **L**idocaine, **E**pinephrine, **A**tropine, or **N**aloxone (mnemonic: **LEAN**) through the tracheal tube.[14] But any *vascular* route of drug administration is preferable to the *tracheal* route because drug absorption from the tracheobronchial tree is inconsistent during cardiac arrest (see Chapter 5: "Fluid Therapy and Medications").

Intraosseous Access During CPR and Treatment of Decompensated Shock

Intraosseous cannulation provides access to a noncollapsible marrow venous plexus, which serves as a rapid, safe, and reliable route for administration of drugs, crystalloids, colloids, and blood during resuscitation.[5,10-13,15-26] Intraosseous access often can be achieved in 30 to 60 seconds.[5,15] In this technique the provider uses a rigid needle, preferably a specially designed IO or Jamshidi-type bone marrow needle. Although an IO needle with a stylet is preferable to prevent obstruction of the needle with cortical bone during insertion, you can also use a butterfly or standard hypodermic needle.[16,20]

The site for insertion of an IO needle is often the anterior tibia. Alternative sites include the distal femur, medial malleolus, and anterior superior iliac spine. You can use this vascular access technique in patients of all ages, from preterm neonates through adults (Figure 1).[13,15,18,19,24] In older children and adults, you may insert an IO cannula into the distal tibia, anterior superior iliac spine, distal radius, or distal ulna.[13,17,18] Although the success rate for out-of-hospital IO cannulation tends to be lower in older children, this technique is still a reasonable alternative when you cannot rapidly achieve vascular access.[13,15,18,19]

A sternal IO cannula system for adults is now available. This system, called the First Access for Shock and Trauma (FAST) system, works by means of a hand-driven, push-pull mechanism. The

FAST system enables rapid (mean time, 114 seconds) establishment of IO access in older patients.[27,28]

The IO route is safe for administration of resuscitation drugs, fluids, and blood products.[11,18,19] You can also provide continuous catecholamine infusion by the IO route.[20] Onset of action and drug levels after IO infusion during CPR are comparable to those achieved after vascular administration, including central venous administration.[23] Some experts recommend flushing all IO medications with 5 to 10 mL of normal saline to facilitate delivery into the central circulation. Fluid for rapid volume resuscitation and administration of viscous drugs and solutions may require administration under pressure using an infusion pump, pressure bag, or forceful manual pressure to overcome the resistance of emissary veins.[29,30] Despite concerns that high-pressure infusion of blood might induce hemolysis, this result was not observed in an experimental animal model.[31]

Intraosseous access also allows you to obtain mixed-venous specimens for blood chemistry, blood gas, and type and cross-match studies. Note that administration of sodium bicarbonate through the IO cannula reduces the validity of blood gas results.[32,33]

Complications have been reported in fewer than 1% of patients after IO infusion.[21,34] Complications include fracture of the tibia,[35,36] lower-extremity compartment syndrome or severe extravasation of drugs,[37-40] and osteomyelitis.[21,41] You can avoid some of these complications by using careful technique. Data from animal studies[42-44] and one human follow-up study[45] indicates that local effects of IO infusion on the bone marrow and bone growth are minimal. Although microscopic pulmonary fat and bone marrow emboli have been demonstrated in animal models, they have never been reported in clinical studies. These complications appear to occur just as frequently during cardiac arrest without IO drug administration.[46,47]

Intraosseous Cannulation Devices

Several types of IO needles are available for use in infants and children. One type is the specially designed intraosseous infusion needle; another is the Jamshidi-type bone marrow aspiration needle. The smaller Jamshidi-type needle for infants and young children is also known as the Illinois Sternal Bone Marrow Needle.[48-50] Theoretically the specially designed IO needles are the best choice. But in a laboratory model, investigators found that the Jamshidi-type bone marrow aspiration needle was more user friendly.[50]

Short, wide-gauge spinal needles with internal stylets are *not* recommended for IO use because they bend easily. You can use these needles in an emergency if no alternative is available. Standard hypodermic and butterfly needles have been used successfully, but they may become clogged with bone and bone marrow.[16,20]

Intraosseous Cannulation Technique

Use the following technique for IO cannulation of the tibia and other sites:

1. Using sterile technique, locate the site of cannulation (Figure 1). Identify the tibial tuberosity by palpation. The site for IO cannulation of the tibia is approximately 1 to 3 cm (approximately one finger's width) below this tuberosity, in the middle of the anteromedial surface of the tibia. At this site the tibia usually is immediately beneath the skin surface and is readily palpable as a flat, smooth surface. Do not place an IO needle into a fractured bone.

2. Check the needle to ensure that the bevels of the outer needle and internal stylet are properly aligned.

3. It is preferable to support the leg on a firm surface. From the front of the leg, grasp the medial and lateral edges of the tibia; use the thumb of the nondominant hand on one side and the index and middle (2nd and 3rd) fingers

on the other side. Do not allow any portion of your hand to rest *behind* the insertion site.

4. Palpate the landmarks, and again identify the flat surface of the tibia just below and medial to the tibial tuberosity.

5. Insert the needle through the skin over the flat anteromedial surface of the tibia.

6. Using a gentle but firm twisting motion, advance the needle through the bony cortex of the proximal tibia; direct the needle perpendicular (90°)

to the long axis of the bone (or slightly caudad—ie, toward the toes) to avoid the epiphysial plate (Figure 1E). *Twist, do not just push, the needle.* Some IO needles have threads; these needles must be turned clockwise and screwed into the bone.

7. When placing an IO needle in other locations, aim slightly *away* from the nearest joint space to reduce the risk of injury to the epiphysis or joint.

8. Stop advancing the needle when you feel a sudden decrease in resistance to forward motion. This decrease in

resistance usually indicates entrance into the bone marrow cavity.

9. Unscrew the cap and remove the stylet from the needle. Attempt to aspirate bone marrow. If aspiration is successful, irrigate the needle to prevent obstruction of the needle with marrow. If aspiration is unsuccessful but you believe that the needle is in the bone marrow, attempt to flush the needle (see step 10). If you do not think the needle is in the bone marrow, you may need to advance the needle farther.

FIGURE 1. **A,** Locations for intraosseous infusion (IOI) in an infant. **B,** Locations for IOI in the distal tibia and the femur in older children. **C,** Location for IOI in the iliac crest. **D,** Location for IOI in the distal tibia. **E,** Technique for IOI infusion needle.

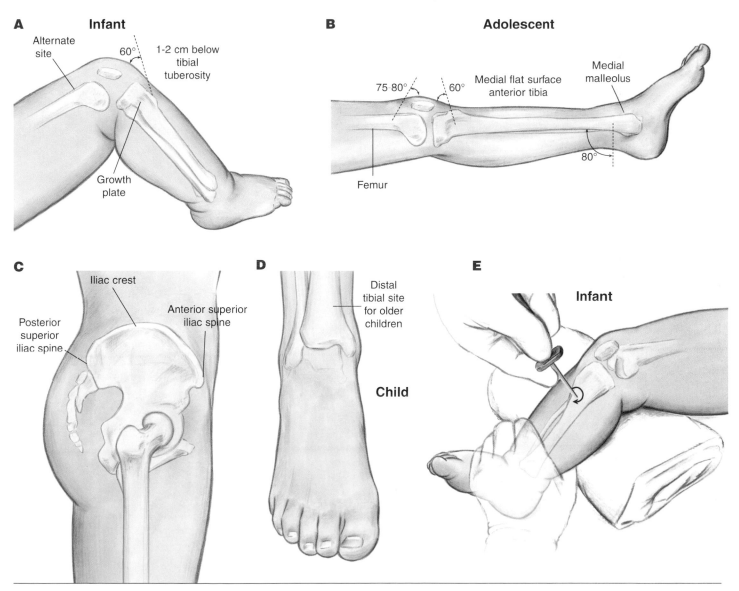

Intraosseous (IO) access is a safe, reliable, rapid, life-saving technique to obtain vascular access during CPR or treatment of severe shock. Use a rigid Jamshidi-type bone marrow needle or a specifically designed IO needle if possible. *Twist* the needle into the bone marrow while applying pressure; do not just push it into the marrow.

The following signs confirm that the needle is in the marrow cavity:

- A sudden decrease in resistance occurs as the needle passes through the bony cortex into the marrow.

- The needle remains upright without support.

- You aspirate marrow through the needle (this sign does not always occur).

- Fluid infuses freely without evidence of subcutaneous infiltration.[20]

Note: Do not place an IO needle into a fractured bone.

10. Stabilize the IO needle, and then slowly inject 10 mL of normal saline through it. Check for any signs of increased resistance to injection, increased circumference of the soft tissues of the calf (or tissues surrounding the cannulated bone), or increased firmness of the tissue. Aspiration at this point may draw blood or serosanguinous fluid (even if no blood return was noted on initial insertion).

11. If the test injection is successful and no signs of infiltration are present, disconnect the syringe, evacuate any air remaining in the connection tubing, and join an infusion set to the needle. Secure the needle and tubing with tape and support them with a bulky dressing.

12. If the test injection is unsuccessful (ie, you observe infiltration of normal saline into the leg tissue), remove the needle and attempt the procedure on another bone. If the first needle penetrated the cortex of the bone, placing another needle in the same extremity will permit fluids and drugs to escape from the original hole into the soft tissues, which could lead to injury. Inserting an IO needle into a fractured bone could cause the same problem.

If the needle becomes obstructed with bone or bone marrow, you can replace it with a second needle. You can pass the second needle through the same cannulation site provided there is no evidence of infiltration. If you observe evidence of infiltration or if the test injection fails, reattempt IO cannulation on another bone (see Critical Concepts: "Intraosseous Access").

Central Venous Access

Central venous administration of drugs during CPR theoretically results in more rapid onset of action and higher peak drug levels than peripheral venous administration. But this difference does not appear to be significant in infants and children.[51-54] Central venous catheters provide more secure access to the circulation, and they permit administration of agents that might injure tissues if they infiltrated from peripheral sites, such as vasopressors, hypertonic sodium bicarbonate, and calcium (see Critical Concepts: "Advantages of Central Venous Cannulation During CPR and Treatment of Decompensated Shock"). For these reasons providers skilled at insertion of these catheters may attempt central venous access during CPR. The femoral, internal jugular, external jugular, or (in older children) subclavian vein may be cannulated. The femoral vein is probably the easiest and safest to cannulate, particularly because providers do not need to interrupt CPR.

When rapid fluid administration is needed, a single-lumen, wide-bore, relatively short

The following characteristics make central venous cannulation advantageous during CPR and treatment of severe shock:

- It provides a secure route of vascular access.

- It is relatively safe for administration of medications that may injure tissues if infiltration occurs.

- It is convenient for blood sampling.

- It enables monitoring of central venous pressure.

catheter will provide lower resistance to flow. Catheter lengths of 5 cm in an infant, 8 cm in a young child, and 12 cm in an older child are usually suitable. If the femoral catheter will also be used to monitor central venous pressure, the tip of the catheter should lie within the vena cava; it can remain below the diaphragm provided the vena cava is unobstructed.[55,56]

Complications of central venous cannulation include local and systemic infection, venous or arterial bleeding, arterial cannulation, thrombosis, phlebitis, pulmonary thromboembolism, pneumothorax, hydrothorax, hemothorax, chylothorax, cardiac tamponade, arrhythmias, air embolism, and catheter-fragment embolism.[3,57-61] The incidence of these complications is affected by the site of access, experience of the clinician, and clinical condition of the patient.[59-61] Pneumothorax, hemothorax, and chylothorax are more likely to occur after attempts to cannulate the subclavian or internal jugular vein on the left side. These complications are more likely because the cupula of the lung is higher on the left side than on the right and because the thoracic duct is located on the left side. Complications of central venous catheterization are more common in infants and children than in adults.

Peripheral Venous Access

Peripheral venous access provides a satisfactory route for administration of drugs or fluid during CPR or treatment of decompensated shock *if* it can be achieved rapidly. During resuscitation you should use the largest catheter you can quickly insert to establish reliable, unobstructed flow.

You can perform peripheral venipuncture in the arm, hand, leg, or foot.[62] But cannulation of small vessels may be difficult when intense vasoconstriction develops during shock or cardiopulmonary arrest. Large peripheral veins, such as the median cubital vein at the elbow or the long saphenous vein at the ankle, are relatively constant in respect to anatomic location, so they may be the best veins to cannulate. Scalp veins are less desirable for vascular access than other sites during resuscitation. Infiltration often occurs when fluids or medications are administered rapidly and forcefully through catheters placed in these small vessels.

Blood flow in peripheral vascular beds will be poor during CPR. Follow drugs administered through a peripheral vein with a rapid flush of isotonic crystalloid (5 to 10 mL) to move the drugs into the central circulation.

Peripheral Venous Cutdown

If peripheral venous, central venous, and intraosseous cannulation are unsuccessful, providers may attempt a venous cutdown to gain vascular access. Percutaneous central venous cannulation is usually easier to achieve, and fewer complications occur than with saphenous vein cutdown.[63] Even in experienced hands a saphenous vein cutdown may take longer than 10 minutes to perform, and access may last no longer than that provided by percutaneous cannulation. Infections are more common with saphenous vein cutdown than with other methods of venous access.[63,64]

Vascular Access in Nonemergent Circumstances

Peripheral Venous Access

Peripheral venous cannulation is the vascular access method of choice in most nonemergent situations. Small-caliber plastic catheters allow easy and reliable venous cannulation in most infants and children.

Peripheral Venous Access Devices

Four types of venous cannulas are used in infants and children:

■ Over-the-needle catheters

■ Catheter-over-wire devices

■ Catheter-through-introducing sheath devices

■ Butterfly needles

Over-the-needle catheters are described here. *Catheter-over-wire* and *catheter-through-sheath* devices are described in "Cannulation of Central Veins" (below). *Butterfly needles* are useful to obtain blood specimens for laboratory analysis, but infiltration tends to occur when they are used for fluid administration. For this reason butterfly needles are used less frequently than over-the-needle catheters.

You can insert an over-the-needle catheter into any vein, including veins in the antecubital fossa, veins in the dorsum of the hands or feet, and the external jugular and saphenous veins. The ideal catheter has a clear hub so that you can see blood flashback when the catheter enters the vein. Over-the-needle catheters are available in a variety of sizes (see the Table).

During catheter insertion in patients with trauma, shock, or cardiopulmonary arrest, some providers prefer to aim the bevel of the needle down.[62] Aiming the bevel down may facilitate entrance into constricted veins. You may temporarily place an over-the-needle catheter into a central vein, especially in small infants, to allow initial drug and fluid administration until a longer catheter is inserted (see "Cannulation of Central Veins," later in this chapter).

TABLE. Equipment for Venous Cannulation

Age (y)	Weight (kg)	Butterfly Needles (gauge)	Over-the-Needle Catheters (gauge)	Venous Catheters				Catheter Introducers			
				French Size	Length (cm)	Wire Diameter [mm (in)]	Needle (gauge)	French Size	Length (cm)	Wire Diameter [mm (in)]	Needle (gauge)
Newborn	4-8	23-25	22, 24	3.0	5-12	0.46 (0.018)	21	4.0	6	0.53 (0.021)	20
								4.5	6		20
Infant <1	5-15	23, 21, 20	22, 24	3.0, 4.0	5-12	0.46 (0.018) to 0.53 (0.021)	21, 20, 18	4.0	13	0.53 (0.021) to 0.64 (0.025)	20
								4.5	13		20
								5.0	13		19
1 to <8	10-30	23, 21, 20	18, 20, 22	4.0-5.0	5-25	0.53 (0.021) to 0.89 (0.035)	20, 18	5.0	13	0.64 (0.025)	19
								5.5	13		19
								6.0	13		19
≥8	25-70	21, 20,18	16, 18, 20	5.0-8.0	5-30	0.89 (0.035)	18, 16	6.0	13	0.64 (0.025) to 0.89 (0.035)	19
								7.0	13		18
								8.0	13		18
								8.5	13		18

Potential Complications of Peripheral Venous Access

Potential complications of peripheral venous access include hematoma formation, cellulitis, thrombosis, phlebitis, pulmonary thromboembolism, air embolism, catheter-fragment embolism, infiltration, and skin slough.[3] Severe complications are relatively infrequent. Infusion of some fluids or medications (eg, calcium, dopamine, or epinephrine) may contribute to the development of vasculitis and subsequent thrombosis. When possible the provider should dilute these substances and administer them through the largest vein available, preferably a central vein.

Central Venous Access

Central venous cannulation is a useful option when you cannot achieve peripheral cannulation. Central venous cannulation provides a more stable and reliable route of venous access than peripheral venous cannulation. Central venous access also allows hemodynamic monitoring and sampling of central venous blood for laboratory studies. Central venous access obviates problems resulting from administration of irritating or vasoconstrictive medications because of the lower risk of extravasation and the dilution of these medications by high-volume central venous blood flow.

Complications of central venous catheterization occur more frequently in infants and children than in adults. The most common complications are thrombosis and suppurative thrombophlebitis. To reduce the risk of complications, limit central venous cannulation to patients with appropriate indications, practice meticulous aseptic technique during catheter insertion and maintenance, and remove the catheter as soon as possible.[3,65,66]

As for all procedures, providers should perform central venous cannulation only when the potential benefits outweigh the risks. A clinician experienced in the technique and knowledgeable of the unique features of central venous anatomy in infants and children should perform or directly supervise the procedure.[59-61,66,67]

Arterial Access

Arterial cannulation enables continuous monitoring of blood pressure and provides a route for blood sampling.[68] But arterial cannulation can produce complications, including localized or generalized infection, air or particulate embolization, and arterial thrombosis. Arterial thrombosis may result in tissue necrosis, tissue ischemia, and growth failure in the affected limb.[69,70] In children the most common complications of radial artery catheterization are minor skin lesions, localized necrosis, and radial artery occlusion.[71] Factors associated with the highest risk of radial artery occlusion are patient age of less than 5 years, cutdown insertion, and duration of cannulation of more than 4 days.[71]

FYI: Evaluation of Collateral Ulnar Blood Flow to the Hand

Modified Allen Test[72]

You can use the modified Allen test to evaluate collateral blood flow from the ulnar artery to the palm. The results indicate whether the collateral flow will be adequate to maintain perfusion of the hand if the radial artery becomes occluded. To perform the Allen test:

1. Compress or clench the child's hand several times.

2. Elevate the hand above the heart and compress or clench the hand tightly.

3. Occlude both the ulnar and radial arteries and lower the hand to the level of the heart.

4. Open the hand, but *do not hyperextend the fingers*. Release pressure over the ulnar artery.

5. Look for reperfusion of the hand (ie, return of color). Results:

   — The result is *negative* if color returns to the hand within 6 seconds while the radial artery remains occluded. A negative result suggests that circulation through the ulnar artery and palmar arch is adequate.

   — The result is *positive* if reperfusion does not occur within 6 seconds. A positive result suggests that flow through the ulnar artery and palmar arch may be inadequate if the radial artery becomes obstructed.

Note: Hyperextension of the fingers frequently produces a *false-positive* result on the Allen test (ie, it inaccurately suggests that collateral flow is inadequate).[73,74] *False-negative* results on the Allen test have been reported in a substantial number of patients shown to have radial artery–dependent palmar flow and inadequate (ulnar) collateral circulation by Doppler flow evaluation.[74,75]

A Doppler study may be more reliable than the modified Allen test.[73]

Doppler Flow Evaluation[74]

1. Place a Doppler probe between the heads of the 3rd and 4th metacarpals on the palm of the hand, perpendicular to the palm.

2. Advance the probe proximally until the pulsatile signal is maximal.

3. Occlude the radial artery while monitoring the Doppler signal. Results:

   — If the pulsatile signal is unchanged or increases in intensity, circulation through the ulnar artery and palmar arch is probably adequate.

   — If the pulsatile signal diminishes in intensity, flow through the ulnar artery and palmar arch will probably be inadequate if the radial artery becomes obstructed.

FIGURE 2. Seldinger technique for catheter placement. **A,** Insert the needle into the target vessel and pass the flexible end of the guidewire into the vessel. **B,** Remove the needle, leaving the guidewire in place. **C,** Using a twisting motion, advance the catheter into the vessel. **D,** Remove the guidewire, and connect the catheter to an appropriate flow device or monitoring device. Modified from Schwartz AJ, Coté CJ, Jobes DR, Ellison N. Central venous catheterization in pediatrics. Scientific exhibit.

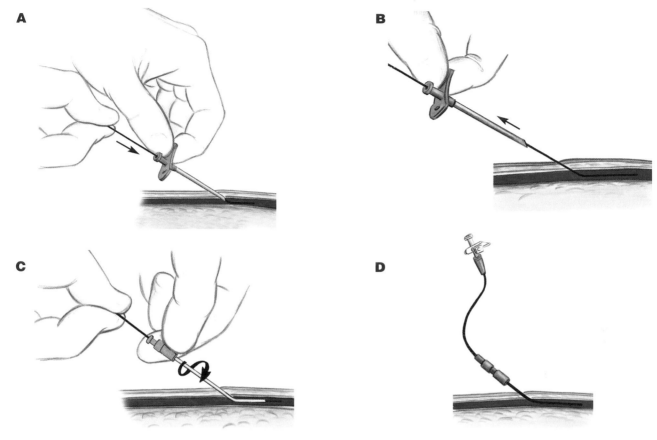

Temporary total occlusion of the radial artery after percutaneous catheterization has been reported in as many as 63% of infants.[76]

The main source of blood flow to the fingers is the superficial palmar arch. In most people (88%) this arch is supplied predominantly by flow from the ulnar artery.[73] Approximately 12% of healthy adults have radial artery–dominant palmar arch flow, and 1.6% of healthy adults have radial artery–dependent flow with no other collateral circulation.[73] This latter group (1.6%) is at high risk for hand ischemia after catheterization of the radial artery, particularly if the artery becomes occluded.

You may evaluate collateral circulation to the hand before radial artery cannulation using a modified Allen test[72] or Doppler flow evaluation[73] (see FYI: "Evaluation

of Collateral Ulnar Blood Flow to the Hand"). Monitor hand perfusion after you insert the catheter into the radial artery. If you observe any evidence of ischemia in the hand, remove the catheter. Consultation with a microvascular surgeon is recommended if evidence of ischemia persists.

Continuous infusion of heparinized saline increases the longevity (patency) of radial artery catheters, and it may decrease the incidence of complications.[77,78] You may infuse papaverine, a smooth muscle–relaxing agent, instead of or in addition to heparin to maintain patency of the artery and to minimize complications. Papaverine is a vasodilator, so you should not use it in patients with a risk of increased intracranial pressure or potential compromise in cerebral perfusion pressure.[79]

Vascular Access Techniques

This section is designed for providers who are expected to achieve vascular access during resuscitation. For other PALS providers, this section is optional.

The Seldinger Technique

The Seldinger (guidewire) technique[66] is especially useful for establishing vascular access in children. This technique allows introduction of catheters (see the Table) into the central venous circulation after initial venous entry is achieved using a small-gauge, thin-walled needle or an over-the-needle catheter.

Once you achieve free flow of blood through the small needle or catheter, thread a flexible guidewire through the needle or catheter into the vessel. Then withdraw the needle or catheter over the guidewire while holding the guidewire in place (Figure 2). To facilitate passage of the catheter or introducing sheath, incise the skin and superficial subcutaneous tissue using a No. 11 blade; insert the blade directly over the site where the guidewire enters the skin. For most catheters you will pass a dilator over the guidewire into the vessel and then remove the dilator before you place the catheter. Finally, pass a large catheter or a catheter-introducing sheath over the guidewire into the vessel and withdraw the guidewire.

Cannulation of Central Veins

Knowledge of anatomic landmarks is essential for successful and safe placement of a central venous catheter. Doppler or ultrasound devices may help you locate central vessels, and they can improve your success rate for central venous cannulation.[80-85]

Central Venous Access Sites

Access to the Inferior Vena Cava Through the Femoral Vein

The femoral vein allows access to the inferior vena cava. Providers frequently use the femoral vein for emergency vascular access because it is relatively easy to cannulate. Fewer complications occur when this site is used,[86-88] and cannulation does not require interruption of compressions or ventilations. The Seldinger technique is probably the most reliable method to access the central venous system through the femoral vein during an emergency. In general the right femoral vein is preferable for cannulation; it is easier to approach from the right side when the operator is right-handed, and the catheter is less likely to migrate into the posterior lumbar venous plexus. Such migration could lead to erosion into the subarachnoid space.[89]

Access to the Superior Vena Cava

The external jugular, internal jugular, axillary, or subclavian veins allow access to the superior vena cava. Only specifically trained, skilled providers should cannulate the internal jugular and subclavian veins. Less experienced providers may attempt cannulation of these veins if a skilled clinician directly supervises the

FIGURE 3. Central veins of the thorax and neck in relation to surrounding anatomy.

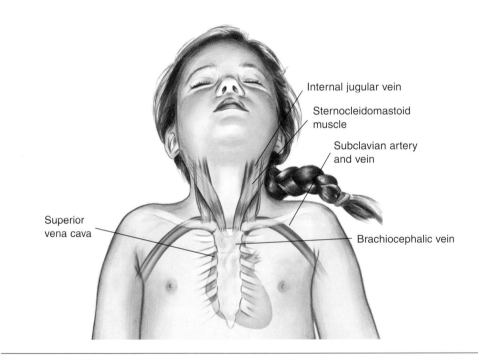

Internal jugular vein

Sternocleidomastoid muscle

Subclavian artery and vein

Superior vena cava

Brachiocephalic vein

FIGURE 4. Femoral vein. **A,** Anatomy. **B,** Cannulation technique.

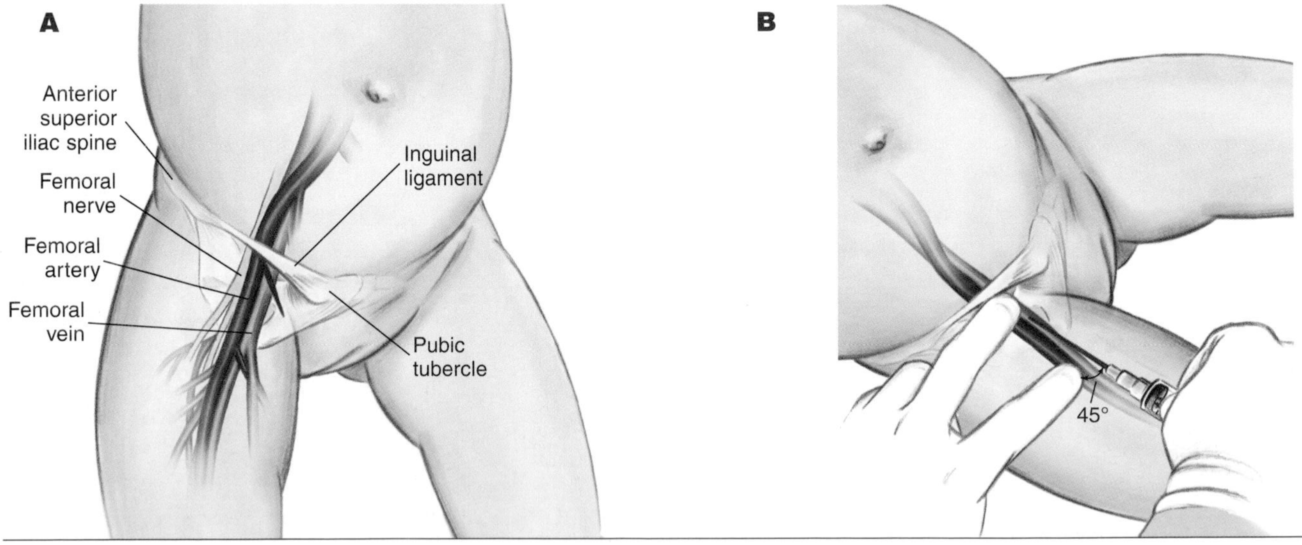

A

Anterior superior iliac spine

Femoral nerve

Femoral artery

Femoral vein

Inguinal ligament

Pubic tubercle

B

45°

procedure. The complication rate is higher when inexperienced providers attempt to cannulate these veins.

Cannulation of the external jugular vein is relatively safe because the vein is superficial and easy to see. The major disadvantages of this site are

- Potential compromise of the airway by extension and rotation of the neck to expose the vein

- A low success rate for central placement of the catheter because the angle of entry of the external jugular vein into the subclavian vein is acute[90,91]

Figure 3 shows the internal jugular vein in relation to the carotid artery, sternocleidomastoid muscle, and clavicle. The right internal jugular vein is preferable to the left because there is less chance that a pneumothorax or injury to the thoracic duct will occur and a greater chance that the catheter will pass directly from the innominate vein into the superior vena cava instead of the right subclavian vein. Three approaches are possible for internal jugular venous cannulation: the posterior, anterior, and central (middle) routes.[3,91] No one approach is clearly superior to the others.[92-96] The high central route appears to be the most widely used, but the operator should choose the route on the basis of his/her experience.

The subclavian vein in infants and children can be cannulated through the infraclavicular route.[97-99] But the complication rate is high when this route is used during emergencies, particularly in infants.[99,100] For this reason the subclavian vein is generally not the route of choice for small children when urgent access is needed. But a skilled provider may prefer the subclavian vein. The procedure does not require immobilization of an extremity, so the catheter will not limit movement of the patient after insertion.

Techniques of Central Venous Access

Note: Whenever possible, wash your hands and use sterile technique to establish *vascular access. During resuscitation vascular access must be achieved as quickly as possible, so some of the following steps may have to be omitted. Always use universal precautions. For elective catheter placement, use full-barrier precautions (masks, caps, sterile gowns, and large sterile drapes) and administer local anesthetic.*

Femoral Venous Catheterization

Following is the suggested procedure for femoral venous catheterization (see Figure 4):

1. Restrain the leg with slight external rotation. Place a small towel or diaper under the buttocks of the infant to flatten the inguinal area. Placing the infant in this position will make the angle of entry less acute and facilitate entry into the vein.

2. Identify the femoral artery by palpation or, if pulses are absent, by finding the midpoint between the anterior superior iliac spine and the symphysis pubis. Note that pulsations in the femoral area during chest compressions may originate from either the femoral vein or femoral artery.[101] If CPR is in progress, attempt needle puncture at the point of pulsation.

3. Using sterile technique, access the femoral vein using a thin-walled needle. Insert the needle one finger's breadth below the inguinal ligament and just medial to the femoral artery. Apply gentle negative pressure to an attached 3-mL syringe and slowly advance the needle. Direct the needle parallel to the arterial pulse (generally toward the umbilicus) at a 45° angle.

Note: Steps 4 through 6 are common to most central venous catheterization sequences.

4. When you observe a free flow of blood into the syringe, separate the syringe from the needle and advance a guidewire through the needle. Remove the needle and advance the appropriate central venous catheter over the guidewire using the Seldinger technique (described earlier in this chapter).

5. Secure the catheter in place with suture material or tape. Evacuate any air remaining in the connecting tubing and attach an infusion set. Apply a sterile, occlusive dressing to the site of catheter insertion.

6. Obtain an x-ray to verify that the tip of the catheter is correctly positioned.

FIGURE 5. Positioning of patient for cannulation of internal or external jugular vein.

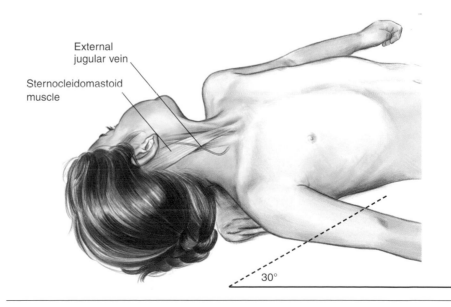

External jugular vein

Sternocleidomastoid muscle

30°

FIGURE 6. Technique for catheterization of internal jugular vein. **A,** Anterior route. **B,** Central route. **C,** Posterior route.

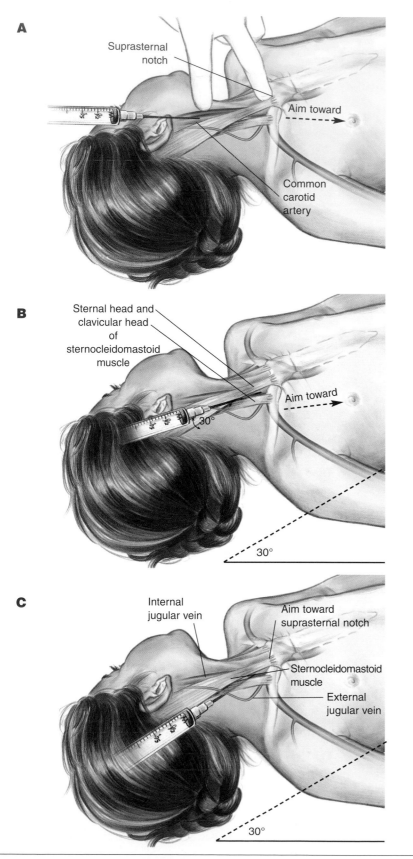

Internal Jugular Vein Catheterization

The following technique is commonly used with the anterior, central, and posterior routes of internal jugular vein cannulation. The right side of the neck is preferable for several reasons: the dome of the right lung and pleura is lower than that on the left, so the risk of pneumothorax is reduced; the path from the right internal jugular vein to the right atrium is more direct; and the risk of injury to the thoracic duct is eliminated.

1. If no cervical spine injury is present, hyperextend the patient's neck by placing a rolled towel transversely beneath the shoulders.

2. Restrain the child in a 30° head-down (Trendelenburg) position with the head turned slightly away from the side to be punctured (Figure 5).[102] The right side is preferable. Auscultate and document bilateral breath sounds before you start the procedure.

3. Identify the sternocleidomastoid muscle and clavicle.

4. Use the Seldinger technique to access the internal jugular vein. If the patient is breathing spontaneously with no positive-pressure support, prevent inadvertent movement of air into the superior vena cava. To prevent this air movement, use your finger to occlude any open needles or catheters during patient inspiration and attempt to thread the guidewire during exhalation. If the guidewire advances into the right atrium, premature atrial contractions may occur. Advance the catheter to the junction of the superior vena cava and right atrium (determine the distance beforehand from surface landmarks).

5. Aspirate blood from each port of the central line. Alternatively, lower the intravenous fluid reservoir below the level of the right atrium and allow blood to flow back freely into the intravenous tubing before you initiate fluid infusion through the catheter.

If blood return does not occur, the catheter may be lodged against the wall of a vessel or against the wall of the right atrium. In that case slightly withdraw the catheter and repeat aspiration. (You may perform this withdrawal/aspiration sequence twice.) If you still do not observe blood return, you must assume that the catheter is not in the vessel. You should remove the catheter and make another attempt.

Note: Follow steps 4 through 6 of "Femoral Venous Catheterization" (above) to complete catheterization of the internal jugular vein. In addition, auscultate and document bilateral breath sounds. Verify on the x-ray that the tip of the catheter is correctly positioned at or above the junction of the superior vena cava and right atrium; rule out pneumothorax and hemothorax.

There are three common approaches for cannulation of the internal jugular vein. The provider should become familiar with one technique rather than randomly attempt all three.

■ *Anterior route.* Use your index and middle (2nd and 3rd) fingers to palpate the carotid artery medially at the anterior border of the sternocleidomastoid muscle. Introduce the needle at the midpoint of this anterior border at a 30° angle to the coronal plane. Direct the needle caudad and toward the ipsilateral nipple (Figure 6A).

■ *Central route.* Identify a triangle formed by the two portions (sternoclavicular heads) of the sternocleidomastoid muscle with the clavicle at its base. Introduce the needle at the apex of this triangle at a 30° to 45° angle to the coronal plane. Direct the needle caudad and toward the ipsilateral nipple. If you do not enter the vein, withdraw the needle to just below the skin surface and redirect the needle directly caudad along the sagittal plane (ie, less lateral). Do *not* direct the needle medially across the sagittal plane because you will likely puncture the carotid artery (Figure 6B).

■ *Posterior route.* Introduce the needle deep into the sternal head of the sternocleidomastoid muscle at the junction of the middle and lower thirds of the posterior margin (eg, just above the point where the external jugular vein crosses this muscle). Direct the needle toward the suprasternal notch (Figure 6C).

Follow steps 4 through 6 of "Femoral Venous Catheterization" to complete the procedure.

External Jugular Vein Catheterization

The external jugular vein provides another portal to the central venous circulation. Although this vein is an excellent site for venous access, it can be difficult to thread a guidewire or catheter into the central circulation because the angle of entry into the subclavian vein is acute.

1. Restrain the child in a 30° head-down (Trendelenburg) position with the head turned away from the side to be punctured (Figure 5). Auscultate and document bilateral breath sounds before you start the procedure. The right side is preferable.

2. Using sterile technique, puncture the skin slightly distal to or beside the visible external jugular vein with a 16- or 18-gauge needle. This puncture will facilitate entry of the catheter through the skin.

3. Use the tip of the middle (3rd) finger of your nondominant hand to temporarily occlude the vein just above the clavicle, mimicking the effect of a tourniquet.

4. Stretch the skin over the vein just below the angle of the mandible. Allow the vein to distend fully and then use the thumb of the nondominant hand to immobilize the vein.

5. For *peripheral* cannulation, insert a short over-the-needle catheter into the vein and proceed as described for peripheral venous cannulation. For *central* venous access, insert a guidewire through the over-the-needle catheter, remove the short catheter, and insert a longer catheter-over-guidewire device

as described for cannulation of the internal jugular vein.

Note: Follow steps 4 through 6 for "Femoral Venous Catheterization" (above) to complete catheterization of the external jugular vein. Auscultate and document breath sounds. If you attempted central venous catheterization, verify on a chest x-ray that the tip of the catheter is correctly positioned at or above the junction of the superior vena cava and right atrium; rule out pneumothorax and hemothorax.

Subclavian Vein Cannulation

1. If no cervical spine injury is present, hyperextend the patient's neck and open the costoclavicular angles by placing a rolled towel directly beneath and parallel with the thoracic spine.

2. Restrain the child in a 30° head-down (Trendelenburg) position with the head turned away from the side to be punctured. Auscultate and document bilateral breath sounds before you start the procedure. The right side is preferable.

3. Identify the junction of the middle and medial thirds of the clavicle.

4. Use a long (1- to 1.5-inch) 25-gauge needle to administer local anesthetic. You may also use this needle to help locate the subclavian vein (see step 6).

5. Flush the needle, catheter, and syringe with sterile saline.

6. Using sterile technique, introduce a thin-walled needle just under the clavicle at the junction of the middle and medial thirds of the clavicle. Slowly advance the needle while applying gentle negative pressure with an attached syringe; direct the needle toward a fingertip placed in the suprasternal notch. The syringe and needle should be parallel with the frontal plane, directed medially and slightly cephalad, beneath the clavicle toward the posterior aspect of the sternal end of the clavicle (ie, the lower end of the fingertip in the sternal notch) (Figure 7). Once you obtain a free flow of blood, indicated by backflash into the syringe,

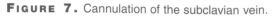

FIGURE 7. Cannulation of the subclavian vein.

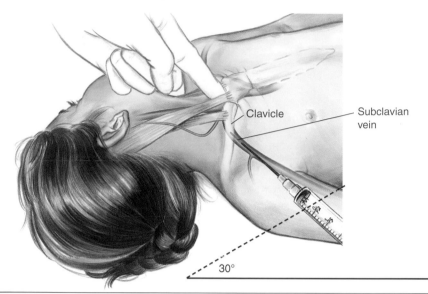

Clavicle

Subclavian vein

30°

rotate the bevel to a caudad position. This position will facilitate placement of the catheter or guidewire into the superior vena cava. Carefully disconnect the syringe while stabilizing the position of the needle. Place a finger over the hub of the needle to prevent entrainment and embolism of air.

7. During a positive-pressure breath or spontaneous exhalation, insert a guidewire through the needle. Advance the guidewire into the right atrium. Entrance of the guidewire into the right atrium often produces premature atrial contractions. If atrial or ventricular arrhythmias occur, withdraw the guidewire a few centimeters. Complete cannulation of the vein using the Seldinger technique.

8. Demonstrate free blood return from all ports of the catheter and, subsequently, free flow of infusate. If blood does not immediately flow back freely, the catheter may be lodged against a vessel wall or the wall of the right atrium. Slightly withdraw the catheter and repeat aspiration. (You may perform this withdrawal/aspiration sequence twice.) If you still do not observe blood return, you must assume that the catheter is not in the vessel and remove the catheter.

9. Once you document free blood return and free flow of infusate, secure the catheter or catheter-introducing sheath in place with suture material. Apply a sterile, occlusive dressing.

10. Auscultate and document bilateral breath sounds.

11. Obtain a chest x-ray to verify that the tip of the catheter is correctly positioned at or above the junction of the superior vena cava and right atrium; rule out pneumothorax and hemothorax.

Saphenous Vein Cutdown

If peripheral venous, central venous, and intraosseous cannulation are unsuccessful, providers may attempt a venous cutdown to gain vascular access.

Site

The long saphenous vein that courses anterior to the medial malleolus at the ankle is the preferred site for cutdown.

Technique

1. Identify a proposed incision site perpendicular to the long axis of the tibia. Choose a site one finger's breadth (approximately 2 cm) superior and anterior to the medial malleolus in children. In infants choose a site one half finger's breadth (approximately 1 cm) anterior and superior to the medial malleolus.

2. Apply a tourniquet proximal to the proposed incision site.

3. Using sterile technique, infiltrate the skin with 1% lidocaine (if the child responds to pain). Make an incision through the skin perpendicular to the long axis of the tibia. Carefully dissect the subcutaneous tissue with the tips of a small, curved hemostat to expose the superficial fascia.

4. Pierce the superficial fascia with the tips of the hemostat and spread it gently, parallel with the long axis of the tibia. Pass the hemostat to the bone with the tips down. Twist the tips under the presumed area of the vessel and raise the hemostat from the incision site with the tips up. You should lift the saphenous vein with the hemostat. Alternatively, you may dissect the adjacent tissues with the tips of the hemostat to identify the saphenous vein before it is elevated.

5. After you isolate the vein, place a ligature or tie around the distal end of the vein and anchor the vein in place. Place a second ligature or tie around the proximal end of the vein, but leave it untied.

6. Make an anterior venostomy through the vein. Insert a No. 11 scalpel blade perpendicular to the long axis of the vessel into the upper (most superficial) third of the vessel. Thread a catheter into the proximal limb of the vein through the venostomy site. Tie the proximal ligature around the vein and catheter to hold the catheter in place. Tie the distal ligature around the vein. Alternatively, catheterize the exposed vein under direct visualization using an over-the-needle catheter. With this technique it is often helpful to point the bevel of the needle down so that the tip is less likely to penetrate the posterior wall of the vein.

Figure 8. Radial artery. **A,** Anatomy. **B,** Cannulation.

A

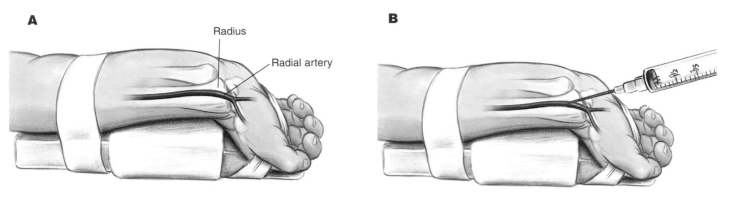

Radius

Radial artery

B

7. Remove the tourniquet. Evacuate any air remaining in the connecting tubing and attach an infusion set. Suture the incision site and apply a sterile, occlusive dressing.

Arterial Access

Site

Arterial catheters can be placed percutaneously in the radial, axillary, femoral, dorsalis pedis, and posterior tibial arteries.[3,103] The radial and femoral arteries are the preferred sites. Do not cannulate a temporal artery: severe cerebral thromboembolic complications may occur, presumably as a result of embolization of air or other material into the internal carotid circulation.[104,105]

Technique

This section describes the technique for cannulation of the radial artery[106-108] (Figure 8). A similar technique is used for cannulation of other arteries.

Location of the Radial Artery

You may use a Doppler flow probe to locate the radial artery and confirm catheter placement.[109] For small infants you may place a fiberoptic light source under the wrist to locate the radial artery (or under the foot to locate the dorsalis pedis artery).

Cannulation of the Radial Artery

You may use the following procedure to cannulate the radial artery:

1. Dorsiflex the hand at the wrist 45° to 60° and secure both the hand and lower forearm to a board. Place a roll of gauze behind the wrist to maintain dorsiflexion. Tape down the hand, leaving all fingers exposed so that perfusion of the hand can be assessed (Figure 8). Temporarily tape the thumb aside to prevent movement during attempts at arterial cannulation.

2. Locate the radial pulse just proximal to the head of the radius.

3. Anesthetize the skin with 1% lidocaine (if the child responds to pain).

4. Using sterile technique, puncture the skin at the site of maximal pulsation with a 20-gauge needle. Advance a 20- to 24-gauge, heparin-flushed catheter at a 30° angle until blood appears in the hub. Three techniques of arterial cannulation are frequently used:

   — Pass the catheter and needle through the artery to transfix it. Withdraw the needle and then withdraw the catheter very slowly until there is a free flow of blood. Slowly advance the catheter into the lumen of the artery.

   — Using a catheter-over-needle device, puncture only the anterior wall of the artery (ie, slowly advance the needle until blood appears). Carefully lower the needle to a 10° angle. Ascertain that blood flow is continuing and slowly advance

the catheter over the needle into the lumen of the artery. The catheter should advance with little resistance, and blood return should be brisk.

   — Insert a catheter using the Seldinger (guidewire) technique.

5. Once you advance the catheter into the artery, attach the catheter to a T-connector to permit continuous infusion of saline (you may use heparinized saline 1 to 5 U/mL).

6. Apply antibiotic ointment, an occlusive dressing, and adhesive tape to the puncture site.

Remove the catheter immediately if any evidence of tissue ischemia develops. Immediately consult a microvascular surgeon if evidence of ischemia continues after you remove the catheter.[110,111]

Summary Points

Vascular access is a critical component of pediatric advanced life support. Base your priorities and site of vascular access on the patient's clinical status. For CPR and treatment of decompensated shock, the highest priority is prompt availability.

■ Intravascular or intraosseous access is the preferred route for medication and drug delivery in cardiopulmonary emergencies.

■ Immediate intraosseous access is recommended in cases of decompensated shock and cardiopulmonary arrest, particularly if the provider lacks experience in pediatric central venous access techniques.

■ Central venous catheterization can be used in children in emergencies, but it requires significant expertise. Many complications and delays may occur even in expert hands.

Case Scenario

Note: Vascular access is a technique that requires a small amount of cognitive information. This information is reviewed in "Summary Points," the discussion of the introductory case scenario (below), and "Review Questions." If your clinical responsibilities include establishing vascular access in seriously ill or injured children, you should develop experience and expertise in the prerequisite *psychomotor* skills. This chapter does not contain case scenarios beyond the introductory scenario. Indications for and approach to vascular access are included in Chapter 7, "Case Scenarios in the Management of Shock."

Introductory Case Scenario

A 2-month-old girl arrives at the Emergency Department in cardiac arrest. Other providers promptly begin ventilation and perform chest compressions. You need to establish vascular access to administer fluids and medications.

Review Questions and Answers

■ *What is the optimal site for immediate vascular access for this infant?*

The optimal site for immediate vascular access for this infant is the site that will enable prompt administration of medications and fluids. You may attempt central venous access or peripheral venous access. But if you are not immediately successful, you should establish intraosseous access.

■ *If resuscitative efforts are successful, what is the optimal site for vascular access during the postresuscitation period?*

Central venous access would be appropriate during postresuscitation stabilization for this infant. If no one with expertise in establishing central venous access is available, peripheral venous access is acceptable.

Review Questions

1. A 3-year-old child presents in cardiopulmonary arrest after being found in a bathtub. CPR is provided. An intraosseous needle and tracheal tube are in place, and you have confirmed tracheal tube position. What is the preferred route for administration of epinephrine for this child?

    a. tracheal tube

    b. subclavian catheter

    c. intramuscular injection

    d. intraosseous access

    The correct answer is d. Intraosseous or intravenous access is the preferred route for administration of medication during resuscitation. Medication administered by the IO or IV route will produce drug delivery times and drug levels equivalent to those achieved by central venous administration.

    Answer a is incorrect because drug absorption is less predictable after tracheal administration than after IV or IO administration. If IV or IO access has not been established, you may use the tracheal route.

    Answer b is incorrect because insertion of a subclavian catheter at this time would introduce unjustifiable risk. You would also need to stop chest compressions to insert this catheter.

    Answer c is incorrect because intramuscular absorption is unreliable during states of profound shock and cardiac arrest.

2. Which of the following, *if present*, is a reliable and practical indicator of successful placement of an intraosseous needle?

    a. aspiration of bone marrow

    b. insertion of the needle until the hub meets the skin

    c. ability to draw an arterial blood gas sample through the IO needle

    d. demonstration of the needle in the bone on an x-ray

    The correct answer is a. Aspiration of bone marrow is the most reliable and practical indicator of these choices, although it is not always observed. Other reliable indicators are a sudden decrease in resistance as the needle passes through the bony cortex into the marrow cavity, the observation that the needle remains upright without support, and free infusion of fluid with no evidence of subcutaneous infiltration (such as swelling or induration of the tissues surrounding the bone).

    Answer b is incorrect because in most patients the needle should not be inserted to the hub. Some length of the needle will remain outside the skin.

    Answer c is incorrect because IO cannulation accesses a venous plexus. Although you may be able to aspirate blood, the blood would not be an arterial sample.

    Answer d is incorrect because x-rays are neither needed nor practical to confirm placement during emergencies.

3. Which of the following is a potential complication of femoral venous catheterization?

    a. pneumothorax

    b. deep venous thrombosis

    c. hemothorax

    d. aneurysm formation

    The correct answer is b. Deep venous thrombosis may develop after catheterization of any central vein, including the femoral vein.

    Answers a and **c** are incorrect because pneumothorax and hemothorax are potential complications of subclavian or internal jugular catheterization. These complications should not occur when you place a short catheter into the femoral vein.

    Answer d is incorrect because aneurysm formation is a potential complication of arterial, not venous, puncture.

References

1. Rosetti VA, Thompson BM, Aprahamian C, Darin JC, Mateer JR. Difficulty and delay in intravascular access in pediatric arrests [abstract]. *Ann Emerg Med*. 1984;13:406.

2. Carcillo JA, Davis AL, Zaritsky A. Role of early fluid resuscitation in pediatric septic shock. *JAMA*. 1991;266:1242-1245.

3. Stovroff M, Teague WG. Intravenous access in infants and children. *Pediatr Clin North Am*. 1998;45:1373-1393.

4. Lillis KA, Jaffe DM. Prehospital intravenous access in children. *Ann Emerg Med*. 1992; 21:1430-1434.

5. Glaeser PW, Losek JD, Nelson DB, Bonadio WA, Smith DS, Walsh-Kelly C, Hennes H. Pediatric intraosseous infusions: impact on vascular access time. *Am J Emerg Med*. 1988;6:330-332.

6. Redding JS, Asuncion JS, Pearson JW. Effective routes of drug administration during cardiac arrest. *Anesth Analg*. 1967;46: 253-258.

7. Davison R, Barresi V, Parker M, Meyers SN, Talano JV. Intracardiac injections during cardiopulmonary resuscitation: a low-risk procedure. *JAMA*. 1980;244:1110-1111.

8. Pun KK. Cardiac tamponade after intracardiac injection. *Anaesth Intensive Care*. 1984;12:66-67.

9. Vijay NK, Schoonmaker FW. Cardiopulmonary arrest and resuscitation. *Am Fam Physician*. 1975;12:85-90.

10. Kanter RK, Zimmerman JJ, Strauss RH, Stoeckel KA. Pediatric emergency intravenous access: evaluation of a protocol. *Am J Dis Child*. 1986;140:132-134.

11. Fiser DH. Intraosseous infusion. *N Engl J Med*. 1990;322:1579-1581.

12. Banerjee S, Singhi SC, Singh S, Singh M. The intraosseous route is a suitable alternative to intravenous route for fluid resuscitation in severely dehydrated children. *Indian Pediatr*. 1994;31:1511-1520.

13. Glaeser PW, Hellmich TR, Szewczuga D, Losek JD, Smith DS. Five-year experience in prehospital intraosseous infusions in children and adults. *Ann Emerg Med*. 1993;22:1119-1124.

14. Johnston C. Endotracheal drug delivery. *Pediatr Emerg Care*. 1992;8:94-97.

15. Miner WF, Corneli HM, Bolte RG, Lehnhof D, Clawson JJ. Prehospital use of intraosseous infusion by paramedics. *Pediatr Emerg Care*. 1989;5:5-7.

16. Daga SR, Gosavi DV, Verma B. Intraosseous access using butterfly needle. *Trop Doct*. 1999;29:142-144.

17. Waisman M, Waisman D. Bone marrow infusion in adults. *J Trauma*. 1997;42:288-293.

18. Guy J, Haley K, Zuspan SJ. Use of intraosseous infusion in the pediatric trauma patient. *J Pediatr Surg*. 1993;28:158-161.

19. Anderson TE, Arthur K, Kleinman M, Drawbaugh R, Eitel DR, Ogden CS, Baker D. Intraosseous infusion: success of a standardized regional training program for prehospital advanced life support providers. *Ann Emerg Med*. 1994;23:52-55.

20. Berg RA. Emergency infusion of catecholamines into bone marrow. *Am J Dis Child*. 1984;138:810-811.

21. Heinild S, Sodergaard T, Tudvad F. Bone marrow infusions in childhood: experiences from 1000 infusions. *J Pediatr*. 1947;30: 400-412.

22. Meola F. Bone marrow infusions as a routine procedure in children. *J Pediatr*. 1944;25: 13-16.

23. Andropoulos DB, Soifer SJ, Schreiber MD. Plasma epinephrine concentrations after intraosseous and central venous injection during cardiopulmonary resuscitation in the lamb. *J Pediatr*. 1990;116:312-315.

24. Ellemunter H, Simma B, Trawoger R, Maurer H. Intraosseous lines in preterm and full term neonates. *Arch Dis Child Fetal Neonatal Ed*. 1999;80:F74-F75.

25. Goldstein B, Doody D, Briggs S. Emergency intraosseous infusion in severely burned children. *Pediatr Emerg Care*. 1990;6:195-197.

26. Macgregor DF, Macnab AJ. Intraosseous fluids in emergencies [letter]. *Pediatrics*. 1990;85:386-387.

27. Macnab A, Christenson J, Findlay J, Horwood B, Johnson D, Jones L, Phillips K, Pollack C, Jr, Robinson DJ, Rumball C, Stair T, Tiffany B, Whelan M. A new system for sternal intraosseous infusion in adults. *Prehosp Emerg Care*. 2000;4:173-177.

28. Calkins MD, Fitzgerald G, Bentley TB, Burris D. Intraosseous infusion devices: a comparison for potential use in special operations. *J Trauma*. 2000;48:1068-1074.

29. Orlowski JP, Porembka DT, Gallagher JM, Lockrem JD, VanLente F. Comparison study of intraosseous, central intravenous, and peripheral intravenous infusions of emergency drugs. *Am J Dis Child*. 1990;144: 112-117.

30. Warren DW, Kissoon N, Sommerauer JF, Rieder MJ. Comparison of fluid infusion rates among peripheral intravenous and humerus, femur, malleolus, and tibial intraosseous sites in normovolemic and hypovolemic piglets. *Ann Emerg Med*. 1993;22:183-186.

31. Plewa MC, King RW, Fenn-Buderer N, Gretzinger K, Renuart D, Cruz R. Hematologic safety of intraosseous blood transfusion in a swine model of pediatric hemorrhagic hypovolemia. *Acad Emerg Med*. 1995;2:799-809.

32. Johnson L, Kissoon N, Fiallos M, Abdelmoneim T, Murphy S. Use of intraosseous blood to assess blood chemistries and hemoglobin during cardiopulmonary resuscitation with drug infusions. *Crit Care Med*. 1999;27: 1147-1152.

33. Abdelmoneim T, Kissoon N, Johnson L, Fiallos M, Murphy S. Acid-base status of blood from intraosseous and mixed venous sites during prolonged cardiopulmonary resuscitation and drug infusions. *Crit Care Med*. 1999;27:1923-1928.

34. Rosetti VA, Thompson BM, Miller J, Mateer JR, Aprahamian C. Intraosseous infusion: an alternative route of pediatric intravascular access. *Ann Emerg Med*. 1985;14:885-888.

35. Katz DS, Wojtowycz AR. Tibial fracture: a complication of intraosseous infusion. *Am J Emerg Med*. 1994;12:258-259.

36. La Fleche FR, Slepin MJ, Vargas J, Milzman DP. Iatrogenic bilateral tibial fractures after intraosseous infusion attempts in a 3-month-old infant. *Ann Emerg Med*. 1989;18:1099-1101.

37. Vidal R, Kissoon N, Gayle M. Compartment syndrome following intraosseous infusion. *Pediatrics*. 1993;91:1201-1202.

38. Moscati R, Moore GP. Compartment syndrome with resultant amputation following intraosseous infusion [letter]. *Am J Emerg Med*. 1990;8:470-471.

39. Galpin RD, Kronick JB, Willis RB, Frewen TC. Bilateral lower extremity compartment syndromes secondary to intraosseous fluid resuscitation. *J Pediatr Orthop*. 1991;11: 773-776.

40. Simmons CM, Johnson NE, Perkin RM, van Stralen D. Intraosseous extravasation complication reports. *Ann Emerg Med*. 1994;23: 363-366.

41. Rosovsky M, FitzPatrick M, Goldfarb CR, Finestone H. Bilateral osteomyelitis due to intraosseous infusion: case report and review of the English-language literature. *Pediatr Radiol*. 1994;24:72-73.

42. Pollack CVJ, Pender ES, Woodall BN, Tubbs RC, Iyer RV, Miller HW. Long-term local effects of intraosseous infusion on tibial bone marrow in the weanling pig model. *Am J Emerg Med*. 1992;10:27-31.

43. Dedrick DK, Mase C, Ranger W, Burney RE. The effects of intraosseous infusion on the growth plate in a nestling rabbit model. *Ann Emerg Med*. 1992;21:494-497.

44. Brickman KR, Rega P, Schoolfield L, Harkins K, Weisbrode SE, Reynolds G. Investigation of bone developmental and histopathologic changes from intraosseous infusion. *Ann Emerg Med.* 1996;28:430-435.

45. Fiser RT, Walker WM, Seibert JJ, McCarthy R, Fiser DH. Tibial length following intraosseous infusion: a prospective, radiographic analysis. *Pediatr Emerg Care.* 1997;13:186-188.

46. Orlowski JP, Julius CJ, Petras RE, Porembka DT, Gallagher JM. The safety of intraosseous infusions: risks of fat and bone marrow emboli to the lungs. *Ann Emerg Med.* 1989;18:1062-1067.

47. Fiallos M, Kissoon N, Abdelmoneim T, Johnson L, Murphy S, Lu L, Masood S, Idris A. Fat embolism with the use of intraosseous infusion during cardiopulmonary resuscitation. *Am J Med Sci.* 1997;314:73-79.

48. Wagner MB, McCabe JB. A comparison of four techniques to establish intraosseous infusion. *Pediatr Emerg Care.* 1988;4:87-91.

49. Glaeser PW, Losek JD. Intraosseous needles: new and improved. *Pediatr Emerg Care.* 1988;4:135-136.

50. Halm B, Yamamoto LG. Comparing ease of intraosseous needle placement: Jamshidi versus Cook. *Am J Emerg Med.* 1998;16:420-421.

51. Hedges JR, Barsan WB, Doan LA, Joyce SM, Lukes SJ, Dalsey WC, Nishiyama H. Central versus peripheral intravenous routes in cardiopulmonary resuscitation. *Am J Emerg Med.* 1984;2:385-390.

52. Kuhn GJ, White BC, Swetnam RE, Mumey JF, Rydesky MF, Tintinalli JE, Krome RL, Hoehner PJ. Peripheral vs central circulation times during CPR: a pilot study. *Ann Emerg Med.* 1981;10:417-419.

53. Emerman CL, Pinchak AC, Hancock D, Hagen JF. Effect of injection site on circulation times during cardiac arrest. *Crit Care Med.* 1988;16:1138-1141.

54. Fleisher G, Caputo G, Baskin M. Comparison of external jugular and peripheral venous administration of sodium bicarbonate in puppies. *Crit Care Med.* 1989;17:251-254.

55. Lloyd TR, Donnerstein RL, Berg RA. Accuracy of central venous pressure measurement from the abdominal inferior vena cava. *Pediatrics.* 1992;89:506-508.

56. Berg RA, Lloyd TR, Donnerstein RL. Accuracy of central venous pressure monitoring in the intraabdominal inferior vena cava: a canine study. *J Pediatr.* 1992;120:67-71.

57. Wellmann KF, Reinhard A, Salazar EP. Polyethylene catheter embolism. Review of the literature and report of a case with associated fatal tricuspid and systemic candidiasis. *Circulation.* 1968;37:380-392.

58. Grabenwoeger F, Bardach G, Dock W, Pinterits F. Percutaneous extraction of centrally embolized foreign bodies: a report of 16 cases. *Br J Radiol.* 1988;61:1014-1018.

59. Nicolson SC, Sweeney MF, Moore RA, Jobes DR. Comparison of internal and external jugular cannulation of the central circulation in the pediatric patient. *Crit Care Med.* 1985;13:747-749.

60. Cobb LM, Vinocur CD, Wagner CW, Weintraub WH. The central venous anatomy in infants. *Surg Gynecol Obstet.* 1987;165:230-234.

61. Stenzel JP, Green TP, Fuhrman BP, Carlson PE, Marchessault RP. Percutaneous central venous catheterization in a pediatric intensive care unit: a survival analysis of complications. *Crit Care Med.* 1989;17:984-988.

62. Filston HC, Johnson DG. Percutaneous venous cannulation in neonates and infants: a method for catheter insertion without "cutdown." *Pediatrics.* 1971;48:896-901.

63. Newman BM, Jewett TC Jr, Karp MP, Cooney DR. Percutaneous central venous catheterization in children: first line choice for venous access. *J Pediatr Surg.* 1986;21:685-688.

64. Iserson KV, Criss EA. Pediatric venous cutdowns: utility in emergency situations. *Pediatr Emerg Care.* 1986;2:231-234.

65. Maki DG, Ringer M. Evaluation of dressing regimens for prevention of infection with peripheral intravenous catheters. Gauze, a transparent polyurethane dressing, and an iodophor-transparent dressing. *JAMA.* 1987;258:2396-2403.

66. Seldinger SI. Catheter replacement of the needle in percutaneous arteriography: a new technique. *Acta Radiol.* 1953;39:368-376.

67. Puntis JW, Holden CE, Smallman S, Finkel Y, George RH, Booth IW. Staff training: a key factor in reducing intravascular catheter sepsis. *Arch Dis Child.* 1991;66:335-337.

68. Saladino R, Bachman D, Fleisher G. Arterial access in the pediatric emergency department. *Ann Emerg Med.* 1990;19:382-385.

69. Hack WW, Vos A, Okken A. Incidence of forearm and hand ischaemia related to radial artery cannulation in newborn infants. *Intensive Care Med.* 1990;16:50-53.

70. Guy RL, Holland JP, Shaw DG, Fixsen JA. Limb shortening secondary to complications of vascular cannulae in the neonatal period. *Skeletal Radiol.* 1990;19:423-425.

71. Miyasaka K, Edmonds JF, Conn AW. Complications of radial artery lines in the paediatric patient. *Can Anaesth Soc J.* 1976;23:9-14.

72. Allen EV. Thromboangiitis obliterans: methods of diagnosis of chronic occlusive arterial lesions distal to the wrist with illustrative cases. *Am J Med Sci.* 1929;178:237-239.

73. Mozersky DJ, Buckley CJ, Hagood CO Jr, Capps WF Jr, Dannemiller FJ Jr. Ultrasonic evaluation of the palmar circulation: a useful adjunct to radial artery cannulation. *Am J Surg.* 1973;126:810-812.

74. Kamienski RW, Barnes RW. Critique of the Allen test for continuity of the palmar arch assessed by doppler ultrasound. *Surg Gynecol Obstet.* 1976;142:861-864.

75. Little JM, Zylstra PL, West J, May J. Circulatory patterns in the normal hand. *Br J Surg.* 1973;60:652-655.

76. Sellden H, Nilsson K, Larsson LE, Ekstrom-Jodal B. Radial arterial catheters in children and neonates: a prospective study. *Crit Care Med.* 1987;15:1106-1109.

77. Butt W, Shann F, McDonnell G, Hudson I. Effect of heparin concentration and infusion rate on the patency of arterial catheters. *Crit Care Med.* 1987;15:230-232.

78. Hack WW, Vos A, van der Lei J, Okken A. Incidence and duration of total occlusion of the radial artery in newborn infants after catheter removal. *Eur J Pediatr.* 1990;149:275-277.

79. Heulitt MJ, Farrington EA, O'Shea TM, Stoltzman SM, Srubar NB, Levin DL. Double-blind, randomized, controlled trial of papaverine-containing infusions to prevent failure of arterial catheters in pediatric patients. *Crit Care Med.* 1993;21:825-829.

80. Legler D, Nugent M. Doppler localization of the internal jugular vein facilitates central venous cannulation. *Anesthesiology.* 1984;60:481-482.

81. Bratton SL, Ramamoorthy C, Eck JB, Sorensen GK. Teaching successful central venous cannulation in infants and children: audio Doppler versus anatomic landmarks. *J Cardiothorac Vasc Anesth.* 1998;12:523-526.

82. Mallory DL, McGee WT, Shawker TH, Brenner M, Bailey KR, Evans RG, Parker MM, Farmer JC, Parillo JE. Ultrasound guidance improves the success rate of internal jugular vein cannulation. A prospective, randomized trial. *Chest.* 1990;98:157-160.

83. Denys BG, Uretsky BF. Anatomical variations of internal jugular vein location: impact on central venous access. *Crit Care Med.* 1991;19:1516-1519.

84. Denys BG, Uretsky BF, Reddy PS. Ultrasound-assisted cannulation of the internal jugular vein. A prospective comparison to the external landmark-guided technique. *Circulation.* 1993;87:1557-1562.

85. Alderson PJ, Burrows FA, Stemp LI, Holtby HM. Use of ultrasound to evaluate internal jugular vein anatomy and to facilitate central venous cannulation in paediatric patients. *Br J Anaesth*. 1993;70:145-148.

86. Stenzel JP, Green TP, Fuhrman BP, Carlson PE, Marchessault RP. Percutaneous femoral venous catheterizations: a prospective study of complications. *J Pediatr*. 1989;114:411-415.

87. Kanter RK, Gorton JM, Palmieri K, Tompkins JM, Smith F. Anatomy of femoral vessels in infants and guidelines for venous catheterization. *Pediatrics*. 1989;83:1020-1022.

88. Kanter RK, Zimmerman JJ, Strauss RH, Stoeckel KA. Central venous catheter insertion by femoral vein: safety and effectiveness for the pediatric patient. *Pediatrics*. 1986;77:842-847.

89. Lavandosky G, Gomez R, Montes J. Potentially lethal misplacement of femoral central venous catheters. *Crit Care Med*. 1996;24:893-896.

90. Taylor EA, Mowbray MJ, McLellan I. Central venous access in children via the external jugular vein. *Anaesthesia*. 1992;47:265-266.

91. Defalque RJ. Percutaneous catheterization of the internal jugular vein. *Anesth Analg*. 1974;53:116-121.

92. Rao TL, Wong AY, Salem MR. A new approach to percutaneous catheterization of the internal jugular vein. *Anesthesiology*. 1977;46:362-364.

93. Coté CJ, Jobes DR, Schwartz AJ, Ellison N. Two approaches to cannulation of a child's internal jugular vein. *Anesthesiology*. 1979;50:371-373.

94. Prince SR, Sullivan RL, Hackel A. Percutaneous catheterization of the internal jugular vein in infants and children. *Anesthesiology*. 1976;44:170-174.

95. Hall DM, Geefhuysen J. Percutaneous catheterization of the internal jugular vein in infants and children. *J Pediatr Surg*. 1977;12:719-722.

96. Krausz MM, Berlatzky Y, Ayalon A, Freund H, Schiller M. Percutaneous cannulation of the internal jugular vein in infants and children. *Surg Gynecol Obstet*. 1979;148:591-594.

97. Filston HC, Grant JP. A safer system for percutaneous subclavian venous catheterization in newborn infants. *J Pediatr Surg*. 1979;14:564-570.

98. Eichelberger MR, Rous PG, Hoelzer DJ, Garcia VF, Koop CE. Percutaneous subclavian venous catheters in neonates and children. *J Pediatr Surg*. 1981;16(suppl 1):547-553.

99. Venkataraman ST, Orr RA, Thompson AE. Percutaneous infraclavicular subclavian vein catheterization in critically ill infants and children. *J Pediatr*. 1988;113:480-485.

100. Groff DB, Ahmed N. Subclavian vein catheterization in the infant. *J Pediatr Surg*. 1974;9:171-174.

101. Niemann JT, Rosborough JP, Ung S, Criley JM. Hemodynamic effects of continuous abdominal binding during cardiac arrest and resuscitation. *Am J Cardiol*. 1984;53:269-274.

102. Sulek CA, Gravenstein N, Blackshear RH, Weiss L. Head rotation during internal jugular vein cannulation and the risk of carotid artery puncture. *Anesth Analg*. 1996;82:125-128.

103. Greenwald BM, Notterman DA, DeBruin WJ, McCready M. Percutaneous axillary artery catheterization in critically ill infants and children. *J Pediatr*. 1990;117:442-444.

104. Simmons MA, Levine RL, Lubchenco LO, Guggenheim MA. Warning: serious sequelae of temporal artery catheterization. *J Pediatr*. 1978;92:284.

105. Prian GW. Complications and sequelae of temporal artery catheterization in the high-risk newborn. *J Pediatr Surg*. 1977;12:829-835.

106. Todres ID, Rogers MC, Shannon DC, Moylan FM, Ryan JF. Percutaneous catheterization of the radial artery in the critically ill neonate. *J Pediatr*. 1975;87:273-275.

107. Cole FS, Todres ID, Shannon DC. Technique for percutaneous cannulation of the radial artery in the newborn infant. *J Pediatr*. 1978;92:105-107.

108. Randel SN, Tsang BH, Wung JT, Driscoll JMJ, James LS. Experience with percutaneous indwelling peripheral arterial catheterization in neonates. *Am J Dis Child*. 1987;141:848-851.

109. Morray JP, Brandford HG, Barnes LF, Oh SM, Furman EB. Doppler-assisted radial artery cannulation in infants and children. *Anesth Analg*. 1984;63:346-348.

110. LaQuaglia MP, Upton J, May JWJ. Microvascular reconstruction of major arteries in neonates and small children. *J Pediatr Surg*. 1991;26:1136-1140.

111. Chaikof EL, Dodson TF, Salam AA, Lumsden AB, Smith RB. Acute arterial thrombosis in the very young. *J Vasc Surg*. 1992;16:428-435.

Case Scenarios in Shock

Learning Objectives

After completing this chapter the PALS provider should be able to

- Describe the clinical signs of shock in infants and children

- Describe the clinical classification of shock

- Differentiate between decompensated and compensated shock

- Discuss the clinical signs of hypovolemic, cardiogenic, and distributive (septic) shock in infants and children

- Describe the initial management of hypovolemic, cardiogenic, and distributive (septic) shock in infants and children

Introduction

This chapter differs significantly from other chapters in this book in that it presents in-depth case scenarios to allow you to apply what you have learned. The scenarios emphasize important aspects of assessment and management of pediatric shock. They also provide opportunities to integrate additional components of pediatric advanced life support, including rapid cardiopulmonary assessment, assessment and support of respiratory function, and decisions about establishment of vascular access. The explanations for acceptable actions in these scenarios are more comprehensive than the explanations in many chapters. These comprehensive explanations reinforce core PALS course content.

After you read each case scenario, think about the case in the same way you would think through the evaluation case scenario in the PALS course. The following sequence may be helpful:

1. Perform an initial rapid cardiopulmonary assessment, identify impending respiratory failure or shock, and classify the patient's physiological status into 1 of 5 categories:

   - Stable
   - Respiratory distress
   - Potential or actual respiratory failure
   - Shock (compensated or decompensated; etiologic classification of shock)
   - Cardiopulmonary failure

2. Plan treatment, including specific interventions recommended by algorithms, guidelines, or drug therapy tables. Identify the monitors you would use in your scope of practice. Identify the critical errors to avoid (eg, failing to treat symptomatic bradycardia with oxygen and to ensure adequate ventilation; placing a chest tube for decreased breath sounds on the left after tracheal intubation without checking for intubation of the right main bronchus).

3. Evaluate your performance by reading the acceptable actions, the rationale for those actions, and the unacceptable actions.

4. If you missed critical steps, review the appropriate sections in Chapters 1 through 6.

Case Scenario 1

A 3-month-old girl arrives in the Emergency Department. Her parents say that the infant has had "nearly continuous vomiting and diarrhea" during the previous 8 hours. Her parents are uncertain if she has urinated during this time because her diapers have been filled with watery diarrhea. The infant became ill yesterday with occasional episodes of vomiting and diarrhea. These symptoms are worse today. On examination the infant appears listless with little response to verbal or painful stimulation. She is breathing without retractions or respiratory distress. Her heart rate is 210 bpm, respiratory rate is 50 breaths/min, blood pressure is 54/38 mm Hg, and axillary temperature is 97°F (36.1°C). You palpate weak brachial and femoral pulses, but you cannot palpate distal pulses. Extremities are cool and mottled below the elbows and knees, and capillary refill time in the foot is >8 seconds. Auscultation reveals clear lungs with good distal air entry.

Acceptable Actions

The following actions are generally acceptable for assessment and management of this infant with shock:

- Use universal precautions.

- Perform rapid cardiopulmonary assessment; identify decompensated hypovolemic shock.

- Administer oxygen, initiate cardiorespiratory monitoring, and keep the infant warm; attach a pulse oximeter if available.

- Quickly establish vascular access with vascular or intraosseous (IO) cannulation.

- Administer isotonic fluid as rapidly as possible (5 to 10 minutes) in boluses of 20 mL/kg.

- Reassess the patient after each fluid bolus; give additional boluses as indicated by assessment of systemic perfusion.

- Conduct a bedside glucose test to rule out hypoglycemia as a cause of shock or as a contributing factor to poor clinical status.

- Obtain laboratory studies.

Rationale for Acceptable Actions

Perform rapid cardiopulmonary assessment; identify decompensated shock.

Initial cardiopulmonary assessment includes evaluation of **A**irway and **B**reathing. These functions are adequate on initial examination, but the infant is tachypneic. Evaluation of **C**irculation consists of both direct and indirect cardiovascular assessments (see Critical Concepts: "Cardiovascular Assessment for Shock"). For the indirect assessment, you will evaluate end-organ function to assess end-organ perfusion. Throughout the initial assessment, evaluate the infant's **general appearance** and responsiveness and look for changes in response to therapy.

Shock is a clinical condition in which tissue perfusion is inadequate to meet metabolic demands. Although shock often occurs with low cardiac output, patients with sepsis may have normal or increased cardiac output. In any form of shock, cardiac output and organ perfusion are *inadequate relative to metabolic needs*. In this scenario, the

Critical Concepts:
Cardiovascular Assessment for Shock

- *Direct* cardiovascular assessment:
  — Heart rate
  — Pulses (proximal and distal), noting quality
  — Blood pressure, noting pulse pressure
- *Indirect* cardiovascular assessment (evaluation of end-organ perfusion):
  — Brain: alertness, responsiveness
  — Skin: color, temperature, capillary refill (presuming warm ambient temperature)
  — Kidneys: urine output

infant's cardiac output is probably low because of severe hypovolemia and dehydration. When cardiac output decreases, cardiovascular compensatory mechanisms increase heart rate and vascular resistance in the peripheral circulation and splanchnic organs (kidney and gut) to maintain perfusion pressure and blood flow to the heart and brain.

The clinical manifestations of these compensatory mechanisms in this scenario include tachycardia, poor peripheral pulses, delayed capillary refill, cool extremities, narrow pulse pressure, and hypotension. These symptoms are *direct* findings consistent with shock. Tachycardia is an early and sensitive indicator of shock, but it is not *specific* to shock. There are many nonspecific causes of tachycardia, such as pain, fear, anger, and fever. If any of these nonspecific causes were responsible for the tachycardia, you would likely find bounding or at least easily palpable distal pulses. The absence of peripheral pulses in this infant is consistent with low stroke volume and increased systemic vascular resistance.

Rapid assessment of end-organ perfusion includes a brief neurologic evaluation and

assessment of skin blood flow (see Critical Concepts: "Priorities for Rapid Assessment of Circulation"). Brief neurologic evaluation by the **AVPU** approach (**A**lert, responsive to **V**oice, responsive to **P**ain, **U**nresponsive) indicates that this infant has signs of significantly altered mental status; she is **U**nresponsive. The infant's unresponsiveness could be caused by neurologic disease, injury, or infection. But in this case it is most consistent with poor cerebral perfusion due to shock.

To assess peripheral perfusion, feel the temperature of the patient's extremities, and evaluate capillary refill and skin color. Often you can identify a line of demarcation between warm and cool skin; monitor skin temperature to assess response to treatment. Normally capillary refill takes less than 2 seconds. Cool skin and prolonged capillary refill are consistent with shock. But a cold ambient temperature (as you might find in a radiology suite or outdoors) or increased sympathetic tone (due to anger, fear, or pain) can also cause these signs. This infant's cool extremities, prolonged capillary refill, and mottled skin are consistent with shock.

Decreased urine output may be caused by inadequate renal perfusion resulting from dehydration. Often the history provided

Critical Concepts:
Priorities for Rapid Assessment of Circulation

- Observe mental status, general appearance, and response to stimulation (AVPU score).

- Evaluate heart rate. Palpate central and distal pulses, noting rate and quality; feel skin temperature; evaluate capillary refill.

- Evaluate end-organ function/perfusion.

- Measure blood pressure soon.

- Measure urine output later.

by the parents about the frequency of wet diapers suggests poor urine output. But in this case scenario the parents could not differentiate watery diarrhea from urine output.

If blood pressure is normal but signs of poor perfusion are present, the child is in *compensated* shock. If hypotension is present with signs of poor perfusion, the child is in *decompensated* shock. This infant is hypotensive with a systolic blood pressure less than the 5th percentile for age (see Critical Concepts: "Identifying Hypotension in Infants and Children"). Hypotension is a *late* finding in most types of shock. Hypotension develops when physiological attempts to maintain blood pressure by increasing heart rate, cardiac contractility, and peripheral vascular tone are no longer effective. This infant's condition is life threatening.

For more information about rapid cardiopulmonary assessment, see Chapter 2.

Administer oxygen, initiate cardiorespiratory monitoring, and keep the infant warm; attach a pulse oximeter if available.

Monitor the infant's heart rate continuously; heart rate should decrease gradually as shock is treated. This infant's peripheral perfusion may be inadequate for pulse oximetry. Nonetheless pulse oximetry may provide another assessment of tissue perfusion. With effective therapy the pulse oximeter will detect pulsatile perfusion.

Quickly establish vascular access with vascular or IO cannulation.

Vascular access is vital for drug and fluid administration. But it may be difficult to achieve in the pediatric patient, particularly if shock is present. For treatment of decompensated shock the preferred access site is the one most readily available. If CPR is in progress the preferred access site is the one most readily available that will not require interruption of CPR. Although peripheral or central venous access is sufficient for fluid resuscitation in most patients, you should establish IO access if you cannot rapidly achieve reliable venous access. Moreover, in decompensated shock *immediate* IO access is appropriate. Attempting peripheral vascular access in an unstable patient with poor perfusion and peripheral vasoconstriction wastes precious time.

Administer isotonic fluid as rapidly as possible (5 to 10 minutes) in boluses of 20 mL/kg.

The initial treatment of hypovolemic shock is rapid infusion of 20 mL/kg isotonic crystalloid, such as normal saline or Ringer's lactate, over 5 to 20 minutes. Ideally you should infuse this fluid for this infant within 5 to 10 minutes. Bolus infusion over 10 to 20 minutes may be appropriate for children with myocardial dysfunction or less severe compromise in systemic perfusion. Reassess the patient after each bolus to determine the need for additional fluids. For optimal resuscita-

tion most patients in decompensated shock will need at least 40 to 80 mL/kg isotonic fluids (2 to 4 boluses of 20 mL/kg each) during the first 1 to 2 hours of therapy. (For more information about fluid resuscitation see Chapter 5.)

This infant is probably dehydrated because of the vomiting and diarrhea; she should respond well to fluid resuscitation. But if dehydration and shock are complicated by poor myocardial function (cardiogenic shock) or sepsis (distributive shock), the infant's systemic perfusion may improve minimally or transiently after fluid administration. Be alert for signs that the infant's shock is more than simple hypovolemic shock.

If the infant has *cardiogenic* shock caused by poor myocardial function, volume resuscitation could result in pulmonary edema, compromising respiratory function. You will identify the pulmonary edema when you repeat the rapid cardiopulmonary assessment after each fluid bolus. Infants and children with cardiogenic shock often require drug therapy to increase cardiac output. (For more information about medications to support cardiac output, see Chapter 5.)

This infant could have bacterial enteritis with *septic shock*. This type of shock causes maldistribution of blood flow and increased capillary permeability. Infants with septic shock typically require much *more* fluid than indicated by the initial history and estimated fluid losses. Again, repeating your clinical examinations will help you determine the ongoing need for fluid administration and help you detect any adverse effects.

Do not infuse large volumes of dextrose-containing fluids during resuscitation. Excess amounts of these fluids will cause hyperglycemia, which will induce a rise in serum osmolality and osmotic diuresis. Electrolyte imbalances (eg, hyponatremia) could develop.

Because some of the signs and symptoms that occur with shock can be caused by

Critical Concepts:
Identifying Hypotension in Infants and Children

Hypotension is a systolic blood pressure (SBP) below the 5th percentile for age.

Age	Minimum (5th Percentile) SBP (mm Hg)
<1 month	60
1 month to 1 year	70
>1 year	70 + (2 × age in years)
≥10 years	90

hypoglycemia, you should determine the patient's glucose concentration. Administer glucose (0.5 to 1 g/kg) if the concentration is low, and monitor serum glucose concentration closely. The patient may require a continuous infusion of glucose-containing fluids in addition to the bolus resuscitation fluids.

Unacceptable Actions

The following actions are unacceptable for treatment of the infant in this scenario:

- Failing to use universal precautions
- Failing to identify decompensated hypovolemic shock
- Treating the rapid heart rate with drugs or cardioversion
- Performing airway intervention (other than oxygen administration) before establishing vascular access
- Repeatedly attempting peripheral IV or central venous access instead of attempting IO access
- Administering a hypotonic or glucose-containing fluid for the shock resuscitation boluses
- Giving inadequate volume or giving it too slowly
- Failing to reassess the infant after each fluid bolus

Case Scenario 2

A mother brings her 4-year-old girl to the pediatrician's office. The child has a history of increasing lethargy, fever, and "dizziness" when she tries to stand up. There is no history of vomiting or diarrhea. Her intake has been poor over the last 12 hours. Typical chickenpox lesions developed 5 days ago; over the last 18 hours several lesions on her abdomen have become red, tender, swollen, and confluent.

On physical examination the child is supine, listless, and confused; she looks very ill. The child responds to voice and painful stimulation. But she does not know where she is, and she does not seem to understand what people are saying. She is breathing rapidly and quietly; her airway appears

patent. Heart rate is 175 bpm, respiratory rate is 60 breaths/min, rectal temperature is 39.4°C (103°F), and blood pressure is 90/30 mm Hg. Auscultation reveals clear lungs with good distal air entry. Extremities are warm and bright red, central pulses are full and bounding, and peripheral pulses are easily palpable. Capillary refill is <1 second. The skin lesions on her abdomen are bright red and tender.

Acceptable Actions

The following actions are generally acceptable for assessment and management of this child with shock:

- Use universal precautions.
- Perform rapid cardiopulmonary assessment; identify compensated shock.
- Administer oxygen; initiate ECG and pulse oximetry monitoring.
- Activate the emergency response system if appropriate.
- Establish intravascular access, administer isotonic crystalloid bolus, and reassess the patient.
- Conduct a bedside glucose test and obtain blood for laboratory studies, including blood cultures.
- Start IV antibiotics.

Rationale for Acceptable Actions

Perform rapid cardiopulmonary assessment; identify compensated shock.

Rapid cardiopulmonary assessment of this girl reveals adequate **A**irway and **B**reathing. Direct **C**ardiovascular evaluation reveals tachycardia and adequate systolic blood pressure with excellent central pulses and palpable distal pulses. Assessment of end-organ perfusion indicates that this child is responsive to voice and painful stimulation and that her skin is adequately perfused, but she is confused.

This child has evidence of **compensated shock**. The presence of metabolic acidosis confirms the diagnosis (test for it during the clinical exam). The child's fever,

tachypnea, tachycardia, and presumably infected skin lesions are consistent with *septic shock*.

The pathophysiology of *septic shock* is quite different from that of hypovolemic or cardiogenic shock. This difference results in a unique clinical presentation (see Critical Concepts: "Pathophysiology and Clinical Presentation of Septic Shock"). Complex compensatory mechanisms often enable the child with septic shock to maintain cardiac output that is normal or higher than normal. Shock can develop rapidly in patients with sepsis because blood flow is maldistributed (see below). A rapid heart rate and low systemic vascular resistance help to maintain normal or high cardiac output. Although the ventricular ejection fraction is typically low in septic shock, compensatory ventricular dilation and low systemic vascular resistance enable maintenance of adequate stroke volume *provided intravascular volume is maintained*. For this reason early, aggressive volume administration is important to treat septic shock; inadequate intravascular volume rapidly leads to hypotension and low stroke volume.

In septic shock systemic vascular resistance is typically low because vasodilation develops, particularly in the vascular beds of skin and skeletal muscle. This vasodilation results in maldistribution of cardiac output. Some tissue beds receive excessive blood flow (eg, skeletal muscle and skin), and other tissue beds receive inadequate blood flow (eg, splanchnic organs).

As a result skin perfusion may be excellent with warm, bright red distal extremities and brisk capillary refill. The increased skeletal muscle flow "steals" blood from the splanchnic (ie, intestinal, liver, and renal) vascular beds, causing low urine output and metabolic acidosis. Because blood flow is inadequate to meet metabolic demand in some tissue beds, metabolic acidosis develops. The presence of metabolic acidosis strongly suggests that some organs or tissue beds are ischemic.

Critical Concepts:
Pathophysiology and Clinical Presentation of Septic Shock

- Cardiac output may be normal, increased, or decreased (often increased, particularly early).

  — Blood flow is maldistributed. Perfusion of the skin and skeletal muscles is often excellent, but perfusion in some tissue beds may be inadequate. Metabolic acidosis indicates inadequate perfusion in some tissue beds.

  — Hypotension may develop early in the clinical course despite apparently excellent skin perfusion. Hypotension occurs secondary to inappropriate vasodilation and inadequate vascular response to endogenous or exogenous vasoconstrictors. Vasodilation causes a wide pulse pressure, a common finding in sepsis.

- Early signs of sepsis include the following:

  — Fever or hypothermia

  — Tachycardia and tachypnea

  — Confusion with agitation or lethargy

  — Widened pulse pressure and vasodilation

  — Metabolic acidosis

  — Leukocytosis, leukopenia or increased bands (immature white blood cells)

Administer oxygen; initiate ECG and pulse oximetry monitoring.

This child's clinical status is precarious. Although she is in compensated shock, she may rapidly deteriorate despite therapy. Administer oxygen and prepare to maintain her airway and support ventilation if needed. Initiate continuous ECG monitoring. If therapy is appropriate, her heart rate should decrease toward normal.

Activate the emergency response system if appropriate.

If a child with septic shock presents in an outpatient clinic or office, you should stabilize the patient and arrange transfer. If septic shock develops while the patient is in hospital, you should assemble support staff, equipment, and medications to stabilize the patient and arrange transfer to an appropriate location.

Establish intravascular access, administer isotonic crystalloid bolus, and reassess patient.

Although the girl in this scenario has excellent skin perfusion and normal systolic blood pressure, she is tachycardic with altered mental status. She also has a wide pulse pressure with low systemic vascular resistance. These clinical signs are typical of septic shock.

Patients with septic shock have increased capillary permeability. As you provide fluid resuscitation, you should anticipate the development of systemic edema. Pulmonary edema also may develop, but it occurs more often with *inadequate* fluid resuscitation. If pulmonary edema is present, vigorous fluid resuscitation is needed to correct the perfusion deficit and reduce capillary leak. You should prepare to support oxygenation and ventilation; perform intubation if indicated. If significant pulmonary edema develops, the patient may require mechanical ventilatory support with supplementary oxygen and positive end-expiratory pressure (PEEP).

Unacceptable Actions

The following actions are unacceptable for treatment of the child in this scenario:

- Failing to use universal precautions

- Administering IM ceftriaxone and allowing the mother to transport the child by car

- Treating the heart rate with cardioversion

- Performing an airway intervention (other than oxygen) before addressing vascular access and volume resuscitation

- Administering a hypotonic or glucose-containing fluid

- Giving inadequate volume or giving it too slowly

- Failing to reassess the child after you administer fluid boluses

- Failing to recognize signs of deterioration

- Transferring the child's care to ambulance personnel without reassessing her

Case Scenario 2 Progression

You establish IV access with a 20-gauge angiocatheter placed in the child's left antecubital vein. You then rapidly infuse 20 mL/kg normal saline. The child's glucose concentration (by bedside test) is 150 mg/dL. The child becomes more alert, and ambulance personnel transport her to the nearest healthcare facility. Despite IV antibiotics and administration of 60 mL/kg normal saline over the next hour, the child deteriorates. She becomes unresponsive to voice and barely responsive to painful stimulation. Her distal pulses are no longer palpable, and her extremities are cold. Heart rate ranges from 170 to 180 bpm, and blood pressure decreases to 70/25 mm Hg. The child's respiratory rate and respiratory status remain unchanged.

Aggressive fluid resuscitation is certainly an important part of the treatment for septic shock. But many patients with *decompensated shock* need a vasopressor infusion to improve blood pressure. For these patients you should initially infuse dopamine at 5 µg/kg per minute. Increase the rate to 15 µg/kg per minute within 10 minutes. Continue to provide repeated fluid boluses during dopamine infusion.

Children with any type of shock may deteriorate despite appropriate initial therapy. This potential for deterioration is especially common in children with septic shock. Frequent reassessment is important for optimal care of the child in shock.

For more information about fluid therapy and medications to support cardiac output, including an algorithm for resuscitation of the child with septic shock, see Chapter 5.

Case Scenario 3

A mother brings her 6-month-old son to an urgent care center at 11:00 PM. The infant was normal when the mother went to work and left him with her boyfriend. As soon as the mother came home, she knew her son didn't look right. The infant has no history of feeding problems, vomiting, or diarrhea. He has had no known contact with anyone who was ill and no recent history of upper respiratory illness.

On initial assessment the infant is breathing rapidly without increased effort; he is flaccid and unresponsive to painful stimulation. His heart rate is 210 bpm, blood pressure is 75/45 mm Hg, respiratory rate is 40 breaths/min and unlabored, and rectal temperature is 99°F (37.2°C). His lungs are clear on auscultation, and he has a regular cardiac rhythm with a short systolic ejection murmur. His skin is pale and his distal extremities are cold; capillary refill time is >4 seconds. Peripheral pulses are barely palpable; his brachial pulse is present but weak.

Acceptable Actions

The following actions are generally acceptable for assessment and management of this infant with shock:

- Use universal precautions.
- Perform rapid cardiopulmonary assessment; identify compensated shock.
- Initiate cardiorespiratory monitoring, provide oxygen, and support the airway as necessary. Because the infant is unresponsive to painful stimulation, he is likely unable to protect his airway. Elective intubation is appropriate.
- Establish vascular or IO access, administer isotonic crystalloid bolus, and reassess.
- Give additional boluses as indicated by systemic perfusion.

- Conduct a bedside glucose test; attempt to identify the cause of the infant's condition (consider reversible causes, including the 4 H's and 4 T's).

Rationale for Acceptable Actions

Perform rapid cardiopulmonary assessment; identify compensated shock.

Initial cardiopulmonary assessment reveals tachycardia, poor peripheral pulses, and normal blood pressure in an infant with altered mental status and poor skin perfusion. His airway is open, and his respiratory effort and air entry are adequate. But he is unresponsive to painful stimulation. Support his airway while you prepare for elective intubation. There is no information about urine output. These findings are consistent with *compensated shock.*

Initiate cardiorespiratory monitoring, provide oxygen, and support the airway as necessary.

This infant boy has shock without a fever or any apparent cause suggested by the history. Reassessment and further physical examination are warranted to identify and treat reversible causes of this child's condition. Check the serum glucose concentration, and consider other causes of deterioration.

Establish vascular or IO access, administer an isotonic crystalloid bolus, and reassess. Attempt to identify the cause of the infant's condition.

Establish vascular or IO access. Infuse isotonic crystalloid in rapid (<20 minutes) boluses of 20 mL/kg; reassess after each bolus. If systemic perfusion does not improve, administer additional boluses while attempting to identify and treat reversible causes of the shock.

The most likely cause of shock in this infant is hypovolemia (secondary to nonaccidental trauma) or sepsis. Both hypovolemic and septic shock require rapid volume resuscitation to avoid decompensation.

Unacceptable Actions

The following actions are unacceptable for treatment of the infant in this scenario:

- Failing to use universal precautions
- Administering IM ceftriaxone and allowing the mother to transport the child by car
- Treating the heart rate with cardioversion
- Giving inadequate volume or giving it too slowly
- Using hypotonic or glucose-containing fluid for volume resuscitation
- Failing to consider the diagnosis of inflicted injuries
- Transporting the patient without reassessing him

Case Scenario 3 Progression

You open the airway and provide oxygen; other providers prepare for elective intubation. You achieve vascular access with a 22-gauge catheter placed in the greater saphenous vein. You then rapidly infuse 20 mL/kg isotonic crystalloid (normal saline or Ringer's lactate) over 10 minutes. The infant's heart rate initially decreases to 190 bpm, and peripheral perfusion improves with more readily palpable distal pulses. But the infant's neurologic status does not change. The infant's anterior fontanelle is now bulging and taut. You remove his shirt and pants. Multiple bruises are present over all 4 extremities and his abdomen. Funduscopic examination reveals extensive bilateral retinal hemorrhages. During evaluation and fluid therapy the infant remains unresponsive; he then has a focal tonic-clonic seizure with apnea.

You perform tracheal intubation, confirm tube placement, and provide effective ventilation using a manual resuscitator while awaiting transport. The infant's seizure stops after treatment with lorazepam. On reassessment his perfusion is worse: heart rate is 210 bpm, and blood pressure is 60/40 mm Hg. A second 20 mL/kg rapid bolus of normal saline results in better perfusion with a decrease in heart rate to

190 bpm and an increase in blood pressure to 70/45 mm Hg. After a third 20 mL/kg bolus of normal saline, the infant's heart rate decreases to 160 bpm, blood pressure increases to 80/50 mm Hg, and peripheral perfusion improves. His blood glucose concentration is 120 mg/dL; hematocrit is 23%. After stabilization the infant is transferred to a pediatric trauma center. The retinal hemorrhages strongly suggest abuse. A head CT scan shows large bilateral subdural hematomas, confirming abuse. A pediatric surgeon subsequently drains the hematomas.

This scenario is a classic case of severe but occult child abuse. The infant presented with clinical signs of hypovolemic shock, but no cause was initially apparent from his history. Careful clinical examination revealed evidence of trauma and persistent altered mental status, which are consistent with severe injury.

This child has a massive head injury with subdural hematomas. This presentation is also consistent with hypovolemic shock due to other types of trauma (eg, splenic laceration, liver laceration, and femur fracture). For this reason you should obtain CT scans of the chest and abdomen and skeletal x-rays.

Children with inflicted injury often come to medical attention many hours after the injury. The injured child may not have eaten for many hours, so the child may have hypoglycemia. Providers should check the serum glucose concentration (it was normal in this infant). Moreover, delayed resuscitation in any form of shock results in progressive ischemia and multiple organ dysfunction. For this reason cardiac, liver, and renal dysfunction may be out of proportion to the original injury.

Children who sustain *unintentional* injuries such as those occurring in motor vehicle crashes are generally transported to a trauma center, and their history and diagnosis are usually well established. Children with *inflicted* injuries are not necessarily taken to a trauma center. These children often have clinical signs that do not match the reported history, and the diagnosis may not be apparent during primary assessment. You should always consider child abuse as a potential cause of shock or neurologic deterioration that is inadequately explained by the history.

Case Scenario 4

A 3-month-old girl presents with a several-day history of vomiting and watery diarrhea. She is brought to the Emergency Department after feeding poorly and vomiting several times overnight. Her parents are unsure if she has urinated because she had watery diarrhea several times overnight. On examination the infant appears listless with little response to verbal or painful stimulation. She has increased respiratory effort with mild retractions. Her heart rate is 210 bpm, respiratory rate is 50 breaths/min, blood pressure is 55/40 mm Hg, and axillary temperature is 97°F (36.1°C). Auscultation reveals fair distal air entry and scattered inspiratory crackles at the base of each lung. The infant has a rapid, regular cardiac rhythm without murmur. Her brachial and femoral pulses are weak but palpable, and the distal pulses are not palpable. Extremities are cool and mottled below the elbows and knees, and capillary refill time in the foot is >8 seconds. The infant's liver is firm and palpable 6 cm below the costal margin; it crosses the midline into the left upper quadrant.

Acceptable Actions

The following actions are generally acceptable for assessment and management of this infant with shock:

- Use universal precautions.
- Perform rapid cardiopulmonary assessment; identify decompensated shock.
- Administer oxygen and initiate cardiorespiratory monitoring; attach a pulse oximeter if available.
- Attempt rapid intravascular access; if unsuccessful, attempt IO access.
- Consider administration of 10 mL/kg isotonic crystalloid bolus.

- Reassess the patient after each fluid bolus.
- Conduct a bedside glucose test and obtain blood samples for other laboratory studies (eg, arterial blood gas analysis).
- Obtain a chest x-ray.
- Consider inotropic support (medications to improve myocardial contractility).
- Consult a pediatric cardiologist.

Rationale for Acceptable Actions

Perform rapid cardiopulmonary assessment; identify decompensated shock.

Initial cardiopulmonary assessment includes evaluation of **A**irway and **B**reathing. The airway is open, but breathing is labored. In a patient with poor perfusion this combination of findings is a "red flag" for cardiogenic shock. **C**ardiovascular assessment reveals severe tachycardia, weak peripheral pulses, and hypotension. Evaluation of end-organ perfusion reveals prolonged capillary refill with cool extremities and depressed mental status. These findings are consistent with decompensated shock. Potential types of shock are cardiogenic shock and septic shock (secondary to pneumonia).

Administer oxygen and initiate cardiorespiratory monitoring; attach a pulse oximeter if available.

Administer supplementary oxygen, initiate monitoring, and provide or maintain warmth. Evaluate the ECG (see Chapter 8). Attempts to measure oxygen saturation by pulse oximetry may be unsuccessful because the peripheral pulses are so weak. But return of the pulse oximetry signal may indicate improved perfusion in response to therapy.

Attempt rapid intravascular access; if unsuccessful, attempt IO access.

This child needs immediate vascular access for fluid therapy and medications.

Consider administration of 10 mL/kg isotonic crystalloid bolus. Reassess the patient after each bolus.

You should consider giving a fluid bolus to improve systemic perfusion. The large liver, mild respiratory distress (retractions), and pulmonary congestion in this infant suggest cardiogenic shock, which may warrant less vigorous volume resuscitation and early inotropic support. It would be reasonable to administer an initial fluid bolus of 10 mL/kg and give additional boluses as indicated by the patient's response. The patient's work of breathing may increase, so you should prepare to intubate the child and provide mechanical ventilation with PEEP to maintain oxygenation and ventilation.

Case Scenario 4 Progression

You place a 22-gauge peripheral angiocatheter in an antecubital vein and conduct a bedside glucose test (concentration is 80 mg/dL). You administer a 10 mL/kg isotonic fluid bolus and obtain a chest x-ray. After the fluid bolus the patient's respiratory effort increases with grunting respirations. Perfusion does not improve, and the chest x-ray reveals a large heart and probable pulmonary edema. A 12-lead ECG reveals sinus tachycardia with the rate varying between 195 and 215 bpm. You perform rapid sequence tracheal intubation, confirm tracheal tube placement, and provide mechanical ventilation with oxygen and 6 cm H_2O PEEP. An echocardiogram reveals ventricular dilation and poor myocardial contractility. You infuse vasoactive drugs to improve cardiac function and admit the infant to the PICU.

Although the fluid bolus did not correct this infant's poor perfusion and may have contributed to the deterioration in respiratory status, it is the most appropriate treatment for the most common causes of shock: hypovolemia and sepsis. In patients with cardiogenic shock, a reasonable approach is to give smaller fluid boluses and carefully reassess the patient after each

bolus. Patients with all forms of shock require adequate preload (ie, end-diastolic volume). Whenever you provide fluid therapy, you should anticipate the development of pulmonary edema and deterioration in pulmonary function and prepare to provide assisted ventilation.

The findings of the clinical examination and chest x-ray are consistent with decompensated *cardiogenic shock*. This child has sinus tachycardia documented by a 12-lead ECG and poor myocardial contractility documented by clinical findings and an echocardiogram. The presence of a large, firm liver, respiratory distress with labored respirations and grunting, and the large heart and pulmonary edema (reported

on the chest x-ray) indicate heart failure with systemic and pulmonary congestion. Findings of the clinical exam suggest poor myocardial contractility, which the echocardiogram confirms. These findings are consistent with severe cardiomyopathy or acute myocarditis.

Although hypovolemic and septic shock are the most common forms of shock, you should consider other forms of shock, such as cardiogenic, obstructive, spinal, and anaphylactic shock (see FYI: "Anaphylactic and Obstructive Shock"). Cardiogenic shock is often thought to result from poor myocardial contractility only. But cardiogenic shock may result from other causes, including arrhythmias and poisoning.

FYI: Anaphylactic and Obstructive Shock

Anaphylactic shock may develop as part of an acute multisystem allergic response to various antigens. It is mediated by immunoglobulin E (IgE) and IgG4 subclass antibodies. Insect stings, drugs, and foods are the most common causes of anaphylaxis. Manifestations of anaphylaxis include laryngeal edema, bronchospasm, urticaria, abdominal pain, vomiting, diarrhea, and shock. Treatment includes early administration of IM epinephrine[1] with supplementary oxygen, airway management, inhaled adrenergic agonists for laryngeal edema and bronchospasm, and prompt fluid resuscitation. In this form of shock mast cells release histamine and vasoactive mediators. Early administration of H_1 and H_2 blockers and corticosteroids (eg, 1 to 2 mg/kg of methylprednisolone) is indicated.

Obstructive shock can result from a tension pneumothorax, cardiac tamponade, or a massive pulmonary embolus that obstructs blood flow. Obstructive shock also may develop in neonates with ductal-dependent congenital obstruction

of the left or right ventricle. The patient's history and clinical presentation should suggest one of these processes. For example, sudden development of shock after chest trauma suggests a tension pneumothorax or cardiac tamponade. Similarly, sudden onset of shock in a mechanically ventilated patient with acute respiratory distress syndrome requiring high ventilator pressures suggests a tension pneumothorax.

Clinical evidence of obstructive shock consists of poor perfusion, increased heart rate, and narrow pulse pressure. The patient may also have a large liver, asymmetric breath sounds, or muffled heart sounds. Jugular vein distention may be present, but it is often difficult to assess in infants and young children. Jugular vein distention is not a reliable sign of obstructive shock. A chest x-ray is often helpful, but the cardiac silhouette may be normal in the presence of cardiac tamponade.

Treatments for obstructive shock focus on relief of the obstruction.

Increased work of breathing often distinguishes cardiogenic shock from hypovolemic and septic shock, which are characterized by quiet tachypnea.

Unacceptable Actions

The following actions are unacceptable for treatment of the infant in this scenario:

- Failing to use universal precautions

- Failing to identify decompensated shock

- Failing to recognize myocardial dysfunction as a factor contributing to shock

- Treating the heart rate with cardioversion

- Repeating fluid boluses despite lack of improvement after the first bolus and the clinical and x-ray evidence of cardiogenic shock and respiratory distress

- Failing to support oxygenation and ventilation when deterioration occurs

- Failing to add vasoactive drug therapy when the child fails to respond to volume therapy and support of oxygenation and ventilation

- Administering hypotonic or glucose-containing fluid boluses

Case Scenario 5: For the Experienced Provider

A 2-year-old boy is admitted to the PICU after cardiac arrest due to submersion (near-drowning). Bystander CPR resulted in return of a spontaneous pulse. Initial arterial blood gas analysis (conducted in the Emergency Department) revealed a P_{O_2} of 54 mm Hg, pH of 7.01, and P_{CO_2} of 25 mm Hg. Because the child's poor perfusion and low blood pressure did not respond to fluid bolus therapy, an IV dopamine drip was started and titrated to a dose of 20 µg/kg per minute.

In the PICU the toddler's cardiopulmonary status improves nicely over the next 6 hours in response to aggressive medical management. Ventilator settings are titrated to a

rate of 20 ventilations per minute, peak inspiratory pressure of 35 cm H_2O, PEEP of 12 cm H_2O, and F_{IO_2} of 0.70. Arterial blood gas values improve to a P_{O_2} of 82 mm Hg, pH of 7.31, and P_{CO_2} of 27 mm Hg. Findings on the chest x-ray are consistent with diffuse acute respiratory distress syndrome.

The child's cardiovascular status improves with the addition of continuous infusions of epinephrine at 0.3 µg/kg per minute and dobutamine at 20 µg/kg per minute; the dopamine was discontinued. Heart rate is 164 bpm, blood pressure is 94/60 mm Hg, central venous pressure is 8 mm Hg, peripheral pulses are excellent, and capillary refill time is 3 to 4 seconds. An arterial catheter is in place, providing continuous monitoring of intra-arterial pressure. An echocardiogram reveals low-normal shortening fraction and ejection fraction.

After several hours of stability the boy's arterial blood pressure suddenly drops to 53/25 mm Hg, heart rate decreases to 82 bpm, and central venous pressure increases to 14 mm Hg. Peripheral pulses are no longer palpable, peripheral perfusion is markedly worse, and extremities are now cold below the elbows and knees. Central pulses are weak but palpable. Rectal temperature is 36.5°C (97.7°F).

Acceptable Actions

The following actions are acceptable for assessment and treatment of this toddler with shock:

- Evaluate respiratory status during mechanical ventilation; consider **DOPE** causes of sudden deterioration (**D**isplaced tracheal tube, **O**bstructed tube, **P**neumothorax, **E**quipment failure).

- Consider potential reversible causes of deterioration (the **4 H's** and **4 T's**) and treat appropriately.

- Consider causes of the triad of hypotension, increased central venous pressure, and decreased heart rate.

- Check glucose, electrolytes, and blood gases.

- Order a chest x-ray.

Rationale for Acceptable Actions

Evaluate respiratory status during mechanical ventilation; consider "DOPE" causes of sudden deterioration.

The physician, PICU nurse, and respiratory care practitioner immediately evaluate the boy's respiratory status on the ventilator and consider the **DOPE** mnemonic. The medical team should also consider reversible causes of deterioration, recalled by the **4 H's** and **4 T's** and treat these appropriately (see Critical Concepts: "Reversible Causes of Deterioration in the Infant or Child").

The triad of low blood pressure, high central venous pressure, and a fall in heart rate is consistent with poor myocardial contractility, extrinsic cardiac compression (tension pneumothorax, cardiac tamponade, or excessive PEEP), or obstruction of pulmonary arterial flow (severe pulmonary hypertension or massive pulmonary embolus). In the setting of obstructed pulmonary artery flow or extrinsic cardiac compression, the heart rate often increases initially and then falls as shock progresses. In the setting of severe myocardial dysfunction or loss of the inotropic or vasopressor infusion, the heart rate and blood pressure fall rapidly and central venous pressure typically rises. The team should rule out these causes of deterioration (see Critical Concepts: "Reversible Causes of Deterioration in the Infant or Child").

Case Scenario 5 Progression

The boy's pulse oximeter is not functioning because he has very poor distal perfusion. But his chest is moving well with no changes in expired tidal volume or peak inspiratory pressure (per indications on the mechanical ventilator control panel). You send samples to the laboratory for analysis of arterial blood gases, serum glucose, and electrolytes. You also perform a bedside glucose screen.

Breath sounds are present and equal bi-laterally, but you order a chest x-ray because the clinical findings do not reliably rule out a pneumothorax. Manual ventilation produces bilateral chest expansion with good breath sounds, which makes a significant tension pneumothorax unlikely. Glucose concentration (by bedside test) is 145 mg/dL. The arterial blood is bright red (ie, well oxygenated), so severe hypoxemia is unlikely.

A PICU nurse checks the entire IV administration system and discovers a leak in a 3-way stopcock through which the vasopressors are infusing. This response to unintended discontinuation of the vasoactive drugs suggests the possibility of severe postischemic myocardial dysfunction. The nurse reconnects the IV tubing and infuses catecholamine at a faster rate until blood pressure increases to 100/50 mm Hg. She then tapers the infusion rate to the previous rate while monitoring blood pressure over the next half hour.

Unacceptable Actions

The following actions are unacceptable for treatment of this toddler with acute deterioration in the PICU after global ischemia due to submersion:

- Failing to use universal precautions
- Delaying therapy to await results of laboratory studies (note that it is reasonable to await the results of the chest x-ray for this scenario)
- Failing to look for common reversible causes of acute deterioration in the child
- Treating the high heart rate with cardioversion

Critical Concepts:
Reversible Causes of Deterioration in the Infant or Child

1. **Causes of acute deterioration in the intubated child: DOPE mnemonic**
   - Displacement of the tube
   - Obstruction of the tube
   - Pneumothorax
   - Equipment failure
2. **The 4 H's and 4 T's**
   - Hypoxemia
   - Hypovolemia
   - Hypothermia
   - Hyperkalemia, hypokalemia, and other metabolic disorders, including hypoglycemia
   - Tamponade
   - Tension pneumothorax
   - Toxins, poisons, or drugs
   - Thromboembolism
3. **Potential causes of the triad of ↓BP, ↑CVP, and change in HR**
   - Poor myocardial contractility (congestive heart failure); may be complicated by acute loss of vasoactive drug infusion
   - Extrinsic cardiac compression or obstruction of venous return
     — Tension pneumothorax
     — Cardiac tamponade
     — Excessive PEEP or air trapping (eg, in a patient with status asthmaticus who receives mechanical ventilation)
   - Obstruction of pulmonary arterial flow
   - Severe pulmonary hypertension
   - Massive pulmonary embolus

Summary Points

Shock is a clinical condition in which tissue perfusion is inadequate to meet metabolic demands. In many forms of shock (eg, hypovolemic and cardiogenic), cardiac output is low. In septic shock cardiac output is often normal or increased, but the blood flow is maldistributed.

Recognition of shock requires both direct and indirect cardiovascular assessments. Direct assessments include monitoring of heart rate, evaluation of the strength of central and peripheral pulses, and monitoring of blood pressure. Indirect assessments include evaluation of end-organ function (brain, skin, and kidneys) to determine if end-organ perfusion is adequate. The presence of lactic acidosis combined with clinical signs and symptoms consistent with shock confirms the diagnosis.

The patient's history and clinical signs often suggest the cause of shock. But you should always consider occult trauma (ie, child abuse) as a cause of shock, particularly when the history is inconsistent with clinical signs.

The initial treatment of shock depends on the child's clinical status. If **A**irway and **B**reathing are adequate, the initial priority for treatment of shock is *vascular access*. For compensated shock, peripheral venous cannulation is the preferred technique. For decompensated shock, the preferred access site is the one most readily available. The most readily attainable vascular access site depends on the provider's experience and expertise and the clinical circumstances. But you should generally establish IO access as soon as possible for decompensated shock. Administer fluid boluses and medications to support cardiac output as needed (see Critical Concepts: "Summary Shock Information").

Critical Concepts: Summary Shock Information

Assessment of Shock

■ Initial cardiopulmonary assessment:

— **Appearance:** Note mental status, tone, and response to stimulation.

— **Airway:** Typically open.

— **Breathing:** Note rate and respiratory effort. Quiet tachypnea (to compensate for metabolic acidosis) is characteristic of hypovolemic and septic shock. Increased work of breathing suggests cardiogenic shock.

— **Circulation:** Check for direct and indirect signs of inadequate perfusion (see below).

Cardiovascular Assessment for Shock

■ *Direct* cardiovascular assessment:

— Heart rate

— Pulses (proximal and distal), capillary refill

— Blood pressure

■ *Indirect* cardiovascular assessment (evaluation of end-organ perfusion):

— Brain: Alertness, responsiveness

— Skin: Color, temperature, capillary refill (presuming warm ambient temperature)

— Kidneys: Urine output

Classification of Shock

■ Classification of physiologic status:

— Stable

— Respiratory distress

— Respiratory failure

— Shock

• Compensated

• Decompensated

— Cardiopulmonary failure

— Cardiopulmonary arrest

■ Signs of decompensated shock:

— If blood pressure is obtained: Clinical signs of poor perfusion accompanied by systolic hypotension

— If blood pressure is unavailable: Signs of shock (ie, prolonged capillary refill, cool extremities, tachycardia, and decreased level of consciousness) with no distal pulses

■ Types of shock and key characteristics:

— Hypovolemic: Most common; peripheral vasoconstriction, narrow pulse pressure and history consistent with volume deficit/loss

— Distributive (septic): Wide pulse pressure; hypothermia or hyperthermia

— Cardiogenic: Pulmonary edema, systemic edema, or both; increased work of breathing; grunting; narrow pulse pressure

— Other: Consider special resuscitation circumstances

Management of Shock

■ Initial treatment

— Ensure adequate **A**irway and **B**reathing; give oxygen.

— Circulation: Establish vascular access; obtain rapid IV or IO access for decompensated shock.

— Fluid therapy: 20 mL/kg Rapid bolus of isotonic crystalloid (you may modify if you suspect cardiogenic shock or severe myocardial dysfunction).

— Reassess cardiovascular and pulmonary function.

— Administer additional fluid therapy as needed; consider inotropic agents and vasoactive drugs.

Reference

1. Project Team of the Resuscitation Council (UK). The emergency medical treatment of anaphylactic reactions. *J Accid Emerg Med.* 1999;16:243-247.

Review Questions

1. **You are caring for a child with decompensated shock. Which one of the following lists the appropriate *initial priorities* for therapy?**

   a. check and support airway and breathing, administer oxygen, and establish vascular access to enable fluid and drug administration

   b. perform a thorough head-to-toe examination and obtain x-rays if you suspect injury

   c. establish intra-arterial access to enable continuous monitoring of blood pressure and blood sampling for arterial blood gas and serum glucose analyses

   d. perform a complete neurologic evaluation to determine if head trauma is present

   The correct answer is a. Check and support airway and breathing, administer oxygen, and establish vascular access to enable fluid and drug administration.

   Answer b is incorrect. Although you must ultimately perform a thorough examination, you should support airway, breathing, and circulation first.

   Answer c is incorrect. Although the ability to monitor blood pressure and to sample blood is desirable, it is of less immediate importance than supporting the airway, breathing, and circulation.

   Answer d is incorrect because the neurologic evaluation is not as high a priority as support of the airway, breathing, and circulation.

2. **Which of the following best describes the advantages of IO access over other techniques for rapid vascular access in decompensated shock?**

   a. providers can use readily available plastic over-the-needle catheters for IO access

   b. the risk of infection is lower with the IO route than with IV access

   c. the IO route provides more direct access to the heart than a central venous route

   d. providers can quickly establish reliable access, and the technique is easy to master

   The correct answer is d. PALS providers can easily master the technique of IO access. With practice and experience, providers typically achieve access within seconds.

   Answer a is incorrect because plastic over-the-needle catheters are not stiff or strong enough to penetrate through the bone into the marrow.

   Answer b is incorrect because there is no evidence that IO access poses less risk of infection than peripheral or central venous access.

   Answer c is incorrect. Drugs delivered by the IO, peripheral venous, and central venous routes reach the central circulation in roughly the same time if the drugs are followed by a saline flush.

3. **Which of the following is the best definition of shock?**

   a. a clinical state characterized by low cardiac output

   b. a clinical state characterized by a capillary refill time >3 seconds

   c. a clinical state characterized by hypotension

   d. a clinical state characterized by tissue perfusion that is inadequate to meet metabolic demands

   The correct answer is d. Shock is a clinical state characterized by tissue perfusion that is inadequate to meet metabolic demands.

   Answer a is incorrect because shock may occur with low, normal, or high cardiac output.

   Answer b is incorrect because delayed capillary refill (>3 seconds), although abnormal, does not "define" shock and is not specific for shock.

   Answer c is incorrect because shock may be present with normal, high, or low blood pressure. Shock that occurs with blood pressure that is normal for age is *compensated* shock. Shock that occurs with hypotension is *decompensated* shock.

4. **Which one of the following characteristics of early septic shock differs from typical characteristics of hypovolemic or cardiogenic shock?**

   a. decreased urine output

   b. inadequate tissue perfusion

   c. normal or above normal cardiac output

   d. abnormal neurologic status

   The correct answer is c. Cardiac output often is normal or above normal in early septic shock. This phenomenon is frequently called "high cardiac output shock." The patient often has warm extremities with bounding pulses, but hypotension may be present.

   Answer a is incorrect because urine output decreases whenever renal perfusion is compromised. Decreased urine output may occur with hypovolemic, cardiogenic, or septic shock.

   Answer b is incorrect because tissue perfusion is inadequate to meet metabolic demand in all forms of shock.

   Answer d is incorrect because abnormal neurologic status is evidence of inadequate perfusion of the brain. This symptom may occur with hypovolemic, cardiogenic, or septic shock.

Rhythm Disturbances

Introductory Case Scenario

A previously healthy 4-year-old girl presents to the Emergency Department with a 2-week history of flulike symptoms, including lethargy, fever, and dizziness. The child responds to your voice but is listless and confused. Her skin is pale and mottled, and distal extremities are cool. The child's airway is patent. Her respiratory rate is 40 breaths/min, but breathing is not labored. Her pulse is approximately 240 bpm and weak. Her temperature is 37°C (98.6°F), and her blood pressure is 70/50 mm Hg. Capillary refill time is 4 to 6 seconds. You administer 100% oxygen using a nonrebreathing face mask and attach an ECG monitor. As you attach the pulse oximeter, the child suddenly collapses and becomes unresponsive, apneic, and pulseless.

- What is your initial assessment and how would you classify this child's physiologic status?

- Which algorithm would you follow as you initiate treatment?

- As you begin treatment, what risk factors for special resuscitation circumstances do you recognize?

Learning Objectives

After completing this chapter the PALS provider should be able to

- Recognize unstable conditions requiring urgent intervention, such as those that produce shock with hypotension, poor end-organ perfusion (with altered consciousness) or sudden collapse, and conditions with high risk for deterioration to arrest rhythms

- Differentiate supraventricular tachycardia (SVT) from sinus tachycardia (ST)

- Describe initial stabilization of the child with an unstable arrhythmia

- Describe indications for vagal maneuvers and use of this technique for treatment of SVT with adequate perfusion

- Describe when and how to provide electrical therapy for arrhythmias:
  - Defibrillation attempts
  - Synchronized cardioversion attempts
  - Pacing

- Describe indications for automated external defibrillation and use of an automated external defibrillator (AED)

- Select appropriate medications for treatment of symptomatic bradycardia (rhythms that are too slow), tachycardia (rhythms that are too fast), and arrest rhythms (those associated with collapse and no pulses)

Introduction

In contrast to cardiac arrest in adults, cardiopulmonary arrest in infants and children is rarely sudden and is more often caused by progression of respiratory distress and failure or shock than by primary cardiac arrhythmias.[1] Most pediatric victims of cardiac arrest demonstrate asystole or bradyarrhythmia, often with a wide QRS complex.[1,2] Pediatric prehospital arrest is generally characterized by progression from respiratory distress with hypoxia and hypercarbia to apnea with associated bradycardia and then cardiac arrest with asystole.[1,3,4] For most seriously ill or injured children, the goals of pediatric advanced life support are to prevent development of cardiac arrest by establishing a patent airway, supporting effective ventilation and oxygenation, and stabilizing circulation.

If a previously well child experiences a *sudden witnessed collapse,* however, primary arrhythmic cardiac arrest may be the cause. High risk for arrhythmia is associated with myocarditis, a sudden sharp blow to the chest (eg, *commotio cordis*), underlying congenital or acquired cardiac disease, a history of arrhythmias, prolonged QT syndrome, severe electrolyte abnormality, profound hypothermia, and drug intoxication.[5-7] If an unexpected arrhythmia is associated with shock or sudden collapse, a defibrillation attempt may be appropriate, and the PALS provider should identify and treat potential reversible causes.

This chapter describes simple, broad categories of arrhythmias (eg, pulse too slow, too fast, or absent), reviews algorithms for assessment and treatment of these arrhythmias, describes important ALS interventions, and concludes with a summary of the medications used in emergency treatment of arrhythmias. Special circumstances associated with rhythm disturbances, such as profound hypothermia, electrocution injury, heart transplant and complex congenital heart disease, may require specialized advanced provider interventions. Extensive discussion of these circumstances is beyond the scope of this chapter.

The Electrocardiogram

The surface ECG is a graphic representation of the sequence of myocardial depolarization and repolarization. Each normal cardiac cycle consists of a P wave, a QRS complex, and a T wave (see Figure 1). Electrical depolarization begins in the sino-atrial node at the junction of the superior vena cava and right atrium and advances through atrial tissue to the atrioventricular (AV) node, where conduction velocity slows temporarily. It then progresses via the bundle of His and the Purkinje system to depolarize the ventricular myocardium (see Figure 2). The first deflection on the surface ECG (P wave) represents depolarization of both atria. The time required for depolarization to pass through the atria, the AV node, and the His-Purkinje system is represented by the PR interval. The QRS complex represents depolarization of the ventricular myocardium. Ventricular repolarization is characterized on the surface ECG as the ST segment and T wave (see Figure 3).

FIGURE 1. The electrocardiogram.

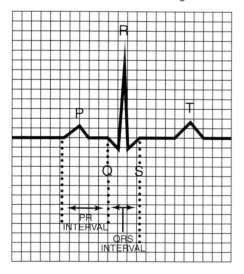

FIGURE 2. The cardiac conduction system.

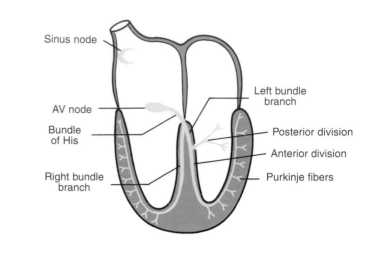

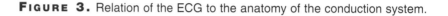

FIGURE 3. Relation of the ECG to the anatomy of the conduction system.

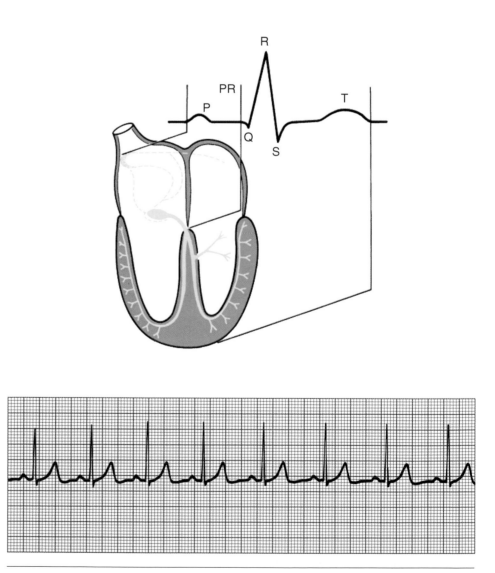

TABLE 1. Heart Rates* in Normal Children

Age	Awake Rate	Mean	Sleeping Rate
Newborn to 3 mo	85 to 205	140	80 to 160
3 mo to 2 years	100 to 190	130	75 to 160
2 to 10 years	60 to 140	80	60 to 90
More than 10 years	60 to 100	75	50 to 90

*Heart rate is measured in beats per minute.
Reproduced from Gillette et al[12] with permission.

The normal heart rate is influenced by the child's age, activity level, and clinical condition. The normal heart rate range gradually declines with age[8-12] (see Table 1), and there is wide variation in the normal heart rate within every age group. The child's temperature, emotional state, and sleep-awake state also influence heart rate.

Children with evidence of respiratory or cardiovascular instability should have continuous ECG monitoring. When arrhythmias are present, a 12-lead ECG is often necessary to supplement continuous bedside (3-lead) monitoring. Monitoring heart rate and rhythm can be helpful in both selection and modification of therapy. Appropriate changes in heart rate or rhythm following interventions may indicate that the patient is responding to therapy. Lack of change or worsening of heart rate or arrhythmia can indicate deterioration in the patient's condition and the need to modify therapy.

The ECG impulse is conducted from the patient to the cardiac monitor through cables attached to the patient with disposable adhesive monitoring pads or metal electrodes and straps. On a normal ECG of good quality, the P waves, QRS complexes, and T waves are visible; the tachometer is triggered by the R wave but not the T wave; and artifact is absent. Place conventional electrodes at the periphery of the anterior chest to avoid interference with cardiopulmonary examination and chest compressions should these become

necessary. Typically you should place electrodes on the shoulders or the lateral chest surfaces; place the ground electrode on the abdomen or thigh (see Figure 4). ECG tracings also can be obtained through transcutaneous monitor/defibrillation/pacing adhesive electrodes on most monitor/defibrillators and some AEDs.

ECG Artifact

The ECG provides information about the *electrical* activity of the heart but not the effectiveness of myocardial contractility or quality of tissue perfusion. Therapy must always be guided by clinical assessment (eg, evaluation of responsiveness, capillary refill, end-organ perfusion, blood pressure) correlated with information derived from the ECG. Artifacts and electrode misplacement or displacement may account for discrepancies between the clinical examination and ECG data. Five of the most common ECG artifacts are

- A straight line (resembling asystole) or a wavy line (resembling coarse fibrillation) may be caused by a loose wire or monitoring electrode
- A tall T wave may be mistaken by the heart rate monitor for an R wave, causing the heart rate to be "double counted" so that the digital heart rate displayed on the monitor will be twice the intrinsic heart (and pulse) rate (see Figure 5A)
- Incorrect lead placement may obscure the P waves (may resemble heart block)
- Muscle or 60-cycle electrical interference artifact (resembling VF; see Figure 5B)
- Motion artifact (chest percussion/physiotherapy or patting the infant can mimic ventricular arrhythmia [see Figure 5C])

Principles of Therapy

Rhythm disturbance in a child should be treated as an emergency if it produces shock with hypotension, poor end-organ perfusion (such as loss of consciousness), or sudden collapse, or if it is at high risk for deteriorating into an arrest rhythm. Many children with rhythm disturbances should be evaluated by a pediatric cardiologist or cardiac rhythm specialist, but this consultation should not delay initiation of emergency treatment.

Cardiac output is the product of heart rate and stroke volume. Within physiologic limits, as the heart rate increases, cardiac output increases. A very slow heart rate can cause shock from inadequate cardiac

FIGURE 4. Placement of electrodes for ECG monitoring.

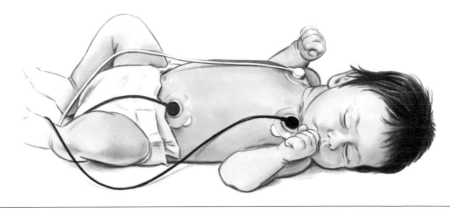

FIGURE 5. **A,** ECG with a tall T wave counted by the monitor tachometer as an R wave. As a result, the digital heart rate displayed is twice the patient's actual intrinsic heart rate. **B,** Asystole with superimposed muscle artifact followed by 60-cycle (60 Hz) artifact resembling VF. **C,** Artifact resembling VT produced by chest physiotherapy. The lower tracing of the arterial waveform demonstrates pulses associated with an underlying sinus rhythm but the ECG artifact caused by chest physiotherapy resembles VT.

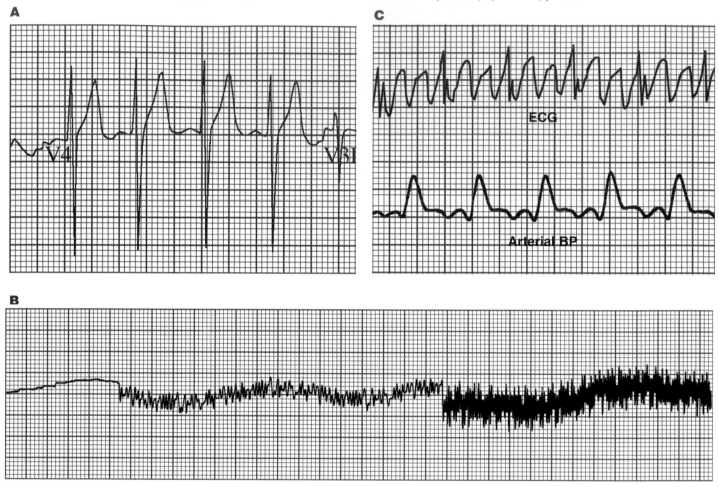

output. Extremely rapid heart rates can compromise stroke volume and cardiac output. When the heart rate becomes so rapid that there is insufficient time for diastolic filling, stroke volume falls. Coronary artery perfusion occurs during diastole; a very rapid heart rate decreases diastole and reduces coronary artery perfusion. A fast heart rate also increases myocardial oxygen demand. A very fast heart rate combined with inadequate cardiac output and poor myocardial blood flow can lead to cardiogenic shock. For assessment of systemic perfusion and signs of shock, see Chapter 2: "Recognition of Respiratory Failure and Shock" and Chapter 7: "Case Scenarios in the Management of Shock."

Classification of Abnormal Rhythms

The PALS provider must be able to broadly classify rhythms by their effect on the pulse, pulse rate, and systemic perfusion (see Critical Concepts: "Broad Classification of Pediatric Arrhythmias"). The urgency of treatment is dictated by the patient's clinical condition.

Hypoxemia is the most frequent cause of *slow rhythms* associated with cardiovascular instability. To treat a symptomatic slow rhythm you should quickly establish a patent airway and provide adequate ventilation and oxygenation. If the slow rhythm persists despite adequate oxygenation and ventilation, medications are needed

to increase heart rate and improve perfusion (ie, sympathomimetics) or to inhibit vagal stimulation (ie, anticholinergics). Patients who do not respond to these interventions may require transcutaneous or transvenous pacing.

SVT and VT are examples of *fast rhythms* associated with cardiovascular instability. *Synchronized cardioversion* is usually the most rapid and effective treatment when these tachyarrhythmias are symptomatic and life-threatening (see below). In synchronized cardioversion the electric shock is synchronized (timed) to be delivered with the patient's R wave. Synchronized cardioversion is the treatment of choice for unstable SVT or VT *with* a detectable pulse and evidence of poor perfusion. It

Critical Concepts:
Broad Classification of Pediatric Arrhythmias

In the setting of an acute emergency, cardiac rhythm disturbances should be broadly classified according to their effect on the central pulses:

- **Slow** pulse rate = bradyarrhythmia
- **Fast** pulse rate = tachyarrhythmia
- **Absent** pulse = pulseless arrest (collapse rhythm)

The cardinal signs of instability associated with arrhythmias are shock with hypotension, poor end-organ perfusion, altered consciousness, and sudden collapse. The rhythm is potentially unstable if it is likely to deteriorate to an arrest rhythm.

Critical Concepts:
Potentially Reversible Causes of Arrest: The 4 H's and 4 T's

Whenever a life-threatening arrhythmia or cardiac arrest develops, the PALS provider should attempt to identify and treat reversible causes of arrest or those requiring a modification of the PALS approach. These reversible causes and special resuscitation circumstances can be recalled with the 4 H's and 4 T's mnemonic:

- **H**ypoxemia
- **H**ypovolemia
- **H**ypothermia
- **H**yper-/**H**ypokalemia and metabolic disorders, including acidosis (some refer to this as a fifth "H"— **H**ydrogen ion—and calcium and magnesium imbalances)

*(Note additional **H**'s for bradycardia: **h**ead injury, **h**eart block, and **h**eart transplant.)*

- **T**amponade (cardiac)
- **T**ension pneumothorax
- **T**oxins/poisons/drugs
- **T**hromboembolism

Remember these H's and T's because they will be referenced throughout this chapter.

may also be used electively in children with stable VT or SVT under the direction of an appropriate specialist.

Collapse rhythms result in absent pulses. VF, pulseless VT, asystole, and all forms of pulseless electrical activity (PEA) are collapse rhythms. VF and pulseless VT require early defibrillation. *Defibrillation is the sudden depolarization of the myocardium that terminates VF or pulseless VT.* The term *return of spontaneous circulation* is used if organized cardiac electrical activity resumes and there is evidence of detectable perfusion (eg, a pulse, blood pressure tracing, etc). If the VF or VT persists despite attempted defibrillation, additional pharmacologic therapy is needed. The PALS provider should identify and treat potentially reversible causes of cardiac arrest (see Critical Concepts: "Potentially Reversible Causes of Arrest: The 4 H's and 4 T's") and modify therapy according to any special resuscitation circumstances that are present (eg, poisoning, severe electrolyte imbalance).

Nonpharmacologic Interventions

The recommended nonpharmacologic interventions used to treat rhythm disturbances are either electrical (defibrillation, synchronized cardioversion, and pacing) or mechanical (vagal maneuvers, pericardiocentesis). Medications for clinically important cardiac rhythm disturbances are briefly discussed as part of the treatment algorithms and then summarized in Table 2 (at the end of this chapter). As

this book went to press, there was no published data on the efficacy of the precordial thump for cardioversion of VT in children. Interventions such as extracorporeal membrane oxygenation (ECMO) and mechanical support of the circulation have been used in the treatment of cardiac arrest, but these therapies are beyond the scope of this text.

Defibrillation

Defibrillation is the treatment for VF or pulseless VT (see FYI: "Management of VT With and Without Pulses"). *Defibrillation* is the sudden depolarization of a critical mass of myocardial cells that terminates VT or VF long enough to allow natural organized myocardial pacemaker activity (automaticity) to resume. Defibrillation does not "jump start" the heart. Instead, a successful shock completely "stuns" the heart into electrical silence, so a brief period of asystole usually follows the shock. Then intrinsic cardiac automaticity can resume if sufficient stores of high-energy phosphates remain in the myocardium (see Figure 6). Attempted defibrillation (shocks) may have 3 outcomes:

- The shock terminates VT/VF and natural automaticity *does* return, and a perfusing rhythm ultimately resumes (see Figure 6).
- The shock terminates VT/VF but automaticity *does not* return, so asystole results.
- The shock does not terminate VT/VF. Persistent VF will eventually progress to electrical silence (ie, asystole).

Termination of fibrillation requires the passage of sufficient electric *current* (amperes or flow of electrons or ions) through the heart. Voltage is the "force" generated by the defibrillator unit that "pushes" that current flow. The *energy* (measured in joules) delivered to the heart is a product of *voltage* (volts), the *current* (amps), and *duration* of the shock (per second). Current delivery to the heart is also influenced by the *waveform* of the current (how the electric current varies with time during delivery of the shock)

FIGURE 6. VF converted to organized rhythm after defibrillation (successful shock).

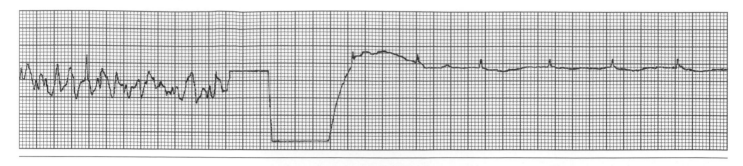

and *resistance* to current flow or *trans-thoracic impedance* (measured in ohms). If transthoracic impedance is high, more energy is required to force sufficient current across the heart to achieve defibrillation or cardioversion.

Transthoracic impedance is *decreased* by a high energy dose, large paddle/electrode pad size, low-impedance (conductive) electrode-skin interface, an increased number of shocks, short intervals between shocks, and firm paddle/electrode pressure. Transthoracic impedance may be *increased* by a low energy dose, small paddle/electrode pad size, poor electrode-skin interface, a lower number of shocks, long intervals between shocks, and inadequate paddle/electrode pressure.[13-18] The shape and size of the child's chest, the size of the heart, and the phases of ventilation can also influence transthoracic impedance.

Ventilation, oxygenation, chest compressions, and pharmacologic therapies may improve the metabolic environment of the myocardium and increase the likelihood of defibrillation even when the heart is refractory to initial shocks.[19,20] Shocks administered in combination with vasopressors or antiarrhythmic medications can be delivered in the sequence "*drug-CPR-shock-drug-CPR-shock*," etc. Alternatively shocks may be delivered in clusters of 3 to decrease transthoracic impedance and increase current flow to the heart. These clusters are separated by drug administration and 30 to 60 seconds of CPR in the sequence "*drug-CPR-shock-shock-shock, drug-CPR-shock-shock-shock*," etc.

FYI: Management of VT With and Without Pulses

VT WITH pulses is treated with attempted synchronized cardioversion (synchronized shock). *VT WITHOUT pulses* is treated like VF with attempted defibrillation (unsynchronized shock). Unsynchronized electrical shocks during repolarization (T wave) can possibly (but rarely) trigger VF or asystole. This is analogous to the "R on T" phenomenon that occurs when a premature ventricular contraction during the T wave precipitates VF. The consequence of delivering a shock during the T wave could inadvertently convert a serious (life-threatening) *organized* rhythm to a lethal *disorganized* rhythm.

When *VT WITH a pulse* is present, use synchronized cardioversion. *VT WITHOUT a pulse* is *not* an effective rhythm (it is not a perfusing rhythm), so the risk of worsening the rhythm has been eliminated. The AHA recommends treating pulseless VT like VF. This encourages rapid delivery of the shock and avoids delays in therapy to analyze the rhythm and attach the 3-lead monitoring cable for synchronization. It also streamlines management and simplifies teaching.

Paddle/Electrode Pad Size

The size of the defibrillator paddle or electrode pad is one determinant of transthoracic impedance: the larger the size, the lower the impedance and the greater the current flow.[21-23] When selecting a paddle or electrode pad, choose the largest size that will allow good contact with the skin over the entire paddle/pad surface but without contact between the 2 paddles/electrodes. Small ("infant") paddles (4.5 cm) should be used for patients up to 1 year of age or 10 kg. This age and weight corresponds to a body length of approximately 30 inches (77 cm) measured with a length-based resuscitation tape. Use large ("adult") paddles (8 to 13 cm) for patients older than 1 year or weighing more than 10 kg or longer than

approximately 30 inches (77 cm). Because the electric current will follow the path of least resistance, the electrode gel or gel pads from one paddle/pad must not touch the gel or gel pads of the other paddle/pad. Such contact could cause bridging, creating a short circuit with current flow between the paddles/electrodes and insufficient delivery of current to the heart.[24]

Electrode Position

Place the paddles/electrode pads so that the heart is between them. Place one paddle on the upper right side of the chest below the clavicle and the other to the left of the left nipple in the anterior axillary line directly over the heart. Alternatively, place paddles or self-adhesive monitor/defibrillator pads in an anterior-posterior position with one just to the left of the sternum and the other over the back.[25] In dextrocardia, position electrode pads in a mirror image of the standard placement. Anterior-posterior placement may be necessary if the patient is an infant and only large paddles are available.

Electrode Interface

The skin acts as a resistor that raises impedance between the paddles/pads and the heart. Apply firm pressure to create good contact between the paddle/pad and the skin. Placing paddles directly on the patient's bare skin without using additional conducting material produces very high chest impedance, decreasing the delivered current.[15] A large amount of hair on the chest may prevent good skin-electrode contact.[26] To improve delivery of current, use a low-impedance interface medium (eg, electrode cream or paste, self-adhesive monitor/defibrillator pads). Saline-soaked gauze pads are not recommended because they often create a bridge between electrodes. Sonographic gels are poor conductors and should not be used. Alcohol pads actually raise impedance and pose a fire hazard, and they can produce chest burns. Repeated shocks may also cause skin burns despite the use of an appropriate electrode interface.[27]

Energy Dose

The optimum energy dose for defibrillation in infants and children has not been established and may vary according to patient- and disease-specific factors. Although the available data has not established a relationship between energy dose per kilogram and successful defibrillation, weight-based pediatric defibrillation doses have been used for more than 20 years. A starting dose of approximately 2 J/kg is recommended.[23,28] If VF persists after the initial shock with 2 J/kg, use a dose of 2 to 4 J/kg and immediately reattempt defibrillation. If a third attempt is necessary, use a dose at 4 J/kg.

When shocks are delivered in rapid succession, transthoracic impedance decreases and current delivered to the heart increases.

The interval between the first and second and the second and third shocks should be just long enough to check the rhythm. If VT/VF persists after 3 defibrillation attempts, additional increases in energy dose are unlikely to increase the efficacy of defibrillation but may increase the patient's risk for myocardial injury. If a shock terminates VF but VF *recurs,* repeat the shock at the dose that terminated fibrillation. Try to identify and treat reversible causes of persistent or recurrent VF or pulseless VT, such as drug intoxication, metabolic disturbance (eg, hyperkalemia), or hypothermia.

Waveforms

Until recently external defibrillators used a monophasic waveform (either damped sinusoidal or truncated exponential). Newer conventional defibrillators and AEDs may use alternative biphasic waveforms that may terminate fibrillation at lower energy doses than monophasic defibrillators.[29] Information on the equivalence of effect with lower energy dosing is accumulating rapidly. Extrapolation of adult evidence suggests that the effective biphasic energy dose may be less than the monophasic energy dose of 2 to 4 J/kg currently recommended for children less than 8 years of age. But the data is inadequate to recommend a biphasic AED energy dose for treatment of VF/pulseless VT in children. As this textbook goes to press, the AHA recommends a monophasic energy dose of 2 to 4 J/kg; when using alternative waveforms, administer a dose that has been shown to produce an equivalent survival rate.

Safety

Electric shocks are potentially dangerous to the operator and others who might have contact with the patient or come in contact with the electric current.[30] Before each defibrillation attempt, make sure that no one is touching the patient. This can be done with a "clear the patient" message announcing that shocks will be delivered. Use a consistent chant such as the following[31]:

1. "I'm going to shock on the count of four. One—I'm clear." Check to make sure that you are not touching the patient, the bed or stretcher, or equipment other than the paddle handles or electrodes.

2. "Two—you're clear." Check to be sure that no one is touching the patient or equipment attached to the patient, such as the tracheal tube, resuscitation bag, and IV solutions.

3. "Three—oxygen's clear." Delivery of a shock while high-concentration oxygen flows across the patient's chest might produce a small spark that could ignite in an oxygen-rich environment.

4. "Four—everybody's clear." Press the SHOCK button to discharge the defibrillator.

For the universal steps in operating a defibrillator, see Critical Concepts: "Typical Defibrillation Sequence." For information about labeling of defibrillator buttons, see FYI: "Defibrillator Buttons."

Testing and Maintenance

The stored and delivered energies of some defibrillators may vary substantially at the very low doses required for infants. Most defibrillators are accurate over a wide range of delivered energies.[22] All defibrillators should be maintained according to the manufacturer's recommendations.

Automated External Defibrillators

Use of AEDs

AEDs are commonly used in the prehospital setting for adults in sudden collapse. The computerized device is attached to the patient with adhesive electrodes. The AED evaluates the victim's ECG to determine if a "shockable" rhythm is present, charges to the appropriate dose, and when activated by the operator, delivers a shock. The AED provides synthesized voice prompts to assist the operator.

In the prehospital setting AEDs are operated by nurses, paramedics, emergency medical technicians, police, rescue personnel, and lay rescuers. The results of

Critical Concepts: Typical Defibrillation Sequence

When VF or pulseless VT is identified, make rapid defibrillation your priority. Provide ongoing CPR. Interrupt CPR only to deliver defibrillatory shocks. The steps in a typical defibrillation sequence are as follows:

■ Apply conductive medium to appropriate-size paddles or attach adhesive electrode pads.

■ POWER ON the defibrillator. Do NOT activate the "sync" mode.

■ Select an energy dose of 2 J/kg and charge the defibrillator.

■ Briefly stop chest compressions and ensure that the paddles/electrodes are in good contact with the chest and are in the proper position.

■ Verify the rhythm (VF/VT) on the monitor.

■ Ensure that no one is touching the patient, the bed or stretcher, or equipment, and make sure that oxygen flow is not directed over the patient's chest ("clear" the victim).

■ Apply firm pressure to the paddles while simultaneously depressing the discharge buttons or discharge the shock from the defibrillator/monitor if "hands-off" pads are used.

■ Assess the rhythm on the monitor; if VF/VT persists, follow the steps below.

■ If VF/VT persists, use an energy dose of 2 to 4 J/kg, charge the defibrillator, "clear" the patient, and deliver the second shock. If VF/VT persists, use a dose of 4 J/kg for the third shock.

■ If cardiac arrest persists after 3 shocks, resume CPR for approximately 1 minute. Administer a vasopressor to increase the likelihood of a response to additional shocks. If VF persists after administration of a vasopressor and an additional shock, consider giving antiarrhythmics.

■ Attempt to identify and treat reversible causes of VF/pulseless VT.

■ If the rhythm becomes organized, confirm that it is a perfusing rhythm and not a form of PEA. If you do not detect a pulse, resume CPR.

FYI: Defibrillator Buttons

The buttons on most commercial defibrillators are labeled with the numbers 1-2-3. These numbers usually indicate the following functions:

1 = Turns on the defibrillator power switch

2 = Selects the energy dose

3 = Charges the defibrillator to the indicated energy

To deliver a shock, you must simultaneously press the 2 SHOCK buttons located on the paddles or press the button on the defibrillator control panel.

All healthcare providers should become familiar with the defibrillator that they are likely to use in their clinical practice.

---

several studies have shown that the widespread availability of AEDs in the hands of trained lay rescuers has shortened the time to defibrillation and improved survival rates for adult victims of prehospital cardiac arrest.[32-34] AEDs are also used in hospitals.

Experience with AEDs in children is very limited. The sensitivity and specificity of the AED VF-recognition algorithms for children need further study. The available data suggests that AEDs can accurately detect VF in children of all ages,[35-37] but questions have been raised about the ability of the AED to correctly distinguish between tachycardic nonarrest rhythms and VF/VT in infants.[37]

Additionally, AEDs were designed to deliver only adult energy doses. Intense interest in these topics prompted the AHA, in conjunction with the International Liaison Committee on Resuscitation, to conduct an evaluation of the AED rhythm analysis data and the technical advances that have been made by the AED manufacturers.[37a] The conclusions of that review and the ILCOR recommendations for pediatric use of AEDs are listed on page 57 of this text.

All healthcare providers should be trained in the use of an AED, including special resuscitation circumstances (see Critical Concepts: "Special Circumstances That May Require Modification of AED Use") and AED troubleshooting. Until data on the safety and efficacy of AEDs suggests the equivalency of these devices with manual defibrillators, healthcare providers who routinely care for children at risk for arrhythmias and cardiac arrest (eg, in-hospital setting) should continue to use defibrillators that can deliver appropriate and adjustable pediatric energy doses.

Critical Steps in AED Use

In the prehospital setting, use of AEDs for children 1 to 8 years of age with sudden collapse cardiac arrest carries a Class IIb recommendation.

The steps for AED use are as follows (see Figure 7):

■ *POWER ON* the AED (turn it on).

■ *Attach* child electrode pads to the patient's chest (right upper sternal border, left chest under the arm at the level of the left nipple). If the child is 8 years of age or older attach *adult* pads.

■ *"Clear"* the patient *and analyze* the rhythm.

■ If a shock is indicated, *"clear"* the patient *and* deliver a *shock*.

Critical Concepts:
Special Circumstances That May Require Modification of AED Use

1. *Children less than 1 year of age or less than approximately 9 kg in weight:* For these children the use of AEDs is a Class Indeterminate recommendation (see text).

2. *Victim in standing water:* Remove the victim from the water and dry the victim's chest.

3. *Victim with implanted defibrillator/ pacemaker:* Do not place an electrode pad directly over the implanted device because the device may block current and reduce delivery of current to the heart.

4. *Victim with a transdermal medication patch:* Do not place an electrode pad directly over a medication patch. If the patch is in the way, remove the patch and wipe the victim's skin before attaching the AED.

If needed, repeat shocks to a total of 3 shocks; after 3 shocks or when the AED indicates *"no shock indicated,"* check the airway, breathing, and circulation, and provide the steps of CPR as needed for 1 minute, then reanalyze the rhythm and provide additional shocks.

It is important to note that basic life support with rescue breathing and chest compressions remains the initial treatment of choice for victims of all ages in cardiac arrest associated with asphyxia (eg, after submersion).

Synchronized Cardioversion

Synchronized cardioversion is the specifically *timed* delivery of a shock to the heart that successfully terminates the rapid rhythm. Synchronization of delivered energy with the ECG R wave reduces the possibility of inducing VF because it avoids delivery of the electrical impulse during the "vulnerable period" (the T wave) of the cardiac cycle.[38]

Synchronized cardioversion is the treatment of choice for patients with tachyarrhythmias (SVT, VT with pulses, atrial flutter) who have a *perfusing rhythm* and

---

evidence of cardiovascular compromise, such as poor perfusion, hypotension, or heart failure. It may also be used electively in children with stable VT or SVT at the direction of an appropriate cardiology specialist.

The initial energy dose for synchronized cardioversion is 0.5 to 1 J/kg. If tachyarrhythmia persists after the first attempt, double the dose to 1 to 2 J/kg. If the rhythm does not convert to sinus rhythm, reevaluate the diagnosis of SVT versus ST.

Electrical cardioversion can be frightening and painful for a child. Therefore, whenever possible, establish vascular access and provide sedation with analgesia before cardioversion, particularly when the cardioversion is elective. If the patient's condition is unstable, however, *do not delay* synchronized cardioversion to achieve vascular access.

Critical Steps in Synchronized Cardioversion

Provide appropriate support and monitoring of oxygenation and ventilation throughout the procedure. The procedure for synchronized cardioversion is the same as that outlined for defibrillation (see above), with the following exceptions:

Critical Concepts: A Comparison of Defibrillation With Synchronized Cardioversion

Defibrillation	Synchronized Cardioversion
■ *Not* synchronized with ECG	■ *Synchronized* with ECG
■ Used for *pulseless* rhythms (VF and pulseless VT)	■ Used for rhythms *with pulses* (symptomatic VT and SVT with pulses)
■ Dose: 2 J/kg, then	■ Dose: 0.5 to 1 J/kg, then 1 to 2 J/kg (consider sedation)
■ 2 to 4 J/kg, then 4 J/kg*	

Note: Historically the AHA has recommended pediatric defibrillation doses of 2 J/kg, then 4 J/kg for subsequent doses. Internationally, defibrillation doses of 2 J/kg, 2 to 4 J/kg, and 4 J/kg are used for pediatric defibrillation, so these doses were included in the *ECC Guidelines 2000* and the pulseless arrest algorithm. Either dose progression is acceptable.

- Use sedation with analgesia for elective cardioversion attempts unless otherwise contraindicated.

- Attach the ECG leads to the patient (so that the defibrillator/monitor can sense the ECG and time the electrical discharge).

- Make sure that the lead select switch is in the lead I, II, or III position and not in the "paddle" position.

- Place the defibrillator in the *sync* mode before *each* cardioversion attempt. In the sync mode, an indicator on the monitor should mark each detected R wave. If the sync indicator is not seen, adjust the ECG size on the monitor; then change the lead select switch to each of the 3 settings (I, II, III but *not* to the "paddle" position) until you find a lead that consistently displays the sync indicator.

- Depress the discharge buttons and hold until the shock is delivered (this will often require detection of 2 to 3 QRS complexes).

Noninvasive (Transcutaneous) Pacing

Noninvasive transcutaneous pacing has been used to treat adults with bradycardia and asystole,[39] but experience with children is limited.[40-43] Transcutaneous pacing has *not* been effective in improving the survival rate of children with out-of-hospital unwitnessed cardiac arrest.[41] However, in selected cases of bradycardia caused by complete heart block or abnormal sinus node function, emergency transcutaneous pacing may be lifesaving.[44] Pacing is not helpful in children with bradycardia secondary to a postarrest hypoxic/ischemic myocardial insult or respiratory failure.[41]

This form of pacing may be painful in a conscious patient, so its use is reserved for children with profound and refractory symptomatic bradycardia. Alternative forms of noninvasive pacing (transesophageal) and invasive pacing (transthoracic, transvenous) usually require subspecialty con-

sultation and are beyond the scope of this text.

The transcutaneous pacing system consists of an external pacing unit and 2 large adhesive-backed electrodes. Pediatric (small or medium) electrodes are recommended for a child who weighs less than 15 kg.[44] Adult-size electrodes are recommended for the child who weighs more than 15 kg. Place the electrodes so that the electric charge passes from the negative electrode through the heart to the positive electrode. *Place the negative electrode over the heart* on the anterior chest and the positive electrode behind the heart on the back. If the positive electrode cannot be placed on the back, place it on the right side of the anterior chest beneath the clavicle with the negative electrode on the left side of the chest over the fourth intercostal space, in the midaxillary area. Precise placement of electrodes does not appear to be necessary, provided that the negative electrode is placed near the apex of the heart.[45] Do not place the electrode directly over an implanted pacemaker or defibrillator because these devices will block passage of some current to the heart (see FYI: "Transcutaneous Pacing of Patients With Implanted Pacemaker/Defibrillators").

For emergency treatment of bradycardic rhythms, set the transcutaneous pacer to start at a rate of 100 bpm (see Figure 8). Set output at maximum and then rapidly adjust downward to slightly above the minimum level that consistently produces ventricular capture.

Either ventricular fixed-rate or ventricular-inhibited pacing may be provided noninvasively. During ventricular-inhibited pacing, the pacemaker does not deliver an impulse if the patient's intrinsic (spontaneous) ventricular activity is detected at a rate above the present minimum (demand) rate. Adjust pacemaker output to ensure that every impulse results in ventricular depolarization (capture).[39] This means that every pacer spike is followed by a ventricular electrical response and repolarization. If ventricular-inhibited pacing is used, you must also adjust the sensitivity of the pacemaker detector circuit to ensure that the pacemaker senses the patient's intrinsic ventricular electrical activity. The large pacing artifact that often occurs with transcutaneous pacing may make it difficult to determine if ventricular capture (depolarization following the pacer spike) is taking place. You can detect the mechanical effects of the depolarization if you palpate a pulse or observe the arterial pressure tracing from an indwelling arterial catheter.

Vagal Maneuvers

In normal infants and children, the heart rate falls with stimulation of the vagus nerve. In patients with SVT, vagal stimulation may terminate the tachycardia by slowing conduction through the AV node. Several maneuvers stimulate vagal activity. The success rates of these maneuvers in terminating tachyarrhythmias vary, depending on the child's underlying condition, level of cooperation, and age. In infants and young children, the most effective vagal maneuver is the *applica-*

FYI: Transcutaneous Pacing of Patients With Implanted Pacemaker/Defibrillators

If you attempt transcutaneous pacing for a patient with an implanted pacemaker or defibrillator, do not position the pacing electrodes directly over the internal pacemaker or defibrillator device ("box"). The device will block delivery of some current to the heart. As you would for any transcutaneous pacer, place the electrodes so that the electric charge traverses the heart from the negative electrode to the opposite positive electrode.

FIGURE 7. AED treatment algorithm for prehospital care of children 1 to 8 years of age or older for emergency cardiovascular care pending arrival of emergency medical personnel.

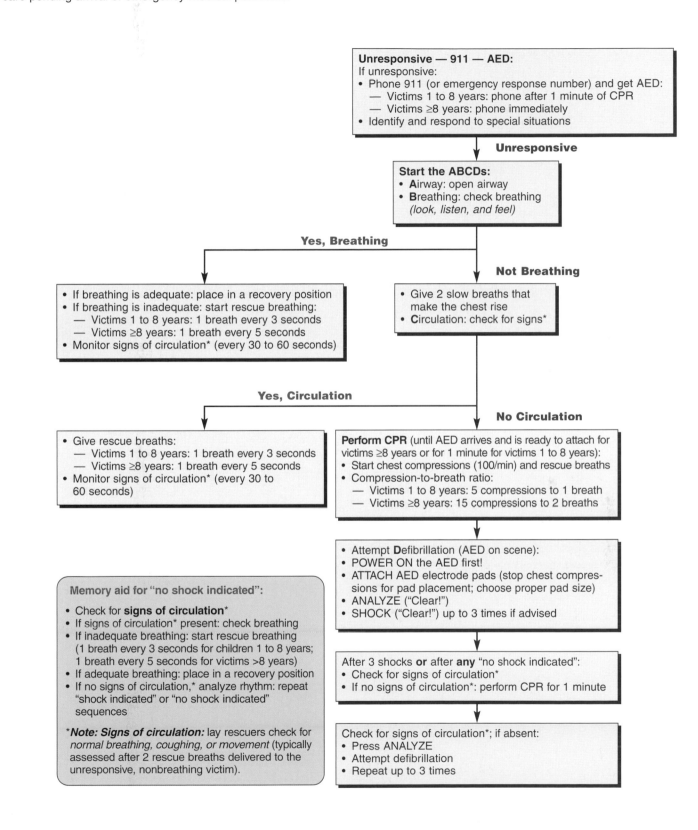

Unresponsive — 911 — AED:
If unresponsive:
- Phone 911 (or emergency response number) and get AED:
  — Victims 1 to 8 years: phone after 1 minute of CPR
  — Victims ≥8 years: phone immediately
- Identify and respond to special situations

Unresponsive

Start the ABCDs:
- **A**irway: open airway
- **B**reathing: check breathing *(look, listen, and feel)*

Yes, Breathing

Not Breathing

- If breathing is adequate: place in a recovery position
- If breathing is inadequate: start rescue breathing:
  — Victims 1 to 8 years: 1 breath every 3 seconds
  — Victims ≥8 years: 1 breath every 5 seconds
- Monitor signs of circulation* (every 30 to 60 seconds)

- Give 2 slow breaths that make the chest rise
- **C**irculation: check for signs*

Yes, Circulation

No Circulation

- Give rescue breaths:
  — Victims 1 to 8 years: 1 breath every 3 seconds
  — Victims ≥8 years: 1 breath every 5 seconds
- Monitor signs of circulation* (every 30 to 60 seconds)

Perform CPR (until AED arrives and is ready to attach for victims ≥8 years or for 1 minute for victims 1 to 8 years):
- Start chest compressions (100/min) and rescue breaths
- Compression-to-breath ratio:
  — Victims 1 to 8 years: 5 compressions to 1 breath
  — Victims ≥8 years: 15 compressions to 2 breaths

- Attempt **D**efibrillation (AED on scene):
- POWER ON the AED first!
- ATTACH AED electrode pads (stop chest compressions for pad placement; choose proper pad size)
- ANALYZE ("Clear!")
- SHOCK ("Clear!") up to 3 times if advised

Memory aid for "no shock indicated":

- Check for **signs of circulation***
- If signs of circulation* present: check breathing
- If inadequate breathing: start rescue breathing (1 breath every 3 seconds for children 1 to 8 years; 1 breath every 5 seconds for victims >8 years)
- If adequate breathing: place in a recovery position
- If no signs of circulation,* analyze rhythm: repeat "shock indicated" or "no shock indicated" sequences

*__Note: Signs of circulation:__ lay rescuers check for *normal breathing, coughing, or movement* (typically assessed after 2 rescue breaths delivered to the unresponsive, nonbreathing victim).

After 3 shocks **or** after **any** "no shock indicated":
- Check for signs of circulation*
- If no signs of circulation*: perform CPR for 1 minute

Check for signs of circulation*; if absent:
- Press ANALYZE
- Attempt defibrillation
- Repeat up to 3 times

FIGURE 8. Initiation of transcutaneous pacing for a child with severe symptomatic bradycardia. The pacemaker is set at a demand rate of 100 bpm with maximum output so capture is achieved immediately. A QRS complex consistently follows each pacer spike.

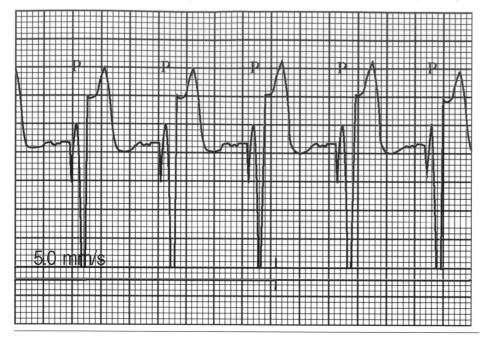

5.0 mm/s

the ventricles and reduces cardiac output. As the heart becomes ischemic, the risk of arrhythmia increases. Cardiac tamponade is most often seen in patients with penetrating trauma or following open heart surgery. The treatment of cardiac tamponade is pericardial drainage with the pericardiocentesis procedure described in Chapter 10: "Trauma Resuscitation and Spinal Immobilization."

Some patients with cardiac tamponade will improve substantially with a combination of volume bolus and pericardial drainage. Elective pericardiocentesis should be performed by specialists who are trained and skilled in the procedure; monitoring and sedation with analgesia are appropriate. Emergency pericardiocentesis may be performed in the setting of impending or actual pulseless arrest when there is strong suspicion of pericardial tamponade.

tion of ice to the face.[46,47] One method of doing this is to mix crushed ice with water in a plastic bag or glove (Figure 9). While recording the ECG, apply the ice water mixture to the infant's face for only 10 to 15 seconds. Do not obstruct ventilation (ie, cover only the forehead, the eyes, and the bridge of the nose). If this method is successful, SVT will terminate in seconds. If the patient is stable, you may repeat the attempt. If the second attempt fails, select another method or provide pharmacologic therapy. If the patient is unstable, attempt vagal maneuvers only while making preparations for pharmacologic or electrical cardioversion. Do not delay cardioversion.

Other vagal maneuvers (ie, carotid sinus massage or the Valsalva maneuver) may be effective, and they appear to be safe based on data obtained largely in older children, adolescents, and adults.[48-50] Children can perform a *Valsalva maneuver* by blowing through an obstructed straw.[49] Some methods to induce vagal activity, such as application of external ocular pressure and carotid massage, may cause complications and should not be used.

Be sure to obtain a 12-lead ECG before and after the maneuver and record and monitor the ECG continuously during the vagal maneuver.

Emergency Pericardiocentesis

Pericardial tamponade results when fluid filling the pericardial sac compresses the heart, prevents adequate venous refill of

Assessment and Management of Symptomatic Pediatric Arrhythmias
Bradyarrhythmias: "TOO SLOW"

Bradycardia is a heart rate that is slow (typically less than 60 bpm) compared with normative heart rates for the patient's

FIGURE 9. Ice water is applied to the infant's face for vagal stimulation in an attempt to terminate SVT. Note that the bag of ice water does *not* cover the nares or mouth and does not obstruct ventilation.

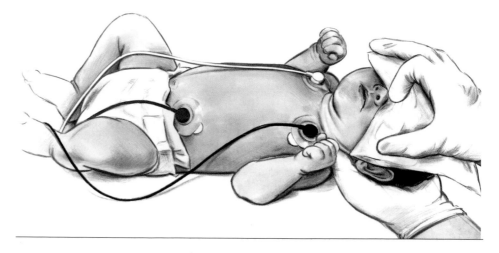

age. Clinically significant bradycardia is defined as a heart rate less than 60 bpm associated with poor systemic perfusion. Bradyarrhythmias are the most common prearrest rhythm in the pediatric patient[51-53] and are often associated with hypoxemia, hypotension, and acidosis. These conditions slow conduction through the sinus node and AV junction (see FYI: "ECG Characteristics of Bradycardia").

Sinus bradycardia (see Figure 10A), sinus node arrest with a slow junctional (Figure 10B) or ventricular escape rhythm, and various degrees of AV block are examples of bradyarrhythmias.[53] Other causes of symptomatic bradycardia are excessive vagal stimulation (eg, induced by suctioning or tracheal intubation), hypothermia, toxins and drugs (eg, digoxin, calcium channel blocker, or β-blocker overdose), congenital heart block, congenital heart surgery with associated heart block, heart transplant, inflammatory myocarditis, and central nervous system insults (eg, increased intracranial pressure or brainstem inflammation/ compression).

All slow rhythms that result in shock or life-threatening hemodynamic instability require immediate treatment with support of the airway, oxygenation, and ventilation. In addition, the provider must identify and treat reversible causes (see Critical Concepts: "Potential Causes of Bradycardia ").

Management of Symptomatic Bradycardia

General Principles

Most clinically significant bradycardic rhythms in infants and children are caused by hypoxemia, so immediate support of airway, ventilation, and oxygenation is warranted. Chest compressions are indicated for a heart rate less than 60 bpm associated with poor systemic perfusion (see Figure 11 and Critical Concepts: "Overview of Pediatric Bradycardia Algorithm").

Drug Therapy

Epinephrine. Administer epinephrine if symptomatic bradycardia persists despite effective oxygenation and ventilation. Epinephrine may be given IV or IO in a dose of 0.01 mg/kg (0.1 mL/kg of 1:10 000 solution) or tracheally in a dose of 0.1 mg/kg (0.1 mL/kg of 1:1000 solution)—or so-called "high-dose epinephrine." The action of catecholamines may be reduced by acidosis and hypoxemia,[54,55] making support of the airway, ventilation, oxygenation, and perfusion (with chest compressions) essential. A continuous epinephrine infusion (0.1 to 0.2 μg/kg per minute titrated to effect; higher doses may be required)

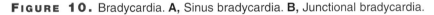

FIGURE 10. Bradycardia. **A,** Sinus bradycardia. **B,** Junctional bradycardia.

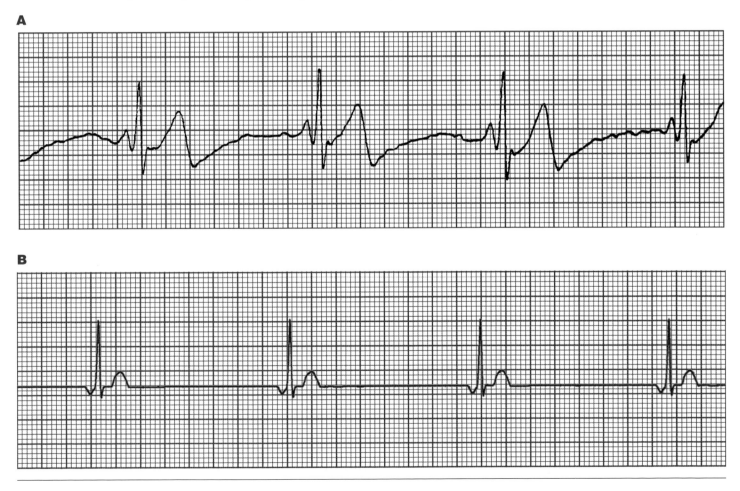

or dopamine (2 to 20 µg/kg per minute) may be useful.

Atropine. If vagal stimulation or cholinergic drug toxicity is suspected, administer atropine. Atropine sulfate is a parasympatholytic drug that accelerates sinus or atrial pacemakers and enhances AV conduction. If bradycardia is known or strongly suspected to be caused by increased vagal tone or primary AV heart block, administer atropine preferentially after establishment of oxygenation and ventilation. Atropine or atropine-like drugs are often used prophylactically in young children to prevent vagally mediated bradycardia during tracheal intubation attempts. Although atropine may be used to treat bradycardia accompanied by poor perfusion or hypotension, epinephrine may be more effective in treating such bradycardia.

The recommended IV/IO dose of atropine is 0.02 mg/kg, with a minimum dose of 0.1 mg and a maximum single dose of 0.5 mg in a child and 1 mg in an adolescent.[56] The dose may be repeated in 5 minutes to a maximum total dose of 1 mg in a child and 2 mg in an adolescent. (See Chapter 5: "Fluid Therapy and Medications for Cardiac Arrest and Shock.") If IV access is not readily available, atropine (0.02 mg/kg) may be administered tracheally,[57] although absorption into the circulation may be unreliable and a larger dose may be required.[58] Note that small doses of atropine may produce para-

Critical Concepts: Potential Causes of Bradycardia

Clinically significant bradycardia is defined as a heart rate less than 60 bpm associated with poor systemic perfusion (ie, the heart rate is too slow for the clinical condition). The initial treatment of this bradycardia is immediate support of the airway and provision of oxygenation, ventilation, and chest compressions. The provider should identify and treat potential reversible causes of refractory bradycardia, including the H's and T's and additional causes, including the following.*

- **H**ypoxemia
- **H**ypothermia
- **H**ead injury (treat increased intracranial pressure)
- **H**eart block (consider atropine, chronotropic drugs, and early pacing)
- **H**eart transplant (sympathetic and vagal denervation)
- **T**oxins/poisons/drugs (especially organophosphates, β-blockers and clonidine)
- **I**ncreased vagal tone. Administer atropine if bradycardia may be caused by increased vagal tone, cholinergic drug toxicity (eg, organophosphates), or AV block.

*Note that this mnemonic is modified from the 4 H's and 4 T's.

doxical bradycardia[56]; for this reason a minimum dose of 0.1 mg is recommended. Large intravascular doses may be required in special resuscitation circumstances such as organophosphate poisoning. Tachycardia may follow administration of atropine, but the agent is generally well tolerated in the pediatric patient.

Pacing

Appropriately trained and equipped providers may consider early pacing for the treatment of symptomatic bradycardia. Pacing is *not* helpful in children with asystole or with bradycardia secondary to a postarrest hypoxic/ischemic myocardial insult or respiratory failure.[41] External pacing may provide a bridge for children with profound refractory symptomatic bradycardia, particularly when caused by underlying congenital or acquired heart disease, producing complete heart block or sinus node dysfunction.[42-44] Many monitor/defibrillators also have the capability for transcutaneous pacing. If transcutaneous pacing is successful, a cardiology consultation is indicated to consider alternative forms of pacing that will limit discomfort and to ensure a more reliable method of ongoing cardiac pacing.

A review of alternative forms of pacing such as transesophageal, transthoracic, or transvenous pacing is beyond the scope of this text. (See the section "Noninvasive [Transcutaneous] Pacing" under "Nonpharmacologic Interventions.")

Tachyarrhythmias: "TOO FAST"

This section discusses the major categories of tachyarrhythmias and presents assessment and management algorithms. A tachyarrhythmia is a rapid heart rate that may or may not be appropriate for the child's clinical condition. All rapid rhythms that result in shock and life-threatening hemodynamic instability require immediate treatment.

The pediatric tachycardia algorithms assume that the PALS provider who encounters an infant or a child with a rapid heart rate and pulse has access to the technology to assess the rhythm (see Critical Concepts: "Initial Evaluation of Tachyarrhythmias"). The treatment approach assumes that *the child has a pulse* and signs of perfusion. The provider then selects the tachycardia algorithm based on the quality of the child's perfusion. The pediatric tachycardia algorithm for infants and children with

FIGURE 11. Pediatric bradycardia algorithm.

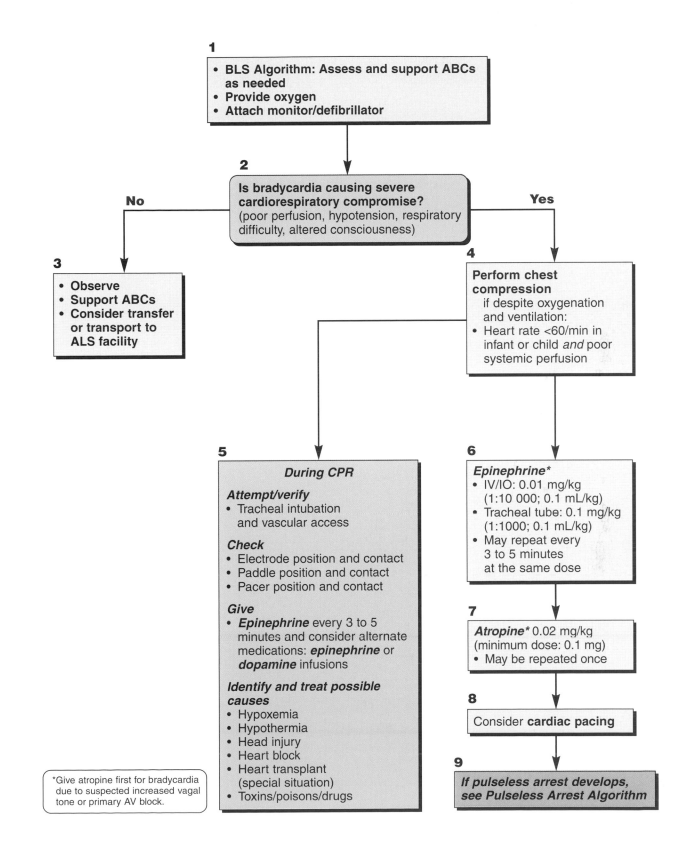

1
- **BLS Algorithm: Assess and support ABCs as needed**
- **Provide oxygen**
- **Attach monitor/defibrillator**

2
Is bradycardia causing severe cardiorespiratory compromise?
(poor perfusion, hypotension, respiratory difficulty, altered consciousness)

No

Yes

3
- **Observe**
- **Support ABCs**
- **Consider transfer or transport to ALS facility**

4
Perform chest compression
if despite oxygenation and ventilation:
- Heart rate <60/min in infant or child *and* poor systemic perfusion

5
During CPR

Attempt/verify
- Tracheal intubation and vascular access

Check
- Electrode position and contact
- Paddle position and contact
- Pacer position and contact

Give
- *Epinephrine* every 3 to 5 minutes and consider alternate medications: *epinephrine* or *dopamine* infusions

Identify and treat possible causes
- Hypoxemia
- Hypothermia
- Head injury
- Heart block
- Heart transplant (special situation)
- Toxins/poisons/drugs

6
*Epinephrine**
- IV/IO: 0.01 mg/kg (1:10 000; 0.1 mL/kg)
- Tracheal tube: 0.1 mg/kg (1:1000; 0.1 mL/kg)
- May repeat every 3 to 5 minutes at the same dose

7
*Atropine** 0.02 mg/kg (minimum dose: 0.1 mg)
- May be repeated once

8
Consider **cardiac pacing**

9
If pulseless arrest develops, see Pulseless Arrest Algorithm

*Give atropine first for bradycardia due to suspected increased vagal tone or primary AV block.

Critical Concepts: Overview of Pediatric Bradycardia Algorithm

Note to providers: Refer to the numbered boxes and ovals in the algorithm.

Box 1: Assess the patient. Assess and support the ABCs as needed; attach a continuous ECG monitor (with transcutaneous pacer/defibrillator capability if available) and a pulse oximeter. Although a 12-lead ECG may be useful, a precise ECG diagnosis of the bradyarrhythmia is not immediately required. Do not delay therapy if severe symptoms are present.

Box 2: Determine if bradycardia is associated with severe cardiorespiratory compromise. Clinically significant bradycardia is defined as a heart rate of less than 60 bpm associated with evidence of poor systemic perfusion, such as shock with hypotension or poor end-organ perfusion, respiratory difficulty, hypoventilation, or altered consciousness.

Box 3: If the bradycardia is *not* associated with evidence of poor perfusion, plan to reassess the patient and observe and support the ABCs. Arrange for further evaluation as needed.

Box 4: If bradycardia *is* associated with severe cardiorespiratory compromise despite effective oxygenation and ventilation, provide chest compressions.

Box 5: During therapy, attempt tracheal intubation and verify tracheal tube position with primary and secondary confirmation techniques. *Hypoxemia* is the leading cause of rhythms that are too slow. Check all equipment and ensure effective oxygenation and ventilation. Establish vascular access. Check paddle/electrode position and contact to ensure that there are no artifacts and that the ECG tracing is accurate. Give epinephrine every 3 to 5 minutes and consider infusing alternative medications (see below). Identify and treat the following potentially reversible causes and special circumstances:

- **Hypoxemia:** Give oxygen.

- **Hypothermia:** Treat with simple warming techniques.

- Head injury with elevated intracranial pressure or brainstem compromise. Provide oxygenation and ventilation, and if signs of herniation are present, provide mild hyperventilation (see "Head Injury, Herniation Syndromes" in Chapter 10).

- Heart block may result from a variety of congenital or acquired conditions. Consider electrical pacing and consultation with an expert.

- Heart transplant recipients often have "denervated hearts," so they may require large doses of sympathomimetics or electrical pacing. Anticholinergic medication may not be effective because transplanted hearts lack vagal innervation.

- Toxins/poisons/drugs may require a specific antidote or modification of ALS. Bradyarrhythmias may develop after poisoning by organophosphates, calcium channel blockers, β-blockers (see Chapter 12), digoxin, and clonidine.

Box 6: Administer epinephrine. Epinephrine may improve heart rate and blood pressure. Administer a dose of 0.01 mg/kg (0.1 mL/kg of 1:10 000 solution) by the IV or IO route or 0.1 mg/kg (0.1 mL/kg of 1:1000 solution) by the tracheal route. For persistent bradycardia, consider continuous infusion of epinephrine (0.1 to 0.2 µg/kg per minute) or dopamine (2 to 20 µg/kg per minute); titrate infusion dose to clinical response.

Box 7: Consider atropine. If you think the bradycardia is caused by increased vagal tone or primary AV heart block, administer atropine preferentially. Administer an IV/IO dose of 0.02 mg/kg (minimum 0.1 mg and maximum single dose of 0.5 mg for a child and 1 mg for an adolescent).[56] You may repeat the dose in 5 minutes (maximum total dose of 1 mg for a child and 2 mg for an adolescent). Larger doses may be required for organophosphate poisoning.[58] If IV access is not available, administer atropine (0.02 mg/kg) tracheally[57] (absorption unreliable[58]). Tachycardia may develop.

Box 8: Consider cardiac pacing. In selected cases of bradycardia caused by complete heart block or abnormal sinus node function, emergent pacing may be lifesaving.[42-44]

Box 9: If pulseless arrest or other rhythms develop, refer to the appropriate algorithm with continued support of adequate ventilation and oxygenation.

---

evidence of poor perfusion should be used if the child shows signs of severe cardiorespiratory compromise thought to be related to the tachyarrhythmia:

- Shock with hypotension or poor end-organ perfusion

- Altered consciousness

- Sudden collapse with rapid detectable pulsatile perfusion (pulse or evidence of perfusion)

Sinus Tachycardia

ST is defined as a rate of sinus node discharge higher than normal for the patient's age that typically develops in response to the body's need for increased cardiac output or oxygen delivery. ST is a nonspecific clinical sign rather than a true arrhythmia (see Figure 12). Hypoxemia, hypovolemia (blood loss), hyperthermia (fever), metabolic stress, toxins/poisons/drugs, and pain or anxiety are common causes of ST.

FIGURE 12. ST (heart rate 180 bpm) in a febrile 10-month-old infant. QRS duration is normal for age (less than 0.08 second). There is a history of fever compatible with a high heart rate, P waves are present and normal, and there is mild heart rate variability with a constant PR interval.

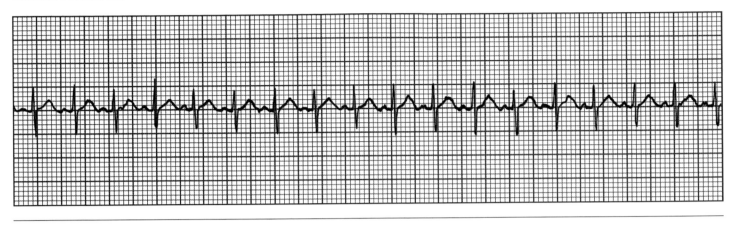

Pericardial tamponade, tension pneumothorax, and thromboembolism are less common causes.

Management of ST

To correct ST you should treat the underlying cause. Because tachycardia is a *symptom*, you should not attempt to decrease heart rate by pharmacologic or electrical interventions. Continuous ECG monitoring will confirm a decrease in heart rate to more normal levels if treatment of the underlying cause is appropriate.

Supraventricular Tachycardia

SVT is the most common tachyarrhythmia that produces cardiovascular compromise during infancy. SVT (see Figure 13) is a rapid and regular rhythm that can appear intermittently and can recur, often with paroxysms (eg, abrupt onset). It is most commonly caused by a reentry mechanism that involves an accessory pathway or the AV conduction system. In infants SVT generally produces a heart rate greater than 220 bpm and sometimes as high as 300 bpm. Lower rates are observed in children. In most infants with SVT (60%), the heart rate is greater than 230 bpm.[59] In more than 90% of children with SVT, the QRS complex is narrow (ie, ≤0.08 second).[60]

Although SVT is initially well tolerated in most infants and older children, it can lead to congestive heart failure, cardio-

vascular collapse, and clinical evidence of shock, particularly if myocardial function is impaired.[61,62] Cardiopulmonary function during episodes of SVT is affected by the child's age, duration of SVT, prior ventricular function, and ventricular rate. Older children will typically complain of lightheadedness, dizziness, or chest discomfort, or simply note the fast heart rate. In infants, however, very rapid rates may go undetected for long periods until cardiac output is significantly impaired. This deterioration in cardiac function results from the combination of increased myocardial oxygen demand and limitation in

myocardial oxygen delivery during the short diastolic phase associated with very rapid heart rates.

If baseline myocardial function is impaired (eg, in a child with congenital heart disease or a cardiomyopathy), SVT can produce signs of shock in a relatively short time. It may be difficult to differentiate SVT as the primary cause of shock from ST as an appropriate compensatory response to a shock state of another etiology.

The following characteristics may aid in differentiation of ST and SVT (see Critical Concepts: "Comparison of ST and SVT"):

Critical Concepts: Initial Evaluation of Tachyarrhythmias

Answer 2 initial questions when evaluating the circulatory status of a seriously ill patient with a rapid heart rate:

- **Does the patient have a pulse and signs of circulation?**

  If the patient has a rapid pulse, continue with the tachycardia algorithm. If the patient has no pulse, initiate the pulseless arrest algorithm.

- **Is perfusion adequate or poor?**

  — If *perfusion is adequate* and the rhythm is *rapid*, proceed

to the algorithm for tachycardia *with adequate perfusion* and consider consulting a pediatric cardiology specialist.

— If there is evidence of *shock or poor perfusion, proceed immediately to the algorithm for tachycardia with poor perfusion* for emergency treatment.

It is appropriate to consult with a pediatric cardiology specialist, but do not delay initial therapy and stabilization.

FIGURE 13. SVT in a 10-month-old infant with no history of fever, pain, medications, or dehydration. The heart rate is approximately 300 bpm with no beat-to-beat variability. There is no history that would explain ST, and P waves are not normal.

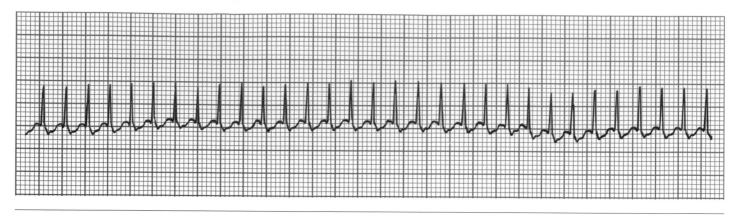

- The child with ST usually has a history consistent with shock unrelated to the cardiac rhythm (eg, dehydration or hemorrhage); the child with SVT has a history that is incompatible or inconsistent with ST (ie, no causes of shock such as trauma or dehydration, no fever or pain that could explain a high heart rate) and may have a history of vague signs of distress.

- P waves may be difficult to identify in both ST and SVT once the ventricular rate exceeds 200 bpm. If P waves can be identified, in ST they are normal and uniform in appearance, and they are usually upright in leads I and aVF. In SVT, P waves are often absent or abnormal. If present, they are negative in leads II, III, and aVF.

- In ST the heart rate usually varies with activity or stimulation. In SVT the heart rate rarely deviates from the baseline rate, regardless of activity or stimulation.

- In ST the heart rate slows gradually if the cause of ST is treated. Frequently there is beat-to-beat variability (variable R-R interval) with a constant PR interval. In SVT the onset and termination are abrupt, and there is minimal beat-to-beat variability during the tachycardia.

- In infants with ST, the heart rate is usually less than 220 bpm; in children with ST, the heart rate is less than 180 bpm. In infants with SVT, the heart rate is typically greater than 220 bpm;

in children with SVT, the heart rate is greater than 180 bpm.

Wide-QRS SVT (ie, SVT with aberrant conduction producing a QRS greater than 0.08 second) is uncommon. Correct diagnosis and differentiation of SVT with aberrant conduction from VT requires careful analysis of at least one 12-lead ECG that may be supplemented by information from an esophageal lead. Both SVT and VT can cause hemodynamic instability, so evidence of shock is not helpful for differentiating them. For simplicity of training the noncardiology specialist, emergency treatment of wide-complex tachycardias should initially be directed toward VT (see "Management of VT").

Management of SVT

General Principles and Cardioversion

Treat SVT with *poor perfusion* (eg, congestive heart failure with poor peripheral perfusion, increased work of breathing, and altered level of consciousness, or shock with hypotension) with immediate electrical or chemical cardioversion. Support the ABCs and obtain a 12-lead ECG to confirm the diagnosis if it can be done quickly. Synchronized electrical cardioversion is recommended, although adenosine may be administered if IV or IO access is immediately available. Cardioversion should *not* be delayed to establish vascular access if the patient's condition is unstable. During preparation for electrical or chemical cardioversion, you

---

Critical Concepts: Comparison of ST and SVT

ST	SVT
■ History compatible with ST (eg, fever, injury, dehydration, pain)	■ History incompatible with ST (no history of dehydration, fever) or nonspecific
■ P waves present/normal	■ P waves absent/abnormal
■ Heart rate often varies with activity	■ Heart rate does not vary with activity
■ Variable R-R with constant PR	■ Abrupt rate changes
■ Infants: heart rate usually less than 220 bpm	■ Infants: heart rate usually greater than 220 bpm
■ Children: heart rate usually less than 180 bpm	■ Children: heart rate usually greater than 180 bpm

may attempt a brief trial of vagal maneuvers, but these efforts should not delay cardioversion.

SVT with *adequate perfusion* is more common and less emergent. After evaluation of a 12-lead ECG, consider vagal maneuvers and establish vascular access to administer adenosine. It is advisable to consult a pediatric cardiology specialist. If synchronized cardioversion is planned, provide sedation with analgesia. During evaluation, try to identify any alternative causes for high heart rate.

Drug Therapy

Adenosine. Adenosine is the drug of choice for treatment of SVT in children. Adenosine temporarily blocks conduction through the AV node—for only about 10 seconds. With continuous ECG monitoring, administer 0.1 mg/kg (maximum initial dose: 6 mg) as a rapid IV bolus. Adenosine has a very short half-life and is rapidly metabolized by an enzyme on the surface of red blood cells (adenosine deaminase), so it must be administered within seconds (see FYI: "Causes of Adenosine 'Failure' to Convert SVT"). To enhance delivery of the drug to its site of action in the heart, use a rapid flush technique (see Critical Concepts: "Technique for Rapid Administration of Adenosine").

A higher dose may be required for peripheral venous administration than administration into a central vein.[63,64] If the drug is effective, you will see an immediate conversion of rhythm (see Figure 14). If there is no effect, the dose may be doubled (0.2 mg/kg; maximum second dose: 12 mg). Experimental data and a case report indicate that adenosine may also be given by the IO route.[65,66]

Adenosine is *not* effective for atrial flutter, atrial fibrillation, atrial tachycardia, or VT that is not caused by reentry at the AV node. But it may enhance diagnosis

FYI: Causes of Adenosine "Failure" to Convert SVT

A common cause of adenosine cardioversion "failure" is that the drug is administered too slowly or with inadequate IV flush. Adenosine is effective for SVT caused by reentry at the AV node. It is *not* generally effective for atrial flutter, atrial fibrillation, or tachycardias caused by mechanisms other than reentry at the AV node.

of these disturbances, especially if the ECG is recorded during administration of adenosine.

Other agents. Many other interventions (eg, digoxin, short-acting β-blockers, overdrive pacing) have been used under expert consultation for treatment of SVT in children in various settings. Immediate synchronized cardioversion or administration of adenosine provides the highest likelihood of success and the broadest therapeutic index for the general PALS provider until expert consultation can be obtained. At that time drugs such as amiodarone, procainamide, or lidocaine may be considered (see "Management of VT," on the next page).

The calcium channel blocking agent verapamil should *not* be used routinely to treat SVT in infants because refractory hypotension and cardiac arrest have been reported after its administration.[67,68] Use of verapamil in children is also discouraged because it may cause hypotension and myocardial depression.[69] If used in children older than 1 year, infuse verapamil in a dose of 0.1 mg/kg.

Ventricular Tachycardia

VT is uncommon in the pediatric age group. When VT with pulses is present,

FIGURE 14. SVT converting to sinus rhythm with administration of adenosine.

Drug administered

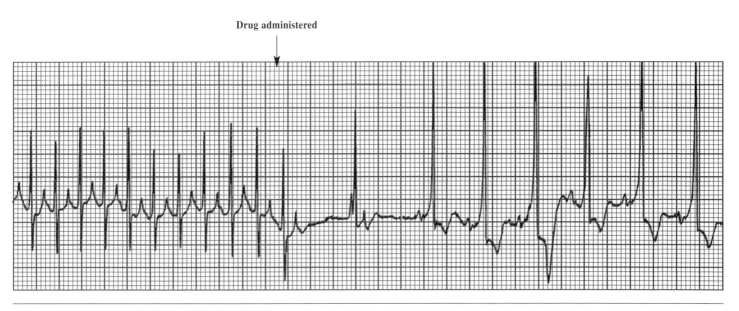

Critical Concepts:
Technique for Rapid Administration of Adenosine

Adenosine has a very short half-life (less than 10 seconds) and must be administered as rapidly as possible and followed immediately with a rapid saline flush. The following is one rapid administration technique:

1. Draw adenosine dose into a 1-mL to 3-mL syringe.

2. Prepare a normal saline flush in a separate (2-mL to 5-mL) syringe.

3. Record ECG continuously during drug administration.

4. Locate the injection port *nearest* the patient. Use central vascular access if available. Alternatively, place 2 adjacent stopcocks as close to the catheter entry into the patient as possible.

5. Place adenosine and flush syringes into the same injection port or into adjacent stopcocks.

6. Clamp the IV line just above the injection site (away from the patient) to ensure that the medication flows

only *toward* the patient. If using 2 adjacent stopcocks, turn the stopcock farther from the patient closed to the distal tubing, and open both stopcocks between the syringes and the patient.

7. While maintaining pressure on the flush syringe plunger (to prevent retrograde flow of medication into that syringe), push adenosine *as rapidly as possible to the patient.*

8. With the finger of one hand still maintaining pressure on the adenosine syringe plunger (to prevent the flush from flowing into the adenosine syringe), *immediately* push the normal saline flush *as rapidly as possible.*

9. If conversion is unsuccessful, double the dose of adenosine (0.2 mg/kg) and repeat steps 2 through 8. The maximum recommended single dose is 12 mg. Adenosine may also be administered via the IO route.[65,66]

the ventricular rate may vary from near normal to more than 200 bpm (see Foundation Facts: "ECG Characteristics of Ventricular Tachycardia"). Rapid ventricular rates often compromise stroke volume and cardiac output and may deteriorate into pulseless VT or VF.

Most children who develop VT have underlying structural heart disease, prolonged QT syndrome, or myocarditis/cardiomyopathy. Other potential causes of VT are acute hypoxemia, acidosis, electrolyte imbalance, and toxins/drugs/poisons (eg, tricyclic antidepressants). For simplicity of approach, previously undiagnosed wide-QRS tachycardia in an infant or a child should be treated as VT until proved otherwise (see Figure 15A).

You should attempt to identify torsades de pointes (see Figure 15B and FYI: "Torsades de Pointes") and VT *without* pulses because these forms of VT require specific treatment (eg, magnesium and defibrillation, respectively) that differs from that provided for VT with a pulse.

Management of VT

General Principles and Cardioversion

Defibrillation is the treatment for both VT *without palpable pulses* and VF. Support the airway, oxygenation, and ventilation and provide chest compressions until the defibrillator is charged, but *do not delay defibrillation.* Management of this form of VT is summarized later in this chapter.

If VT is present *with a pulse and poor perfusion* (eg, signs of congestive heart failure with diminished peripheral perfusion, increased work of breathing, and altered level of consciousness or hypotension), provide immediate *synchronized cardioversion.* If the patient's condition is unstable, do not delay cardioversion to establish vascular access (IV or IO). While the defibrillator or cardioverter is prepared and throughout stabilization, support the airway, oxygenation, and ventilation as needed, and begin continuous ECG monitoring. It may also be helpful to obtain a 12-lead ECG to confirm the rhythm diagnosis. If IV or IO access is established or readily available, provide adequate sedation with analgesia (see Chapter 15: "Sedation"). Attempt to identify and treat the underlying cause of VT (eg, electrolyte imbalance or drug toxicity). If VT with pulses is refractory to electrical cardioversion, the use of pharmacologic agents (eg, amiodarone, procainamide, or lidocaine) may promote cardioversion (see Figure 16 and Critical Concepts:

Foundation Facts:
ECG Characteristics of Ventricular Tachycardia

- Ventricular rate is at least 120 bpm and regular.

- The QRS is wide (greater than 0.08 second).

- P waves are often not identifiable. When present they may not be related to the QRS (AV dissociation). At slower rates the atria may be depolarized in a retrograde manner, and there will be a 1:1 ventricular-to-atrial association.

- T waves are typically opposite in polarity to the QRS.

- It may be difficult to differentiate SVT with aberrant conduction from VT. Fortunately, aberrant conduction is present in less than 10% of children with SVT.

Figure 15. Ventricular tachycardia. **A,** VT in a child with muscular dystrophy and known cardiomyopathy. The ventricular rhythm is rapid and regular at a rate of 158 bpm (greater than the minimum 120 bpm characteristic of VT). The QRS is wide (greater than 0.08 second), and there is no evidence of atrial depolarization. **B,** Torsades de pointes in a child with hypomagnesemia.

A

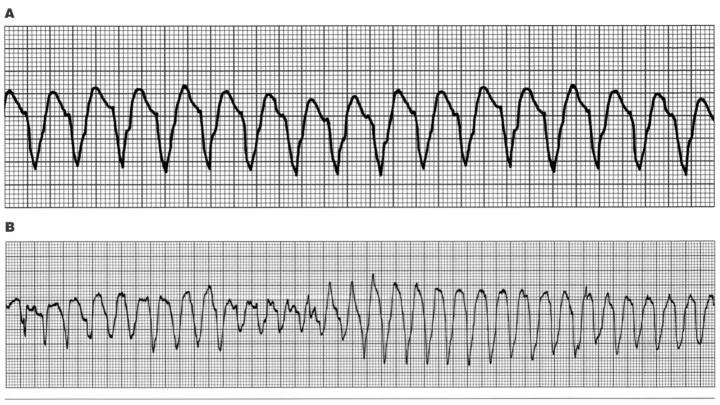

B

"Overview of Pediatric Algorithm for Tachycardia With Poor Perfusion").

VT with *adequate perfusion* is less common and less emergent (see Figure 17 and Critical Concepts: "Overview of Pediatric Algorithm for Tachycardia With Adequate Perfusion") than VT with poor perfusion. After evaluating a 12-lead ECG, establish vascular access to administer medications. Consultation with a pediatric cardiology specialist is strongly recommended. At this time you may also consider synchronized cardioversion with adequate sedation and analgesia. Also attempt to identify and treat reversible causes of the arrhythmia.

Drug Therapy

Amiodarone. Amiodarone and procainamide can both be used to treat a wide range of atrial and ventricular arrhythmias in adults and children, including SVT[73,74] and VT.[74] Amiodarone inhibits α- and β-adrenergic receptors, producing vasodilation and AV nodal suppression (this slows conduction through the AV node). It inhibits the outward potassium current so it prolongs the QT duration. Amiodarone also inhibits the sodium channels, which slows conduction in the ventricles and prolongs QRS duration. These effects may be beneficial in some patients but may also increase the risk for polymorphic VT.[75]

FYI: Torsades de Pointes

Torsades de pointes ("to turn on a point") is a distinctive form of polymorphic VT. The ECG is characterized by QRS complexes that change in amplitude and polarity (see Figure 15B) so they appear to rotate around an isoelectric line. This arrhythmia is seen in conditions distinguished by a long QT interval, including congenital conditions (eg, electrolyte channel abnormalities causing the congenital long-QT syndromes) and drug toxicity. Type IA antiarrhythmics (eg, procainamide, quinidine, and disopyramide), type III antiarrhythmics (eg, sotalol and amiodarone), and tricyclic antidepressants are all reported causes of torsades de pointes. Additional causes are medication interactions such as that between cisapride (which is no longer available) and inhibitors of the cytochrome P450 system (eg, clarithromycin or erythromycin).[70] Magnesium sulfate is the treatment of choice for torsades de pointes. Give in a rapid IV/IO infusion of 25 to 50 mg/kg (up to 2 g) over 10 to 20 minutes.[71,72]

Critical Concepts: Overview of Pediatric Algorithm for Tachycardia With Poor Perfusion

Note to providers: Refer to numbered boxes and ovals in the algorithm.

Box 1: Basic life support. When tachycardia is associated with poor perfusion (shock with hypotension, poor end-organ perfusion, congestive heart failure, change in level of consciousness, or sudden collapse), assess and support the airway, oxygenation, and ventilation as needed.

Box 2: Assess the pulse to determine if a pulse is palpable. If invasive monitoring is already established, assess the arterial pressure waveform. You may also use Doppler assessment of pulses.

Box 3: If *NO* pulse is present, initiate **CPR** and activate the pediatric pulseless arrest algorithm (this appears later in the chapter).

Box 4: If pulses *are* present, continue to provide oxygen and ventilation as needed. Attach a continuous ECG monitor (with transcutaneous pacer/defibrillator capability if available) and a pulse oximeter.

Box 5: Quickly evaluate QRS duration. Although a 12-lead ECG may be useful, initial therapy does not require a precise ECG diagnosis of the tachyarrhythmia causing poor perfusion. You can calculate QRS width from a rhythm strip. If QRS duration is *normal for the patient's age* (approximately 0.08 second or less), ST or SVT is likely to be present. If QRS duration is *wide for the patient's age* (greater than approximately 0.08 second), VT is probably present.

Box 6: During evaluation of the tachycardia, support the airway, breathing, oxygenation, and ventilation, and verify that the ECG monitor is attached correctly with a tracing free of artifact. During treatment consult a pediatric cardiology specialist if possible. Prepare for synchronized cardioversion. Identify and treat potentially reversible causes

and conditions most likely to produce tachyarrhythmias:

- **Hyper**thermia can be treated with simple cooling techniques. Some ectopic pacemaker foci (eg, junctional ectopic tachycardia) may respond to cooling.

- Hyper-/hypokalemia and other metabolic disorders, including hypomagnesemia, may cause ventricular arrhythmias.

- Toxins: particularly tricyclic antidepressants, may require targeted therapy (see Chapter 12).

- Ensure effective pain control.

Box 7: Evaluate the narrow-complex tachycardia. Use the subsequent boxes to determine if the tachyarrhythmia is probable ST or SVT.

Box 8: Probable ST: History is compatible with ST (eg, the patient has fever, dehydration, pain), P waves are present and normal, heart rate varies with activity or stimulation, R-R is variable but PR is constant, and heart rate is less than 220 bpm for an infant or less than 180 bpm for a child. Treatment is directed at the cause of ST.

Box 9: Probable SVT: History is incompatible with ST (no fever or dehydration or other identifiable causes of ST) or nonspecific; P waves are absent or abnormal; heart rate does not vary with activity or stimulation; rate changes abruptly; heart rate is greater than 220 bpm for an infant or greater than 180 bpm for a child.

Box 10: For SVT **consider vagal maneuvers** (see "Nonpharmacologic Interventions"). Do not delay cardioversion in the unstable patient. For an infant consider applying ice water to the face without obstructing ventilation. You can ask a child to blow through an obstructed straw to induce a vagal response. Do not apply ocular pressure.

Box 11: If SVT with poor perfusion persists, provide immediate electrical or chemical cardioversion. *Record and*

monitor the ECG continuously during any cardioversion. **Provide immediate synchronized electrical cardioversion** with 0.5 to 1 J/kg. If this is ineffective you may increase the dose to 1 to 2 J/kg. Provide sedation with analgesia if it will not delay cardioversion. If vascular access and medications are *immediately* available, provide chemical cardioversion with **adenosine** IV/IO (0.1 mg/kg, maximum initial dose: 6 mg as a rapid IV bolus with a *rapid* flush technique; if no effect, administer double the dose: 0.2 mg/kg, maximum 12 mg).

If tachycardia persists, **see Box 14,** obtain a 12-lead ECG, consult a pediatric cardiologist, and consider alternative medications based on the expertise and medication available.

Box 12: Evaluate the wide-complex tachycardia. Wide-complex tachycardia is treated as VT unless a 12-lead ECG or other source identifies a supraventricular origin.

Box 13: Treat probable VT: For urgent treatment of a wide-complex tachycardia with pulses but poor perfusion, provide immediate synchronized cardioversion with 0.5 to 1 J/kg. Provide sedation with analgesia if possible, but do not delay cardioversion in the unstable patient. If the rhythm persists, double the dose (to 1 to 2 J/kg) and reattempt cardioversion.

Box 14: Consider alternative medications: amiodarone (5 mg/kg IV over 20 to 60 minutes) OR procainamide (15 mg/kg IV over 30 to 60 minutes) OR lidocaine 1 mg/kg IV bolus. Administer lidocaine for wide-complex tachycardia only. Amiodarone or procainamide are alternative agents for use in children with SVT and VT. Note: *Do not routinely administer amiodarone and procainamide together or with other medications that prolong the QT interval.*

FIGURE 16. Pediatric tachycardia algorithm for infants and children with rapid rhythm and poor perfusion.

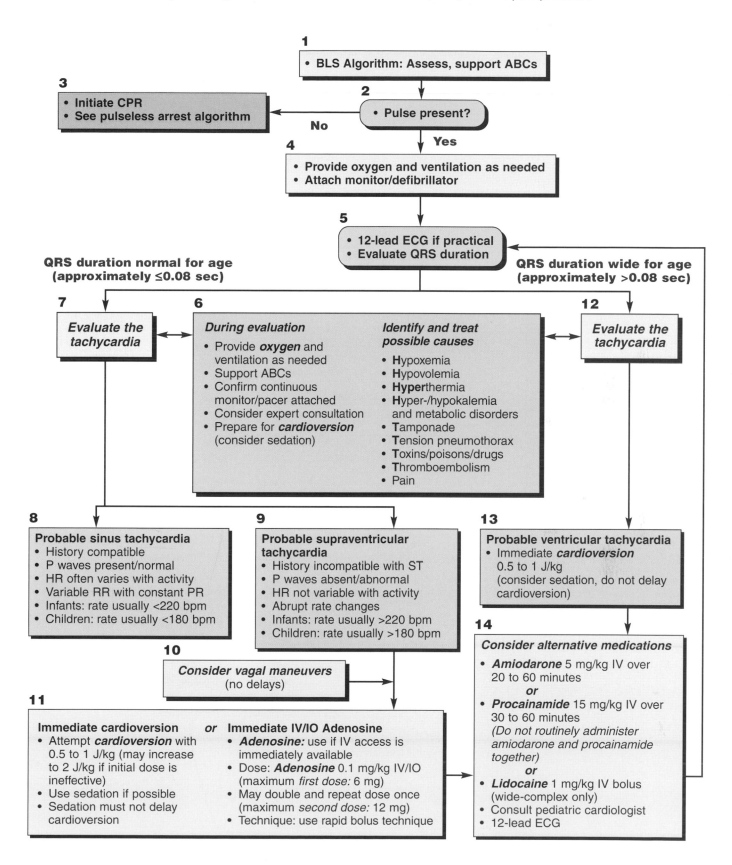

Critical Concepts: Overview of Pediatric Algorithm for Tachycardia With Adequate Perfusion

Note to providers: Refer to numbered boxes and ovals in the algorithm.

Box 1: When tachycardia is present but *systemic perfusion is adequate*, you have more time to evaluate the rhythm and the patient. Assess and support the airway, oxygenation, and ventilation as needed, and evaluate the character of the pulse. Attach a **continuous ECG monitor** (with transcutaneous pacer/defibrillator capability if available) and pulse oximeter. Evaluate a 12-lead ECG if practical.

Box 2: Evaluate QRS duration. If QRS duration is *normal for the child's age* (approximately 0.08 second or less), ST or SVT is probably present (see **Boxes 3, 4,** and **5**). If QRS duration is *wide* for age (greater than approximately 0.08 second), VT is probably present (see **Box 10**).

Box 3: If **QRS duration is normal** for age, evaluate the rhythm and attempt to determine if the rhythm represents ST or SVT.

Box 4: Probable ST: History is compatible with ST (eg, the patient has fever, dehydration, pain), P waves are present and normal, heart rate varies with activity or stimulation, R-R is variable but PR is constant, and heart rate is less than 220 bpm for an infant or less than 180 bpm for a child. Treatment is directed at the cause of ST.

Box 5: Probable SVT: History is incompatible with ST (no fever, dehydration, or other identifiable cause of ST) or nonspecific, P waves are absent or abnormal, heart rate does not vary with activity or stimulation, rate changes abruptly, heart rate is greater than 220 bpm for an infant or greater than 180 bpm for a child.

Box 6: During evaluation of tachycardia, support the airway, breathing, oxygenation, and ventilation as needed and verify that the continuous ECG monitor/pacer is attached correctly and that the tracing is free of artifact. If the rhythm is consistent with SVT or VT with stable perfusion, consult a pediatric cardiology specialist. Prepare to provide *synchronized cardioversion* with appropriate sedation with analgesia. Identify and treat potentially reversible causes and conditions, especially

- Hyperthermia and pain

- Hyper-/hypokalemia and other metabolic disorders, including hypomagnesemia

- Toxins/drugs, particularly tricyclic antidepressants

Box 7: For SVT, **consider vagal maneuvers.** In the stable patient with SVT, put ice water on the face of the infant without obstructing ventilation, or ask the child to blow through an obstructed straw. Perform continuous ECG monitoring and recording before, during, and after these attempted vagal maneuvers. Do not apply ocular pressure or provide carotid massage.

Box 8: For SVT resistant to attempted vagal maneuvers, establish vascular access and prepare for electrical or chemical cardioversion. For most common forms of SVT caused by a reentrant pathway involving the AV node, *adenosine* is the drug of choice.[62-64]

Box 9: Attempt **synchronized electrical cardioversion** with 0.5 to 1 J/kg for SVT or VT unresponsive to initial measures. Increase the dose to 1 to 2 J/kg if the initial dose is ineffective. When making preparations for synchronized cardioversion, consult an expert. If the patient is conscious, provide sedation with analgesia

before elective cardioversion. Obtain a 12-lead ECG after conversion.

Box 10: Probable VT: If QRS duration is wide for age (greater than approximately 0.08 second), assume that the rhythm is VT. Less than 10% of infants and children with SVT present with aberrant conduction and a wide complex, so SVT is unlikely. During evaluation and preparation for treatment, support the airway, oxygenation, and ventilation; establish vascular access; and evaluate for treatable causes (see **Box 6**).

Box 11: Consider alternative medications: Depending on local circumstances, synchronized cardioversion or medications may be appropriate for the stable patient. Careful evaluation of a 12-lead ECG and early consultation with a pediatric cardiology specialist are appropriate. If chemical cardioversion is provided, consider administering amiodarone (5 mg/kg IV over 20 to 60 minutes) OR procainamide (15 mg/kg IV over 30 to 60 minutes) OR lidocaine 1 mg/kg IV bolus. Lidocaine is recommended for wide-complex tachycardia only. Infuse loading doses slowly in the stable patient to avoid hypotension. Do not routinely administer amiodarone and procainamide together or with other medications that prolong the QT interval. If these initial efforts do not terminate the rapid rhythm, reevaluate the rhythm.

FIGURE 17. Pediatric tachycardia algorithm for infants and children with rapid rhythm and adequate perfusion.

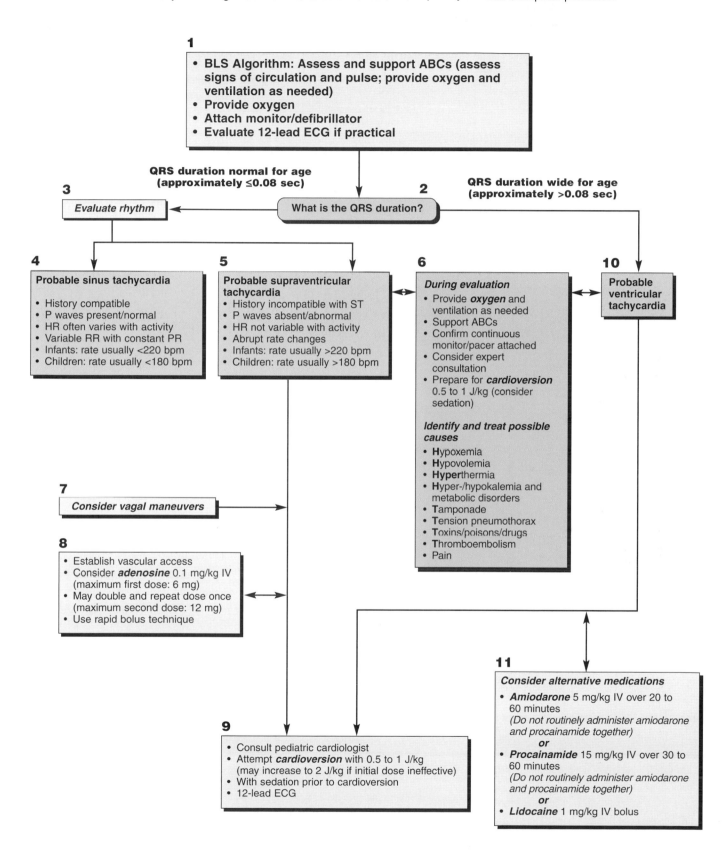

For both supraventricular and ventricular arrhythmias associated with shock, a loading dose infusion of 5 mg/kg over 20 to 60 minutes is recommended, depending on the need to achieve a rapid drug effect.[73,76-80] Repeat doses of 5 mg/kg may be given up to a maximum of 15 mg/kg per day as needed. The major side effect of IV amiodarone is hypotension.[73,78] Amiodarone should *not* routinely be administered in combination with another agent that prolongs the QT interval (eg, procainamide).

Because of amiodarone's complex pharmacology, poor oral absorption, long half-life, and potential for long-term adverse effects, a pediatric cardiologist or similarly experienced provider should direct long-term amiodarone therapy. Administration of amiodarone for children with VT and a pulse is a Class IIb recommendation.

Procainamide. Procainamide is a sodium channel blocking antiarrhythmic agent that prolongs the effective refractory period of both the atria and ventricles and depresses conduction velocity within the conduction system. By slowing intraventricular conduction, procainamide prolongs the QT, QRS, and PR intervals. Procainamide is effective in the treatment of atrial fibrillation, atrial flutter, and SVT.[81,82] Because procainamide paradoxically shortens the effective refractory period of the AV node and increases AV nodal conduction, it may cause an increased heart rate when it is used to treat ectopic atrial tachycardia and atrial fibrillation.[83] Procainamide may be useful in the treatment of postoperative junctional ectopic tachycardia,[84] and it has also been used to treat or suppress VT.[85]

Despite a long history of use, there is little data comparing the effectiveness of procainamide with other antiarrhythmic agents used in children.[86,87] Procainamide must be given by slow infusion to avoid toxicity from heart block, myocardial depression, and prolongation of the QT interval (which predisposes to torsades de pointes tachycardia). Infuse the loading dose of 15 mg/kg over 30 to 60 minutes with continuous monitoring of the ECG and frequent blood pressure monitoring. Because procainamide

---

Critical Concepts: Avoid Concurrent Use of Drugs That Prolong the QT Interval

Both amiodarone and procainamide are antiarrhythmic medications that prolong the QT interval. Rapid administration of both drugs causes vasodilation and hypotension with potential for heart block, and both may increase risk for polymorphic VT. Avoid concurrent use of drugs that prolong the QT interval.

---

must be infused slowly, it is generally not used in the treatment of pulseless VT or VF. Procainamide, like amiodarone, may increase the risk of polymorphic VT and generally should not be used in combination with another agent (eg, amiodarone) that prolongs the QT interval (see Critical Concepts: "Avoid Concurrent Use of Drugs That Prolong the QT Interval").

Lidocaine. Lidocaine is a sodium channel blocker that decreases automaticity and suppresses wide-complex ventricular arrhythmias.[88] It is not used for narrow complex supraventricular arrhythmias, and the data suggests that it is not very effective unless the ventricular arrhythmia is associated with focal myocardial ischemia.[89,90] Lidocaine is an alternative agent for treatment of stable VT and pulseless VT. Provide a loading dose of 1 mg/kg of lidocaine. For treatment of pulseless VT, follow with an infusion of 20 to 50 µg/kg per minute. If there is a delay of more than 15 minutes between the bolus dose and the start of an infusion, consider giving a second bolus of 0.5 to 1 mg/kg to reestablish therapeutic concentrations. Lidocaine toxicity may be observed in patients with high plasma concentrations, persistently low cardiac output, and hepatic or renal failure.

Bretylium. Bretylium is no longer considered an appropriate first-line agent for VT with poor perfusion because of the

prevalence of hypotension associated with its infusion,[91] lack of demonstrable effectiveness in treatment of VT,[92] and the absence of published studies of its use in children.

Vasopressin. Vasopressin is a promising vasopressor agent (see Chapter 7: "Case Scenarios in the Management of Shock") for treatment of shock-refractory VF and VT in adults. A small case series suggests that vasopressin in doses of 0.4 to 1 U/kg per dose may have an emerging role in shock-refractory VF in children,[93] although it has not been well studied in the specific setting of pediatric cardiac arrest or shock-refractory VF. Vasopressin may also be used in very low doses (0.005 to 0.01 U/kg per hour) as a vasopressor for children with circulatory shock.[94,95]

Reevaluation

If VF/pulseless VT persists, carefully evaluate a 12-lead ECG to verify the rhythm diagnosis and identify and treat reversible causes or special resuscitation circumstances. Early consultation with a pediatric cardiology specialist is appropriate.

Pulseless Arrest: "COLLAPSE RHYTHMS"

Patients with collapse rhythms have no detectable pulses or signs of perfusion. VF, pulseless VT, asystole, and all forms of PEA are collapse rhythms. All collapse rhythms are associated with the *absence of signs of circulation:* adequate breathing (ie, other than agonal respirations), coughing, or movement in response to stimulation. The most common arrest rhythm recorded in pediatric cardiac arrest victims is asystole or some form of bradyarrhythmia, often with a wide QRS complex.[1,2]

It is imperative to identify nonasystolic causes of arrest. Some patients with pulseless electrical activity may have reversible causes of arrest that will respond to treatment. It is also important to identify VF and pulseless ventricular arrhythmias because in many studies the survival rate from VF/pulseless VT arrest is higher than the survival rate from asystole or other nonperfusing rhythms.[51,96-98] This higher survival rate may not be observed in submersion victims, in whom VF/pulseless VT has been associated with extremely poor prognosis.[99]

The prevalence of ventricular arrhythmia reported in pediatric victims of cardiac arrest varies with inclusion and exclusion study criteria, range of patient age (VF is a more common arrest rhythm in adolescents than infants), cause of arrest, EMS

Critical Concepts:
Collapse Rhythms

- Collapse rhythms produce cardiac arrest with no pulse and no signs of perfusion.

- If collapse is sudden, especially with known risk factors for cardiac disease, VF/pulseless VT is more likely than asystole. Prepare for immediate rhythm analysis and a possible defibrillation attempt.

- If arrest occurs with risk factors for hypoxia or ischemia preceding the arrest (eg, submersion, trauma, asphyxia, apnea), brady-asystole is far more likely than VF/pulseless VT, and the emphasis should be on early support of airway and oxygenation.

response interval (the longer the response, the more likely that asystole will be present), and whether bystander CPR was performed. VF has been reported in 3% to 20% of out-of-hospital pediatric and adolescent cardiac arrest victims.[2,51,96,97] The higher incidence of VF is reported when adolescents are included and SIDS victims are excluded.[51] In the same EMS system VF was present in only 3% of children from 0 to 8 years of age with nontraumatic arrest but was observed in 17% of victims from 8 to 30 years of age.[100]

The pharmacology of drugs used for resuscitation is summarized in Chapter 5: "Fluid Therapy and Medications for Shock and Cardiac Arrest." Chapter 5 presents therapeutic considerations, indications, doses, routes of administration, precautions, and recommended forms of medications used in resuscitation. This chapter presents the algorithm approach to sequential assessment and management of the collapse rhythms.

Asystole

Asystole is a form of pulseless arrest associated with absent cardiac electrical activity represented by a straight (flat) line on the ECG (see Figure 18). You must clinically confirm the absence of signs of circulation (no pulse, no spontaneous respirations, no response to stimulation) because a "flat line" ECG can also be

caused by a loose ECG lead. If possible you should confirm asystole in more than one ECG lead to identify artifact or very fine VF that might be masquerading as asystole.

Management of Asystole
General Principles

Asystole is the most common rhythm observed in infants and children presenting with out-of-hospital cardiac arrest. The etiology of the arrest is almost always a combination of hypoxia and ischemia, and the prognosis for intact neurologic survival is poor. Prompt bystander CPR with prompt ALS support of oxygenation and ventilation are initial resuscitation interventions.

Defibrillation and transthoracic pacing are *not* effective for asystole and are *not* recommended.[101] Attempts at ineffective therapies may delay initiation of attempts to improve oxygenation and ventilation and initiate catecholamine/pressor therapy, which may be effective. During initial resuscitation, attempt to identify and treat potential reversible causes.

Drug Therapy

To enable IV drug therapy, establish vascular access. Epinephrine increases coronary perfusion pressure associated with return of spontaneous circulation.[102,103] The recommended initial resuscitation

FIGURE 18. Agonal rhythm progressing to asystole. Only 2 QRS complexes representing terminal ventricular complexes are seen. These complexes are followed by the absence of organized electrical activity. This rhythm will be associated with the absence of a pulse and the absence of any signs of circulation. To minimize the risk of artifact and to look for very fine VF, confirm aystole in more than one lead if possible.

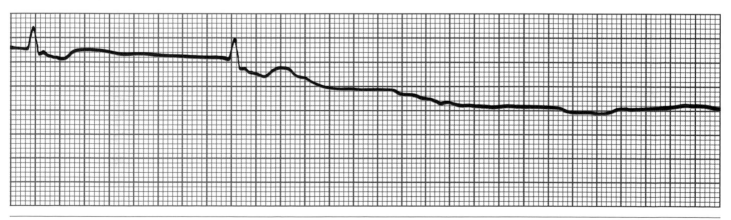

dose of epinephrine for all cases of cardiac arrest is 0.01 mg/kg (0.1 mL/kg of 1:10 000 solution) by the IV or IO route or 0.1 mg/kg (0.1 mL/kg of 1:1000 solution) by the tracheal route. For ongoing arrest repeat doses every 3 to 5 minutes. The same dose of epinephrine is recommended for second and subsequent doses for unresponsive asystolic arrest.

High-dose epinephrine improves myocardial and cerebral blood flow in animals in cardiac arrest. But many randomized controlled studies in adults and animal models and a few less rigorous pediatric investigations have demonstrated that initial or rescue high-dose epinephrine (0.1 to 0.2 mg/kg or 0.1 to 0.2 mL/kg of 1:1000 solution) does not improve outcome.[96,104-117] Great interpatient variability in catecholamine pharmacokinetics and response is well established.[118-125] High-dose epinephrine may be considered for special resuscitation circumstances that suggest a catecholamine-resistant condition (eg, anaphylaxis, known α- or β-blocker overdose, severe sepsis already being treated with high-dose pressors). Increased myocardial oxygen consumption during CPR and a postarrest hyperadrenergic state with postarrest myocardial dysfunction are potential adverse effects of high-dose epinephrine.

Pulseless Electrical Activity

PEA is a rhythmic display of electrical activity other than VF or VT that does not produce a palpable arterial pulse. Although electrical activity without a palpable pulse implies the absence of cardiac output, this might not reflect the true cardiac condition in PEA. Research with cardiac ultrasonography and indwelling pressure catheters in adults has confirmed that a pulseless patient with electrical activity may have associated mechanical contractions. These contractions are too weak to produce an arterial pressure that can be detected by manual palpation or sphygmomanometry. The critical point is that PEA may be reversible if it is identified early and treated appropriately. Unless a specific cause can be identified and an intervention performed to improve the condition, the rhythm will

likely degenerate quickly into an agonal ventricular rhythm or asystole.

Immediate assessment of blood flow by Doppler ultrasound may reveal an actively contracting heart and some blood flow, a condition originally termed "pseudo-EMD."[126,127] To improve cardiac output in these patients, you must identify and treat the causes of PEA. You can recall the potential causes with the 4 H's and 4 T's mnemonic (see Critical Concepts: "Potentially Reversible Causes of Pulseless Electrical Activity"). The outcome of PEA is poor unless the specific cause can be promptly identified and treated.

Management of PEA

General Principles

Aggressively treat any patient with PEA and a Doppler-detectable blood flow. These patients need volume expansion, norepinephrine, dopamine, or some combination of the 3 therapies. Identify and correct reversible causes of PEA, particularly those compromising venous return to the heart (tension pneumothorax, cardiac tamponade, severe hypovolemia). Many causes

---

Critical Concepts:
Potentially Reversible Causes of Pulseless Electrical Activity

The 4 H's and 4 T's mnemonic lists the potentially reversible causes of PEA:

- Hypoxemia
- Hypovolemia
- Hypothermia
- Hyper-/hypokalemia and other metabolic disorders (including acidosis and calcium and magnesium imbalances)
- Tamponade
- Tension pneumothorax
- Toxins/poisons/drugs
- Thromboembolism

Critical Concepts:

Note to providers: Medications for treatment of pulseless cardiac arrest are presented in detail in Chapter 5 and are mentioned here only in the context of the treatment algorithm. Refer to the numbered boxes and ovals in the algorithm.

Box 1: Confirm the absence of a pulse and other signs of perfusion. Continue to support the airway, oxygenation, and ventilation. If invasive monitoring is established, look for signs of pulsatile blood flow (eg, arterial pressure waveform, pulse oximeter waveform). Attach a continuous ECG monitor with transcutaneous defibrillator/pacer capability if available.

Box 2: Quickly determine if VF or pulseless VT is present. If VF/VT is present, then a defibrillation attempt is your first priority. If PEA is detected, your priority is to support circulation while you try to identify and treat reversible causes.

Box 3: Throughout treatment of pulseless arrest, support the airway, oxygenation, and ventilation. The first cycle through the algorithm is projected to take approximately 3 minutes. **Check** paddle/electrode size, position, and skin contact, and verify that the monitor/defibrillator/pacer (if available) is correctly attached and that the tracing is free of artifact. To detect fine VF, confirm asystole in 2 leads if possible. **Attempt intubation and verify** tracheal tube position (with primary and secondary confirmation techniques) and establish vascular access. Prepare to administer and flush medications. In all cases of pulseless arrest refractory to initial

of PEA involve obstruction of venous return to the heart or hypovolemia. Administer a 20 mL/kg rapid fluid bolus and evaluate the response. Consider pericardiocentesis if you suspect tamponade is present and the patient fails to respond to

Overview of Pediatric Pulseless Arrest Algorithm

intervention, administer an initial dose of IV/IO **epinephrine** (0.01 mg/kg or 0.1 mL/kg of 1:10 000 solution) or if vascular access is not established, provide tracheal epinephrine (0.1 mg/kg or 0.1 mL/kg of 1:1000 solution). Attempt to **identify and treat potentially reversible causes** of pulseless arrest:

- **H**ypoxemia: If the victim is intubated and receiving positive-pressure ventilation before cardiac arrest, use the *DOPE* mnemonic (**D**isplacement of tracheal tube, **O**bstruction of tracheal tube, **P**neumothorax, and **E**quipment failure) to identify causes of deterioration.

- **H**ypovolemia: Provide a rapid 20 mL/kg bolus of isotonic crystalloid.

- **H**ypothermia may predispose the ventricle to ectopy, slow conduction through the conduction system and myocardium, and result in a collapse rhythm. Severe hypothermia (core temperature less than 32.2°C) may require rapid rewarming techniques.

- **H**yper-/hypokalemia and metabolic disorders: Correct severe electrolyte imbalance (potassium, calcium, magnesium) and acidosis (hydrogen).

- **T**amponade: May initially present with tachycardia, narrow pulse pressure, distended neck veins, thready pulses, and poor perfusion, usually accompanied by other signs of inadequate venous return to the heart, heart failure, and low cardiac output. Treat with a combination of volume bolus and pericardiocentesis.

- **T**ension pneumothorax: Treat tension pneumothorax with needle decompression.

- **T**oxins/poisons/drugs may require specific therapies (eg, sodium bicarbonate therapy for tricyclic antidepressant overdose). For information see Chapter 12.

- **T**hromboembolism that is severe enough to cause a collapse rhythm is rare and difficult to treat, the result of severe obstruction to cardiac output to the lungs.

Box 4: **VF/pulseless VT: attempt defibrillation.** The most important treatment for VF/pulseless VT is immediate defibrillation. The initial shock should be approximately 2 J/kg, then 2 to 4 J/kg, and then 4 J/kg if VF/VT persists. Note that alternative shock waveforms and higher doses have not been extensively studied under these conditions in infants and children, but alternative waveforms may be used if they are documented to produce survival *equivalent to conventional waveforms.*

Box 5: If VF/VT is refractory to 3 defibrillation attempts, **administer epinephrine** and continue support of oxygenation and ventilation. The recommended initial IV/IO resuscitation dose of epinephrine for cardiac arrest is 0.01 mg/kg (0.1 mL/kg of 1:10 000 solution) or 0.1 mg/kg (0.1 mL/kg of 1:1000 solution) by the tracheal route. For ongoing arrest, repeat doses every 3 to 5 minutes are recommended. The same dose of epinephrine is recommended for second and subsequent doses for unresponsive asystolic and pulseless arrest. Consider a higher dose for some special resuscitation circumstances.

Box 6: **Attempt defibrillation** with 4 J/kg 30 to 60 seconds after administration of each medication if VF/VT persists. The pattern of therapy should be "drug-CPR-shock (repeat)" or "drug-CPR-shock-shock-shock (repeat)."

Box 7: **Administer antiarrhythmic therapy** if VF/VT persists or recurs. Consider amiodarone (5 mg/kg IV/IO rapid bolus) OR lidocaine (1 mg/kg IV/IO bolus). Administer magnesium (25 to 50 mg/kg IV/IO; maximum: 2 g) for torsades de pointes or hypomagnesemia.

Box 8: **Attempt defibrillation** with 4 J/kg 30 to 60 seconds after administration of each medication if VF/VT persists. The sequence should be "drug-CPR-shock (repeat)" or "drug-CPR-shock-shock-shock (repeat)." If there is no response to therapy, reassess the ECG and seek and treat reversible causes (**Boxes 2** and **3**).

Box 9: If the patient is *not* in VF/VT, determine if the rhythm is asystole or PEA. Both collapse rhythms are treated with **epinephrine** (0.01 mg/kg, or 0.1 mL/kg of 1:10 000 solution) every 3 to 5 minutes. If PEA is present, attempt to rapidly identify and treat reversible causes. Because most rapidly reversible causes of PEA involve obstruction of venous return to the heart, administer a 20 mL/kg rapid fluid bolus. Administer calcium or magnesium when hypocalcemia or hypomagnesemia is present or when appropriate for treatment of drug overdose.

Box 10: **Continue CPR** for up to 3 minutes and then reassess cardiac rhythm (**Box 2**), confirm appropriate interventions, and consider alternative medications and special resuscitation circumstances (**Box 3**).

initial interventions. In out-of-hospital studies of resuscitation, the return of spontaneous circulation before the patient arrives in the Emergency Department is associated with an improved chance for long-term survival.[52,97,128]

Supportive management of PEA is the same as that for asystole: deliver chest compressions combined with advanced airway support and support of oxygenation and ventilation and administer epinephrine every 3 to 5 minutes.

Drug Therapy

Epinephrine is the recommended drug for attempted resuscitation of PEA or asystole. Although calcium has historically been used to treat asystole, experimental data does not support its routine administration for PEA or asystole.[129,130] Calcium is indicated for the treatment of documented hypocalcemia and hyperkalemia,[131] particularly in hemodynamically compromised patients. Calcium should also be considered for treatment of hypermagnesemia[132] and calcium channel blocker overdose.[133]

Ventricular Fibrillation

VF is a chaotic, disorganized series of depolarizations (Figure 19A and B) that result in a quivering myocardium incapable of producing blood flow. VF is an uncommon terminal event in the pediatric age group and is documented in only about 10% of children in whom a terminal rhythm is recorded.

Management of VF/Pulseless VT

General Principles and Defibrillation

Prompt defibrillation is the definitive treatment for both VF and pulseless VT.[134,135] Support ventilation and oxygenation and provide chest compressions until the defibrillator arrives and is charged. In adults and animals with prolonged VF cardiac arrest, correction of hypoxemia and acidosis with excellent CPR and administration of vasopressors may increase return of spontaneous circulation after defibrillation.[136] This support may convert fine, low-amplitude VF to coarse, higher-amplitude VF that is more responsive to defibrillation attempts. Therefore, attempt immediate defibrillation, but establish vascular access as soon as possible. If 3 defibrillation attempts (shocks) fail, administer a vasopressor (epinephrine), provide CPR, and attempt defibrillation again within 30 to 60 seconds of administering the drug (drug-CPR-shock). Identify and treat contributing or reversible causes (eg, hypoxemia, hypovolemia, hypothermia), metabolic causes (eg, hyperkalemia, hypomagnesemia, hypocalcemia), toxins/drugs (eg, tricyclic antidepressants, digoxin, or toxicity from the combination of cisapride and macrolide antibiotics),[70] pericardial tamponade, tension pneumothorax, and thromboembolism.[137]

Drug Therapy

Epinephrine (adrenaline) increases coronary perfusion pressure associated with return of spontaneous circulation,[102,103] enhances the contractile state of the heart, stimulates spontaneous contractions, and increases the vigor and intensity of VF, improving the chance for successful defibrillation.[138] Epinephrine is recommended for VF unresponsive to defibrillation attempts or during CPR until a defibrillator is available. The recommended resuscitation dose of epinephrine for cardiac arrest is 0.01 mg/kg (0.1 mL/kg of 1:10 000 solution) IV or IO or 0.1 mg/kg (0.1 mL/kg of 1:1000 solution) by the tracheal route. For ongoing arrest, repeat doses every 3 to 5 minutes. As noted above (see "Management of Asystole"), there is no evidence that high initial or rescue doses of epinephrine improve the patient's chance of survival more than standard doses of epinephrine.

You may consider alternative vasopressors (eg, vasopressin 0.4 to 1.0 U/kg and α-agonists),[93] but these drugs have not been shown to be superior to epinephrine in the setting of pulseless arrest in infants and children.

If VF or pulseless VT persists or recurs after administration of epinephrine and 3 shocks, give an antiarrhythmic (eg, amiodarone or lidocaine), then attempt defibrillation again within 30 to 60 seconds. Note that the sequence of treatment after the initial 3 shocks is "drug-CPR-shock, drug-CPR-shock." Thirty to 60 seconds of CPR is recommended following administration of each medication to allow the drug to reach the central circulation before the next defibrillation attempt. It is also acceptable to attempt defibrillation in clusters of 3 shocks separated by 1 minute of CPR and drug administration. This "drug-CPR-shock-shock-shock, drug-CPR-shock-shock-shock" pattern is an acceptable alternative pattern of resuscitation and may decrease transthoracic impedance to electrical energy.

The antiarrhythmic drugs used to treat VT are the same as those used to treat VF. These drugs are discussed in "Management of VT" and Chapter 5: "Fluid Therapy and Medications for Shock and Cardiac Arrest." Unique aspects of antiarrhythmic therapy for pulseless arrest are presented below (see Figure 20).

Amiodarone. Amiodarone has been effective for treatment of children with VT,[79,80] and in adults it can prevent the recurrence of VF after a successful shock.[139] In the setting of pulseless arrest, provide a rapid bolus loading dose of 5 mg/kg. Repeat doses of 5 mg/kg may be given to a maximum of 15 mg/kg per day if needed. Hypotension is the most significant potential side effect of rapid IV administration.[79,140-142] The use of amiodarone is based on adult data on "shock-resistant VT/VF"[139] and experience with its use in children in the nonarrest setting in the ICU.[73,76] Administration of amiodarone in children with VF and pulseless VT is a Class Indeterminate recommendation. Concurrent use of other medications that prolong the QT interval is not recommended.

Lidocaine. Lidocaine is a sodium channel blocker that decreases automaticity and suppresses wide-complex ventricular arrhythmias.[143] Although lidocaine has long been recommended for treatment of ventricular arrhythmias in infants and children, the data suggests that it is not very effective unless the arrhythmia is associated with focal myocardial ischemia.[89,90] Administer lidocaine with a loading dose of 1 mg/kg, followed by an infusion of 20 to 50 µg/kg per minute. If there is a delay of more than 15 minutes between the bolus dose and the start of an infusion, consider giving a second bolus of 0.5 to 1 mg/kg to rapidly restore therapeutic concentrations.

Magnesium. Data supports the use of magnesium sulfate (25 to 50 mg/kg, up to 2 g) in patients with hypomagnesemia or torsades de pointes VT.[71,72]

FIGURE 19. Ventricular fibrillation. **A,** Coarse VF. High-amplitude waveforms vary in size, shape, and rhythm, representing chaotic ventricular electrical activity with no identifiable P, QRS, or T waves. **B,** Fine VF. Electrical activity is reduced from previous (A) rhythm strip.

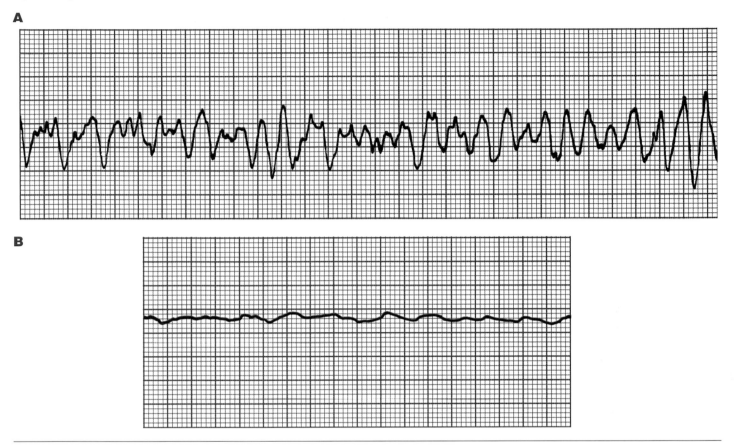

Sodium bicarbonate. Sodium bicarbonate is recommended for the treatment of symptomatic patients with hyperkalemia,[144] a tricyclic antidepressant overdose, or an overdose of other sodium channel blocking agents[145] (see Chapter 12: "Toxicology"). Routine use of sodium bicarbonate during pulseless arrest outside of these special resuscitation circumstances is not recommended.

Calcium. Administration of calcium is indicated for treatment of documented hypocalcemia and hyperkalemia,[131] particularly in patients with hemodynamic compromise. Ionized hypocalcemia is relatively common in critically ill children, particularly those with sepsis[146,147] or after cardiopulmonary bypass. Also consider calcium for treatment of hypermagnesemia[132] and calcium channel blocker overdose.[133] Routine use of calcium except in these

special resuscitation circumstances is not recommended.

Bretylium. Bretylium is no longer considered an appropriate first-line agent for pulseless arrest due to VF/VT because of the prevalence of hypotension associated with bretylium infusion,[92] the lack of demonstrable effectiveness in VT,[88,91] tachycardia,[88,91] and the absence of published studies of its use in children.

Procainamide is a sodium channel blocking antiarrhythmic agent that prolongs the effective refractory period of both atria and ventricles and depresses the conduction velocity within the conduction system. By slowing intraventricular conduction, it prolongs the QT and PR intervals. Procainamide has been used to treat or suppress VT.[85] Because it must be given by slow infusion to avoid toxicity from

heart block, myocardial depression, and prolongation of the QT interval (which predisposes to torsades de pointes tachycardia), its use as a bolus in pulseless arrest is not recommended.

Vasopressin. The results of one study of the use of vasopressin in treatment of pediatric circulatory shock and cardiac arrest have only recently been published (bolus dose 0.4 to 1.0 U/kg per dose).[93]

Summary Points

- The clinical signs of "instability" associated with arrhythmias are shock with hypotension or poor end-organ perfusion, altered consciousness, or sudden collapse.

- Pediatric arrhythmias are classified as "too slow" (bradycardia), "too fast" (tachycardia), or a "collapse" (arrest) rhythm.

FIGURE 20. Pediatric pulseless arrest algorithm.

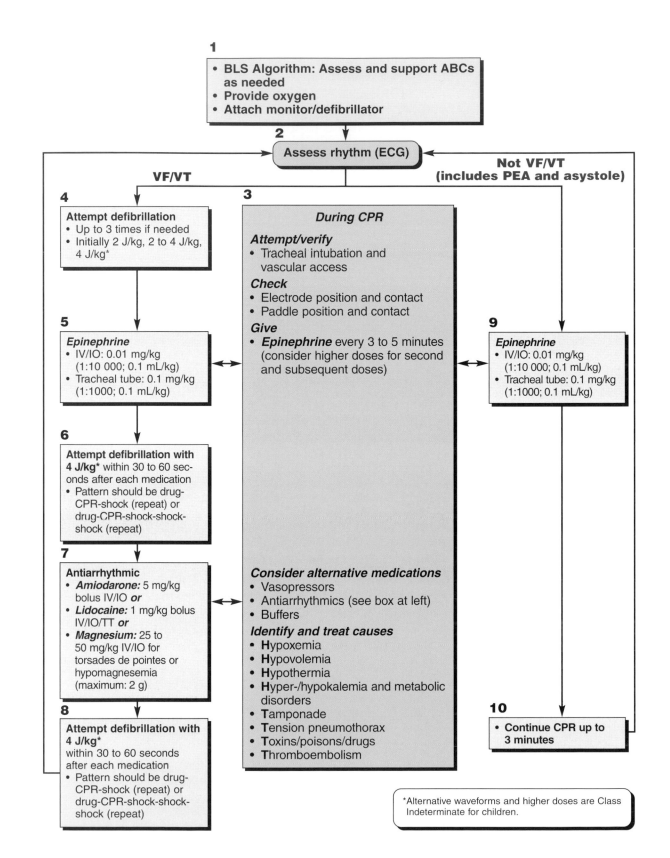

1
- BLS Algorithm: Assess and support ABCs as needed
- Provide oxygen
- Attach monitor/defibrillator

2
Assess rhythm (ECG)

VF/VT

Not VF/VT (includes PEA and asystole)

4
Attempt defibrillation
- Up to 3 times if needed
- Initially 2 J/kg, 2 to 4 J/kg, 4 J/kg*

3
During CPR

Attempt/verify
- Tracheal intubation and vascular access

Check
- Electrode position and contact
- Paddle position and contact

Give
- *Epinephrine* every 3 to 5 minutes (consider higher doses for second and subsequent doses)

5
Epinephrine
- IV/IO: 0.01 mg/kg (1:10 000; 0.1 mL/kg)
- Tracheal tube: 0.1 mg/kg (1:1000; 0.1 mL/kg)

9
Epinephrine
- IV/IO: 0.01 mg/kg (1:10 000; 0.1 mL/kg)
- Tracheal tube: 0.1 mg/kg (1:1000; 0.1 mL/kg)

6
Attempt defibrillation with **4 J/kg*** within 30 to 60 seconds after each medication
- Pattern should be drug-CPR-shock (repeat) or drug-CPR-shock-shock-shock (repeat)

7
Antiarrhythmic
- *Amiodarone:* 5 mg/kg bolus IV/IO *or*
- *Lidocaine:* 1 mg/kg bolus IV/IO/TT *or*
- *Magnesium:* 25 to 50 mg/kg IV/IO for torsades de pointes or hypomagnesemia (maximum: 2 g)

Consider alternative medications
- Vasopressors
- Antiarrhythmics (see box at left)
- Buffers

Identify and treat causes
- **H**ypoxemia
- **H**ypovolemia
- **H**ypothermia
- **H**yper-/hypokalemia and metabolic disorders
- **T**amponade
- **T**ension pneumothorax
- **T**oxins/poisons/drugs
- **T**hromboembolism

8
Attempt defibrillation with **4 J/kg***
within 30 to 60 seconds after each medication
- Pattern should be drug-CPR-shock (repeat) or drug-CPR-shock-shock-shock (repeat)

10
- Continue CPR up to 3 minutes

*Alternative waveforms and higher doses are Class Indeterminate for children.

- The PALS provider may differentiate between ST and SVT based on the child's history, the presence and appearance of P waves, heart rate variability, and rate.

- Special resuscitation circumstances associated with symptomatic arrhythmias may require modification of conventional PALS approaches (eg, wide-complex tachycardia induced by a known tricyclic antidepressant overdose is treated with sodium bicarbonate therapy).

- It is important to identify (using the 4 H's and 4 T's mnemonic) and treat reversible causes of symptomatic arrhythmias.

- General management of arrhythmias is as follows:
  — Administer oxygen, support ventilation if needed.
  — Perform chest compressions if heart rate is less than 60 bpm associated with poor perfusion or if tachycardia is associated with profound hypotension.
  — Obtain a rhythm strip or ECG if appropriate.
  — Identify and treat potentially reversible causes of arrhythmia.

- The main difference between treatment of perfusing VT and nonperfusing VT is the activation of synchronized cardioversion for a perfusing rhythm and defibrillation for pulseless VT.

- Specific therapies for arrhythmias are as follows:
  — *Symptomatic bradycardia:* oxygenation, epinephrine; consider atropine, consider pacing.
  — *SVT:* Determine the need for electrical versus pharmacologic interventions. Adenosine is recommended if IV/IO access is available; use the rapid 2-syringe technique. Consider vagal maneuvers for SVT with adequate perfusion.
  — *Wide-complex tachycardia with pulses:* Consider cardioversion or alternative medications: amiodarone or procainamide or lidocaine.

  — *VF/pulseless VT:* Attempt defibrillation immediately (up to 3 shocks if needed), then epinephrine (use "drug-CPR-shock" or "drug-CPR-shock-shock-shock" pattern; then consider amiodarone or lidocaine; for torsades or hypomagnesemia, give magnesium.

Case Scenarios
Introductory Case Scenario and Review Questions

A previously healthy 4-year-old girl presents to the Emergency Department with a 2-week history of flulike symptoms, including lethargy, fever, and dizziness. The child responds to your voice but is listless and confused. Her skin is pale and mottled, and distal extremities are cool. The child's airway is patent. Her respiratory rate is 40 breaths/min, but breathing is not labored. Her pulse is approximately 240 bpm and weak. Her temperature is 37°C (98.6°F), and her blood pressure is 70/50 mm Hg. Capillary refill time is 4 to 6 seconds. You administer 100% oxygen using a nonrebreathing face mask and attach an ECG monitor. As you attach the pulse oximeter, the child suddenly collapses and becomes unresponsive, apneic, and pulseless.

Case Scenario 1 Review Questions and Answers

- *What is your initial assessment of this child and how would you classify her physiologic status?*

  This child initially presents with symptoms of decompensated shock, including tachycardia, poor perfusion, lethargy (altered level of consciousness), and hypotension. Her condition rapidly deteriorates with *sudden collapse* and loss of pulses. She is now in cardiopulmonary arrest.

- *Which algorithm would you follow as you initiate treatment?*

  In your initial evaluation you would use the algorithm for pediatric tachycardia with poor perfusion. You should

switch to the pediatric pulseless arrest algorithm when the child collapses.

- *As you initiate therapy, what risk factors for the presence of special resuscitation circumstances do you recognize?*

  Marked tachycardia progressing to *sudden collapse* suggests the presence of a possible shockable rhythm, such as pulseless VT or VF. A "quick look" ECG is indicated to determine if a defibrillation attempt is indicated. Provide support of the airway, oxygenation, ventilation, and circulation while the emergency response team is activated and a monitor/defibrillator/pacer is attached.

  The child's history of a 2-week progression from mild symptoms to decompensated shock to sudden collapse is consistent with myocarditis (acquired cardiac disease). As you initiate CPR and treatment, perform a rapid survey to identify and treat reversible causes (ie, the 4H's and 4T's: Hypoxemia, Hypovolemia, Hypo- or Hyperthermia, Hyper-/Hypokalemia and metabolic disturbances, Tension pneumothorax, Tamponade, Toxins/poisons/drugs, Thromboembolism).

- *What key psychosocial support measures should you consider during and after the resuscitation attempt?*

  Every member of the healthcare team should provide support to the family, but additional support can be provided by nonmedical staff, such as social workers and chaplains who are familiar with family support issues and trained to help (see Chapter 16: "Coping With Death and Dying").

Case Scenario 2

You are called to see a 9-month-old infant with cyanosis, coughing, retractions, grunting, and lethargy. The infant's respiratory rate is 90 breaths/min with wheezing. The infant is sleepy but coughs and responds to painful stimuli. You ensure that the airway is patent; then you provide the infant with 100% oxygen. The cyanosis worsens, and the infant develops shallow, irregular respirations with an occasional gasp; the infant no longer responds to painful stimulation. The ECG monitor shows narrow complexes at a rate of 40 bpm. The infant has a weak pulse (40 bpm), and the pulse oximeter displays a rate of 40 bpm with oxygen saturation of 80%.

Case Scenario 2 Acceptable Actions

- Use universal precautions.

- Open the airway and provide effective bag-mask ventilation with 100% oxygen and monitor HR response.

- Perform tracheal intubation if within the scope of care and confirm tracheal tube placement.

- Reassess the patient's response to effective ventilation and oxygenation.

- Provide chest compressions if there is no response to effective oxygenation and ventilation and heart rate remains less than 60 bpm with poor perfusion.

- Consider appropriate medications (epinephrine is the drug of choice; consider atropine if you suspect vagal etiology) for persistent bradycardia.

- Attempt to identify and treat potentially reversible causes of bradycardia.

- Consider pacing for refractory bradycardia.

- Address family presence and coping with the stress of pediatric emergencies.

Case Scenario 2 Rationale for Acceptable Actions

The bradycardia algorithm emphasizes support of effective oxygenation and ventilation as the first priority. If there is no response to approximately 30 seconds of effective assisted ventilation and the heart rate is less than 60 bpm with poor perfusion, begin chest compressions and give epinephrine. If bradycardia persists, consider atropine and pacing. There is no history of profound hypothermia, head injury, heart block, heart transplant, or toxins/poisons/drugs. Nothing suggests excessive vagal stimulation as the cause of arrest, which might lead to earlier con-

sideration of use of anticholinergic (eg, atropine) medications.

Unacceptable Actions

- Failing to use universal precautions

- Failing to provide bag-mask ventilation

- Giving medications before providing support of the airway, oxygenation, and ventilation

- Failing to confirm tracheal tube placement (if within scope of care) or effectiveness of ventilation

- Failing to provide chest compressions and assess for special resuscitation circumstances if there is no response to effective oxygenation and ventilation

- Failing to acknowledge family need for support

Case Scenario 2 Progression

The patient is tracheally intubated (position confirmed), and effective ventilation and a dose of epinephrine are provided. The oxyhemoglobin saturation according to the pulse oximeter improves to 100%, and heart rate increases to 120 bpm with a narrow complex. There is continued respiratory distress but improved perfusion. There is no evidence of heart block on the ECG. The family and primary care providers are informed of the event and necessary interventions, and support is provided to family and bedside providers.

Case Scenario 3

You are called to see a 2-year-old child with a 2-day history of fever, vomiting, diarrhea, and lethargy. The child's airway is clear and the respiratory rate is mildly elevated at 30 breaths/min but unlabored. The child is lethargic and barely withdraws to painful stimulus. His extremities are cool and clammy, and capillary refill time is more than 5 seconds. The child's central pulse is weak and rapid with a rate of 170 bpm. You provide 100% oxygen and attach an ECG monitor as you shout for help and begin to assess and support the ABCs.

The child's blood pressure is 60/30 mm Hg. A 12-lead ECG shows QRS duration is less than 0.08 second at a rate of 170 bpm with normal P waves, heart rate varying with activity, and a variable R-R with constant PR interval. The pulse oximeter indicates a pulse rate of 170 bpm with a saturation reading of 100%. Breath sounds are clear and equal. There is no improvement in perfusion or response to stimulation with initial oxygen therapy.

Case Scenario 3 Acceptable Actions

- Follow universal precautions.

- Ensure effective ventilation and provide 100% oxygen; attach ECG monitor.

- Obtain vascular access (eg, IO) if within the scope of care.

- Provide a rapid fluid bolus of isotonic fluid (20 mL/kg).

- Reassess response to fluid bolus and provide additional boluses as appropriate.

- Recognize ST and differentiate between it and SVT.

- Obtain a bedside glucose analysis.

- Address family presence and coping with the stress of pediatric emergencies.

Case Scenario 3 Rationale for Acceptable Actions

This child's history of vomiting, diarrhea, and fever suggests shock with a likely component of hypovolemia. Weak and rapid pulses combined with cool extremities and delayed capillary refill are consistent with shock. Lethargy and a poor response to stimulation with a low blood pressure indicate decompensated shock (blood pressure is lower than 70 mm Hg + 2 times the child's age in years).

The algorithm for tachycardia with poor perfusion is appropriate. The ECG indicates a narrow complex and a heart rate of less than 180 bpm, normal P waves, heart rate variability with activity, and variable R-R with constant PR, suggesting that ST is likely. According to the child's history, hypovolemia or sepsis (or both) is the probable cause; this is compatible with ST. In this case *hypovolemia* and fever (*hyperthermia*) with possible sepsis are the likely causes. Establishment of vascular access and volume resuscitation are indicated.

Unacceptable Actions

- Failing to follow universal precautions
- Failing to recognize decompensated shock most likely related to hypovolemia
- Failing to prioritize management of shock
- Treating ST initially as SVT with medications or electrical cardioversion
- Failing to reassess the patient's response to volume resuscitation
- Using hypotonic crystalloid or glucose-containing fluid without suspicion or documentation of hypoglycemia
- Failing to acknowledge family stress or to deal with the issue of the family's presence during resuscitation

Case Scenario 3 Progression

After administration of 3 boluses of isotonic crystalloid, the child's pulse rate improves to 150 bpm, capillary refill time improves to less than 3 seconds, and the child is now awake and verbally responding to family members. Blood pressure is 80/40 mm Hg.

Case Scenario 4

(This case scenario is intended for advanced providers who work in intensive care, Emergency Department, critical care, or transport settings.)

The same 2-year-old child from Case Scenario 3 who presented with hypovolemic shock and sepsis syndrome has now been admitted to an intensive care/monitored setting. In the first 12 hours the child required 240 mL/kg of isotonic crystalloid boluses, a dopamine infusion of 10 µg/kg per minute, tracheal intubation with confirmation of exhaled CO_2, and mechanical ventilation with moderate settings.

Central venous and arterial catheters have been placed. Initial vital signs after these interventions are temperature of 39°C (102.2°F), heart rate of 170 bpm with narrow QRS complexes, respiratory rate of 25 breaths/min (mechanical ventilator set at 25 breaths/min), blood pressure of 90/50 mm Hg, oxyhemoglobin saturation of 98% on 40% O_2, and exhaled CO_2 of 35 mm Hg (normal is 30 to 40 mm Hg). The child is lethargic, responsive only to painful stimulus, and has a capillary refill time of 3 seconds. Central and peripheral pulses are rapid and palpable, and arterial waveform measurements correlate with noninvasive (oscillometric) blood pressure measurements.

The monitors suddenly alarm for heart rate of less than 60 bpm, damped arterial waveform of 50/30 mm Hg deteriorating to flat line, pulse oximeter SpO_2 of 80% that deteriorates until it does not detect a pulse, and exhaled CO_2 of 70 mm Hg that falls to 0. Pulses are not palpable, and breath sounds are decreased on the right. You increase inspired O_2 to 100% as you shout for help and assess and support the ABCs.

Case Scenario 4 Initial Acceptable Actions and Rationale

This child is in pulseless arrest. Immediately provide manual ventilation through the tracheal tube with 100% oxygen and perform a rapid survey to assess for airway displacement, tracheal tube obstruction, pneumothorax, and equipment failure (DOPE mnemonic). Assess the response to manual ventilation and begin chest compressions, following the pulseless arrest algorithm. Attach a monitor/defibrillator/pacer. In this scenario a tension pneumothorax seems a likely cause of the sudden deterioration. The sudden decompensation suggests acute *cardiopulmonary failure*, although you should rule out a complication of positive-pressure ventilation.

Case Scenario 4 Progression

The ECG monitor suggests PEA at a rate of less than 40 bpm. You detach the mechanical ventilator circuit from the child and provide manual ventilation with 100% O_2. The tracheal tube is securely taped at 13 cm at the lips and has not moved since admission. A colleague begins chest compressions; between compressions you detect no pulses, arterial waveform, or exhaled CO_2. Exhaled CO_2 is 15 mm Hg measured by capnography during vigorous chest compressions but 0 mm Hg when chest compressions are held. A suction catheter passes easily through the tracheal tube to at least 1 cm beyond the tip. The lungs are more difficult to ventilate (stiffer) than previously, and the right side of the chest is not moving well with manual ventilation with a bag-mask device. The neck veins are distended, but the trachea appears midline. The dopamine infusion is connected and infusing properly. There is no improvement in perfusion or response to stimulation with initial manual bag–tracheal tube ventilation.

Case Scenario 4 Additional Acceptable Actions and Rationale

This child demonstrates an organized ECG rhythm with no pulses and no evidence of perfusion consistent with PEA. The low exhaled CO_2 is consistent with cardiac arrest, but chest compressions are moving blood to the lungs and the tracheal tube is still intact. The increased resistance to ventilation and decreased breath sounds and chest expansion over the right chest suggest a tension pneumothorax as the cause of the PEA. In children, neck vein distention and tracheal deviation are late and unreliable signs of pneumothorax.

This child needs immediate needle decompression of the right chest with continued CPR and preparation for epinephrine and crystalloid bolus. Reassess cardiopulmonary status after this intervention.

TABLE 2. Drugs and Electrical Therapy Used in PALS for Rhythm Disturbances

Drug	Indications/Precautions	Dosage
Adenosine	*Indications:* Drug of choice for treatment of symptomatic SVT *Precautions:* Very short half-life (use rapid injection technique)	IV/IO: — Continuous ECG monitoring — 0.1 mg/kg rapid IV push Follow with 5 mL NS flush — May double (0.2 mg/kg) for second dose — Maximum first dose: 6 mg — Maximum second dose: 12 mg
Amiodarone	*Indications:* Wide range of atrial and ventricular arrhythmias and shock-refractory VF/VT *Precautions:* May cause bradycardia and hypotension; may prolong QT interval and increase risk for polymorphic VT; *do not* routinely combine with other medications that prolong QT interval (eg, procainamide)	*For perfusing VT and SVT:* 5 mg/kg IV/IO over 20 to 60 minutes (repeat as needed to maximum: 15 mg/kg per day) *For shock-refractory pulseless VT/VF:* 5 mg/kg rapid IV/IO bolus
Atropine sulfate	*Indications:* Vagally induced symptomatic bradycardia; symptomatic bradycardia refractory to oxygenation, ventilation, and epinephrine *Precautions:* Low dose may cause paradoxical bradycardia; tracheal absorption may be unreliable	IV/IO/tracheal: 0.02 mg/kg per dose; may double for second dose — Minimum dose: 0.1 mg — Maximum single dose, child: 0.5 mg (maximum total dose: 1 mg) — Maximum single dose, adolescent: 1 mg (maximum total dose: 2 mg)
Calcium chloride (10% solution = 27.2 mg/mL of elemental calcium)	*Indications:* Symptomatic hypocalcemia, hyperkalemia, calcium channel blocker overdose *Precautions:* Rapid IV push may result in bradycardia or asystole; do not mix with buffer; infiltration may cause skin to slough	IV/IO: 20 mg/kg (0.2 mL/kg of 10% solution) slow push — Repeat for documented conditions
Calcium gluconate (10% solution = 9 mg/mL of elemental calcium)	*Indications:* Symptomatic hypocalcemia, hyperkalemia, calcium channel blocker overdose *Precautions:* Rapid IV push may result in bradycardia or asystole; do not mix with buffer; infiltration may cause skin to slough	IV/IO: 60 to 100 mg/kg (0.6 to 1 mL/kg of 10% solution) slow push — Repeat for documented conditions
Synchronized cardioversion attempt	*Indications:* Tachyarrhythmias (SVT, VT, atrial fibrillation, atrial flutter) with symptoms of cardiovascular compromise *Precautions:* Activate sync mode; provide sedation with analgesia when possible	Initial energy (shock) level: 0.5 to 1 J/kg — Second and subsequent energy levels: 1 to 2 J/kg
Defibrillation attempt	*Indications:* VF/pulseless VT *Precautions:* Do not delay; use largest paddle size with good skin contact and no bridging	Deliver up to 3 shocks: — 2 J/kg; 2 to 4 J/kg; 4 J/kg — Subsequent energy level: 4 J/kg
Epinephrine for bradycardia*	*Indications:* Symptomatic bradycardia refractory to oxygenation and ventilation *Precautions:* May produce profound vasoconstriction, tachyarrhythmias, hypertension; do not mix with buffer	IV/IO: 0.01 mg/kg (0.1 mL/kg of 1:10 000) Tracheal: 0.1 mg/kg (0.1 mL/kg of 1:1000)

Drug	Indications/Precautions	Dosage
Epinephrine for asystolic or pulseless arrest*	*Indications:* Pulseless arrest: asystole, PEA, shock-refractory VF/VT *Precautions:* May produce profound vasoconstriction, tachyarrhythmias, hypertension; do not mix with buffer; avoid use in cocaine-related VT	**First dose:** IV/IO: 0.01 mg/kg (0.1 mL/kg of 1:10 000) Tracheal: 0.1 mg/kg (0.1 mL/kg of 1:1000) **Subsequent doses:** — Repeat every 3 to 5 minutes during CPR — Consider a higher dose (0.1 mg/kg, 0.1 mL/kg of 1:1000) for special conditions
Epinephrine infusion	*Indications:* Refractory hypotension or persistent brady-cardia *Precautions:* May produce profound vasoconstriction, tachyarrhythmias, hypertension; do not mix with buffer; avoid use in cocaine-related VT	0.1 to 1 µg/kg per minute Titrate to desired effect
Lidocaine bolus*	*Indications:* Alternative treatment for wide-complex tachycardias or VF/pulseless VT *Precautions:* High doses may cause myocardial depression and seizures; do not use if rhythm is wide-complex bradycardia (ventricular escape beats)	IV/IO/tracheal bolus: 1 mg/kg May repeat every 5 to 15 minutes
Lidocaine infusion	*Indications:* Alternative for recurrent VT/VF or ventricular ectopy, especially if associated with ischemic heart disease *Precautions:* High doses may cause myocardial depression and seizures; do not use if rhythm is wide-complex bradycardia (ventricular escape beats)	IV/IO infusion: 20 to 50 µg/kg per minute — Administer bolus of 1 mg/kg when initiating infusion if bolus has not been given within previous 15 minutes
Magnesium sulfate	*Indications:* Torsades de pointes VT or symptomatic hypomagnesemia *Precautions:* May cause hypotension with rapid bolus	Rapid IV/IO infusion: 25 to 50 mg/kg (maximum 2 g) over 10 to 20 minutes
Procainamide	*Indications:* Alternative treatment for recurrent or refractory VT, SVT *Precautions:* Hypotension, bradycardia, and QT prolongation *Do not routinely administer with amiodarone*	Loading dose: 15 mg/kg IV over 30 to 60 minutes
Sodium bicarbonate	*Indications:* Hyperkalemia, sodium channel blocker toxicity, and severe metabolic acidosis (documented or suspected after prolonged arrest) with adequate ventilation *Precautions:* Infuse slowly; may produce CO_2; therefore, ventilation must be adequate; do not mix with catecholamines or calcium	1 mEq/kg per dose Infuse slowly and only if ventilation is adequate

*For tracheal administration, dilute medication with normal saline to a volume of 3 to 5 mL and follow with several positive-pressure ventilations.

Review Questions

1. **A 3-year-old unresponsive, apneic child is brought to the ED. The EMTs transporting the child tell you that the child became pulseless on arrival at the hospital. The child is receiving CPR, including positive-pressure ventilation with bag and mask and 100% oxygen and chest compressions. You confirm that apnea is present and that ventilation is producing bilateral breath sounds and chest expansion while a colleague confirms the absence of spontaneous central pulses and other signs of circulation. Another colleague attaches the ECG monitor and reports that VF is present. Which of the following therapies is most appropriate for this child at this time?**

   a. establish IV/IO access and administer amiodarone 5 mg/kg

   b. establish IV/IO access and administer lidocaine 1 mg/kg

   c. attempt defibrillation at 2 J/kg

   d. establish IV/IO access and administer epinephrine 0.01 mg/kg

   The correct answer is c. The first therapy you should provide for VF or pulseless VT is immediate defibrillation. For infants and children the first energy dose is 2 J/kg. If that dose is ineffective, attempt defibrillation at 2 to 4 J/kg.

   Answers a and **b** are incorrect because you should not delay the defibrillation attempt. Although vascular access should be established quickly, you can wait until the first 3 shocks are delivered if needed. Administration of amiodarone or lidocaine is not recommended unless or until VF/pulseless VT persists despite 3 shocks, a dose of epinephrine, and a fourth shock.

   Answer d is incorrect because you should not delay the defibrillation attempt. You can wait to establish vascular access until after the delivery of the first 3 shocks if needed. Give epinephrine if VF/pulseless VT persists after 3 shocks.

2. **You are attempting resuscitation of an infant or a child with severe symptomatic bradycardia and no evidence of vagal etiology. The bradycardia persists despite establishment of an effective airway, oxygenation, and ventilation. Which of the following is the first drug you should administer?**

   a. atropine

   b. dopamine

   c. adenosine

   d. epinephrine

   The correct answer is d. Epinephrine is the first drug recommended for treatment of severe symptomatic bradycardia that is unresponsive to establishment of airway, oxygenation, and ventilation.

   Answer a is incorrect because atropine should be administered after epinephrine unless you suspect that the bradycardia is vagally induced.

   Answer b is incorrect because dopamine is not recommended in the initial treatment algorithm for severe symptomatic bradycardia. Dopamine provides only indirect release of catecholamines that can stimulate heart rate. Epinephrine, a catecholamine with direct effects, should initially be administered for severe symptomatic bradycardia unresponsive to establishment and support of airway, oxygenation, and ventilation.

   Answer c is incorrect because adenosine blocks AV conduction. Adenosine is used to treat SVT. It is not recommended for treatment of severe symptomatic bradycardia.

3. **A 9-month-old infant presents with a respiratory rate of 45 breaths/min and a heart rate of 250 bpm with narrow (less than 0.08 second) QRS complexes. The infant is receiving 100% oxygen by face mask, and an IV catheter is in place. The infant's systolic blood pressure is 64 mm Hg and palpable with faint pulses. Capillary refill time is 5 to 6 seconds. The infant responds only to painful stimulation, and he has no history of vomiting or diarrhea. Which of the following is the most appropriate initial treatment for this infant?**

   a. attempt immediate defibrillation

   b. administer a 20 mL/kg fluid bolus of normal saline over 20 minutes or less

   c. administer adenosine 0.1 mg/kg rapid bolus (2-syringe technique)

   d. administer verapamil

   The correct answer is c. The narrow-complex heart rate of 250 bpm suggests that the infant is in SVT; in infants ST rarely produces a heart rate greater than 220 bpm. Adenosine is the drug of choice for treatment of SVT because it blocks conduction through the AV node and interrupts SVT, enabling the return of normal sinus rhythm. Because the infant is unstable with hypotension and signs of poor perfusion, either synchronized cardioversion (0.5 to 1 J/kg initially) or immediate administration of adenosine by rapid push (using the 2-syringe technique) is appropriate. IV access is immediately available, so you should administer adenosine. If IV access or adenosine is unavailable or cannot immediately be obtained, synchronized cardioversion is the treatment of choice.

Answer a is incorrect because defibrillation shocks may convert SVT to VF or asystole. Defibrillation also uses higher initial and subsequent energy doses (2 J/kg initially) than synchronized cardioversion.

Answer b is incorrect because volume resuscitation will not resolve the basic problem of SVT.

Answer d is incorrect because routine use of verapamil, a calcium channel blocker, is not recommended for infants (less than 1 year of age). Refractory hypotension and cardiac arrest have been reported with administration of verapamil in this age group.

4. **You are preparing to attempt synchronized cardioversion for a child with SVT. What is the recommended** *initial* **energy dose for synchronized cardioversion for infants and children?**

   a. 0.05 to 0.1 J/kg

   b. 0.5 to 1 J/kg

   c. 2 to 4 J/kg

   d. 6 to 10 J/kg

   The correct answer is b. A starting dose of 0.5 to 1 J/kg is recommended for attempted cardioversion. If the patient remains in a rhythm requiring cardioversion, double the energy dose to 1 to 2 J/kg.

   Answer a is incorrect because a dose of 0.05 to 0.1 J/kg is too low for routine cardioversion. If a child is known to be receiving a drug such as digitalis, a low initial cardioversion dose may be used. But digitalis therapy is a special resuscitation circumstance, and the initial dose would still be higher than 0.05 to 0.1 J/kg.

   Answer c is incorrect because an initial dose of 2 to 4 J/kg is too high for routine cardioversion. If VF occurs, attempt defibrillation with an initial dose of 2 J/kg. The recommended

dose for a second defibrillation attempt is 2 to 4 J/kg.

Answer d is incorrect because 6 to 10 J/kg is much higher than the dose recommended for attempted cardioversion in infants and children.

5. **You are participating in the attempted resuscitation of a 3-year-old child in pulseless VT. You have attempted defibrillation 3 times without converting the VT to a perfusing rhythm. The airway is secure and ventilation is effective. Attempts at IV access have been unsuccessful, but IO access has been established. You have been unable to identify any reversible cause of the VT. You administer epinephrine IO, circulate it for 30 to 60 seconds, and attempt defibrillation a fourth time, but VT persists. Which of the following drugs should you administer next?**

   a. epinephrine 0.1 mg/kg by tracheal tube (1:1000 solution, 0.1 mL/kg)

   b. adenosine 0.1 mg/kg IV push

   c. epinephrine 0.1 mg/kg IO (1:1000 solution, 0.1 mL/kg)

   d. lidocaine 1 mg/kg IO or amiodarone 5 mg/kg IO

   The correct answer is d. Lidocaine and amiodarone are listed in the pediatric pulseless arrest algorithm under the pulseless VT/VF branch (left side). If 3 shocks, IV/IO epinephrine, and a fourth shock are unsuccessful, you may administer lidocaine or amiodarone. These drugs may successfully treat VT because they decrease automaticity and may suppress ventricular ectopy.

   Answer a is incorrect because it is too soon for the next epinephrine dose. The vascular or IO route is preferred for resuscitative medications, and IO access is available in this patient. Each drug should be

followed by 30 to 60 seconds of CPR and additional defibrillation attempts.

Answer b is incorrect because adenosine is recommended for SVT *with pulses,* not for pulseless VT.

Answer c is incorrect because it is too soon for the next dose of epinephrine, and this dose is high dose. The standard IV dose of epinephrine is 0.01 mg/kg or 0.1 mL/kg of 1:10 000 solution (not 0.1 mL/kg of 1:1000 solution). The standard dose should be given unless special resuscitation circumstances exist.

6. **You are assisting at a statewide track-and-field event in a professional sports facility. You see a teenage girl collapse while running. She is unresponsive when you arrive at her side. Other bystanders have called for EMS support and are performing well-coordinated CPR. They report that the teen has no known health problems, but she is now apneic and pulseless. Which of the following actions is most likely to improve her chance of survival?**

   a. you take over mouth-to-mouth resuscitation

   b. you attach and operate an AED as soon as one is available

   c. you provide crowd control

   d. you get a blanket to keep the patient warm

   The correct answer is b. Although primary cardiac events are uncommon causes of cardiopulmonary arrest in the young, they do occur and are more common in adolescents than in infants and children. This scenario describes an adolescent with an apparent primary cardiac event during strenuous exertion. With sudden cardiac arrest the

(Continued on next page)

most likely rhythm is VF or pulseless VT. The most effective treatment for VF/pulseless VT is defibrillation, so you should attach the AED as soon as possible. Because this victim is older than 1 year, use of an AED is a Class IIb recommendation.

Answer a is incorrect because you should not interfere with well-coordinated CPR.

Answer c is incorrect because crowd control, although helpful, will not contribute to this girl's chance of survival.

Answer d is incorrect because the therapies that will have the greatest impact on this girl's chance of survival are prompt bystander CPR and early defibrillation.

References

1. Young KD, Seidel JS. Pediatric cardiopulmonary resuscitation: a collective review. *Ann Emerg Med*. 1999;33:195-205.

2. Sirbaugh PE, Pepe PE, Shook JE, Kimball KT, Goldman MJ, Ward MA, Mann DM. A prospective, population-based study of the demographics, epidemiology, management, and outcome of out-of-hospital pediatric cardiopulmonary arrest [published correction appears in *Ann Emerg Med*. 1999;33:358]. *Ann Emerg Med*. 1999;33:174-184.

3. Richman PB, Nashed AH. The etiology of cardiac arrest in children and young adults: special considerations for ED management. *Am J Emerg Med*. 1999;17:264-270.

4. Adgey AA, Johnston PW, McMechan S. Sudden cardiac death and substance abuse. *Resuscitation*. 1995;29:219-221.

5. Zaritsky A, Nadkarni V, Hazinski MF, Foltin G, Quan L, Wright J, Fiser D, Zideman D, O'Malley P, Chameides L. Recommended guidelines for uniform reporting of pediatric advanced life support: the pediatric Utstein Style: a statement for healthcare professionals from a task force of the American Academy of Pediatrics, the American Heart Association, and the European Resuscitation Council. Writing Group. *Circulation*. 1995;92:2006-2020.

6. Ackerman MJ. The long QT syndrome. *Pediatr Rev*. 1998;19:232-238.

7. Zaritsky A, Nadkarni V, Getson P, Kuehl K. CPR in children. *Ann Emerg Med*. 1987;16:1107-1111.

8. Alimurung MM, Joseph LG, Nadas AS, Massell BF. Unipolar precordial and extremity electrocardiogram in normal infants and children. *Circulation*. 1951;4:420-429.

9. Ziegler RF. *Electrocardiographic Studies in Normal Infants and Children*. Springfield, Ill: Charles C Thomas Publishing; 1951.

10. Furman RA, Halloran WR. Electrocardiogram in the first two months of life. *J Pediatr*. 1951;39:307-319.

11. Tudbury PB, Atkinson DW. Electrocardiograms of 100 normal infants and young children. *J Pediatr*. 1950;34:466-481.

12. Gillette PC, Garson A Jr, Porter CJ, McNamara DG. Dysrhythmias. In: Adams FH, Emmanouildies GC, Riemenschneider TA, eds. *Moss' Heart Disease in Infants, Children and Adolescents*. Baltimore, Md: Williams & Wilkins; 1989.725-741.

13. Kerber RE, Kouba C, Martins J, Kelly K, Low R, Hoyt R, Ferguson D, Bailey L, Bennett P, Charbonnier F. Advance prediction of transthoracic impedance in human defibrillation and cardioversion: importance of impedance in determining the success of low-energy shocks. *Circulation*. 1984;70:303-308.

14. Kerber RE, Grayzel J, Hoyt R, Marcus M, Kennedy J. Transthoracic resistance in human defibrillation: influence of body weight, chest size, serial shocks, paddle size and paddle contact pressure. *Circulation*. 1981;63:676-682.

15. Sirna SJ, Ferguson DW, Charbonnier F, Kerber RE. Factors affecting transthoracic impedance during electrical cardioversion. *Am J Cardiol*. 1988;62:1048-1052.

16. Lerman BB, DiMarco JP, Haines DE. Current-based versus energy-based ventricular defibrillation: a prospective study. *J Am Coll Cardiol*. 1988;12:1259-1264.

17. Dalzell GW, Cunningham SR, Anderson J, Adgey AA. Initial experience with a microprocessor controlled current based defibrillator. *Br Heart J*. 1989;61:502-505.

18. Kerber RE, Martins JB, Kelly KJ, Ferguson DW, Kouba C, Jensen SR, Newman B, Parke JD, Kieso R, Melton J. Self-adhesive preapplied electrode pads for defibrillation and cardioversion. *J Am Coll Cardiol*. 1984;3:815-820.

19. Cobb LA, Fahrenbruch CE, Walsh TR, Copass MK, Olsufka M, Breskin M, Hallstrom AP. Influence of cardiopulmonary resuscitation prior to defibrillation in patients with out-of-hospital ventricular fibrillation. *JAMA*. 1999;281:1182-1188.

20. Yakaitis RW, Ewy GA, Otto CW, Taren DL, Moon TE. Influence of time and therapy on ventricular defibrillation in dogs. *Crit Care Med*. 1980;8:157-163.

21. Atkins DL, Sirna S, Kieso R, Charbonnier F, Kerber RE. Pediatric defibrillation: importance of paddle size in determining transthoracic impedance. *Pediatrics*. 1988;82:914-918.

22. Atkins DL, Kerber RE. Pediatric defibrillation: current flow is improved by using "adult" electrode paddles. *Pediatrics*. 1994;94:90-93.

23. Chameides L, Brown GE, Raye JR, Todres DI, Viles PH. Guidelines for defibrillation in infants and children: report of the American Heart Association target activity group: cardiopulmonary resuscitation in the young. *Circulation*. 1977;56:502A-503A.

24. Caterine MR, Yoerger DM, Spencer KT, Miller SG, Kerber RE. Effect of electrode position and gel-application technique on predicted transcardiac current during transthoracic defibrillation. *Ann Emerg Med*. 1997;29:588-595.

25. Garcia LA, Kerber RE. Transthoracic defibrillation: does electrode adhesive pad position alter transthoracic impedance? *Resuscitation*. 1998;37:139-143.

26. Bissing JW, Kerber RE. Effect of shaving the chest of hirsute subjects on transthoracic impedance to self-adhesive defibrillation electrode pads. *Am J Cardiol*. 2000;86:587-589.

27. McNaughton GW, Wyatt JP, Byrne JC. Defibrillation: a burning issue in coronary care units! *Scott Med J.* 1996;41:47-48.

28. Gutgesell HP, Tacker WA, Geddes LA, Davis S, Lie JT, McNamara DG. Energy dose for ventricular defibrillation of children. *Pediatrics.* 1976;58:898-901.

29. Cummins RO, Hazinski MF, Kerber RE, Kudenchuk P, Becker L, Nichol G, Malanga B, Aufderheide TP, Stapleton EM, Kern K, Ornato JP, Sanders A, Valenzuela T, Eisenberg M. Low-energy biphasic waveform defibrillation: evidence-based review applied to emergency cardiovascular care guidelines: a statement for healthcare professionals from the American Heart Association Committee on Emergency Cardiovascular Care and the Subcommittees on Basic Life Support, Advanced Cardiac Life Support, and Pediatric Resuscitation. *Circulation.* 1998;97:1654-1667.

30. Gibbs W, Eisenberg M, Damon SK. Dangers of defibrillation: injuries to emergency personnel during patient resuscitation. *Am J Emerg Med.* 1990;8:101-104.

31. Defibrillation. Cummins RO, ed. *Textbook of Advanced Cardiac Life Support.* Dallas, Tex: American Heart Association; 1994.

32. Cummins RO, Eisenberg MS, Litwin PE, Graves JR, Hearne TR, Hallstrom AP. Automatic external defibrillators used by emergency medical technicians: a controlled clinical trial. *JAMA.* 1987;257:1605-1610.

33. Weaver WD, Hill D, Fahrenbruch CE, Copass MK, Martin JS, Cobb LA, Hallstrom AP. Use of the automatic external defibrillator in the management of out-of-hospital cardiac arrest. *N Engl J Med.* 1988;319:661-666.

34. Sedgwick ML, Watson J, Dalziel K, Carrington DJ, Cobbe SM. Efficacy of out of hospital defibrillation by ambulance technicians using automated external defibrillators: the Heartstart Scotland Project. *Resuscitation.* 1992;24:73-87.

35. Atkins DL, Hartley LL, York DK. Accurate recognition and effective treatment of ventricular fibrillation by automated external defibrillators in adolescents. *Pediatrics.* 1998;101 (pt 1):393-397.

36. Cecchin F, Perry JC, Berul CI, Jorgenson DB, Brian DW, Lyster T, Snider DE, Zimmerman AA, Lupinetti FM, Rosenthal GL, Rule D, Atkins DL. Accuracy of automatic external defibrillator analysis algorithm in young children [abstract]. *Circulation.* 1999;100 (suppl I):I-663.

37. Hazinski MF, Walker C, Smith J, Deshpande J. Specificity of automatic external defibrillator rhythm analysis in pediatric tachyarrhythmias [abstract]. *Circulation.* 1997;96(suppl I):I-561.

37a. Automated External Defibrillators for Children: an Update. An Advisory Statement by the Pediatric Advanced Life Support Task Force of the International Liaison Committee on Resuscitation (ILCOR). *Circulation* 2003. In press.

38. Lown B. Electrical reversion of cardiac arrhythmias. *Br Heart J.* 1967;29:469-489.

39. Zoll PM, Zoll RH, Falk RH, Clinton JE, Eitel DR, Antman EM. External noninvasive temporary cardiac pacing: clinical trials. *Circulation.* 1985;71:937-944.

40. Dalsey WC, Syverud SA, Hedges JR. Emergency department use of transcutaneous pacing for cardiac arrests. *Crit Care Med.* 1985;13:399-401.

41. Quan L, Graves JR, Kinder DR, Horan S, Cummins RO. Transcutaneous cardiac pacing in the treatment of out-of-hospital pediatric cardiac arrests. *Ann Emerg Med.* 1992;21:905-909.

42. Cummins RO, Haulman J, Quan L, Graves JR, Peterson D, Horan S. Near-fatal yew berry intoxication treated with external cardiac pacing and digoxin-specific FAB antibody fragments. *Ann Emerg Med.* 1990;19:38-43.

43. Kissoon N, Rosenberg HC, Kronick JB. Role of transcutaneous pacing in the setting of a failing permanent pacemaker. *Pediatr Emerg Care.* 1989;5:178-180.

44. Beland MJ, Hesslein PS, Finlay CD, Faerron-Angel JE, Williams WG, Rowe RD. Non-invasive transcutaneous cardiac pacing in children. *Pacing Clin Electrophysiol.* 1987;10:1262-1270.

45. Falk RH, Ngai ST. External cardiac pacing: influence of electrode placement on pacing threshold. *Crit Care Med.* 1986;14:931-932.

46. Sreeram N, Wren C. Supraventricular tachycardia in infants: response to initial treatment. *Arch Dis Child.* 1990;65:127-129.

47. Aydin M, Baysal K, Kucukoduk S, Cetinkaya F, Yaman S. Application of ice water to the face in initial treatment of supraventricular tachycardia. *Turk J Pediatr.* 1995;37:15-17.

48. Ornato JP, Hallagan LF, Reese WA, Clark RF, Tayal VS, Garnett AR, Gonzalez ER. Treatment of paroxysmal supraventricular tachycardia in the emergency department by clinical decision analysis. *Am J Emerg Med.* 1988;6:555-560.

49. Lim SH, Anantharaman V, Teo WS, Goh PP, Tan AT. Comparison of treatment of supraventricular tachycardia by Valsalva maneuver and carotid sinus massage. *Ann Emerg Med.* 1998;31:30-35.

50. Waxman MB, Wald RW, Sharma AD, Huerta F, Cameron DA. Vagal techniques for termination of paroxysmal supraventricular tachycardia. *Am J Cardiol.* 1980;46:655-664.

51. Mogayzel C, Quan L, Graves JR, Tiedeman D, Fahrenbruch C, Herndon P. Out-of-hospital ventricular fibrillation in children and adolescents: causes and outcomes. *Ann Emerg Med.* 1995;25:484-491.

52. Hickey RW, Cohen DM, Strausbaugh S, Dietrich AM. Pediatric patients requiring CPR in the prehospital setting. *Ann Emerg Med.* 1995;25:495-501.

53. Walsh CK, Krongrad E. Terminal cardiac electrical activity in pediatric patients. *Am J Cardiol.* 1983;51:557-561.

54. Huang YG, Wong KC, Yip WH, McJames SW, Pace NL. Cardiovascular responses to graded doses of three catecholamines during lactic and hydrochloric acidosis in dogs. *Br J Anaesth.* 1995;74:583-590.

55. Preziosi MP, Roig JC, Hargrove N, Burchfield DJ. Metabolic acidemia with hypoxia attenuates the hemodynamic responses to epinephrine during resuscitation in lambs. *Crit Care Med.* 1993;21:1901-1907.

56. Dauchot P, Gravenstein JS. Effects of atropine on the electrocardiogram in different age groups. *Clin Pharmacol Ther.* 1971;12:274-280.

57. Howard RF, Bingham RM. Endotracheal compared with intravenous administration of atropine. *Arch Dis Child.* 1990;65:449-450.

58. Lee PL, Chung YT, Lee BY, Yeh CY, Lin SY, Chao CC. The optimal dose of atropine via the endotracheal route. *Ma Tsui Hsueh Tsa Chi.* 1989;27:35-38.

59. Fisher DJ, Gross DM, Garson A Jr. Rapid sinus tachycardia: differentiation from supraventricular tachycardia. *Am J Dis Child.* 1983;137:164-166.

60. Kugler JD, Danford DA. Management of infants, children, and adolescents with paroxysmal supraventricular tachycardia. *J Pediatr.* 1996;129:324-338.

61. Olley PH. Cardiac arrhythmias. In: Keith JD, Rowe RD, Vald P, eds. *Heart Disease in Infancy and Childhood.* New York, NY: Macmillan Publishing Co, Inc; 1978, 279-280.

62. Gikonyo BM, Dunnigan A, Benson DW Jr. Cardiovascular collapse in infants: association with paroxysmal atrial tachycardia. *Pediatrics.* 1985;76:922-926.

63. Losek JD, Endom E, Dietrich A, Stewart G, Zempsky W, Smith K. Adenosine and pediatric supraventricular tachycardia in the emergency department: multicenter study and review. *Ann Emerg Med.* 1999;33:185-191.

64. Overholt ED, Rheuban KS, Gutgesell HP, Lerman BB, DiMarco JP. Usefulness of adenosine for arrhythmias in infants and children. *Am J Cardiol.* 1988;61:336-340.

65. Getschman SJ, Dietrich AM, Franklin WH, Allen HD. Intraosseous adenosine: as effective as peripheral or central venous administration? *Arch Pediatr Adolesc Med.* 1994;148:616-619.

66. Friedman FD. Intraosseous adenosine for the termination of supraventricular tachycardia in an infant. *Ann Emerg Med.* 1996;28:356-358.

67. Epstein ML, Kiel EA, Victorica BE. Cardiac decompensation following verapamil therapy in infants with supraventricular tachycardia. *Pediatrics.* 1985;75:737-740.

68. Kirk CR, Gibbs JL, Thomas R, Radley-Smith R, Qureshi SA. Cardiovascular collapse after verapamil in supraventricular tachycardia. *Arch Dis Child.* 1987;62:1265-1266.

69. Rankin AC, Rae AP, Oldroyd KG, Cobbe SM. Verapamil or adenosine for the immediate treatment of supraventricular tachycardia. *Q J Med.* 1990;74:203-208.

70. van Haarst AD, van't Klooster GA, van Gerven JM, Schoemaker RC, van Oene JC, Burggraaf J, Coene MC, Cohen AF. The influence of cisapride and clarithromycin on QT intervals in healthy volunteers. *Clin Pharmacol Ther.* 1998;64:542-546.

71. Banai S, Tzivoni D. Drug therapy for torsade de pointes. *J Cardiovasc Electrophysiol.* 1993;4:206-210.

72. Fazekas T, Scherlag BJ, Vos M, Wellens HJ, Lazzara R. Magnesium and the heart: antiarrhythmic therapy with magnesium. *Clin Cardiol.* 1993;16:768-774.

73. Perry JC, Fenrich AL, Hulse JE, Triedman JK, Friedman RA, Lamberti JJ. Pediatric use of intravenous amiodarone: efficacy and safety in critically ill patients from a multicenter protocol. *J Am Coll Cardiol.* 1996;27:1246-1250.

74. Naccarelli GV, Wolbrette DL, Patel HM, Luck JC. Amiodarone: clinical trials. *Curr Opin Cardiol.* 2000;15:64-72.

75. Mattioni TA, Zheutlin TA, Dunnington C, Kehoe RF. The proarrhythmic effects of amiodarone. *Prog Cardiovasc Dis.* 1989;31:439-446.

76. Perry JC, Knilans TK, Marlow D, Denfield SW, Fenrich AL, Friedman RA. Intravenous amiodarone for life-threatening tachyarrhythmias in children and young adults. *J Am Coll Cardiol.* 1993;22:95-98.

77. Raja P, Hawker RE, Chaikitpinyo A, Cooper SG, Lau KC, Nunn GR, Cartmill TB, Sholler GF. Amiodarone management of junctional ectopic tachycardia after cardiac surgery in children. *Br Heart J.* 1994;72:261-265.

78. Scheinman MM, Levine JH, Cannom DS, Friehling T, Kopelman HA, Chilson DA, Platia EV, Wilber DJ, Kowey PR. Dose-ranging study of intravenous amiodarone in patients with life-threatening ventricular tachyarrhythmias. The Intravenous Amiodarone Multicenter Investigators Group. *Circulation.* 1995;92:3264-3272.

79. Figa FH, Gow RM, Hamilton RM, Freedom RM. Clinical efficacy and safety of intravenous amiodarone in infants and children. *Am J Cardiol.* 1994;74:573-577.

80. Pongiglione G, Strasburger JF, Deal BJ, Benson DW Jr. Use of amiodarone for short-term and adjuvant therapy in young patients. *Am J Cardiol.* 1991;68:603-608.

81. Hjelms E. Procainamide conversion of acute atrial fibrillation after open-heart surgery compared with digoxin treatment. *Scand J Thorac Cardiovasc Surg.* 1992;26:193-196.

82. Boahene KA, Klein GJ, Yee R, Sharma AD, Fujimura O. Termination of acute atrial fibrillation in the Wolff-Parkinson-White syndrome by procainamide and propafenone: importance of atrial fibrillatory cycle length. *J Am Coll Cardiol.* 1990;16:1408-1414.

83. Mehta AV, Sanchez GR, Sacks EJ, Casta A, Dunn JM, Donner RM. Ectopic automatic atrial tachycardia in children: clinical characteristics, management and follow-up. *J Am Coll Cardiol.* 1988;11:379-385.

84. Walsh EP, Saul JP, Sholler GF, Triedman JK, Jonas RA, Mayer JE, Wessel DL. Evaluation of a staged treatment protocol for rapid automatic junctional tachycardia after operation for congenital heart disease. *J Am Coll Cardiol.* 1997;29:1046-1053.

85. Singh BN, Kehoe R, Woosley RL, Scheinman M, Quart B. Multicenter trial of sotalol compared with procainamide in the suppression of inducible ventricular tachycardia: a double-blind, randomized parallel evaluation. Sotalol Multicenter Study Group. *Am Heart J.* 1995;129:87-97.

86. Luedtke SA, Kuhn RJ, McCaffrey FM. Pharmacologic management of supraventricular tachycardias in children, part 1: Wolff-Parkinson-White and atrioventricular nodal reentry. *Ann Pharmacother.* 1997;31:1227-1243.

87. Luedtke SA, Kuhn RJ, McCaffrey FM. Pharmacologic management of supraventricular tachycardias in children, part 2: atrial flutter, atrial fibrillation, and junctional and atrial ectopic tachycardia. *Ann Pharmacother.* 1997;31:1347-1359.

88. Chow MS, Kluger J, DiPersio DM, Lawrence R, Fieldman A. Antifibrillatory effects of lidocaine and bretylium immediately postcardiopulmonary resuscitation. *Am Heart J.* 1985;110:938-943.

89. Wesley RC Jr, Resh W, Zimmerman D. Reconsiderations of the routine and preferential use of lidocaine in the emergent treatment of ventricular arrhythmias. *Crit Care Med.* 1991;19:1439-1444.

90. Armengol RE, Graff J, Baerman JM, Swiryn S. Lack of effectiveness of lidocaine for sustained, wide QRS complex tachycardia. *Ann Emerg Med.* 1989;18:254-257.

91. Kowey PR, Levine JH, Herre JM, Pacifico A, Lindsay BD, Plumb VJ, Janosik DL, Kopelman HA, Scheinman MM. Randomized, double-blind comparison of intravenous amiodarone and bretylium in the treatment of patients with recurrent, hemodynamically destabilizing ventricular tachycardia or fibrillation. The Intravenous Amiodarone Multicenter Investigators Group. *Circulation.* 1995;92:3255-3263.

92. Chandrasekaran S, Steinberg JS. Efficacy of bretylium tosylate for ventricular tachycardia. *Am J Cardiol.* 1999;83:115-117, A9.

93. Mann K, Berg RA, Nadkarni V. Beneficial effects of vasopressin in prolonged pediatric cardiac arrest: a case series. *Resuscitation.* 2002;52:149-156.

94. Katz K, Lawler J, Wax J, O'Connor R, Nadkarni V. Vasopressin pressor effects in critically ill children during evaluation for brain death and organ recovery. *Resuscitation.* 2000;47:33-40.

95. Liedal JL, Meadow W, Nachman J, Koogler T, Kahana MD. Use of vasopressin in refractory hypotension in children with vasodilatory shock; five cases of review of the literature. *Pediatr Crit Care Med.* 2002;3:15-18.

96. Dieckmann RA, Vardis R. High-dose epinephrine in pediatric out-of-hospital cardiopulmonary arrest. *Pediatrics.* 1995;95:901-913.

97. Losek JD, Hennes H, Glaeser P, Hendley G, Nelson DB. Prehospital care of the pulseless, nonbreathing pediatric patient. *Am J Emerg Med.* 1987;5:370-374.

98. Coffing CR, Quan L, Graves JR, et al. Etiologies and outcomes of the pulseless, nonbreathing pediatric patient presenting with ventricular fibrillation [abstract]. *Ann Emerg Med.* 1992;21:1046.

99. Quan L, Gore EJ, Wentz K, Allen J, Novack AH. Ten-year study of pediatric drownings and near-drownings in King County, Washington: lessons in injury prevention. *Pediatrics.* 1989;83:1035-1040.

100. Appleton GO, Cummins RO, Larson MP, Graves JR. CPR and the single rescuer: at what age should you "call first" rather than "call fast"? *Ann Emerg Med.* 1995;25:492-494.

101. Losek JD, Hennes H, Glaeser PW, Smith DS, Hendley G. Prehospital countershock treatment of pediatric asystole. *Am J Emerg Med.* 1989;7:571-575.

102. Niemann JT, Criley JM, Rosborough JP, Niskanen RA, Alferness C. Predictive indices of successful cardiac resuscitation after prolonged arrest and experimental cardiopulmonary resuscitation. *Ann Emerg Med.* 1985;14:521-528.

103. Sanders AB, Ewy GA, Taft TV. Prognostic and therapeutic importance of the aortic diastolic pressure in resuscitation from cardiac arrest. *Crit Care Med.* 1984;12:871-873.

104. Stiell IG, Hebert PC, Weitzman BN, Wells GA, Raman S, Stark RM, Higginson LA, Ahuja J, Dickinson GE. High-dose epinephrine in adult cardiac arrest. *N Engl J Med.* 1992;327:1045-1050.

105. Brown CG, Martin DR, Pepe PE, Stueven H, Cummins RO, Gonzalez E, Jastremski M. A comparison of standard-dose and high-dose epinephrine in cardiac arrest outside the hospital. The Multicenter High-Dose Epinephrine Study Group. *N Engl J Med.* 1992;327:1051-1055.

106. Callaham M, Madsen CD, Barton CW, Saunders CE, Pointer J. A randomized clinical trial of high-dose epinephrine and norepinephrine vs standard-dose epinephrine in prehospital cardiac arrest. *JAMA.* 1992;268:2667-2672.

107. Lipman J, Wilson W, Kobilski S, Scribante J, Lee C, Kraus P, Cooper J, Barr J, Moyes D. High-dose adrenaline in adult in-hospital asystolic cardiopulmonary resuscitation: a double-blind randomised trial. *Anaesth Intensive Care.* 1993;21:192-196.

108. Lindner KH, Ahnefeld FW, Prengel AW. Comparison of standard and high-dose adrenaline in the resuscitation of asystole and electromechanical dissociation. *Acta Anaesthesiol Scand.* 1991;35:253-256.

109. Sherman BW, Munger MA, Foulke GE, Rutherford WF, Panacek EA. High-dose versus standard-dose epinephrine treatment of cardiac arrest after failure of standard therapy. *Pharmacotherapy.* 1997;17:242-247.

110. Choux C, Gueugniaud PY, Barbieux A, Pham E, Lae C, Dubien PY, Petit P. Standard doses versus repeated high doses of epinephrine in cardiac arrest outside the hospital. *Resuscitation.* 1995;29:3-9.

111. Woodhouse SP, Cox S, Boyd P, Case C, Weber M. High dose and standard dose adrenaline do not alter survival, compared with placebo, in cardiac arrest. *Resuscitation.* 1995;30:243-249.

112. Gueugniaud PY, Mols P, Goldstein P, Pham E, Dubien PY, Deweerdt C, Vergnion M, Petit P, Carli P. A comparison of repeated high doses and repeated standard doses of epinephrine for cardiac arrest outside the hospital. European Epinephrine Study Group. *N Engl J Med.* 1998;339:1595-1601.

113. Berg RA, Otto CW, Kern KB, Hilwig RW, Sanders AB, Henry CP, Ewy GA. A randomized, blinded trial of high-dose epinephrine versus standard-dose epinephrine in a swine model of pediatric asphyxial cardiac arrest. *Crit Care Med.* 1996;24:1695-1700.

114. Berg RA, Otto CW, Kern KB, Sanders AB, Hilwig RW, Hansen KK, Ewy GA. High-dose epinephrine results in greater early mortality after resuscitation from prolonged cardiac arrest in pigs: a prospective, randomized study. *Crit Care Med.* 1994;22:282-290.

115. Ronco R, King W, Donley DK, Tilden SJ. Outcome and cost at a children's hospital following resuscitation for out-of-hospital cardiopulmonary arrest. *Arch Pediatr Adolesc Med.* 1995;149:210-214.

116. Kuisma M, Suominen P, Korpela R. Paediatric out-of-hospital cardiac arrests: epidemiology and outcome. *Resuscitation.* 1995;30:141-150.

117. Carpenter TC, Stenmark KR. High-dose epinephrine is not superior to standard-dose epinephrine in pediatric in-hospital cardiopulmonary arrest. *Pediatrics.* 1997;99:403-408.

118. Fisher DG, Schwartz PH, Davis AL. Pharmacokinetics of exogenous epinephrine in critically ill children. *Crit Care Med.* 1993;21:111-117.

119. Berg RA, Donnerstein RL, Padbury JF. Dobutamine infusions in stable, critically ill children: pharmacokinetics and hemodynamic actions. *Crit Care Med.* 1993;21:678-686.

120. Padbury JF, Agata Y, Baylen BG, Ludlow JK, Polk DH, Goldblatt E, Pescetti J. Dopamine pharmacokinetics in critically ill newborn infants. *J Pediatr.* 1987;110:293-298.

121. Habib DM, Padbury JF, Anas NG, Perkin RM, Minegar C. Dobutamine pharmacokinetics and pharmacodynamics in pediatric intensive care patients. *Crit Care Med.* 1992;20:601-608.

122. Martinez AM, Padbury JF, Thio S. Dobutamine pharmacokinetics and cardiovascular responses in critically ill neonates. *Pediatrics.* 1992;89:47-51.

123. Berg RA, Padbury JF. Sulfoconjugation and renal excretion contribute to the interpatient variation of exogenous catecholamine clearance in critically ill children. *Crit Care Med.* 1997;25:1247-1251.

124. Zaritsky A, Lotze A, Stull R, Goldstein DS. Steady-state dopamine clearance in critically ill infants and children. *Crit Care Med.* 1988;16:217-220.

125. Notterman DA, Greenwald BM, Moran F, DiMaio-Hunter A, Metakis L, Reidenberg MM. Dopamine clearance in critically ill infants and children: effect of age and organ system dysfunction. *Clin Pharmacol Ther.* 1990;48:138-147.

126. Paradis NA, Martin GB, Goetting MG, Rivers EP, Feingold M, Nowak RM. Aortic pressure during human cardiac arrest: identification of pseudo-electromechanical dissociation. *Chest.* 1992;101:123-128.

127. Berg RA, Hilwig RW, Kern KB, Ewy GA. "Bystander" chest compressions and assisted ventilation independently improve outcome from piglet asphyxial pulseless "cardiac arrest." *Circulation.* 2000;101:1743-1748.

128. Kyriacou DN, Arcinue EL, Peek C, Kraus JF. Effect of immediate resuscitation on children with submersion injury. *Pediatrics.* 1994;94(pt 1):137-142.

129. Stueven HA, Thompson B, Aprahamian C, Tonsfeldt DJ, Kastenson EH. Lack of effectiveness of calcium chloride in refractory asystole. *Ann Emerg Med.* 1985;14:630-632.

130. Stueven HA, Thompson B, Aprahamian C, Tonsfeldt DJ, Kastenson EH. The effectiveness of calcium chloride in refractory electromechanical dissociation. *Ann Emerg Med.* 1985;14:626-629.

131. Bisogno JL, Langley A, Von Dreele MM. Effect of calcium to reverse the electrocardiographic effects of hyperkalemia in the isolated rat heart: a prospective, dose-response study. *Crit Care Med.* 1994;22:697-704.

132. Bohman VR, Cotton DB. Supralethal magnesemia with patient survival. *Obstet Gynecol.* 1990;76(pt 2):984-986.

133. Ramoska EA, Spiller HA, Winter M, Borys D. A one-year evaluation of calcium channel blocker overdoses: toxicity and treatment. *Ann Emerg Med.* 1993;22:196-200.

134. Bossaert L, Van Hoeyweghen R. Bystander cardiopulmonary resuscitation (CPR) in out-of-hospital cardiac arrest. The Cerebral Resuscitation Study Group. *Resuscitation.* 1989;17(suppl):S55-S69.

135. Nichol G, Stiell IG, Laupacis A, Pham B, De Maio VJ, Wells GA. A cumulative meta-analysis of the effectiveness of defibrillator-capable emergency medical services for victims of out-of-hospital cardiac arrest. *Ann Emerg Med.* 1999;34(pt 1):517-525.

136. Berg RA, Hilwig R, Kern K, Ewy G. Precountershock cardiopulmonary resuscitation improves readiness for defibrillation in a swine model of prehospital ventricular fibrillation [abstract]. *Crit Care Med.* 2001;29:A73.

137. Eisenberg M, Bergner L, Hallstrom A. Epidemiology of cardiac arrest and resuscitation in children. *Ann Emerg Med.* 1983;12:672-674.

138. Otto CW, Yakaitis RW, Blitt CD. Mechanism of action of epinephrine in resuscitation from asphyxial arrest. *Crit Care Med.* 1981;9:321-324.

139. Kudenchuk PJ, Cobb LA, Copass MK, Cummins RO, Doherty AM, Fahrenbruch CE, Hallstrom AP, Murray WA, Olsufka M, Walsh T. Amiodarone for resuscitation after out-of-hospital cardiac arrest due to ventricular fibrillation. *N Engl J Med.* 1999;341:871-878.

140. Kosinski EJ, Albin JB, Young E, Lewis SM, LeLand OS Jr. Hemodynamic effects of intravenous amiodarone. *J Am Coll Cardiol.* 1984;4:565-570.

141. Mason JW. Amiodarone. *N Engl J Med.* 1987;316:455-466.

142. Raeder EA, Podrid PJ, Lown B. Side effects and complications of amiodarone therapy. *Am Heart J.* 1985;109(pt 1):975-983.

143. Bigger JT Jr, Mandel WJ. Effect of lidocaine on the electrophysiological properties of ventricular muscle and Purkinje fibers. *J Clin Invest.* 1970;49:63-77.

144. Ettinger PO, Regan TJ, Oldewurtel HA. Hyperkalemia, cardiac conduction, and the electrocardiogram: a review. *Am Heart J.* 1974;88:360-371.

145. Hoffman JR, Votey SR, Bayer M, Silver L. Effect of hypertonic sodium bicarbonate in the treatment of moderate-to-severe cyclic antidepressant overdose. *Am J Emerg Med.* 1993;11:336-341.

146. Cardenas-Rivero N, Chernow B, Stoiko MA, Nussbaum SR, Todres ID. Hypocalcemia in critically ill children. *J Pediatr.* 1989;114: 946-951.

147. Zaritsky A. Cardiopulmonary resuscitation in children. *Clin Chest Med.* 1987;8:561-571.

Postarrest Stabilization and Transport

Introductory Case Scenario

A 1-year-old child with a history of developmental delay and seizure disorder presents after a prolonged seizure (more than 30 minutes) with vomiting and aspiration. The child was flaccid, cyanotic, apneic, and profoundly bradycardic (heart rate of 40 bpm with poor perfusion) and required 10 minutes of resuscitation with bag-mask ventilation, tracheal intubation, chest compressions, and intraosseous (IO) epinephrine. These efforts led to return of adequate heart rate and perfusion. The seizures have stopped, but the child does not respond to verbal or painful stimuli.

On examination she has bilateral coarse breath sounds that are better on the right side than on the left. Her temperature is 39°C, heart rate is 160 bpm (sinus rhythm), respiratory rate is 30 breaths/min with manual ventilation, blood pressure is 90/60 mm Hg, capillary refill time is less than 2 seconds, and pupils are 6 mm and minimally reactive bilaterally. Pulse oximetry measures 90% oxyhemoglobin saturation while 100% oxygen is given by tracheal tube. Exhaled CO_2 is 50 mm Hg. There are copious, thick secretions from the child's tracheal tube. The referring physician asks you to stabilize the child, perform a CT scan of the brain, and transport her to a tertiary pediatric intensive care unit (PICU).

- How would you approach postarrest stabilization and transport of this child?

- What is your rapid physiologic assessment?

- What are the stabilization and transport treatment priorities for this child?

Learning Objectives

After completing this chapter the PALS provider should be able to

- Describe the initial approach to assessment and stabilization after cardiopulmonary arrest and in preparation for transport

- Describe how initial assessment and treatment priorities for postarrest stabilization are similar to the standard PALS approach with emphasis on common postarrest problems and interventions:
  — Assess and support oxygenation and ventilation
  — Assess and support cardiovascular function and anticipate and treat myocardial dysfunction
  — Control body temperature
  — Assess and support metabolic needs (eg, glucose, electrolytes, acid-base balance)

- Describe factors influencing method and mode of transport within and between hospitals

- Identify potential high-risk problems (eg, tube displacement, tube obstruction, pneumothorax, equipment failure) for children after cardiopulmonary arrest and during transport

- Prioritize communication to providers and families before, during, and after patient stabilization and transport

Principles of Stabilization and Transport

Postarrest care involves stabilization and transport of the patient. Stabilization involves initiating treatment for any reversible cause of arrest and providing continuous ALS. Transport encompasses providing supportive care while moving the patient to a pediatric tertiary care setting and transferring responsibility for the patient's care to the receiving providers (see Figure 1). The PALS principles of rapid cardiopulmonary assessment and support of the ABCs (**A**irway, **B**reathing, and **C**irculation) are continued in postresuscitative care. This care also includes evaluating neurologic function (**D**isability), monitoring **E**xposure and **E**nvironment, and assessing and maintaining a core temperature range. Important aspects of postresuscitation stabilization and transport, including preparation for transport, are emphasized. A detailed presentation of critical care management is beyond the scope of this textbook.

The goals of postarrest stabilization are to preserve brain function, prevent secondary organ injury, assess and treat the cause of illness, and deliver the patient in optimum condition to a tertiary care setting. After resuscitation you must continue to evaluate the child's cardiopulmonary

FIGURE 1. Phases of resuscitation.

Prearrest	Arrest	CPR	Postarrest: Stabilize/Transport
Priority: Prevent respiratory arrest Prevent cardiac arrest	**Priority:** Restore oxygen Restart heart flow Restart brain flow	**Priority:** Maximize heart flow Maximize brain flow Ensure O_2/ventilation	**Priority:** Normal O_2/ventilation Manage heart dysfunction Prevent further organ injury
	No Flow	**Low Flow**	**Low, Normal, or High Flow**
Assess: HR, BP, RR Breath sounds Pulse oximetry Capillary refill	**Assess:** Response Spontaneous respirations Pulse ECG	**Assess:** Palpable pulses Exhaled CO_2 Perfusion, systolic and diastolic BP	**Assess:** HR, pulses, mental status, urine output, cap refill, BP, pulse oximetry, ABGs, exhaled CO_2, venous saturation, lactate, CVP, echocardiogram, imaging
Treat: ABCs, O_2 Fluid bolus Vasoactive meds IV	**Treat:** Prompt CPR Defibrillate if VF	**Treat:** Compress chest hard Assist ventilation Vasopressors	**Treat:** Fluids and drugs (vasopressors, inotropes, vasodilators) Cerebral protection (no hypotension, no hyperglycemia, no hyperthermia)

function for development of postarrest cardiorespiratory failure. Repeat the primary survey and support the airway, ventilation and oxygenation, and perfusion as needed (see Table 1). Then perform a detailed secondary survey to assess the patient's bones, joints, skin, and neurologic status. Obtain a focused patient history.

Postarrest myocardial dysfunction is common.[1-4] Infants and children often exhibit recurrent hypoxemia, hypercapnia, hemodynamic instability, hypothermia and hyperthermia,[5] and altered sensorium during the immediate postresuscitation period. Monitoring and support of the patient in a pediatric tertiary care setting are recommended.[6] Excellent communication between the referring and receiving providers is essential to ensure optimum patient outcome. Appropriate support of the family is also part of a comprehensive care program (see Chapter 16: "Coping With Death and Dying").

General postresuscitation care is required before and during transport and comprises the following:

■ Assess and support cardiopulmonary function (see Critical Concepts: "Postresuscitation Support").

■ Maintain **A**irway patency and administer humidified oxygen titrated to the patient's pulse oximetry and arterial blood gas results if available.

■ Maintain effective **B**reathing and evaluate ventilation.

— Signs of *effective* ventilation include adequate chest expansion (chest rise), adequate breath sounds, and no signs of excessive respiratory effort (eg, use of accessory muscles of respiration, nasal flaring, chest retractions, grunting).

— Signs of *inadequate* ventilation include minimal or unexplained unequal chest expansion, inadequate or unexplained unequal breath sounds, paradoxical (eg, seesaw)

movement of the chest during spontaneous breathing, gasping respirations, and excessive work of breathing.

— If the child is breathing spontaneously, you can evaluate air movement by assessing voice quality; patients in respiratory distress often speak in short phrases.

— Ideally monitor oxygenation continuously with a pulse oximeter. Once perfusion is restored, continuous or frequent monitoring of exhaled CO_2 is recommended. Correlate noninvasive monitors with arterial blood gas results when possible.

■ Assess peripheral **C**irculation and end-organ perfusion by assessing skin temperature, capillary refill, quality of distal pulses, level of consciousness, continuous ECG tracing, degree of metabolic (lactic) acidosis, and urine output. Evaluation of urine output is facilitated by use of an indwelling urinary catheter.

TABLE 1. Summary of Postresuscitation Care

Airway	Tracheal intubation with confirmation of tracheal tube position; repeat confirmation after movement/transport of the patient.
	Secure tube before transport.
	Gastric decompression.
Breathing	100% inspired oxygen.
	Provide mechanical ventilation targeting normal ventilation goals (Pco_2, 35 to 40 mm Hg).
	Monitor pulse oximetry and exhaled CO_2 (or capnography) if available.
Circulation	Ensure adequate intravascular volume (volume titration).
	Optimize myocardial function and systemic perfusion (inotropes, vasopressors, vasodilators).
	Monitor capillary refill, blood pressure, continuous ECG, urine output; measure arterial blood gas and lactate to assess degree of acidosis if available.
	Ideally maintain 2 routes of functional vascular access.
Disability	Perform a rapid secondary survey, including brief neurologic assessment.
	Avoid hyperglycemia, treat hypoglycemia (monitor glucose).
	If seizures are observed, administer anticonvulsant medications.
	Obtain laboratory studies if available: arterial blood gases, glucose, electrolytes, hematocrit, chest radiograph.
Exposure	Avoid and correct hyperthermia (monitor temperature).
	Avoid profound hypothermia (less than 33°C).

Be sure to communicate to the patient's family and to transport and receiving providers the patient's status and interventions performed.

- Support circulation as needed.

- Insert and maintain 2 functional vascular catheters.

- Evaluate blood pressure with a Doppler device, manual sphygmomanometer, automated oscillometric blood pressure measurement device, or invasive arterial catheter. Evaluate blood pressure at least every 5 minutes until the patient is stable and every 15 minutes thereafter. Note that indirect (non-invasive) blood pressure measurements may be inaccurate when systemic perfusion is poor (see Chapter 2: "Recognition of Respiratory Failure and Shock").

- Assess **D**isability (neurologic function); perform serial neurologic examinations to detect signs of intracranial hypertension, seizures, or focal findings that require intervention.

- Monitor **E**xposure and **E**nvironment; assess and maintain a target core temperature range. Treat hyperthermia (Class IIa recommendation for the patient with head injury or reduced cardiac output); allow moderate hypothermia (Class IIb). The beneficial effect of active cooling is currently under investigation (Class Indeterminate). To warm the patient, use warm or thermal reflective blankets or crushable heat packs. In infants and children, the head repre-

sents a relatively large portion of the body surface: covering the head may help prevent significant heat loss.

- Consider administering a fluid bolus and determine the appropriate maintenance fluid rate and composition. Maintain normal glucose levels; avoid hypoglycemia and hyperglycemia.

- Perform a detailed secondary survey.

- Assess for and anticipate postischemic myocardial dysfunction.

- Perform a focused medical history and identify allergies and immunizations, chronic diseases, etc.

- Document and communicate assessments and interventions.

Critical Concepts:
Postresuscitation Support

- **Maintain normal ventilation (Class IIa)**
  - No *routine* hyperventilation (Class III)
  - Reserve hyperventilation for those with signs of impending brain or brainstem herniation

- **Monitor and maintain target temperature**
  - Treat hyperthermia (Class IIa for the patient with a head injury or reduced cardiac output)
  - Allow moderate hypothermia after resuscitation (Class IIb)
  - The effectiveness of active cooling is under investigation (Class Indeterminate)

- **Anticipate postarrest myocardial dysfunction**

- **Maintain normal glucose and electrolyte levels**
  - Avoid hyperglycemia and hypoglycemia
  - Support normal electrolyte balance

Tailor fluid therapy to the patient's condition. One common method of calculating maintenance fluid requirements is based on body weight (see Critical Concepts: "Estimation of Maintenance Fluid Requirements").[7]

Evaluate appropriate laboratory values: serum electrolyte, calcium, and glucose measurements; hemoglobin measurement; and arterial blood gas analysis. Use arterial blood gas analysis to help assess the accuracy of noninvasive monitors (eg, pulse oximetry, detection of exhaled CO_2) to be used during transport. Evaluate the chest radiograph. Consider insertion of a gastric drainage tube to reduce or prevent gastric inflation. Search for and treat the precipitating cause of the arrest (eg,

correct electrolyte imbalance or administer antibiotics if sepsis is the suspected cause).

Postarrest Stabilization
Respiratory Function

After resuscitation of a child, provide supplementary oxygen until you confirm that oxygenation (eg, pulse oximetry, arterial Po_2) and oxygen-carrying capacity (eg, hemoglobin concentration) are adequate. Support oxygenation and ventilation if the patient has evidence of significant respiratory distress with agitation, poor air exchange, cyanosis, or hypoxemia. Tracheal intubation and mechanical ventilation are usually required.

Elective intubation may be appropriate to achieve airway control and perform

diagnostic studies such as CT scanning. After tracheal intubation, confirm tracheal tube position with a clinical examination and a test such as detection of exhaled CO_2 (Class IIa). Chest radiography can facilitate evaluation of tracheal tube location, although head and neck positioning can affect the location of the tip of the tracheal tube. The tip of the tube should be midtrachea, above the carina and below the clavicles (see Foundation Facts: "Evaluation of Tracheal Tube Position With Chest Radiography"). For further information see Chapter 4: "Airway, Ventilation, and Management of Respiratory Distress and Failure."

Intermittent or continuous monitoring of exhaled CO_2 is recommended for ongoing confirmation of tracheal tube placement (Class IIa), particularly if the patient requires transport. Verify proper tracheal tube position immediately before transport because it is difficult to detect tube displacement and reintubate the patient during transport.[8,9] You should also verify tracheal tube position and patency when the patient is moved and if the patient becomes agitated despite mechanical ventilatory support.

If the condition of an intubated patient deteriorates, consider several possibilities that can be recalled by the mnemonic **"DOPE"**: **D**isplacement of the tube from the trachea, **O**bstruction of the tube, **P**neumothorax, and **E**quipment failure. Gastric inflation may also develop, causing discomfort and interfering with ventilation. If gastric inflation develops, insert an orogastric or a nasogastric tube. If the patient is agitated and you have ruled out gastric inflation and the acute causes of deterioration recalled with the DOPE mnemonic, analgesia (eg, fentanyl or morphine) or sedation (eg, lorazepam, midazolam, or ketamine) may be required. Occasionally neuromuscular blocking agents (eg, vecuronium or pancuronium) are combined with analgesics or sedatives to optimize ventilation and minimize the risk of barotrauma or inadvertent dislodgment of the tracheal tube (see Chapter 15: "Sedation").

Critical Concepts:
Estimation of Maintenance Fluid Requirements

Maintenance fluid rate requirements can be estimated using the "4-2-1" formula. Then you can tailor the actual fluid administration rate to the patient's condition:

- *For infants weighing less than 10 kg:* Infuse crystalloid (typically 0.2% saline in 5% dextrose) at a rate of 4 mL/kg per hour.

  Example: The maintenance rate for an 8-kg infant is

  $$4 \text{ mL/kg per hour} \times 8 \text{ kg} = 32 \text{ mL/h}$$

- *For children weighing 10 to 20 kg:* Infuse crystalloid (typically 0.2% saline in 5% dextrose) at a rate of 40 mL/h **plus** 2 mL/kg per hour for each kilogram between 10 and 20 kg.

  Example: The maintenance rate for a 15-kg child is

  $$40 \text{ mL/h} + [2 \text{ mL/kg per hour} \times 5 \text{ kg}] = 50 \text{ mL/h}$$

- *For children weighing more than 20 kg:* Infuse crystalloid at a rate of 60 mL/h plus 1 mL/kg per hour for each kilogram over 20 kg.

  Example: The maintenance rate for a 30-kg child is

  $$60 \text{ mL/h} + [1 \text{ mL/kg per hour} \times 10 \text{ kg}] = 70 \text{ mL/h}$$

- *Shortcut for patients weighing more than 20 kg:* Weight in kg + 40 mL/h[7]

Note: Tailor IV fluid maintenance *rate* and *composition* to the patient. Maintenance sodium for infants and small children is approximately 3 to 5 mEq/kg per day. This calculates to approximately one fourth normal saline at the fluid rates calculated above. Administration of *maintenance* fluid differs from administration of fluid used in acute volume *resuscitation* (ie, hypotonic fluid is avoided during volume resuscitation).

Determine the effectiveness of ventilation with clinical assessment, blood gas analysis, and detection of exhaled CO_2. Clinical assessment comprises evaluation of respiratory rate and effort, general appearance and responsiveness, color, chest wall movement, and breath sounds.

Tachypnea, head bobbing, nasal flaring, intercostal retractions, the use of accessory neck and abdominal muscles, and grunting are signs of increased work of breathing, suggesting that spontaneous respiratory effort or ventilatory support is inadequate. Continued efforts by the patient to breathe "against" the ventilator or asynchronous with it may indicate inadequate minute ventilation. Agitation or lethargy may indicate inadequate oxygenation or ventilation. Central cyanosis (cyanosis of the mucous membranes) is an indication of hypoxemia, although significant hypoxemia may be present without apparent cyanosis. The resolution of cyanosis and the return of pink color to the mucous membranes indicate improved oxygenation.

Chest wall movement and breath sounds in normal lungs should be equal bilaterally. Perform auscultation over the lateral lung fields (axillary areas). If the tube is in the proper tracheal position, breath sounds should be easily auscultated in these areas but absent over the abdomen.[10] A unilateral decrease in breath sounds may indicate right or left main bronchus intubation or may be caused by a mucus plug, foreign-body obstruction, pneumothorax, pleural effusion, or lung consolidation. Rales (crackles), rhonchi, or wheezing may be heard in the presence of pulmonary edema, infection, aspiration, or bronchospasm.

In both hospital and out-of-hospital settings, continuously monitor oxygen saturation and cardiac rate and rhythm, and frequently assess blood pressure, breath sounds, perfusion, and color.

Colorimetric exhaled CO_2 monitors may provide qualitative feedback on the presence and approximate level of exhaled CO_2. In the hospital setting, continuous capnography is helpful during mechanical ventilatory support as a "trend" monitor to guide ventilation support and prevent inadvertent hypoventilation or hyperventilation.[11] Capnography results should be interpreted with caution, however, in patients with significant ventilation-perfusion mismatch or inadequate cardiac output.

Any noninvasive blood gas monitoring device (eg, pulse oximetry, capnography) may provide inaccurate results in the presence of hypothermia, poor peripheral perfusion,[12] or tracheal tube obstruction or displacement—problems that frequently develop in the postresuscitation phase. When possible, correlate the results of invasive arterial Po_2 and Pco_2 to pulse oximetry and end-tidal CO_2 analysis (see FYI: "Monitoring of Blood Gases").

Initial Ventilator Settings

Initial mechanical or manual ventilation of an intubated patient should provide 100% oxygen at a rate appropriate for the child's age and clinical condition (Table 2). Delivered tidal volume should be just enough to cause the chest to rise.

Oxygen. Low cardiac output promotes intrapulmonary shunting and hypoxemia. Because the risk of hypoxemia is high after resuscitation, provide an initial Fio_2 of 1.0 and then titrate to maintain target oxygen saturation or Pao_2.

Tidal volume. The initial tidal volume should be adequate to move the chest, typically 6 to 15 mL/kg. This volume is slightly larger than the 7 to 10 mL/kg noted in the *ECC Guidelines 2000* to allow for a broader range of ventilation needs in a wide variety of infants and

Foundation Facts: Evaluation of Tracheal Tube Position With Chest Radiography

The tip of the tracheal tube should be at the level of the midtrachea, corresponding to the 4th thoracic vertebra on radiography. The tip of the tube should be *above* the 6th thoracic vertebra because that is the typical level of the carina.

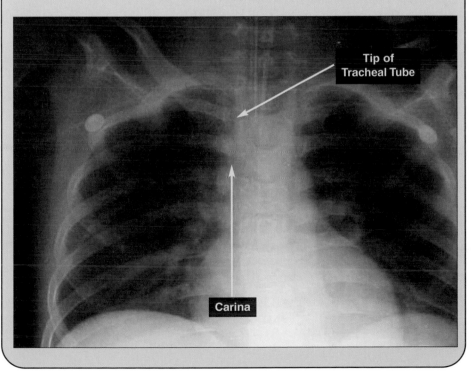

Tip of Tracheal Tube

Carina

children. If there is a large air leak around the tracheal tube, higher tidal volumes or a pressure-controlled mode of ventilation may be required. If a substantial air leak compromises ventilation, it may be necessary to replace the tracheal tube with a larger tube or a cuffed tube. If delivered tidal volume is adequate, chest expansion and breath sounds should be adequate and $Paco_2$ should be appropriate for the patient's clinical condition. Inspiratory time should be a minimum of 0.5 second; for most children, inspiratory time ranges from 0.5 to 1 second.

Peak inspiratory pressure. Initial peak inspiratory pressure should be set at the lowest level that produces adequate chest expansion and good breath sounds. When using a time-cycled, pressure-limited ventilator, adjust peak inspiratory pressure according to the patient's size and lung compliance to ensure adequate ventilation

and chest expansion. When lung compliance is normal, effective ventilation may be achieved at peak inspiratory pressures of approximately 20 cm H_2O and an inspiratory time of 0.6 to 1 second. Higher inspiratory pressures (30 to 35 cm H_2O) are frequently required in the presence of lung disease or decreased lung compliance. Adjust mechanical ventilatory parameters to limit long-term exposure to peak inspiratory pressures greater than 35 cm H_2O. Short-term use of higher pressures may be necessary in special resuscitation circumstances (eg, aspiration, asthma).

Respiratory rate. When providing mechanical ventilatory support for a patient with normal lungs, administer 100% oxygen at a typical rate of 20 to 30 breaths/min for infants, 16 to 20 breaths/min for children, and 8 to 12 breaths/min for adolescents. These rates are slightly different than those cited in the *ECC Guidelines 2000* because the rates listed here target younger children, older adolescents, and children with pulmonary disease. When lung disease is present, higher rates may be required to ensure adequate ventilation.

Rapid respiratory rates reduce the time available for exhalation. In the presence of asthma, bronchiolitis, or other conditions that cause air trapping, mechanical

ventilation at a rapid rate may result in "stacking" of breaths and high risk of barotrauma, including pneumothorax. Under these conditions provide the target tidal volume at a relatively slow ventilation rate (20 to 25 breaths/min for infants, 12 to 20 breaths/min for children, and 8 to 12 breaths/min for adolescents) and accept persistent mild or moderate hypercarbia (*permissive hypercapnia*[16]). Consider using neuromuscular blocking agents during mechanical ventilation of the patient with air trapping because the child's spontaneous respiratory effort often contributes to greater airway obstruction.

Positive end-expiratory pressure. Tracheal intubation bypasses glottic function and eliminates the physiologic positive end-expiratory pressure (PEEP) created during closure of the glottis in normal coughing, talking, and crying. To maintain adequate functional residual capacity, provide a PEEP of 2 to 5 cm H_2O when initiating mechanical ventilation. Higher levels of PEEP may be required if lung recruitment is desired, as in patients with diffuse alveolar disease or marked ventilation-perfusion mismatch. PEEP increases functional residual capacity, reduces intrapulmonary shunting, and can increase lung compliance. High levels

---

TABLE 2. Initial Ventilator Settings*

Oxygen	100%
Tidal volume[†]	6 to 15 mL/kg
Inspiratory time[†‡]	0.6 to 1 second
Peak inspiratory pressure[‡]	20 to 35 cm H_2O (lowest level that results in adequate chest expansion)
Respiratory rate	Infants: 20 to 30 breaths/min
	Children: 16 to 20 breaths/min
	Adolescents: 8 to 12 breaths/min
PEEP	2 to 5 cm H_2O (adjust to optimize oxygen delivery)

PEEP indicates positive end-expiratory pressure.

*These settings should be adjusted based on clinical assessment and arterial blood gas analysis.

[†]For volume ventilators.

[‡]For time-cycled, pressure-limited ventilators.

of PEEP, however, can produce barotrauma, impede systemic venous return, and distort the geometry of the left ventricle. If PEEP significantly compromises systemic venous return and left ventricular function, the associated fall in cardiac output is likely to reduce oxygen delivery. Optimal PEEP should be determined for each patient.

Circulation

Persistent circulatory dysfunction is often observed after resuscitation from cardiac arrest.[17,18] The clinical signs of circulatory dysfunction are decreased capillary refill, absent or decreased intensity of distal pulses, altered mental status, cool extremities, tachycardia, decreased urine output, and hypotension.

Decreased cardiac output or shock may be secondary to insufficient volume resuscitation, myocardial dysfunction, extremely high or low peripheral vascular tone, or an inappropriate heart rate (ie, too slow or too fast). Treatment of inadequate systemic perfusion involves fluid resuscitation, administration of inotropic agents and vasoactive agents, correction of hypoxia and metabolic disorders, and optimization of heart rate. Continuous monitoring of heart rate, blood pressure, and oxyhemoglobin saturation with pulse oximetry is needed, and clinical evaluation should be repeated at least every 5 minutes.

In children normotension may be observed despite the presence of shock. Hypotension is a late sign of shock and requires urgent and rapid therapy (see Chapters 2, 5, and 7). Cuff blood pressure measurements may be inaccurate in the patient who remains hemodynamically unstable; in these children, consider direct intra-arterial monitoring as soon as feasible.

Urine volume often correlates with the effectiveness of renal and splanchnic perfusion and should be monitored with an indwelling catheter. Although renal failure may result in oliguria, prerenal causes (especially shock) must be ruled out when urine output is inadequate.

Peripheral perfusion, heart rate, and mental status are nonspecific indicators of cardiac output that may be affected by ambient temperature, pain, fear, and neurologic function, as well as cardiac output. If central venous access has been established, continuous or intermittent measurement of central venous (right side of the heart) "filling" pressure may help guide fluid administration and titration of vasopressor support.

Laboratory evaluation of circulation includes blood gas analysis with evaluation of pH to identify metabolic or respiratory acidosis. Evaluation of baseline serum electrolytes and levels of lactic acid, ionized calcium, magnesium, glucose, blood urea nitrogen, and creatinine may be helpful. Persistent metabolic (lactic) acidosis suggests that cardiac output and oxygen delivery are inadequate.

Radiographic evaluation of heart size may aid in the initial and subsequent assessment of intravascular volume. In the absence of congenital or acquired heart disease, a small heart is consistent with hypovolemia and a large heart is consistent with volume overload. Pericardial effusion may also produce cardiomegaly on chest x-ray.

Drugs Used to Maintain Cardiac Output

Although vasoactive and inotropic agents are widely used to maintain cardiac output and blood pressure in the postarrest period (see Table 3), no clinical data documents an advantage of one agent over another in postarrest outcome. Drug pharmacokinetics (drug levels produced by a drug dose) and pharmacodynamics (clinical response to or effects of a given dose) vary from patient to patient and even from hour to hour in the same patient. In addition, many vasoactive agents have different hemodynamic effects at different infusion rates. Optimal use of these agents requires knowledge of the patient's cardiovascular physiology. Noninvasive or invasive hemodynamic monitoring, including measurement of central venous pressure, pulmonary capillary wedge pressure, and cardiac output, may provide helpful information to guide vasoactive therapy.[19] The infusion doses recommended in Table 3 are starting points. To achieve the desired effect, the infusions must be adjusted according to measured patient response.

The agents used to maintain circulatory function can be classified as *inotropes, vasopressors, vasodilators,* and *inodilators* (see FYI: "Classes of Cardiovascular Agents"). Administer all vasoactive agents through a secure vascular catheter to ensure uninterrupted delivery and reduce the risk of infiltration and tissue injury. Do not administer catecholamines with sodium bicarbonate because catecholamines are inactivated by alkaline solutions.

After resuscitation from cardiac arrest or shock, the patient may have hemodynamic compromise secondary to a combination of inadequate intravascular volume, decreased cardiac contractility, increased systemic or pulmonary vascular resistance, or very low systemic vascular resistance

---

FYI: **Classes of Cardiovascular Agents**

Inotropes = Increase cardiac contractility and heart rate

Inodilators = Increase cardiac contractility, decrease afterload, and may not increase myocardial oxygen demand

Vasodilators = Decrease vascular resistance and afterload and myocardial oxygen demand

Vasopressors = Increase vascular resistance and afterload (blood pressure)

(see Critical Concepts: "Support of Systemic Perfusion"). Very low systemic vascular resistance is most common in the patient with septic shock, although recent data shows that most children with *fluid-refractory* septic shock have high rather than low systemic vascular resistance and poor myocardial function.[19] Children with *cardiogenic* shock typically have poor myocardial function and a compensatory increase in systemic and pulmonary vascular resistance as the body attempts to maintain an adequate blood pressure (see Figure 2).

Epinephrine

An infusion of epinephrine can be used for treatment of fluid-refractory shock. Epinephrine is a potent inotrope and is typically infused at a rate sufficient to increase systemic vascular resistance and therefore blood pressure. Epinephrine is also a potent chronotrope (ie, it increases heart rate). It may be useful in patients with hemodynamically significant bradycardia that is unresponsive to oxygenation and ventilation. Epinephrine may be preferable to dopamine in patients with *marked* circulatory instability, particularly in infants (see "Dopamine").

Critical Concepts:
Support of Systemic Perfusion

Four parameters can be manipulated to optimize systemic perfusion following resuscitation:

1. Preload (administer volume)

2. Contractility (administer inotropes or inodilators, correct hypoxia and metabolic disorders)

3. Afterload (administer vasopressors or vasodilators, correct hypoxia)

4. Heart rate (administer antiarrhythmics, correct hypoxia, consider pacing)

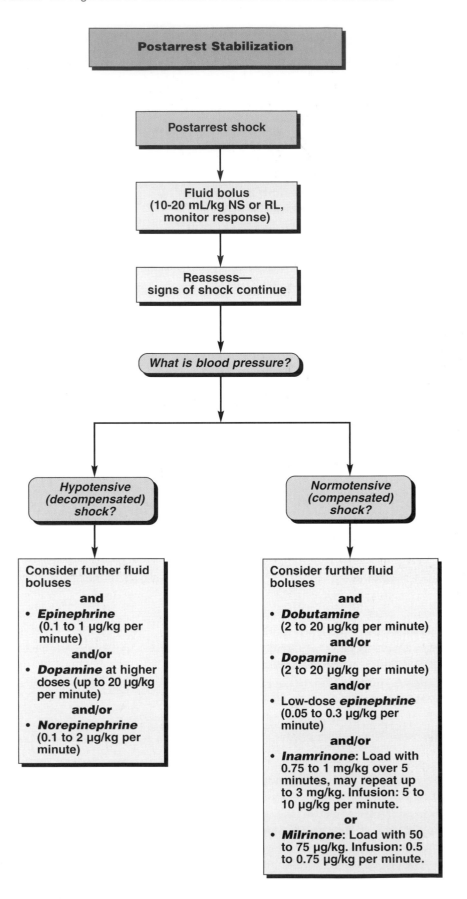

FIGURE 2. Algorithm for stabilization of infants and children after arrest.

Postarrest Stabilization

Postarrest shock

Fluid bolus
(10-20 mL/kg NS or RL, monitor response)

Reassess—signs of shock continue

What is blood pressure?

Hypotensive (decompensated) shock?

Normotensive (compensated) shock?

Consider further fluid boluses
and
- *Epinephrine* (0.1 to 1 µg/kg per minute)
and/or
- *Dopamine* at higher doses (up to 20 µg/kg per minute)
and/or
- *Norepinephrine* (0.1 to 2 µg/kg per minute)

Consider further fluid boluses
and
- *Dobutamine* (2 to 20 µg/kg per minute)
and/or
- *Dopamine* (2 to 20 µg/kg per minute)
and/or
- Low-dose *epinephrine* (0.05 to 0.3 µg/kg per minute)
and/or
- *Inamrinone*: Load with 0.75 to 1 mg/kg over 5 minutes, may repeat up to 3 mg/kg. Infusion: 5 to 10 µg/kg per minute.
or
- *Milrinone*: Load with 50 to 75 µg/kg. Infusion: 0.5 to 0.75 µg/kg per minute.

TABLE 3. PALS Medications for Postresuscitation Stabilization and Maintaining Cardiac Output

Drug	Dose Range	Remarks	Preparation*†
Amrinone (Inamrinone)	*IV/IO loading dose:* 0.75 to 1.0 mg/kg IV over 5 minutes; may repeat 2 times *IV/IO infusion:* 5 to 10 µg/kg per minute	Inodilator	6 × body weight (kg) = mg diluted to total 100 mL; then 1 mL/h infusion delivers 1 µg/kg per minute
Dobutamine	*IV/IO infusion:* 2 to 20 µg/kg per minute	Inotrope; vasodilator	6 × body weight (kg) = mg diluted to total 100 mL; then 1 mL/h infusion delivers 1 µg/kg per minute
Dopamine	*IV/IO infusion:* 2 to 20 µg/kg per minute	Inotrope; chronotrope; renal and splanchnic vasodilator in lower doses; pressor in higher doses	6 × body weight (kg) = mg diluted to total 100 mL; then 1 mL/h infusion delivers 1 µg/kg per minute
Epinephrine	*IV/IO infusion:* 0.1 to 1.0 µg/kg per minute	Inotrope; chronotrope; vasodilator in lower doses and pressor in higher doses	0.6 × body weight (kg) = mg diluted to total 100 mL; then 1 mL/h infusion delivers 0.1 µg/kg per minute
Lidocaine	*IV/IO loading dose:* 1 mg/kg *IV/IO infusion:* 20 to 50 µg/kg per minute	Antiarrhythmic, mild negative inotrope; use lower infusion rate if poor cardiac output or poor hepatic function	60 × body weight (kg) = mg diluted to total 100 mL; then 1 mL/h infusion delivers 10 µg/kg per minute *or* **alternative premix** 120 mg/100 mL at 1 to 2.5 mL/kg per hour
Milrinone	*IV/IO loading dose:* 50 to 75 µg/kg *IV/IO infusion:* 0.5 to 0.75 µg/kg per minute	Inodilator	0.6 × body weight (kg) = mg diluted to total 100 mL; then 1 mL/h infusion delivers 0.1 µg/kg per minute
Norepinephrine	*IV/IO infusion:* 0.1 to 2.0 µg/kg per minute	Vasopressor	0.6 × body weight (kg) = mg diluted to total 100 mL; then 1 mL/h infusion delivers 0.1 µg/kg per minute
Prostaglandin E₁	*IV/IO infusion:* 0.05 to 0.1 µg/kg per minute; titrate to effect: doses as low as 0.01 µg/kg per minute may be effective	Maintains patency of ductus arteriosus in cyanotic congenital heart disease; monitor for apnea, hypotension, and hypoglycemia	0.3 × body weight (kg) = mg diluted to total 50 mL; then 1 mL/h infusion delivers 0.1 µg/kg per minute
Sodium nitroprusside	*IV/IO infusion:* 1 to 8 µg/kg per minute (prepare only in dextrose in water)	Vasodilator; prepare only in dextrose in water (cannot be diluted in normal saline)	6 × body weight (kg) = mg diluted to total 100 mL; then 1 mL/h infusion delivers 1 µg/kg per minute

IV indicates intravenous; IO, intraosseous.

*Most infusions may be calculated based on the "Rule of 6" illustrated in the table. Alternatively a standard concentration may be used to provide a more dilute or more concentrated drug solution, but the individual dose must be calculated for each patient and infusion rate as follows:

$$\text{Infusion rate (mL/h)} = \frac{[\text{Weight (kg)} \times \text{dose (µg/kg per minute)} \times 60 \text{ min/h}]}{\text{Concentration (µg/mL)}}$$

†Diluent may be 5% dextrose in water, 5% dextrose in half-normal saline, normal saline, or Ringer's lactate unless otherwise noted.

Initiate the infusion at 0.1 to 0.3 μg/kg per minute and titrate it up to 1 μg/kg per minute if necessary. Epinephrine may cause tachyarrhythmias, severe hypertension, hyperglycemia, increased lactate concentration,[20] and hypokalemia.

Dopamine

Dopamine is an endogenous catecholamine with complex cardiovascular effects. At low infusion rates (0.5 to 2 μg/kg per minute), dopamine typically increases renal and splanchnic blood flow with little effect on systemic hemodynamics, although increases in blood pressure and cardiac output have been observed in neonates after infusions as low as 0.5 to 1 μg/kg per minute.[21] At infusion rates greater than 5 μg/kg per minute, dopamine can result in both direct stimulation of cardiac β-adrenergic receptors and indirect stimulation through the release of norepinephrine stored in cardiac sympathetic nerves.[22] Because myocardial norepinephrine stores are depleted in chronic congestive heart failure and may be diminished in infants, the inotropic action of dopamine may be reduced when used for these patients.[22]

Dopamine is used to treat fluid-refractory shock and shock following resuscitation, particularly if associated with low systemic vascular resistance[19,23] (Class IIb). Start the infusion at 2 to 5 μg/kg per minute and increase it as needed to 10 to 20 μg/kg per minute in an effort to improve blood pressure, perfusion, and urine output.

Dopamine infusions may produce tachycardia, vasoconstriction, and ventricular ectopy. If dopamine is used for several days, it may adversely affect thyroid function by inhibiting thyrotropin-stimulating hormone release from the pituitary gland.[24]

Dobutamine Hydrochloride

Dobutamine hydrochloride is a synthetic catecholamine with a relatively selective effect on β1-adrenergic receptors and a lesser effect on β2-adrenergic receptors. Because dobutamine increases myocardial contractility and usually decreases peripheral vascular tone, it can improve cardiac output and blood pressure in neonates and children.[25,26] Dobutamine may be particularly useful in treatment of low cardiac output secondary to poor myocardial function,[27] such as after cardiac arrest.[18]

Dobutamine is usually infused in a dose range of 2 to 20 μg/kg per minute. Higher infusion rates may produce tachycardia or ventricular ectopy. Pharmacokinetics and clinical responses to specific doses vary widely among pediatric patients.[25-27]

Norepinephrine

Norepinephrine is a potent inotropic agent that activates peripheral α- and β-adrenergic receptors. It is used for treatment of fluid-refractory shock with low systemic vascular resistance (eg, septic shock, spinal shock, anaphylaxis). At the infusion rates used clinically, α-adrenergic effects predominate, producing both beneficial and adverse effects. Although vasoconstrictors are generally thought to *reduce* renal and splanchnic perfusion, norepinephrine *improves* splanchnic perfusion, renal function, and urine output,[28,29] particularly if combined with dobutamine[20] or dopamine.[30,31] Monitor urine output, systemic perfusion, and pH carefully during norepinephrine infusion.

Norepinephrine is generally infused at rates of 0.1 to 2 μg/kg per minute. Titrate the infusion rate to achieve the desired change in blood pressure and perfusion. Heart rate may actually decrease despite β-adrenergic stimulation. The main toxicities of norepinephrine are hypertension, organ ischemia (including distal extremity vascular beds), and arrhythmias.

Sodium Nitroprusside

Sodium nitroprusside is a vasodilator that reduces tone in all vascular beds by stimulating local nitric oxide production. It is indicated for treatment of shock or low cardiac output states characterized by high vascular resistance and is also used for treatment of severe hypertension. In cardiogenic shock, sodium nitroprusside often stabilizes or even increases arterial pressure because it increases stroke volume substantially while it decreases systemic vascular resistance. Sodium nitroprusside is contraindicated in volume-depleted patients because it is likely to produce hypotension.

Sodium nitroprusside must be prepared in dextrose in water (it cannot be infused with a saline-containing solution), and it should be shielded from light. Infusions are typically started at 1 μg/kg per minute and adjusted as needed up to 8 μg/kg per minute. Nitroprusside undergoes metabolism by endothelial cells and red blood cells, releasing nitric oxide and cyanide. Cyanide is rapidly metabolized in the liver to thiocyanate, provided that hepatic function is adequate. High infusion rates or diminished hepatic function may exceed the ability of the liver to metabolize cyanide, resulting in clinical toxicity.[32] Furthermore, the hepatic metabolite thiocyanate must be renally excreted. Thiocyanate may accumulate in patients with poor renal function, leading to central nervous system dysfunction that ranges from irritability to seizures, abdominal pain, nausea, and vomiting. Measure thiocyanate levels in patients receiving prolonged sodium nitroprusside infusions, particularly if the infusion rate exceeds 2 μg/kg per minute.

Inodilators

This class of agents combines inotropic stimulation of the heart with vasodilation of the systemic and pulmonary vascular beds. Unlike catecholamines, inodilators do not work through activation of adrenergic receptors. Instead, these agents inhibit phosphodiesterase type III, so they produce an increase in the intracellular concentration of cAMP and increased cardiac contractility, increased heart rate, and relaxation of vascular smooth muscle (vasodilation). The vasodilatory effect is most pronounced because phophodiesterase type III is more prevalent in myocytes and vascular smooth muscle than it is in pacemaker cells.

Inodilators are used to treat children with myocardial dysfunction and increased systemic or pulmonary vascular resistance (eg, congestive heart failure, dilated cardiomyopathy, or septic shock with high systemic vascular resistance).[33,34] Like vasodilators, inodilators have the ability to augment cardiac output with little effect on myocardial oxygen demand and often with little change in heart rate. Blood pressure is generally well maintained, provided that the patient has adequate intravascular volume.

The major disadvantage of inodilators is that they have relatively long elimination half-lives. They must be administered with a loading dose followed by an infusion. If the infusion rate is changed without a bolus, 3 half-lives are needed to reach steady-state concentration. If no bolus is provided, hemodynamic effects from a change in infusion rate may not be observed for 18 hours after a change in inamrinone infusion and 4.5 hours after a change in milrinone infusion.[35] If toxicity develops, the adverse effect may persist for several hours until the drug is metabolized.

Inamrinone (formerly amrinone) is given as a loading dose of approximately 0.75 to 1 mg/kg over 5 minutes. If the patient tolerates it, the loading dose may be repeated 2 times to a total of up to 3 mg/kg. An infusion rate of 5 to 10 µg/kg per minute is recommended, although the optimal infusion rate is difficult to predict because there is a 6-fold variation in inamrinone pharmacokinetics in children.[36] In infants under 4 weeks of age and in patients with renal dysfunction,[37] inamrinone clearance is low, leading to a greater risk of toxicity. Increased platelet destruction is a major side effect of inamrinone.[38] Check the platelet count every 12 to 24 hours when you initiate inamrinone therapy.

Milrinone is a newer inodilator agent that is also cleared by the kidney but has a shorter half-life than inamrinone and less effect on platelets.[34,35] Milrinone has been used in children with fluid-refractory septic shock and high systemic vascular resistance.[33,35] Initially give milrinone as a bolus of 50 to 75 µg/kg, followed by an infusion of 0.5 to 0.75 µg/kg per minute.[34,36]

Central Nervous System

Central nervous system dysfunction may be either the cause or result of cardiopulmonary arrest. The key to preserving neurologic function after resuscitation is rapid restoration and support of adequate oxygen delivery to the brain and prevention of secondary neurologic injury.

Perform a brief neurologic assessment (including evaluation of pupil size and response to light, spontaneous movement, movement in response to painful stimuli, and ability to follow commands) and document the findings with each measurement of vital signs. Evaluate the level of consciousness and response to stimulation using a simple neurologic scoring system. The Glasgow Coma Scale (GCS) score and the AVPU scale (**A** = **A**lert; **V** = response to **V**erbal stimulation; **P** = response to **P**ainful stimulation; **U** = **U**nresponsive) are common methods of neurologic assessment and serial evaluation of level of consciousness.

If significant central nervous system depression is present, support adequate oxygenation and ventilation to normocarbia (Class IIa). There is no evidence that *routine* use of hyperventilation is beneficial (see Critical Concepts: "Hyperventilation"), and it may be harmful (Class III).[39]

Seizures may occur at any time after a significant hypoxic-ischemic insult to the brain, such as that following a cardiac arrest. If seizures occur, search for a correctable metabolic cause such as hypoglycemia or an electrolyte disturbance. Because seizures greatly increase cerebral metabolic demand at a time when cerebral blood flow may be compromised, treat postischemic seizures. A benzodiazepine such as lorazepam, diazepam, or midazolam is often effective. No clinical data supports the *routine* administration of an antiepileptic to prevent postarrest seizures. If a patient requires neuromuscular blockade after sustaining a head injury or cardiac arrest, use a cerebral function monitor or continuous electroencephalogram to detect seizure activity. If a cerebral function

Critical Concepts: Hyperventilation

Routine hyperventilation in brain-injured patients and postresuscitation patients is not recommended because it may reduce cerebral blood flow by decreasing cardiac output and increasing cerebral vasoconstriction.[39] Reserve hyperventilation as a response to acute elevations of intracranial pressure or signs of impending brainstem herniation, including asymmetric or fixed dilated pupils, bradycardia, hypertension, and irregular respirations.

monitor is unavailable, you may administer a loading dose of an anticonvulsant in an attempt to prevent unrecognized seizures and further brain injury.

Temperature Management

Mild postarrest or postischemia hypothermia (core temperatures of 33°C to 36°C) may have beneficial effects on neurologic function.[40,41-43] There is insufficient data, however, to recommend the routine use of hypothermia (Class Indeterminate). The PALS guidelines do not recommend active rewarming of postarrest patients with a core temperature of 33°C to 37.5°C (Class IIb). If the core temperature is less than 33°C, the guidelines recommend rewarming the patient to 34°C (Class IIb).

Hyperthermia should be treated after resuscitation. Metabolic demand increases by 10% to 13% for each degree Celsius elevation of temperature above normal. Because increasing metabolic demand may worsen neurologic injury, it is not surprising that the presence of fever after brain injury is associated with worsened neurologic outcome in adults with cerebral ischemia.[44] In the brain-injured or postarrest patient with compromised cardiac output, correct hyperthermia with active cooling to achieve a normal core temperature (Class IIa). Prevent shivering because it will increase metabolic demand. Sedation may be adequate to control shivering, but neuromuscular blockade may be needed (see Critical Concepts: "Temperature Management").

Critical Concepts:
Temperature Management

Treat hyperthermia greater than 37.5°C (99.5°F) (Class IIa)

Allow mild hypothermia: 33°C to 37.5°C (91.3°F to 99.5°F) (Class IIb)

Active cooling therapies are under investigation (Class Indeterminate)

Rewarm the patient if temperature is less than 33°C (91.3°F)

Renal System

Decreased urine output (less than 1 mL/kg per hour for patients weighing up to 30 kg or less than 30 mL/h for patients weighing more than 30 kg) may result from prerenal causes, inadequate systemic perfusion, renal ischemic damage, or a combination of these conditions. If urine output is decreased, determine serum creatinine and blood urea nitrogen values as soon as possible. Provide fluids if there is evidence of volume depletion, and treat myocardial dysfunction with vasoactive drugs (see Chapter 5: "Fluid Therapy and Medications for Shock and Cardiac Arrest"). Avoid nephrotoxic drugs and medications excreted by the renal route, or use them with caution until renal status can be fully evaluated.

Gastrointestinal System

To prevent gastric inflation, insert an orogastric or a nasogastric tube if bowel sounds are absent, abdominal distention is present, or mechanical ventilation is required. Blind nasogastric tube placement is contraindicated in patients with severe facial injuries because intracranial tube migration may occur.[45] An *orogastric* tube can usually be placed safely in these patients.

Supportive Care

Once the patient's cardiopulmonary status is stable, change IO access to IV access and secure all catheters. Support any apparent fractures for comfort. Treat contributing causes of the arrest (infection, poisoning, etc). Because hypoglycemia, hyperglycemia, hypothermia, and hyperthermia are frequently observed, monitor serum glucose level and core body temperature frequently and take corrective measures as needed.[46] Poor outcome is associated with hyperthermia and hyperglycemia[47] after cardiac arrest, so these problems should be treated. Document all interventions and diagnostic studies and communicate the results to the healthcare team and the patient's family.

A summary of guidelines for treatment recommended for stabilization of seriously ill or injured children is presented in Table 1. For suggested equipment, supplies, and drugs for EMS and ALS providers, see the Appendix to Chapter 1.

Family Presence During Resuscitation

According to surveys,[48-53] most family members want to be present during the attempted resuscitation of a loved one. Parents or family members often fail to ask if they can be present, but healthcare providers should offer the opportunity whenever possible.[52,54,55] When family members are present during an in-hospital resuscitation, one healthcare provider should remain with the family to answer questions, clarify information, and offer comfort.[56] (See Chapter 16.)

Termination of Resuscitative Efforts

Most children who experience a cardiac arrest will not survive. If a child fails to respond to at least 2 doses of epinephrine with a return of spontaneous circulation, the child is unlikely to survive.[57-59] In the absence of recurring or refractory VF or VT, history of a toxic drug exposure, or a primary hypothermic insult, resuscitative efforts may be discontinued if there is no return of spontaneous circulation despite ALS interventions. Generally this requires no more than 30 minutes. For further discussion of the ethics of resuscitation, see Chapter 17: "Ethical and Legal Aspects of CPR in Children."

Secondary Transport: Intrahospital and Interhospital

Many children who are seriously ill or injured must undergo a lengthy transport to a PICU. The PALS principles of postresuscitation assessment, monitoring, intervention, stabilization, communication, and documentation apply to transport of the pediatric patient, whether the transport is interhospital or intrahospital. Ideally postresuscitation care is provided by medical personnel with specialized training in pediatric emergency and intensive care.[60-62]

Transport and transfer to a tertiary care setting should be coordinated with the receiving providers to ensure that the child is delivered safely in stable or improved condition.[63] Transport should be supervised by a physician with experience and training in pediatric emergency medicine or pediatric critical care. The mode of transport and composition of the transport team for each EMS and hospital system should be based on the care required by the individual patient.[64] For a list of equipment that should be available for transport of children, see the Appendix to Chapter 1.

Every pediatric tertiary care facility should have an organized pediatric transport system.[60] Ideally the system is regional, with central control by the pediatric tertiary care facility under the direction of a physician trained in pediatric emergency medicine or critical care. Transport of the critically ill or injured infant or child is best performed by a team experienced in such care even if this creates a delay at the referring hospital until an experienced transport team arrives. The transport team should be capable of providing pediatric ALS at the referring hospital and maintaining that level of care during transport.[65]

Both the referring and receiving facilities are responsible for establishing well-defined protocols for specific clinical situations. If EMS protocols include indications for direct transport of pediatric patients to hospitals and facilities equipped to handle their critical care needs, the need for secondary transport will be reduced. Transfer and transport agreements must be completed in advance to prevent needless transport delays.

Once the patient has been resuscitated, the most appropriate method of interhospital transport must be determined. Other decisions to be made concern the selection of the mode of transport, members of the transport team,[66-73] and transport triage.[70-75] Advance preparations must be made for transport,[76] the period immediately before transport, communication,[60] and follow-up after transport.

Mode of Transport

Interhospital transport can be accomplished through the use of a local ambulance, mobile ICU ambulance from the receiving hospital, helicopter, or fixed-wing aircraft. A child with significant respiratory or circulatory compromise requires constant medical supervision, which precludes transport in the parents' vehicle.

Ground ambulances are readily available, relatively inexpensive, and spacious (compared with most transport aircraft). They are operable in most weather conditions and can stop easily if a procedure must be performed. The disadvantages of ground ambulance transport are increased transport time over long distances and the risk of traffic-related delays.

Helicopter transport is fast, allowing rapid arrival at the receiving hospital and avoiding traffic congestion, enabling the referring hospital to transfer care quickly. Monitoring or evaluating the pediatric patient is extremely difficult during helicopter transport, however, and it is usually impossible to perform emergency procedures. Weather conditions preclude flying up to 15% of the time, and the cost is high.

Fixed-wing aircraft are used for only long-distance transport. These aircraft are pressurized and land at controlled sites. Patient monitoring and interventions can be performed more easily in fixed-wing aircraft than in rotor-wing aircraft. The disadvantages are long start-up times (usually offset by the speed of flight) and the need to transfer the patient from hospital to ambulance to aircraft, with a reverse transfer sequence on landing.

Transport Team

The transport team may comprise local EMS personnel, medical personnel from the referring hospital, hospital-based critical care teams who transport patients of all ages, and dedicated pediatric and neonatal transport teams. Local EMS teams rarely have the training, experience, or equipment for long-distance transport of a critically ill or injured child after resuscitation.[77,78] The use of local EMS personnel may also deprive the community of service in the event of other local emergencies.

Healthcare professionals from the referring hospital may be rapidly mobilized, but their involvement on the transport team may deprive their facility of necessary personnel unless they are specifically scheduled for transport. Personnel with limited experience in pediatric prehospital and critical care will find patient management especially difficult in a moving vehicle with limited equipment (eg, portable monitors). Anticipated care during transfer should not exceed the level that the transport team is capable of providing.

Critical care transport teams who transport patients of all ages may or may not have the appropriate training, experience, and equipment for optimum care of a critically ill or injured child.[79] The ability of transport teams in a given area to care for critically ill or injured children should be evaluated *before* this type of care is needed. The most qualified team (as measured by existing pediatric transport guidelines) should be used.[60]

Pediatric critical care transport teams provide optimum transport for critically ill children and often provide continuity of care from transport to the PICU. Unfortunately such teams are not available in all areas, and they may not have access to all types of transport vehicles. If available, such a team should be used for transporting the most unstable children even if the team requires more time to arrive or to stabilize the patient. An exception to this "most-skilled" transport rule would be the child who requires immediate surgical intervention at the tertiary care center (cg, a craniotomy for epidural hematoma).[65]

Transport Triage

No specific criteria are available to reliably determine the need for a pediatric critical care transport team,[74,80,81] although the following are broad criteria:

■ Patients expected to require PICU admission at the receiving hospital. Patients who require that level of monitoring and care on arrival will likely need such care during transport.

■ Patients with a respiratory condition (eg, asthma or croup) with significant potential for deterioration during a long ride.

■ Patients who have recently experienced a life-threatening event (even if they are stable at the time of transport) because the event may recur. Neonates and infants with a history of apnea and any patient who has required aggressive stabilization (eg, after seizure with apnea or shock) are examples.

Advance Preparation for Transport

Every hospital should establish protocols that outline access to the various transport systems *before* a seriously ill or injured child actually requires transport (see Critical Concepts: "Advance Preparation for Interhospital Transport"). Post the names and telephone numbers of facilities equipped to care for critically ill and injured children near the Emergency Department telephone; a list of transport

Critical Concepts:
Advance Preparation for Interhospital Transport

- List of pediatric tertiary care facilities and telephone numbers
- List of pediatric transport systems and telephone numbers
- List (or pack) of pediatric equipment and supplies for patients to include with standard EMS equipment
- Personnel trained and experienced in pediatric care
- Administrative protocols

Critical Concepts:
Responsibilities of Referring Hospital Before Transport

- Copy all patient records and x-rays
- Obtain transport consent (many teams require signatures on their own consent forms)
- Secure vascular access and the tracheal tube
- Stabilize the cervical spine and any fractures
- Prepare blood products if indicated
- Provide the transport team with the laboratory telephone number for pending laboratory results

or arrest, seizure activity, and cardiac arrest). A list of necessary equipment should be prepared in advance, and a more extensive list of equipment should be available if a physician accompanies the patient. Ideally pediatric transport packs, containing equipment of the correct size and medication doses for particular emergency situations, should be prepared in advance.

In some areas of the country, transfer of uninsured patients may be restricted, especially if the nearest available pediatric center is across a state line. Advance preparation for transport must address such administrative matters in written, pre-arranged contracts between the referring and receiving hospitals and preparation of written protocols to initiate appropriate communication between administrators. Arrangements for transport reimbursement should be discussed in advance.

Preparation Immediately Before Transport

If the transport team is not from the referring or receiving hospital, the referring hospital must assist in the efficient transfer of the patient. Some transport teams operate on the basis of implied consent and consider transport part of treatment for a life-threatening emergency without requiring formal consent to transport. Written consent to transport should still be obtained from the patient's legal guardian if possible. Many transport teams request that the parents remain at the referring hospital to give consent directly to the team.

If airway patency or ventilatory status is questionable, secure the airway with a tracheal tube before transport. Tape intravascular lines and the tracheal tube securely in place before transport (see Critical Concepts: "Responsibilities of Referring Hospital Before Transport"). Vascular catheters and tracheal tubes frequently become dislodged during transport, often because they were inadequately secured for a moving environment.[9] The movement and vibrations that occur

systems capable of transporting pediatric patients (if different from the list of receiving hospitals) should be kept in the same location. If there is only one pediatric tertiary care center in the area, list the nearest alternative hospital (even if it is in another state). Because the number of beds in a PICU is usually limited, a backup plan is essential.

Ambulance personnel who transport children should have specific training and ongoing experience in pediatric assessment, stabilization, and resuscitation. All EMTs should be encouraged to complete the PALS course and to maintain their proficiency by helping care for pediatric patients in the Emergency Department. Ambulance equipment should be periodically evaluated to ensure that it is appropriate for the entire range of ages and sizes of pediatric patients and to ensure that lost or missing equipment is immediately replaced (see the Appendix to Chapter 1).[75]

Transport team members should have specific training and experience in pediatric evaluation, stabilization, and resuscitation. Written protocols must be available delineating management of potential crises during transport (eg, respiratory failure

during transport make replacement of dislodged catheters or tracheal tubes difficult. Stabilize the cervical spine and any fractured bones before transport.

Transfer will be more efficient if the referring hospital anticipates the requirements of the transport team and prepares to meet them. Copies of the patient's chart and x-rays should be made *before* the transport team arrives. If blood products may be required during transport, prepare a supply in advance to accompany the patient.

Communication

The initial call to transfer a patient should be made by one physician to another.[76] In fact the transport system should not be activated until the referring physician has discussed the patient's case with the physician who will accept the patient being transferred. The referring physician should consult the patient's chart at the time of the call to give specific details about vital signs, fluids administered, timing of events, etc. In a crisis a brief history of the illness/accident, interventions, and the patient's current clinical status should facilitate decisions about treatment and method of transport. Document the names of the receiving physician and hospital and advice

Foundation Facts:
Transport Information

The following information should be documented and provided to the transport team when available:

- Patient name, address, age, sex, weight, family contact, referring hospital/contact

- Times of injury, admission to ED, admission to operating room, transfer from facility

- History of current illness/injury, including mechanism, AMPLE (**A**llergies, **M**edications, **P**ast history, **L**ast meal, and **E**vents leading to cardiopulmonary arrest) history

- Condition on admission, including vital signs

- Initial diagnostic impression

- Diagnostic studies, including laboratory data, radiographic studies, ECG, specimens

- Treatment rendered, including medications and fluid therapy

- Status of the patient at the time of transport

- Management during transport

- Referring physician (hospital and phone contact)

- Receiving physician (hospital and phone contact)

provided by the receiving physician; transport team personnel may need additional specific information to select the proper equipment for transport. Any potential need for isolation should be discussed at this time so that appropriate arrangements can be made at the receiving hospital.

The referring physician should notify the receiving hospital if the patient's condition changes significantly at any time before

arrival of the transport team. Nurses from both hospitals should request and provide updates on the patient's status. When the transport team arrives, the referring physician should personally provide a current report about the patient directly to the transport team, formally relinquishing care of the patient. If the receiving hospital's transport team is not involved in the transport, the referring physician should telephone the receiving physician immediately before the patient's departure and report the patient's most recent vital signs, current clinical status, and estimated time of arrival at the receiving hospital.

Successful communication between the receiving and referring hospitals is essential for successful transport, and both hospitals must ensure that this communication is successful. The tertiary care center that accepts the patient must be accessible and provide recommendations by telephone. The referring hospital must provide adequate information about the patient for appropriate recommendations to be made.

Copies of all records, laboratory results, and radiographs should be transferred with the patient. Laboratory results pending at the time of transport should be noted and the laboratory phone number included with the patient's record so that the receiving physician can obtain the results.

Post-Transport Documentation and Follow-up

Many transport teams provide an evaluation form for the referring hospital to complete. The receiving physician should contact the referring physician after the transport is complete to identify any problems and to advise the referring providers of the patient's status. The tertiary care center is also responsible for providing personnel at the referring hospital with subsequent follow-up information about the patient's condition, including the ultimate outcome. If such communication does not occur, the referring physician should contact the medical director of the transport system to express any concerns about the trans-

port. Such a discussion can often clarify misunderstandings about matters such as the necessity for interventions or timing of transport. This feedback is necessary to improve the performance of the transport team and referring hospital.

Summary Points

Postarrest resuscitation care involves patient stabilization in the receiving facility, ongoing care within that facility, and transport to an appropriate level of support with tertiary care capability. The PALS principles apply throughout the period of postresuscitation stabilization and transport: rapid cardiopulmonary assessment and support of airway, breathing, circulation, and neurologic function (disability); a systematic approach to sudden deterioration; and recognition of special resuscitation circumstances. The goals of postarrest resuscitation care are preservation of brain function, prevention of secondary organ injury, and delivery of the patient in optimal condition to a tertiary care setting.

The key treatment priorities in the initial approach to assessment and stabilization of patients after cardiopulmonary arrest and in preparation for transport are

1. Assess and reassess

2. Control and support oxygenation and ventilation

3. Assess and support cardiovascular function (anticipate dysfunction)

4. Control temperature and environment

5. Assess and support metabolic needs (eg, glucose, electrolytes, acidosis)

6. Match provider equipment and training to potential interventions during transport

Common and potential high-risk problems after arrest and during transport were identified, and important elements to communicate to providers and families before, during, and after stabilization and transport were presented.

Case Scenarios

Note: These case scenarios are abbreviated. The rationale for acceptable actions and the list of unacceptable actions for all case scenarios in this chapter are presented with Case Scenario 2.

Introductory Case Scenario

A 1-year-old child with a history of developmental delay and seizure disorder presents after a prolonged seizure (more than 30 minutes) with vomiting and aspiration. The child was flaccid, cyanotic, apneic, and profoundly bradycardic (heart rate of 40 bpm with poor perfusion) and required 10 minutes of resuscitation with bag-mask ventilation, tracheal intubation, chest compressions, and IO epinephrine. These efforts led to return of adequate heart rate and perfusion. The seizures have stopped, but the child does not respond to verbal or painful stimuli.

On examination she has bilateral coarse breath sounds that are better on the right side than on the left. Her temperature is 39°C, heart rate is 160 bpm (sinus rhythm), respiratory rate is 30 breaths/min with manual ventilation, blood pressure is 90/60 mm Hg, capillary refill time is less than 2 seconds, and pupils are 6 mm and minimally reactive bilaterally. Pulse oximetry measures 90% oxyhemoglobin saturation while 100% oxygen is given by tracheal tube. Exhaled CO_2 is 50 mm Hg. There are copious, thick secretions from the child's tracheal tube. The referring physician asks you to stabilize the child, perform a CT scan of the brain, and transport her to a tertiary PICU.

Introductory Case Scenario Review Questions and Answers

■ *How would you approach postarrest stabilization and transport of this child?*

The initial PALS approach (ABCDE) to assessment and support of the Airway, Breathing, Circulation, Disability, and Exposure is the same for all patients. The history provided by the child's caregivers for baseline activity, responsive-ness, vital signs, and appearance plays a large role in assisting with your initial rapid physiologic assessment.

■ *What is your rapid physiologic assessment?*

This child has probable respiratory failure following an episode of respiratory arrest and profound bradycardia. Her artificial airway (tracheal tube) appears patent, but she is congested with copious secretions that complicate the management of breathing. Assessment of breath sounds, chest movement, and exhaled CO_2 confirm tracheal tube placement, but appropriate tube depth of insertion needs to be assessed and the tracheal tube secured in midtracheal position. The child's breathing appears labored and requires advanced support. Capillary refill time and blood pressure appear to be within normal limits, but the child is unresponsive to verbal or painful stimulation. You must attempt to determine if the lack of response is caused by shock or postictal (seizure) neurologic depression or another cause.

■ *What are the most important post-arrest stabilization and transport treatment priorities for this child?*

— Assessment and support of the airway, breathing, and circulation, with seizure control during completion of the primary survey (ABCDE)

— Rapid communication with primary caregivers to compare activity with baseline for this child and obtain pertinent history

— Rapid communication with radiology, ICU, and transport provider consultants to prepare for stabilization, evaluation, and transport

— Preparation for support needs during intrahospital and interhospital transport and transfer

— Communication with and support of family members and other providers

Case Scenario 2: Prehospital and Interhospital Transport

A 3-month-old infant was found pale and apneic in his crib by his parents. He had no signs of circulation. One parent initiated CPR while the other called 911. EMS providers arrived in 3 minutes and continued the resuscitative effort, providing effective bag-mask ventilation, chest compressions, and IO epinephrine. There was no history of trauma or obvious traumatic injury. Spontaneous circulation returned after a CPR duration of less than 10 minutes.

The infant has now arrived in the ED of your community hospital. He is limp and unresponsive with no spontaneous movements or response to noxious stimuli. With assisted tracheal tube ventilation, breath sounds are clear with good air entry, and exhaled CO_2 confirms the tracheal tube location. Capillary refill time is 5 seconds, with absent distal pulses and weak central pulses, core temperature of 36°C, heart rate of 170 bpm (sinus tachycardia), and blood pressure of 60/30 mm Hg. The nearest facility with pediatric capability is 20 miles away. The providers and family want the infant to be transported to that facility.

Case Scenario 2 Acceptable Actions

The following acceptable actions are performed to stabilize infants and children after resuscitation and to prepare patients for appropriate transport to definitive care:

■ Follow universal precautions.

■ Assess and support the airway, breathing, and circulation:

— Confirm tracheal tube position, secure tracheal tube, decompress the stomach, and establish adequate vascular access.

— Optimize oxygenation, ventilation, and cardiovascular support.

• Maintain normal ventilation (P_{CO_2}) as measured by arterial blood gas analysis or reflected by capnography. This child has no signs of impending brain herniation to justify hyperventilation.

- Consider treatment with bolus fluid infusion, vasopressors, inotropes, and/or vasodilators to maintain adequate blood pressure and perfusion.

— Monitor for postarrest myocardial dysfunction.

— Monitor the ECG, blood pressure, pulse oximetry, and exhaled CO_2.

■ Obtain and record a rapid, focused history. The AMPLE mnemonic is useful for assessing Allergies, Medications, Past history, Last meal, and Events leading to cardiopulmonary arrest.

■ Perform the secondary survey and attempt to identify potential traumatic injury or special resuscitation circumstances.

— Monitor for seizures.

— Evaluate renal, hepatic and hematologic status, using clotting studies if appropriate.

— Initiate organ-specific treatments as appropriate.

■ Initiate treatment for underlying cause of arrest if appropriate.

■ Avoid postarrest hyperthermia and hyperglycemia or hypoglycemia.

■ Contact the appropriate transport personnel and facility as soon as it is clear that transport is needed. Match the anticipated transport needs of the infant to the equipment and training level of the providers who will accompany the infant.

— Communicate the key elements of the patient's history and any interventions that have been completed or are in progress. Match the level of equipment, monitoring, and therapy with the training and expertise of the providers who will accompany the infant during transport.

■ Prepare for potential common pitfalls and progression of support during transport:

— Confirm vascular access and tube placement and clearly document interventions, assessments, and communications with the referring hospital.

— Look for causes of acute deterioration in airway and breathing (use the DOPE mnemonic: tracheal tube **D**isplacement, tube **O**bstruction, **P**neumothorax, **E**quipment failure).

— Anticipate causes of deterioration in circulation: loss of vascular access, progression of shock requiring vasopressor, inotropic, or vasodilator support.

— Anticipate other complications: seizures, arrhythmias, electrolyte abnormalities, acidosis, hypothermia or hyperthermia, and hypoglycemia or hyperglycemia.

— Arrange for copies of documentation and laboratory/radiographic studies that will assist the receiving facility in caring for the patient.

■ Provide support for family and providers stressed by the ongoing emergency and resuscitation events.

■ Obtain informed consent for transport.

Rationale for Acceptable Actions for All Case Scenarios in Chapter 9

All these case scenarios illustrate how PALS stabilization and transport interventions provide critical links for support of infants and children after resuscitation. The goals during transport and therapy are

■ **Prevention** of further injury

■ Continuous effective **BLS**

■ Continuous effective **ALS**

■ **Communication with the family** and support for the family and providers throughout stabilization, transport, and eventual rehabilitation

Place special emphasis on ensuring that appropriate equipment is available before transport and functioning during transport. ALS-trained providers accompanying the patient during transport should be able to

recognize and intervene when sudden decompensation occurs. Most causes of acute decompensation can be predicted and anticipated. Therefore, **a**nticipate **b**efore **c**omplications occur (ABC). Documentation, communication, and emotional support for families are important.

Unacceptable Actions for Case Scenario 2 and All Case Scenarios in Chapter 9

■ Failing to assess and frequently reassess and support airway, breathing, and circulation. Cardiopulmonary assessment is essential for prompt and appropriate treatment. Frequent reassessments are necessary because the child's clinical condition may change rapidly.

■ Failing to confirm tube placement and failing to adequately secure the tracheal tube

■ Failing to establish adequate vascular access and provide appropriate fluid therapy

■ Failing to monitor the ECG, blood pressure, pulse oximetry, and exhaled CO_2

■ Failing to obtain a rapid, focused AMPLE history. History of an injury, poisoning, acute disease process, or preexisting chronic disease may have important treatment implications.

■ Lack of appropriate communication with transport personnel and referring hospital

■ Lack of preparation for potential common pitfalls or need for support during transport due to progression of circulatory or respiratory dysfunction (see above)

■ Failing to obtain informed consent for transport

■ Failing to provide ongoing support of the family and providers involved in resuscitation

Case Scenario 2 Progression

Following stabilization, vascular lines and tracheal and gastric tubes are secured and appropriate placement of each is confirmed.

After communication and discussion with the tertiary care PICU, a bedside assessment of glucose, electrolyte, and blood gas is completed, fluid bolus and epinephrine infusion are initiated, blood cultures are drawn, and antibiotics empirically provided. A critical-care ground transport team (trained nurse and respiratory care practitioner) is mobilized and arrives within 30 minutes. During transport the infant begins to spontaneously breathe, cough, and resist manual ventilation. The heart rate abruptly drops from 170 bpm to 80 bpm, and the pulse oximeter alarms for low heart rate and an oxyhemoglobin saturation of 80%.

Case Scenario 2
Additional Acceptable Actions

When acute decompensation occurs during transport, the PALS provider must identify and treat the cause by performing the following actions:

- Perform a rapid cardiopulmonary reassessment (ie, assess the ABCs) and confirm that decompensation is real (not an artifact)

- First consider an airway or breathing problem (including DOPE)

- Next consider a circulation problem (eg, worsening shock, need for fluid bolus or vasoactive support)

- Vascular access problem—is the vasopressor infusion still reaching the circulation? Has the pump stopped or been disconnected?

- Then consider other metabolic problems (hypoglycemia, electrolyte abnormalities, acidosis, hypothermia or hyperthermia)

- Commonly decompensation is related to awakening and agitation. If other causes of decompensation are eliminated, sedation is often appropriate.

- Document and communicate assessments, interventions, and consultations as soon as practical

Case Scenario 2
Further Progression and Resolution

Following a rapid cardiopulmonary assessment, bradycardia and desaturation are confirmed, but no problem was identified during assessment with the DOPE mnemonic. Neither seizures nor progression of disease is noted, and breath sounds are bilaterally symmetric. Oxygenation, ventilation, and heart rate improve after the coughing episode. The transport team contacts medical command, administers the recommended sedative, and documents/communicates their assessments and interventions. On arrival the family is informed, and the infant is stabilized in the tertiary PICU.

Case Scenario 3:
Intrahospital Transport

A 7-year-old boy was injured in a motor vehicle crash. On his arrival in the ED his airway was open and breath sounds were equal with good air entry. His skin appeared somewhat mottled with cool distal extremities, but distal pulses were palpable at a rate of 135 bpm.

Now his pupils are equal and reactive to light, he has no response to verbal stimulus, and he demonstrates extensor posture to painful stimulus. His right femur is grossly deformed. There is no other obvious major organ injury, but it is difficult to assess him for pain because his mental status is altered. After orotracheal intubation with simultaneous cervical spine immobilization, he is mechanically ventilated. Two large-bore peripheral IVs and an orogastric tube are placed, and he receives a 20 mL/kg bolus of NS. On reassessment his heart rate is 120 bpm, respiratory rate 25 breaths/min, blood pressure 90/60 mm Hg, SpO_2 100% saturation while receiving 40% O_2, and exhaled CO_2 measured by continuous capnography 30 to 35 mm Hg.

After initial stabilization he must be transported to the CT scanner for further evaluation.

Case Scenario 3
Acceptable Actions

The following actions are acceptable during intrahospital transport of any critically injured child:

- Follow universal precautions and establish continuous cardiorespiratory monitoring and pulse oximetry. Perform repeated cardiopulmonary assessments, including evaluation of blood pressure.

- For injured patients assess and support the ABCs with the following modifications:

  — Assess **A**irway (for this child, confirm tracheal tube location) with simultaneous cervical spine immobilization.

  — Assess and support **B**reathing. Identify and treat pneumothorax.

  — Evaluate **D**isability (neurologic function)

  — Assess and support **C**irculation and control bleeding.

  — Stabilize the patient in the Emergency Department before transport if possible.

- Anticipate complications. Prepare for sudden cardiopulmonary deterioration or arrest due to potential exsanguination, injured viscus, intracranial injury or hemorrhage, pneumothorax, pulmonary contusion, or spinal shock.

- Stabilize all vascular access lines and invasive tubes.

- Mobilize an appropriate transport team that can provide the necessary monitoring and support.

- Anticipate the following equipment needs: battery power for mechanical supports and monitors, adequate portable oxygen supply, appropriate bag-mask device and suction, medications and fluids, documentation forms, and access to medical command in an emergency.

- Communicate with the receiving medical personnel to ensure that appropriate supports are available on arrival.

Case Scenario 3 Progression

During transfer from the gurney to the CT scanner, the child vomits and is briefly agitated. His blood pressure decreases to 70/50 mm Hg, and his heart rate increases to 160 bpm. Oxyhemoglobin saturation as measured by pulse oximetry drops to 80%, and breath sounds decrease bilaterally.

Case Scenario 3 Additional Acceptable Actions

- Perform a rapid cardiopulmonary reassessment (ie, assess the ABCs) to confirm the presence of decompensation and not artifact.

- Suction the airway immediately, disconnect the tracheal tube from the ventilator, and provide manual ventilation.

- First consider an airway or breathing problem (DOPE). If airway and breathing are effective and deterioration continues, assess and support Circulation and ensure control of bleeding. Attempt to identify progressive hemorrhage or third space fluid loss in the area of previous hemorrhage. Consider the need for additional fluid resuscitation. Ensure that vascular access is secure.

- Consider Disability a neurologic problem: spinal shock, intracranial hypertension from intracranial hemorrhage or other causes, and seizures.

- If decompensation continues and is unrelated to evaluation, it may be caused by agitation or pain. Sedation and analgesia may be necessary.

- Communicate and document assessments and interventions.

- Provide information and support to the family and providers.

Case Scenario 3 Further Progression and Resolution

You quickly suction the tracheal tube and provide manual ventilation with 100% O_2. The child's oxyhemoglobin saturation improves to 100%, with equal breath sounds that are coarse bilaterally. The child's exhaled CO_2 is approximately 30 mm Hg.

No seizures or change in pupil symmetry or reaction is noted. The child's heart rate remains 160 bpm, blood pressure is 80/50 mm Hg, and capillary refill time is 4 seconds with weak distal pulses and cool extremities.

You conclude that the child received inadequate volume resuscitation. You provide an IV fluid bolus of 20 mL/kg isotonic crystalloid bolus. The child's heart rate decreases to 110 bpm, blood pressure increases to 100/60 mm Hg, and capillary refill time is now 2 seconds. The radiologic evaluations are complete, and the patient is admitted to the PICU. The entire team documents and communicates their assessments and interventions to the PICU receiving team.

Review Questions

1. **A 6-month-old infant required tracheal intubation for central apnea associated with sepsis. Breath sounds are now equal and oxygen saturation is 100%. Heart rate is now 160 bpm, blood pressure is 50/30 mm Hg with a capillary refill time of 4 seconds, and the infant is mechanically ventilated. No fluid boluses or vasopressors have been given. The nearest tertiary care pediatric facility with ICU capability is 20 miles away. The providers and family want the infant to be transported to that facility. To stabilize this child before transport, which of the following interventions is most appropriate?**

   a. evaluate with the DOPE mnemonic, followed by bilateral chest decompression for potential pneumothorax

   b. provide an immediate bolus of 0.1 mL/kg of 1:10 000 epinephrine to treat decompensated shock

   c. provide an immediate bolus with 20 mL/kg isotonic crystalloid fluid to treat decompensated shock

   d. place the child in a BLS ambulance and transport to the facility to avoid potential delay while awaiting the arrival of an ALS team

   The correct answer is c. Decompensated shock is suggested by the tachycardia, decreased end-organ perfusion, and hypotension. Do not await transport to give the immediate isotonic fluid bolus. See Figure 2, an algorithm for stabilization of infants and children after arrest. In this case initial volume resuscitation seems appropriate.

Answer a is incorrect. Although a DOPE approach to sudden decompensation is appropriate, bilateral pneumothoraces are unlikely, based on clinical signs.

Answer b is incorrect because a pressor should be considered if there is no response to initial fluid boluses; vasopressors are not the first intervention.

Answer d is incorrect because even though rapid transport is desirable, it is most important to initiate treatment for decompensated shock before transport. ALS-trained providers with appropriate equipment should maintain support of the child throughout transport.

2. **Which of the following is the most critical factor for determining the mode and composition of a transport team?**

   a. pediatric risk of mortality score or other standard severity of illness score

   b. cost and availability of insurance reimbursement to the hospital

   c. match equipment and provider training with anticipated patient needs

   d. duration of CPR required before return of spontaneous circulation

   The correct answer is c. Matching equipment and provider training and expertise with anticipated patient needs during transport is the overriding factor that should dictate the mode and composition of the transport team. Weather conditions, distance, and team availability are important in determining ground versus helicopter versus fixed-wing modes and team composition. But anticipated patient needs are the overriding factor in most cases.

Answers a and **d** are incorrect. Although surrogate factors associated with outcome, such as severity of illness scores (eg, PRISM = Pediatric Risk of Mortality score) or duration of CPR, may be used to assist assessment of patient severity of illness, these factors should not override the considerations outlined in answer **c**.

Answer b is incorrect because the method of transport should be determined by patient needs. Reimbursement issues should be identified and addressed before transport.

3. **You accompany a 7-year-old child to the Radiology Department for head CT after an isolated closed head injury that resulted from a 3-foot fall from a jungle gym onto a blacktop. The child briefly lost consciousness at the scene but is now sleepy, although arousable to a loud voice. His GCS score is 13. There is no other obvious injury. His spine has been immobilized, and he is breathing comfortably in room air with good bilateral breath sounds and chest expansion. Which of the following would be the most likely cause of acute decompensation during intrahospital transport of this child?**

   a. airway obstruction due to position, vomitus, or secretions

   b. tension pneumothorax

   c. hyperkalemia with abnormal cardiac rhythm and shock

   d. sudden intra-abdominal hemorrhage with massive bleeding

   The correct answer is a. Airway obstruction due to patient position, vomitus, or secretions is the most likely cause of acute decompensation. Appropriate equipment and trained personnel should be available to rapidly suction the airway and provide assisted ventilation if needed. Until spinal cord injury is ruled out, cervical spine immobilization should be maintained.

Answer b is incorrect because tension pneumothorax is unlikely given the patient presentation. The patient is breathing comfortably in room air with good bilateral breath sounds and chest expansion.

Answer c is also unlikely because no risk factors for hyperkalemia are noted (eg, renal failure).

Answer d is unlikely because sudden, massive intra-abdominal hemorrhage is unlikely, given the mechanism of injury and presentation of the child.

Suggested Reading

AAPMR practice parameter: antiepileptic drug treatment of posttraumatic seizures. Brain Injury Special Interest Group of the American Academy of Physical Medicine and Rehabilitation. *Arch Phys Med Rehabil.* 1998;79:594-597.

American Academy of Pediatrics, Committee on Pediatric Emergency Medicine. In: Seidel JS, Knapp JF, eds. *Childhood Emergencies in the Office, Hospital, and Community.* Elk Grove Village, Ill: American Academy of Pediatrics; 2000.

American Academy of Pediatrics, Committee on Injury and Poison Prevention. Transporting children with special health care needs (RE9852). *Pediatrics.* 1999;104:988-992.

American Heart Association in collaboration with International Liaison Committee on Resuscitation. Guidelines 2000 for Cardiopulmonary Resuscitation and Emergency Cardiovascular Care: International Consensus on Science. *Circulation.* 2000; 102 (suppl 1). Also available as a separate publication.

Barkin RM, ed. Pediatrics in the emergency medical services system. *Pediatr Emerg Care.* 1990; 6:72-77.

Bigatello LM, Patroniti N, Sangalli F. Permissive hypercapnia. *Curr Opin Crit Care.* 2001;7:34-40.

Criteria for prehospital air medical transport: nontrauma and pediatric considerations by the Air Medical Services Committee of the National Association of EMS Physicians (NAEMSP). *Air Med J.* 1994;13:317-318.

Day S, McCloskey K, Orr R, Bolte R, Notterman D, Hackel A. Pediatric interhospital critical care transport: consensus of a national leadership conference. *Pediatrics.* 1991;88:696-704.

Lowell MJ. Justifying cardiac transports. *Air Med J.* 2000;19:37.

McCloskey K, Orr R. Interhospital transport. In: Ludwig S, ed. *Emergency Medical Services for Children: What the Practitioner Needs to Know.* Elk Grove Village, Ill: American Academy of Pediatrics; 1992.

Position paper on the appropriate use of emergency air medical services by the Association of Air Medical Services. *J Air Med Transport.* September 1990;22-23.

Talbert S. Pilot study for predicting appropriate use of air medical helicopters, part I: interfacility transports. *Air Med J.* 2000;19:2:59-65.

References

1. Kern KB, Hilwig RW, Rhee KH, Berg RA. Myocardial dysfunction after resuscitation from cardiac arrest: an example of global myocardial stunning. *J Am Coll Cardiol.* 1996;28:232-240.

2. Tang W, Weil MH, Sun S, Gazmuri RJ, Bisera J. Progressive myocardial dysfunction after cardiac resuscitation. *Crit Care Med.* 1993; 21:1046-1050.

3. Tang W, Weil MH, Sun S, Noc M, Yang L, Gazmuri RJ. Epinephrine increases the severity of postresuscitation myocardial dysfunction. *Circulation.* 1995;92:3089-3093.

4. Gazmuri RJ, Weil MH, Bisera J, Tang W, Fukui M, McKee D. Myocardial dysfunction after successful resuscitation from cardiac arrest. *Crit Care Med.* 1996;24:992-1000.

5. Hickey RW, Kochanek PM, Ferimer H, Graham SH, Safar P. Hypothermia and hyperthermia in children after resuscitation from cardiac arrest. *Pediatrics.* 2000;106:118-122.

6. Pollack MM, Alexander SR, Clarke N, Ruttimann UE, Tesselaar HM, Bachulis AC. Improved outcomes from tertiary center pediatric intensive care: a statewide comparison of tertiary and nontertiary care facilities. *Crit Care Med.* 1991;19:150-159.

7. Barnett AK, Nikiforov S. Calculating the maintenance fluid rate. *Acad Emerg Med.* 2002; 9:96.

8. Hunt RC, Bryan DM, Brinkley VS, Whitley TW, Benson NH. Inability to assess breath sounds during air medical transport by helicopter. *JAMA.* 1991;265:1982-1984.

9. Gausche M, Lewis RJ, Stratton SJ, Haynes BE, Gunter CS, Goodrich SM, Poore PD, McCollough MD, Henderson DP, Pratt FD, Seidel JS. Effect of out-of-hospital pediatric endotracheal intubation on survival and neurological outcome: a controlled clinical trial. *JAMA.* 2000;283:783-790.

10. Andersen KH, Hald A. Assessing the position of the tracheal tube: the reliability of different methods. *Anaesthesia.* 1989;44:984-985.

11. Tobias JD, Lynch A, Garrett J. Alterations of end-tidal carbon dioxide during the intrahospital transport of children. *Pediatr Emerg Care.* 1996;12:249-251.

12. Escalante-Kanashiro R, Tantalean-Da-Fieno J. Capillary blood gases in a pediatric intensive care unit. *Crit Care Med.* 2000;28:224-226.

13. Tobias JD, Meyer DJ. Noninvasive monitoring of carbon dioxide during respiratory failure in toddlers and infants: end-tidal versus transcutaneous carbon dioxide. *Anesth Analg.* 1997;85:55-58.

14. O'Connor TA, Grueber R. Transcutaneous measurement of carbon dioxide tension during long-distance transport of neonates receiving mechanical ventilation. *J Perinatol*. 1998;18: 189-192.

15. Hand IL, Shepard EK, Krauss AN, Auld PA. Discrepancies between transcutaneous and end-tidal carbon dioxide monitoring in the critically ill neonate with respiratory distress syndrome. *Crit Care Med*. 1989;17:556-559.

16. Bigatello LM, Patroniti N, Sangalli F. Permissive hypercapnia. *Curr Opin Crit Care*. 2001; 7:34-40.

17. Lucking SE, Pollack MM, Fields AI. Shock following generalized hypoxic-ischemic injury in previously healthy infants and children. *J Pediatr*. 1986;108:359-364.

18. Kern KB, Hilwig RW, Berg RA, Rhee KH, Sanders AB, Otto CW, Ewy GA. Postresuscitation left ventricular systolic and diastolic dysfunction: treatment with dobutamine. *Circulation*. 1997;95:2610-2613.

19. Ceneviva G, Paschall JA, Maffei F, Carcillo JA. Hemodynamic support in fluid-refractory pediatric septic shock. *Pediatrics*. 1998;102:e19.

20. Levy B, Bollaert PE, Charpentier C, Nace L, Audibert G, Bauer P, Nabet P, Larcan A. Comparison of norepinephrine and dobutamine to epinephrine for hemodynamics, lactate metabolism, and gastric tonometric variables in septic shock: a prospective, randomized study. *Intensive Care Med*. 1997;23:282-287.

21. Padbury JF, Agata Y, Baylen BG, Ludlow JK, Polk DH, Goldblatt E, Pescetti J. Dopamine pharmacokinetics in critically ill newborn infants. *J Pediatr*. 1987;110:293-298.

22. Zaritsky AL. Catecholamines, inotropic medications, and vasopressor agents. In: Chernow B, ed. *The Pharmacologic Approach to the Critically Ill Patient*. 3rd ed. Baltimore, Md: Williams & Wilkins; 1994:387-404.

23. Ushay HM, Notterman DA. Pharmacology of pediatric resuscitation. *Pediatr Clin North Am*. 1997;44:207-233.

24. Van den Berghe G, de Zegher F, Lauwers P. Dopamine suppresses pituitary function in infants and children. *Crit Care Med*. 1994;22: 1747-1753.

25. Berg RA, Donnerstein RL, Padbury JF. Dobutamine infusions in stable, critically ill children: pharmacokinetics and hemodynamic actions. *Crit Care Med*. 1993;21:678-686.

26. Habib DM, Padbury JF, Anas NG, Perkin RM, Minegar C. Dobutamine pharmacokinetics and pharmacodynamics in pediatric intensive care patients. *Crit Care Med*. 1992;20: 601-608.

27. Martinez AM, Padbury JF, Thio S. Dobutamine pharmacokinetics and cardiovascular responses in critically ill neonates. *Pediatrics*. 1992;89:47-51.

28. Martin C, Papazian L, Perrin G, Saux P, Gouin F. Norepinephrine or dopamine for the treatment of hyperdynamic septic shock? *Chest*. 1993;103:1826-1831.

29. Redl-Wenzl EM, Armbruster C, Edelmann G, Fischl E, Kolacny M, Wechsler-Fordos A, Sporn P. The effects of norepinephrine on hemodynamics and renal function in severe septic shock states. *Intensive Care Med*. 1993;19:151-154.

30. Hoogenberg K, Smit AJ, Girbes AR. Effects of low-dose dopamine on renal and systemic hemodynamics during incremental norepinephrine infusion in healthy volunteers. *Crit Care Med*. 1998;26:260-265.

31. Juste RN, Panikkar K, Soni N. The effects of low-dose dopamine infusions on haemodynamic and renal parameters in patients with septic shock requiring treatment with noradrenaline. *Intensive Care Med*. 1998;24: 564-568.

32. Rindone JP, Sloane EP. Cyanide toxicity from sodium nitroprusside: risks and management [published correction appears in *Ann Pharmacother*. 1992;26:1160]. *Ann Pharmacother*. 1992;26:515-519.

33. Barton P, Garcia J, Kouatli A, Kitchen L, Zorka A, Lindsay C, Lawless S, Giroir B. Hemodynamic effects of i.v. milrinone lactate in pediatric patients with septic shock: a prospective, double-blinded, randomized, placebo-controlled, interventional study. *Chest*. 1996;109:1302-1312.

34. Bailey JM, Miller BE, Lu W, Tosone SR, Kanter KR, Tam VK. The pharmacokinetics of milrinone in pediatric patients after cardiac surgery. *Anesthesiology*. 1999;90:1012-1018.

35. Lindsay CA, Barton P, Lawless S, Kitchen L, Zorka A, Garcia J, Kouatli A, Giroir B. Pharmacokinetics and pharmacodynamics of milrinone lactate in pediatric patients with septic shock. *J Pediatr*. 1998;132:329-334.

36. Allen-Webb EM, Ross MP, Pappas JB, McGough EC, Banner WJ. Age-related amrinone pharmacokinetics in a pediatric population. *Crit Care Med*. 1994;22:1016-1024.

37. Lawless ST, Zaritsky A, Miles M. The acute pharmacokinetics and pharmacodynamics of amrinone in pediatric patients. *J Clin Pharmacol*. 1991;31:800-803.

38. Ross MP, Allen-Webb EM, Pappas JB, McGough EC. Amrinone-associated thrombocytopenia: pharmacokinetic analysis. *Clin Pharmacol Ther*. 1993;53:661-667.

39. Muizelaar JP, Marmarou A, Ward JD, Kontos HA, Choi SC, Becker DP, Gruemer H, Young HF. Adverse effects of prolonged hyperventilation in patients with severe head injury: a randomized clinical trial. *J Neurosurg*. 1991; 75:731-739.

40. Bernard SA, Jones BM, Horne MK. Clinical trial of induced hypothermia in comatose survivors of out-of-hospital cardiac arrest. *Ann Emerg Med*. 1997;30:146-153.

41. Marion DW, Leonov Y, Ginsberg M, Katz LM, Kochanek PM, Lechleuthner A, Nemoto EM, Obrist W, Safar P, Sterz F, Tisherman SA, White RJ, Xiao F, Zar H. Resuscitative hypothermia. *Crit Care Med*. 1996;24(suppl): S81-S89.

42. Bernard SA, Ray TW, Buist MD, Jones BM, Silvester W, Gutteridge G, Smith K. Treatment of comatose survivors of out-of-hospital cardiac arrest with induced hypothermia. *N Engl J Med*. 2002;346:557-563.

43. The Hypothermia After Cardiac Arrest Study Group. Mild therapeutic hypothermia to improve the neurologic outcome after cardiac arrest. *N Engl J Med*. 2002;346:548-555.

44. Ginsberg MD, Busto R. Combating hyperthermia in acute stroke: a significant clinical concern. *Stroke*. 1998;29:529-534.

45. Fletcher SA, Henderson LT, Miner ME, Jones JM. The successful surgical removal of intracranial nasogastric tubes. *J Trauma*. 1987;27: 948-952.

46. Seidel J, Tittle S, Hodge DR, Garcia V, Sabato K, Gausche M, Scherer LR, Gerardi M, Baker MD, Weber S, Iakahashi I, Boechler E, Jalalon S. Guidelines for pediatric equipment and supplies for emergency departments. Committee on Pediatric Equipment and Supplies for Emergency Departments. National Emergency Medical Services for Children Resource Alliance. *J Emerg Nurs*. 1998;24:45-48.

47. Van den Berghe G, Wouters P, Weekers F, Verwaest C, Bruyninckx F, Schetz M, Vlasselaers D, Ferdinande P, Lauwers P, Bouillon R. Intensive insulin therapy in critically ill patients. *N Engl J Med*. 2001;345:1359-1367.

48. Barratt F, Wallis DN. Relatives in the resuscitation room: their point of view. *J Accid Emerg Med*. 1998;15:109-111.

49. Boie ET, Moore GP, Brummett C, Nelson DR. Do parents want to be present during invasive procedures performed on their children in the emergency department? A survey of 400 parents. *Ann Emerg Med*. 1999;34:70-74.

50. Doyle CJ, Post H, Burney RE, Maino J, Keefe M, Rhee KJ. Family participation during resuscitation: an option. *Ann Emerg Med*. 1987;16:673-675.

51. Hanson C, Strawser D. Family presence during cardiopulmonary resuscitation: Foote Hospital emergency department's nine-year perspective. *J Emerg Nurs*. 1992;18:104-106.

52. Meyers TA, Eichhorn DJ, Guzzetta CE. Do families want to be present during CPR? A retrospective survey. *J Emerg Nurs*. 1998;24: 400-405.

53. Robinson SM, Mackenzie-Ross S, Campbell Hewson GL, Egleston CV, Prevost AT. Psychological effect of witnessed resuscitation on bereaved relatives. *Lancet*. 1998;352:614-617.

54. Boyd R. Witnessed resuscitation by relatives. *Resuscitation*. 2000;43:171-176.

55. Offord RJ. Should relatives of patients with cardiac arrest be invited to be present during cardiopulmonary resuscitation? *Intensive Crit Care Nurs*. 1998;14:288-293.

56. Eichhorn DJ, Meyers TA, Mitchell TG, Guzzetta CE. Opening the doors: family presence during resuscitation. *J Cardiovasc Nurs*. 1996;10:59-70.

57. Young KD, Seidel JS. Pediatric cardiopulmonary resuscitation: a collective review. *Ann Emerg Med*. 1999;33:195-205.

58. Sirbaugh PE, Pepe PE, Shook JE, Kimball KT, Goldman MJ, Ward MA, Mann DM. A prospective, population-based study of the demographics, epidemiology, management, and outcome of out-of-hospital pediatric cardiopulmonary arrest [published correction appears in *Ann Emerg Med*. 1999;33:358]. *Ann Emerg Med*. 1999;33:174-184.

59. Zaritsky A, Nadkarni V, Getson P, Kuehl K. CPR in children. *Ann Emerg Med*. 1987;16:1107-1111.

60. American Academy of Pediatrics Task Force on Interhospital Transport. *Guidelines for Air and Ground Transport of Neonatal and Pediatric Patients*. Elk Grove Village, Ill: The American Academy of Pediatrics; 1993.

61. Beyer AJ III, Land G, Zaritsky A. Nonphysician transport of intubated pediatric patients: a system evaluation. *Crit Care Med*. 1992;20:961-966.

62. Edge WE, Kanter RK, Weigle CG, Walsh RF. Reduction of morbidity in interhospital transport by specialized pediatric staff. *Crit Care Med*. 1994;22:1186-1191.

63. Henning R. Emergency transport of critically ill children: stabilisation before departure. *Med J Aust*. 1992;156:117-124.

64. Guidelines for the transfer of critically ill patients. Guidelines Committee of the American College of Critical Care Medicine; Society of Critical Care Medicine and American Association of Critical-Care Nurses Transfer Guidelines Task Force. *Crit Care Med*. 1993;21:931-937.

65. Aoki BY, McCloskey K. *Evaluation, Stabilization, and Transport of the Critically Ill Child*. St Louis, Mo: Mosby-Year Book; 1992.

66. Baxt WG, Moody P. The impact of a physician as part of the aeromedical prehospital team in patients with blunt trauma. *JAMA*. 1987;257:3246-3250.

67. Kanter RK, Tompkins JM. Adverse events during interhospital transport: physiologic deterioration associated with pretransport severity of illness. *Pediatrics*. 1989;84:43-48.

68. Kanter RK, Boeing NM, Hannan WP, Kanter DL. Excess morbidity associated with interhospital transport. *Pediatrics*. 1992;90:893-898.

69. McCloskey KA, King WD, Byron L. Pediatric critical care transport: is a physician always needed on the team? *Ann Emerg Med*. 1989;18:247-249.

70. McCloskey KA, Johnston C. Critical care interhospital transports: predictability of the need for a pediatrician. *Pediatr Emerg Care*. 1990;6:89-92.

71. McCloskey KA, Johnston C. Pediatric critical care transport survey: team composition and training, mobilization time, and mode of transportation [published correction appears in *Pediatr Emerg Care*. 1990;6:88]. *Pediatr Emerg Care*. 1990;6:1-3.

72. Macnab AJ. Optimal escort for interhospital transport of pediatric emergencies. *J Trauma*. 1991;31:205-209.

73. Snow N, Hull C, Severns J. Physician presence on a helicopter emergency medical service: necessary or desirable? *Aviat Space Environ Med*. 1986;57(pt 1):1176-1178.

74. Orr RA, Venkataraman ST, Cinoman MI, Hogue BL, Singleton CA, McCloskey KA. Pretransport Pediatric Risk of Mortality (PRISM) score underestimates the requirement for intensive care or major interventions during interhospital transport. *Crit Care Med*. 1994;22:101-107.

75. Rubenstein JS, Gomez MA, Rybicki L, Noah ZL. Can the need for a physician as part of the pediatric transport team be predicted? A prospective study. *Crit Care Med*. 1992;20:1657-1661.

76. Seidel JS, Knapp JF, eds. *Childhood Emergencies in the Office, Hospital, and Community*. Elk Grove Village, Ill: American Academy of Pediatrics; 2000.

77. Seidel JS. Emergency medical services and the pediatric patient: are the needs being met? II: training and equipping emergency medical services providers for pediatric emergencies. *Pediatrics*. 1986;78:808-812.

78. Seidel JS, Hornbein M, Yoshiyama K, Kuznets D, Finklestein JZ, St Geme JW Jr. Emergency medical services and the pediatric patient: are the needs being met? *Pediatrics*. 1984;73:769-772.

79. McCloskey K, Orr R, Hardwick W. Pediatric transport by team transporting patients of all ages [abstract]. *Pediatr Emerg Care*. 1992;8:307.

80. Kissoon N, Frewen TC, Kronick JB, Mohammed A. The child requiring transport: lessons and implications for the pediatric emergency physician. *Pediatr Emerg Care*. 1988;4:1-4.

81. Orr R, Venkataraman S, McCloskey K, King W, Cinoman M. Predicting the need for major interventions during pediatric interhospital transport using pretransport variables [abstract]. *Pediatr Emerg Care*. 1992;8:371.

Trauma Resuscitation and Spinal Immobilization

Introductory Case Scenario

A 7-year-old boy runs into the street. A car traveling at 30 mph (approximately 50 km/h) strikes the child, throwing him approximately 30 feet (10 meters). The child immediately loses consciousness. The child continues to breathe spontaneously, but his breathing is labored. He has an obvious contusion to his forehead and a swollen, deformed left thigh. When EMS arrives the boy is lying prone. He has labored respirations at a rate of 10 breaths/min, a pulse of 160 bpm, and a blood pressure of 90/70 mm Hg. Capillary refill time is >3 seconds in all extremities. Rescuers apply painful stimuli. The child moans, withdraws from stimuli, and localizes pain. But he does not open his eyes in response to painful stimuli.

■ How would you approach initial assessment and stabilization of this child?

■ What is your rapid cardiopulmonary assessment?

■ What are the 3 most important treatment priorities for this child?

Learning Objectives and Definitions

After completing this chapter the PALS provider should be able to

■ Perform a primary survey (initial assessment) with cervical spine immobilization. (*Note:* Problems in bold type may be life threatening; they

require immediate identification and treatment.)

Airway: Assess and support the airway while immobilizing the cervical spine if needed.

— Use a jaw thrust *without* head tilt if you suspect **cervical spine injury.**

— Have suction available at all times.

— Determine need for advanced airway adjuncts.

— Treat **hypoxia** to prevent secondary hypoxic brain injury.

Breathing: Identify causes of respiratory failure and be prepared to treat them.

— **Hypoventilation** due to brain injury.

— Pneumothorax or **tension pneumothorax.**

— Hemothorax.

— Flail chest.

— Pulmonary contusion.

Circulation: Identify signs of **shock**. If present, determine cause and implement appropriate treatment.

— Assess for **hemorrhage**: assess for active external bleeding and internal bleeding (such as occurs after solid organ injury).

— Establish appropriate vascular access and provide volume resuscitation.

— Identify **cardiac tamponade** and determine need for pericardiocentesis.

— Identify **hemodynamic instability**, which may persist despite volume resuscitation: consider occult blood loss and spinal shock.

— Prevent or promptly treat potential causes of secondary brain injury, including **hypovolemia, hypotension,** and **hypoxia.**

Disability: Perform a rapid neurologic assessment to identify conditions that require urgent intervention.

— Apply Glasgow Coma Scale (GCS) (score: 3 to 15).

— Apply AVPU Pediatric Response Scale (score: **A**lert, responsive to **V**erbal stimuli, responsive to **P**ainful stimuli, or **U**nresponsive).

— Examine pupils (look for unequal size, dilation, and sluggish response to light).

— Assess for **epidural hematoma** or **herniation syndrome** requiring urgent surgical intervention.

— Consider indications for assisted ventilation (including GCS score ≤8 and inhalation injuries).

— Immobilize spine if needed.

Exposure and **E**nvironmental control: remove clothing, examine for injuries, measure core temperature, and maintain a neutral thermal environment.

— Prevent and treat significant hypothermia.

■ Perform a secondary survey (focused history and detailed physical examination) and an environmental examination.

Do not be distracted by visible but non–life-threatening injuries initially; treat these injuries after you complete the primary survey. *Note:* Complete presentation of the secondary survey is beyond the scope of the PALS course. Courses such as the Advanced Trauma Life Support (ATLS) Course offered by the American College of Surgeons provide additional training in trauma care.

■ Prioritize the assessment and management of life-threatening injuries.

■ Recognize the potential for and patterns of child abuse and self-destructive behavior.

■ Understand and apply the terminology used to describe initial assessment and stabilization of the injured child in the ATLS Course and the National Highway Traffic Safety Administration (NHTSA) EMS Course (see Critical Concepts: "ATLS and NHTSA Terminology").

Introduction

Trauma is the leading cause of death in children worldwide.[1,2] In industrialized nations trauma is the leading cause of death from the age of 6 months through young adulthood.[3] The 6 most common types of fatal childhood injuries amenable to prevention strategies are motor vehicle passenger injuries, pedestrian injuries, bicycle injuries, submersion, burns, and firearm injuries.[4-7] Prevention of these injuries would substantially reduce infant and child deaths and disability. Chapter 1 discusses injury prevention.

When a child is severely injured, resuscitation must begin as soon as possible, preferably at the scene.[8-11] Early and effective support of airway, ventilation, oxygenation, and perfusion is vital because survival from out-of-hospital cardiac arrest secondary to blunt trauma is poor in children and adults.[12-15]

The principles of resuscitation for the seriously injured child are the same as those for any other pediatric patient. Some

---

Critical Concepts: ATLS and NHTSA Terminology

Primary survey = initial assessment

Secondary survey = focused history and detailed physical examination

The National Highway Traffic Safety Administration (NHTSA) EMS National Standard Curricula uses some terms for the initial assessment and stabilization of the injured patient that differ slightly from those used in the Advanced Trauma Life Support Course (ATLS) offered by the American College of Surgeons. The terms used by the two courses to describe the same rescuer actions are used interchangeably in this chapter to ensure that the provider can apply both sets of terms to the care of the injured child.

Terminology:

Scene survey: Quick assessment to determine safety of scene.

General impression: A quick "from the door," "across the room," or "approaching the victim" assessment to determine if the patient looks "good" or "bad."

Primary survey (ATLS) or initial assessment (NHTSA): Rapid evaluation and stabilization of airway, breathing, circulation, disability (neurologic function), and exposure.

Secondary survey (ATLS) or focused history and detailed physical examination (NHTSA): A complete "head-to-toe" physical examination. The detailed physical examination of the NHTSA includes a *focused history.* Use the AMPLE mnemonic to identify important aspects of the child's history and presenting complaint:

■ **A**llergies

■ **M**edications

■ **P**ast medical history

■ **L**ast meal

■ **E**vents leading up to the current injury

---

aspects of pediatric trauma care require emphasis because improper resuscitation may be a major cause of preventable pediatric trauma-related death.[16-21] Special resuscitation circumstances that require specific interventions are often suggested by the history surrounding the event, knowledge of the common causes of arrest in various age groups, and findings of bedside or rapid diagnostic tests.

Four common errors in pediatric trauma resuscitation are (1) failure to open and maintain the airway with concurrent spinal stabilization and immobilization, (2) failure to provide appropriate oxygenation and ventilation, (3) failure to provide appropriate fluid resuscitation (including for children with brain injury), and (4) failure to recognize and treat hemorrhage.[20-22]

The *primary survey* is designed to identify and treat life-threatening injuries unique to trauma victims. Rapid cardiopulmonary assessment and support of cardiopulmonary

function are fundamental aspects of the primary survey; you should perform these components during the initial minutes of trauma care. At the same time, you should perform a rapid patient examination to detect life-threatening chest or head injuries that may interfere with successful resuscitation. You can perform a definitive evaluation and provide initial treatment of most other injuries after you protect the airway and restore ventilation, oxygenation, and perfusion.

Provide definitive care of injuries after you complete the *secondary survey.* This survey is a detailed "head-to-toe" examination for specific injuries. This secondary survey, which is unique to trauma care, is beyond the scope of this course. In the NHTSA course the secondary survey includes a focused history using the AMPLE mnemonic.

Trauma scoring systems, including the Pediatric Trauma Score (Table 1), are used to classify the severity of the child's injuries and potential for mortality. Children with multisystem trauma have a high risk of death. If possible rescuers should transport these children to a trauma center with expertise in treating pediatric patients.[23-25] A qualified surgeon should be involved early in the course of their resuscitation.

Detailed presentation of pediatric trauma management is beyond the scope of this course and textbook. Advanced courses are taught by the American College of Surgeons (Advanced Trauma Life Support Course),[26] National Association of Emergency Medical Technicians (Pre-Hospital Trauma Life Support Course), American Academy of Pediatrics and American College of Emergency Physicians (Advanced Pediatric Life Support Course),[27] and American Academy of Pediatrics (Pediatric Emergencies for Prehospital Professionals Course).[28] Whenever possible, recommendations in this chapter and the PALS course were made consistent with the recommendations taught in those courses.

Initial Approach to the Pediatric Trauma Victim

Rapid cardiopulmonary assessment and prompt establishment of effective ventilation, oxygenation, and perfusion are the keys to successful treatment of infants and children with any life-threatening illness or injury, including trauma.

In pediatric trauma victims, abnormalities of airway and breathing are far more common than abnormalities of circulation.[31] But circulatory compromise is more lethal, especially when brain injury is present.[32] For this reason pediatric trauma resuscitation emphasizes support of oxygenation and ventilation with restoration of perfusion when shock is present. Although the incidence of secondary spinal cord injury is unknown, continuous spinal immobilization throughout extrication and stabilization is recommended to minimize exacerbation of occult neck and spinal cord injuries.

Critical Concepts: Critical Aspects of Pediatric Trauma Resuscitation

Most pediatric trauma injuries result from blunt, not penetrating, force. Compromise of oxygenation and ventilation are relatively common. Compromise of perfusion is a less common but ominous sign. The 2 major causes of early death in pediatric trauma victims are airway compromise and inadequate volume resuscitation.[20,21]

Most pediatric trauma injuries result from blunt, not penetrating, force. Multisystem blunt trauma in childhood usually includes brain injury, and it may involve the chest and abdomen. The outcome from cardiopulmonary collapse (profound hypotension) and cardiopulmonary arrest associated with *blunt* trauma is poor (see Critical Concepts: "Critical Aspects of Pediatric Trauma Resuscitation").[12-14] Patients who survive out-of-hospital cardiopulmonary arrest associated with trauma generally were previously healthy; they usually have *penetrating* injuries and receive early (out-of-hospital) advanced care, which often includes tracheal intubation, and prompt transport by highly skilled providers to a definitive care facility.[33-36]

Overview of the Primary Survey/Initial Assessment (ABCDE Approach)

Stabilization of the trauma victim involves 2 surveys: the initial *primary survey (initial assessment)* and the *secondary survey (focused history and detailed physical examination)*. The primary survey consists of the initial cardiopulmonary assessment and stabilization of the patient. This survey, also called the ABCDE Approach, involves the following steps (see Critical Concepts: "Components of Primary Survey (Initial Assessment)"):

■ Airway: assess and stabilize

TABLE 1. Pediatric Trauma Score* and Revised Trauma Score†

Pediatric Trauma Score*			
Patient Characteristics	**Coded Value**		
	+2	**+1**	**−1**
Weight (kg)	>20	10-20	<10
Airway	Normal	Maintained	Unmaintained
Systolic blood pressure (mm Hg)	>90	50-90	<50
Central nervous system (level of consciousness)	Awake	Obtunded	Comatose/decerebrate
Open wound	None	Minor	Major/penetrating
Skeletal trauma	None	Closed fractures	Open, multiple fractures

Revised Trauma Score†			
Glasgow Coma Scale Score‡	**Systolic Blood Pressure (mm Hg)**	**Respiratory Rate (breaths/min)**	**Coded Value**
13-15	>89	10-29	4
9-12	76-89	>29	3
6-8	50-75	6-9	2
4-5	1-49	1-5	1
3	0	0	0

*From Tepas et al.[29]
†From Champion et al.[30]
‡Refer to Glasgow Coma Scale Score in the "Disability" section later in this chapter.

- **B**reathing: assess and stabilize
- **C**irculation: assess and stabilize
- **D**isability: evaluate neurologic condition
- **E**xposure and **E**nvironmental control: expose the patient's skin to look for hidden injuries, and take measures to prevent cold stress and hypothermia

The secondary survey involves an abbreviated trauma-specific history, a detailed head-to-toe examination, and a prioritized plan for definitive care. The secondary survey is beyond the scope of this text.

Airway

Airway control involves use of a jaw thrust with cervical spine stabilization. The head tilt–chin lift is contraindicated in trauma patients with possible head or neck injury because it may worsen existing spinal cord injury. If you suspect head or neck injury, immobilize the cervical spine in the field; maintain immobilization during transport to and stabilization in an ALS facility. To immobilize the cervical spine, use the combined jaw thrust/spinal stabilization maneuver[31] (Figure 1).

Rescuers should hold the head and neck firmly in a neutral position to prevent movement of the neck. Do not apply traction to the neck. If 2 rescuers are present, the first rescuer opens the airway with a jaw thrust while the second rescuer ensures stabilization of the head and neck in a neutral position. The prominent occiput of the child frequently causes slight flexion of the neck when the child is placed on a flat surface.[17,37,38] To maintain a neutral position, you may need to place folded linens under the child's torso (to elevate it) or use a backboard that contains a well for the head (see "Immobilizing the Body on a Spine Board," later in this chapter).

Establishment of a patent airway with simultaneous control of the cervical spine is particularly difficult in the pediatric victim of multisystem trauma. Foreign matter such as blood, mucus, and dental fragments easily obstruct the child's narrow airway. You must clear these obstructions by suctioning with a rigid, large-bore device (eg, a Yankauer suction device). Occasionally direct retrieval of a foreign body with pediatric Magill forceps is necessary. The child's tongue is a frequent cause of airway obstruction. If respiratory effort is ade-

quate and the child is unconscious, an oropharyngeal airway may maintain airway patency until you can safely perform tracheal intubation. You should immediately provide high-flow oxygen to the victim.

Rescuers will need to perform tracheal intubation if the airway is compromised, respiratory effort is inadequate, or the victim is comatose (see Critical Concepts: "Potential Indications for Tracheal Intubation of Injured Children"). Providers with appropriate advanced airway expertise should perform *orotracheal* intubation with simultaneous cervical spine immobilization.

Avoid use of *nasotracheal* intubation, especially if you suspect cervical spine injury. Nasotracheal intubation is more likely than orotracheal intubation to require excessive manipulation of the cervical spine. Also avoid nasotracheal intubation if you suspect maxillofacial injury or basilar skull fracture; if the maxillofacial injury is associated with a dural tear, the tracheal tube may migrate intracranially. Nasotracheal intubation may result in introduction of bacteria through the dura.

If you suspect cervical spine injury, maintain cervical spine immobilization during

Critical Concepts:
Components of Primary Survey (Initial Assessment)

Airway: Open the airway using a jaw thrust with cervical spine stabilization. Provide advanced airway support and use adjuncts as needed.

Breathing: Provide effective ventilation and oxygenation. Assess for and treat pneumothorax and hemothorax.

Circulation: Control obvious bleeding. Obtain vascular access for delivery of fluid or blood products.

Disability: Evaluate neurologic response.

Exposure and Environment: Look for external signs of injuries. Control bleeding and maintain normothermia.

FIGURE 1. Simultaneous manual cervical spine immobilization and jaw thrust.

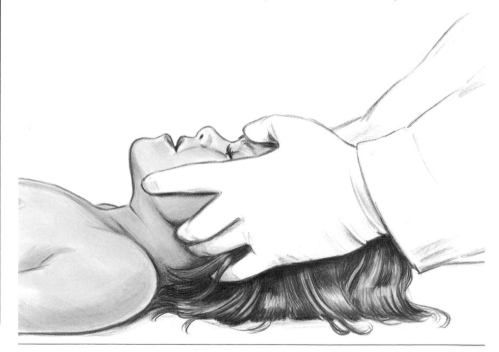

Critical Concepts:
Potential Indications for Tracheal Intubation of Injured Children

- Respiratory arrest or failure (hypoventilation, arterial hypoxemia despite supplemental oxygen therapy, or severe respiratory acidosis)
- Actual or potential airway obstruction
- Coma or significant alteration in mental status (eg, Glasgow Coma Scale [39] or modified Pediatric Glasgow Coma Scale [40-42] of 8 or less; see "Glasgow Coma Scale Score" in the "Disability" section later in this chapter)

- To facilitate acute hyperventilation when appropriate (eg, transtentorial herniation)
- Anticipated need for prolonged ventilatory support (eg, thoracic injuries, pulmonary contusion, or intrahospital or interhospital transport)
- Decompensated shock

Note: Only providers suitably trained and experienced in the intubation of pediatric trauma victims should perform this procedure.

---

the entire tracheal intubation procedure (Figure 2). If the victim is unconscious, cricoid pressure may facilitate tracheal intubation. Cricoid pressure is particularly helpful when movement of the neck must be avoided. Perform secondary confirmation of tracheal tube placement after intubation and throughout transport. Hypoxemia and hypercarbia can complicate intracranial injury; both conditions are

associated with poor outcome (see FYI: "Causes of Respiratory Failure in Children With Head Injury").

Cervical Spine Immobilization During Stabilization

After you open the airway and manually stabilize the spine, you should immobilize the spine with a semirigid collar and head immobilizer. Maintain cervical spine

immobilization throughout resuscitation, stabilization, and transport to definitive care. Rigid cervical collars are available in a wide variety of sizes. These collars can help maintain immobilization of the cervical spine in most children. Place the injured child on a spine board after you immobilize the cervical spine with a rigid cervical collar or rolled towel (see below); further immobilize the child with rolled towels, tape, and straps (see "General Technique of Spinal Immobilization" in this chapter).

Breathing

Provide **B**reathing support as needed. In out-of-hospital emergencies, bag-mask ventilation may adequately support oxygenation and ventilation, particularly when transport time is short. See Chapter 4.

The goal of respiratory support for the injured victim is to restore or maintain normal ventilation and oxygenation (see

---

FIGURE 2. Manual cervical spine immobilization during intubation in trauma. One provider maintains a neutral position of the neck and spine while avoiding compromise of the airway. Another provider performs tracheal intubation. A third rescuer may provide cricoid pressure.

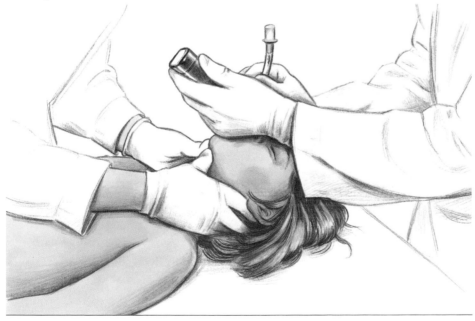

FYI: Causes of Respiratory Failure in Children With Head Injury

Sudden airway obstruction or respiratory arrest may develop rapidly in a child with severe closed head injury. These problems occur through several mechanisms:

- Central neurologic injury leading to a depressed level of consciousness, which leads to obstruction of the upper airway (by the tongue or secretions) or loss of protective airway reflexes [43,44]

- Transection of the upper cervical spinal cord leading to paralysis of respiratory muscles, which leads to respiratory arrest

- Midbrain or medullary contusion affecting the respiratory center, which leads to hypoventilation or apnea

Critical Concepts: "Support of Breathing in the Trauma Victim"). Routine hyperventilation is *not* associated with an improved outcome in trauma patients.[45] Hyperventilation may increase intrathoracic pressure, adversely affecting venous return and cardiac output. Hyperventilation may also compromise cerebral perfusion in areas of the brain that are still responsive to changes in $PaCO_2$. In these areas vasoconstriction of cerebral arteries can lead to further local or global brain ischemia.[46,47] Routine hyperventilation is no longer recommended for children with head trauma and increased intracranial pressure. Use hyperventilation when the victim has signs of increased intracranial pressure and clinical deterioration, such as signs of transtentorial herniation[48] (ie, bradycardia, asymmetric or fixed dilated pupils, decerebrate posturing, or lack of motor response to painful stimulation).

Chest injuries may impair respiratory function. The child's chest wall is very compliant. As a result the child may not have rib fractures or external evidence of chest injury after significant blunt trauma that produces major internal thoracic in-

Critical Concepts:
Support of Breathing in the Trauma Victim

- Routine hyperventilation is not associated with improved outcome in children with head injury. Reserve hyperventilation for children with increased intracranial pressure and signs of clinical deterioration, such as bradycardia or transtentorial herniation.

- Be alert to life-threatening intrathoracic injuries even if there are no external signs of chest trauma.

- Consider gastric decompression using a nasogastric or orogastric tube.

juries. Suspect and treat thoracic injuries if the child has a history of thoracic trauma, upper abdominal trauma, or arrhythmias or if you have difficulty providing effective ventilation. If ventilation is impaired, look for tension pneumothorax, open pneumothorax, hemothorax, or flail chest (see "Special Circumstances in Trauma," later in this chapter).

After you secure the airway, insert a nasogastric or orogastric tube to prevent or relieve gastric inflation. Maxillofacial trauma and suspicion of basilar skull fracture are indications for use of an orogastric tube; a nasogastric tube may migrate intracranially if these injuries are present.[49,50]

Circulation

Circulation support in the trauma victim includes rapid and repeated assessment of systemic perfusion and identification and treatment of compromise (see Critical Concepts: "Assessment and Support of Circulation in the Trauma Victim"). To treat hemorrhagic shock, control external hemorrhage, assess and support systemic perfusion, and restore and maintain blood volume. The best way to control external hemorrhage is with direct pressure. Blind application of hemostatic clamps and use of tourniquets are contraindicated except in cases of traumatic amputation associated with bleeding from a major vessel that does not stop with application of pressure.

Open or closed long-bone and pelvic fractures may bleed extensively. Rescuers should immobilize the extremity or pelvis in an anatomic position using appropriate splints. An angulated or poorly reduced fracture or a vascular injury associated with a fracture may compromise perfusion in extremities.

Circulation Assessment

Signs of shock may be evident immediately after injury, or they may evolve gradually. Hypovolemic shock is most common after trauma. Signs of hypovolemic shock caused by trauma are identical to the signs of hypovolemic shock due to other causes (see Chapter 2). In most cases rescuers

will observe the typical signs of shock (quiet tachypnea, tachycardia, decreased intensity of peripheral pulses, narrow pulse pressure, delayed capillary refill, cool extremities, and altered mental status).

In rare cases *neurogenic shock* develops after trauma. If circulating blood volume is adequate, the child may have hypotension with warm extremities and a wide pulse pressure secondary to loss of vascular tone. Deficient cardiac sympathetic activity causes bradycardia. The extremities will typically become cool if neurogenic shock occurs with hypovolemia (see "Special Circumstances in Trauma" later in this chapter).

Signs of shock may initially be subtle in the child; they may be difficult to distinguish from signs of pain or fear. *Decompensated* shock (ie, poor perfusion with hypotension) due to hemorrhage may not develop until a large portion of the child's blood volume is lost. Hypotension traditionally was assumed to indicate a loss of blood volume of 30% or more.[51] But this assumption was based on animal models; there is minimal human data to support this assumption in children. The shock classification system in Table 2 may help rescuers estimate the degree of blood loss based on the child's clinical presentation.

Volume Resuscitation

If systemic perfusion is inadequate, provide rapid volume replacement with 20 mL/kg isotonic crystalloid (eg, normal saline or lactated Ringer's solution). Obtain blood samples for type and crossmatch tests as quickly as possible after a child with multiple trauma arrives in the ED (Figure 3).

Use of a pressure infusion system or a "wide-open" intravenous system may be necessary to enable rapid administration of fluids and blood products to hypotensive patients. You must establish reliable vascular access quickly in the pediatric trauma patient. Healthcare providers should attempt to secure 2 short, large-bore catheters at peripheral sites such as the antecubital fossae or saphenous veins at

Critical Concepts:
Assessment and Support of Circulation in the Trauma Victim

- Assess for signs of hypovolemic shock, which are the same for all pediatric victims: quiet tachypnea, tachycardia, thready pulses, prolonged capillary refill, and narrow pulse pressure. For more information see Chapter 2.

- Control external bleeding with direct pressure.

- Suspect internal hemorrhage and consider early administration of blood products, especially if shock is refractory to initial fluid boluses.

the ankle, preferably in extremities that are not obviously injured (see Chapter 6: "Vascular Access"). The intraosseous route is acceptable if you cannot rapidly establish an intravenous route.[52-60] If these methods of access are unsuccessful, a skilled provider should attempt percutaneous cannulation of the femoral vein at the groin or saphenous vein cutdown at the ankle if available.

Personnel should notify a qualified surgeon before the arrival of any child with multiple injuries in the ED; this surgeon should be involved in initial evaluation and stabilization. If the child's heart rate, level of consciousness, capillary refill, and other signs of systemic perfusion do not improve, rapidly administer a second bolus (20 mL/kg). If systemic perfusion does not respond to administration of 40 to 60 mL/kg crystalloid (2 to 3 rapid 20 mL/kg boluses), transfuse 10 to 15

mL/kg packed red blood cells. Although type-specific crossmatched blood is preferable, you may use Type O blood in urgent circumstances. O-negative blood is often reserved for girls and women of child-bearing age to prevent Rh isoimmunization. You can give O-positive blood to women past child-bearing age, boys, and men. Warm the blood before transfusion; otherwise rapid administration may result in significant hypothermia. Rapid, large-volume transfusions can result in transient ionized hypocalcemia, so you must monitor the child's serum ionized calcium concentration.[61,62]

If shock persists despite control of external hemorrhage and volume administration, internal bleeding is likely present. Inadequate volume resuscitation is a leading cause of preventable trauma-related mortality in children.[20,21] Signs of intra-abdominal bleeding caused by organ rupture include

---

TABLE 2. Categorization of Hemorrhage and Shock in Pediatric Trauma Patients Based on Systemic Signs of Decreased Organ and Tissue Perfusion

System	Mild Hemorrhage, Compensated Shock, Simple Hypovolemia (<30% blood volume loss)	Moderate Hemorrhage, Decompensated Shock, Marked Hypovolemia (30%-45% blood volume loss)	Severe Hemorrhage, Cardiopulmonary Failure, Profound Hypovolemia (>45% blood volume loss)
Cardiovascular	Mild tachycardia Weak peripheral pulses, strong central pulses Low-normal blood pressure (SBP >70 mm Hg + [2 × age in y]) Mild acidosis	Moderate tachycardia Thready peripheral pulses, weak central pulses Frank hypotension (SBP <70 mm Hg + [2 × age in y]) Moderate acidosis	Severe tachycardia Absent peripheral pulses, thready central pulses Profound hypotension (SBP <50 mm Hg) Severe acidosis
Respiratory	Mild tachypnea	Moderate tachypnea	Severe tachypnea
Neurologic	Irritable, confused	Agitated, lethargic	Obtunded, comatose
Integumentary	Cool extremities, mottling Poor capillary refill (>2 seconds)	Cool extremities, pallor Delayed capillary refill (>3 seconds)	Cold extremities, cyanosis Prolonged capillary refill (>5 seconds)
Excretory	Mild oliguria, increased specific gravity	Marked oliguria, increased blood urea nitrogen	Anuria

SBP indicates systolic blood pressure.

Used/Reproduced with permission from American College of Surgeons' Committee on Trauma, from *Advanced Trauma Life Support® for Doctors (ATLS®) Student Manual, 1997 (6th) Edition*, American College of Surgeons. Chicago: First Impressions, 1997.

FIGURE 3. Approach to fluid resuscitation in a child with multiple injuries.

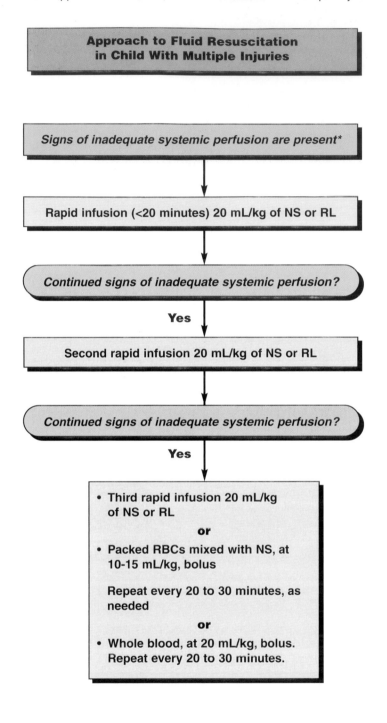

Approach to Fluid Resuscitation in Child With Multiple Injuries

Signs of inadequate systemic perfusion are present*

Rapid infusion (<20 minutes) 20 mL/kg of NS or RL

Continued signs of inadequate systemic perfusion?

Yes

Second rapid infusion 20 mL/kg of NS or RL

Continued signs of inadequate systemic perfusion?

Yes

- **Third rapid infusion 20 mL/kg of NS or RL**

  or

- **Packed RBCs mixed with NS, at 10-15 mL/kg, bolus**

  Repeat every 20 to 30 minutes, as needed

  or

- **Whole blood, at 20 mL/kg, bolus. Repeat every 20 to 30 minutes.**

*In child with severe trauma and life-threatening blood loss:
- Type and cross emergently
- Consider giving O-negative blood without crossmatch
- Consult Trauma Service at once

abdominal tenderness, abdominal distention that does not improve after gastric decompression, and signs of shock. Such bleeding requires continued transfusion therapy, surgical assessment, and urgent surgical exploration.

Hypotension may occur secondary to conditions such as tension pneumothorax, pericardial tamponade, or neurologic insult (eg, spinal cord injury or massive brain or brainstem injury resulting in loss of sympathetic nervous system control of peripheral vascular tone). Providers must identify and treat these sources of hypotension (see Critical Concepts: "Potential Causes of Cardiopulmonary Deterioration in Pediatric Trauma Victims").

Continue fluid volume resuscitation and blood transfusion as long as signs of shock are present. Treatment of shock is particularly important for children with brain injury to prevent secondary brain ischemia. Once intravascular volume and systemic perfusion are restored, avoid excessive fluid administration; excess fluids may produce hypervolemia or extravascular fluid shifts. Isolated head injury rarely causes sufficient blood loss to produce shock. But scalp lacerations may produce significant blood loss in infants and young children.

If shock is present in a child with head injury but you cannot identify a site of external bleeding, an internal source of bleeding is likely. In this case you should rule out intra-abdominal hemorrhage. Isolated long-bone or pelvic fractures may also cause significant blood loss in children. But these fractures rarely produce a volume deficit sufficient to cause hypovolemic shock.[63]

Disability

Evaluation of **D**isability involves rapid assessment of critical neurologic functions. In general you may apply a standard instrument like the Glasgow Coma Scale, a modification of the GCS for infants and children (Table 3), the Adelaide Pediatric Coma Scale (Table 4), or the AVPU Pediatric Response Scale (see Critical Concepts). The GCS has not been validated for use

Critical Concepts:
Potential Causes of Cardiopulmonary Deterioration in Pediatric Trauma Victims

The 4 H's and 4 T's used in the PALS algorithms and the rapid cardiopulmonary assessment capture many potentially reversible causes of acute cardiopulmonary deterioration in pediatric trauma victims. Providers must rapidly identify and treat these problems.

- Hypoxia (eg, secondary to respiratory compromise resulting from neurologic injury, airway obstruction, tension pneumothorax, flail chest, pulmonary contusion, tracheobronchial laceration, or crush injury)

- Hypovolemia (eg, due to uncontrolled or inadequately treated hemorrhage, leading to exsanguination, or coagulopathy)

- Hypothermia

- Hyperkalemia, hypokalemia, and metabolic disorders (eg, serum ionized calcium may be low if multiple transfusions are administered)

- Tamponade or cardiac contusion

- Tension pneumothorax

- Toxins, poisons, and drugs (consider toxidromes, particularly in adolescents)

- Thromboembolism

The 4 C's are additional potential causes of acute deterioration in the trauma victim:

- Central neurologic injury or cervical spinal cord transection

- Cardiovascular injury, particularly direct injury to cardiovascular structures such as the heart, aorta, or pulmonary arteries

- Chest wall disruption (ruptured diaphragm is uncommon; open pneumothorax is possible)

- Comorbid conditions that may contribute to the injury (eg, diving causing head injury and secondary submersion, seizure leading to a fall, or electric shock resulting in a fall)

Critical Concepts:
AVPU Pediatric Response Scale[64]

- **A**lert
- **V**erbal response
- **P**ain response
- **U**nresponsive

Exposure

Exposure involves a head-to-toe physical examination to evaluate for external signs of injury due to blunt or penetrating force. Maintain a neutral thermal environment to prevent hypothermia or hyperthermia.

Special Circumstances in Trauma
Common and Reversible Life-Threatening Chest Injuries

Serious chest injuries are uncommon in pediatric trauma. But some intrathoracic injuries (Figure 4), including tension pneumothorax, massive hemothorax, open pneumothorax, flail chest, blunt cardiac injury, and cardiac tamponade, may pose an immediate threat to life. Providers must treat these injuries rapidly to establish effective ventilation, oxygenation, and perfusion. Likewise, multiple or severe pulmonary contusions with or without bone fractures are a potential threat to life if unrecognized and untreated.

The chest wall of infants and children is extremely compliant; a child may sustain severe blunt chest trauma with no rib fractures or overt evidence of trauma.[65] For this reason providers must suspect injury to underlying thoracic and abdominal organs whenever a child experiences blunt force to the chest; be suspicious even if there are no external chest injuries. Rupture of the diaphragm, aortic transection, and major tracheobronchial disruption are uncommon in children. These injuries suggest severe chest trauma.

in children, but it is familiar to healthcare providers. The Adelaide Coma Scale has been validated in infants and children, but expected scores differ for children of different ages. The AVPU Pediatric Response Scale is less specific but quick to perform; it also has not been validated in children. These scales enable rapid assessments that organize the approach to trauma care and facilitate communication between providers. Serial assessments allow rapid identification of improvement or deterioration in a child's neurologic status provided all members of the team use the scale in the same way.

The response to pain is an important component of critical neurologic function. To evaluate response to a central painful stimulus, apply the stimulus to the trunk above the nipple line or to the neck. To create a reproducible central pain stimulus, rub the sternum with your knuckles or pinch the trapezius. If the patient grabs for your hand, he/she *localizes* the painful stimulus.

To evaluate the patient's ability to *withdraw* from a painful stimulus in all 4 extremities, pinch the *medial* aspect of each arm and leg. If the patient *abducts* each extremity (pulls the extremity *outward* or *away* from the body), he/she *withdraws* from the painful stimulus. Other methods of applying a painful stimulus may elicit *reflex* movement or flexion and extension of the extremities. These responses are difficult to distinguish from the withdrawal response.

TABLE 3. Glasgow Coma Scale[39] for Adults and Modified Glasgow Coma Scale for Infants and Children*

Response	Adult	Child	Infant	Coded Value
Eye opening	Spontaneous	Spontaneous	Spontaneous	4
	To speech	To speech	To speech	3
	To pain	To pain	To pain	2
	None	None	None	1
Best verbal response	Oriented	Oriented, appropriate	Coos and babbles	5
	Confused	Confused	Irritable, cries	4
	Inappropriate words	Inappropriate words	Cries in response to pain	3
	Incomprehensible sounds	Incomprehensible words or nonspecific sounds	Moans in response to pain	2
	None	None	None	1
Best motor response†	Obeys	Obeys commands	Moves spontaneously and purposefully	6
	Localizes	Localizes painful stimulus	Withdraws in response to touch	5
	Withdraws	Withdraws in response to pain	Withdraws in response to pain	4
	Abnormal flexion	Flexion in response to pain	Decorticate posturing (abnormal flexion) in response to pain	3
	Extensor response	Extension in response to pain	Decerebrate posturing (abnormal extension) in response to pain	2
	None	None	None	1
Total score				**3-15**

*Modified from Davis RJ, et al. Head and spinal cord injury. In: Rogers MC, ed. *Textbook of Pediatric Intensive Care.* Baltimore, Md: Williams & Wilkins; 1987. James H, Anas N, Perkin RM. *Brain Insults in Infants and Children.* New York, NY: Grune & Stratton; 1985. Morray JP, et al. Coma scale for use in brain-injured children. *Crit Care Med.* 1984;12:1018. Reproduced with permission from Hazinski MF. Neurologic disorders. In: Hazinski MF, ed. *Nursing Care of the Critically Ill Child.* 2nd ed. St Louis, Mo: Mosby Year Book; 1992.

†If the patient is intubated, unconscious, or preverbal, the most important part of this scale is motor response. Providers should carefully evaluate this component.

The 2 injuries most likely to impede initial stabilization of the pediatric trauma victim are tension pneumothorax and open pneumothorax. Among pediatric trauma victims, tension pneumothorax is relatively common; open pneumothorax is rare (see Table 5).

Tension pneumothorax can result from penetrating or blunt chest trauma. It can complicate positive-pressure ventilation. A pneumothorax is created by leakage of air from the lung into the thoracic cavity. If the pneumothorax is large, it can become a tension pneumothorax. In this condition the underlying lung collapses; the air that accumulates in the chest can compress the heart and great vessels. The child will have severe respiratory distress. Systemic perfusion deteriorates when the intrathoracic pressure rises and the mediastinum shifts to the contralateral side, obstructing venous return to the heart.

Other signs of tension pneumothorax include hyperresonance on percussion, decreased movement of the chest wall, and diminished or absent breath sounds on the side of the pneumothorax. The child may also have distended neck veins and contralateral tracheal deviation (a shift away from the side of the pneumothorax), but these signs occur less frequently in children than adults. The diagnosis of tension pneumothorax should be made clinically so that immediate treatment can be provided

TABLE 4. Adelaide Pediatric Coma Scale[42]

Response	Coded Value
Eye opening	
Spontaneous	4
To speech	3
To pain	2
None	1
Best verbal response	
Oriented	5
Words	4
Vocal sounds	3
Cries	2
None	1
Best motor response*	
Obeys commands	5
Localizes pain	4
Flexion in response to pain	3
Extension in response to pain	2
None	1
Total score	**3-14**
Normal aggregate score	
0-6 months	9
6-12 months	11
1-2 years	12
2-5 years	13
>5 years	14

*If the patient is intubated, unconscious, or preverbal, the most important part of this scale is motor response. Providers should carefully evaluate this component.

Critical Concepts:
Secondary Survey (Focused History and Detailed Physical Assessment)

The *secondary survey* involves an abbreviated trauma-specific history; a detailed, head-to-toe examination for injuries; laboratory studies; and radiographic evaluation. Use the AMPLE mnemonic to recall the components of the focused history:

- **A**llergies

- **M**edications: long and short term, last dose and time of recent medications

- **P**ast medical history: significant underlying problems, past surgeries, immunization status (tetanus)

- **L**ast meal: time and nature of last drink or food (including breast or bottle feeding in infants)

- **E**vents leading to current injury: key events, mechanism of injury, hazards at scene, treatment to date, estimated time of arrival

Note: Obtain the AMPLE history before sedation or rapid sequence intubation.

---

without delay to await a confirmatory chest x-ray.

Urgent treatment of tension pneumothorax requires needle decompression followed by placement of a chest tube. If signs of respiratory distress or shock are present in a child with suspected tension pneumothorax, perform decompression *before* you obtain a confirmatory chest x-ray. Immediate needle decompression may alleviate respiratory distress so that tracheal intubation is unnecessary. To perform needle decompression, insert a needle or over-the-needle catheter through the second intercostal space in the midclavicular line, just above the third rib. See the Appendix for a description of this procedure.

An *open pneumothorax* or "sucking chest wound" results from an open chest wound that allows free flow of air into and out of the chest. Air may accumulate in the pleural space, reducing ventilation and cardiac output. Treat associated respiratory distress with positive-pressure ventilation. Cover the wound with an occlusive dressing such as petrolatum-impregnated gauze. Tape the dressing on three sides to prevent inflow of air through the chest during spontaneous inhalation; leave the fourth side unsecured to allow egress of entrapped air during exhalation. A suitably trained provider should then insert a chest tube unless the defect is so large that it requires immediate surgical repair.

Figure 4. Potential causes of impaired breathing in the trauma victim. **A,** Flail chest. **B,** Hemopneumothorax. **C,** Tension pneumothorax. **D,** Open pneumothorax.

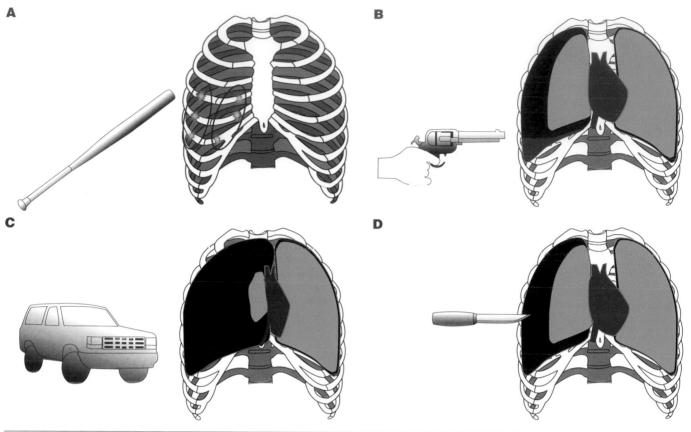

Flail chest results from multiple fractures of adjacent ribs. These fractures cause instability of a portion of the chest wall. This instability may cause respiratory failure. Flail chest requires positive-pressure ventilation. The patient may need a chest tube if a pneumothorax or hemothorax is present.

Other potentially life-threatening complications of chest trauma include massive hemothorax, blunt cardiac injury, and cardiac tamponade. Hemothorax may produce signs of shock (as a result of blood loss) and respiratory failure. Hemothorax requires initial aggressive treatment of respiratory compromise and shock and urgent placement of a chest tube by a suitably trained provider.

Cardiac tamponade may occur with penetrating chest trauma, but it rarely occurs with blunt trauma. Traumatic tamponade results from compression of the heart by blood filling the pericardial sac; this

Table 5. Life-Threatening Chest Injuries and Initial Management

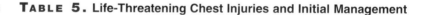

Injury*	Initial Management
Tension pneumothorax	Support ABCs, perform rapid decompression of pleural space, and insert chest tube
Hemothorax	Support ABCs, perform decompression of pleural space, insert chest tube, and give fluid bolus
Flail chest	Support ABCs and give positive-pressure ventilation (chest tube may be needed for associated pneumothorax or hemothorax)
Pericardial tamponade	Support ABCs, drain pericardium, and give fluid bolus
Open pneumothorax	Support ABCs, place occlusive dressing, perform decompression of pleural space, and insert chest tube

*Listed in order from most to least prevalent.

compression prevents adequate venous refill of the ventricles. In some cases a combination of intravenous volume loading and pericardial drainage may temporarily improve systemic perfusion. A

provider skilled in pericardiocentesis and ultrasonography should perform the procedure urgently using appropriate monitoring, sedation, and analgesia. Emergent pericardiocentesis may be performed in patients with impending or actual pulseless arrest if there is a strong suspicion of pericardial tamponade. See the Appendix for a description of pericardiocentesis.

Blunt cardiac injury (including myocardial contusion and valvular or ventricular rupture) is less common in children than in adults. But providers should suspect this injury in cases of blunt chest trauma associated with hypotension. Providers may use echocardiography to confirm blunt cardiac injury. Treatment of hypotension in patients with blunt cardiac injury requires cautious volume loading and ECG monitoring. Arrhythmias and cardiac dysfunction may develop, so close observation is warranted (see Chapter 8).

Identification of Life-Threatening Abdominal Injuries

During the primary survey look for external signs of intra-abdominal injury, such as contusions, abrasions, lap-belt marks on the abdomen, and abdominal distention. Inadequately treated hemorrhage (inadequate volume resuscitation) is a leading cause of preventable mortality in pediatric trauma victims,[20,21] so providers must identify and treat abdominal hemorrhage. Signs of intra-abdominal hemorrhage are often subtle; intra-abdominal injury does not usually cause massive hemorrhage. Injuries of the chest and abdomen that cause hemodynamic instability require immediate evaluation by a qualified surgeon to determine how to manage these injuries. Children with major intra-abdominal hemorrhage (>30% loss of blood volume) often have multisystem injury with respiratory distress or failure and shock.

Spinal Injury

In the United States approximately 3.8% of children admitted to a hospital after trauma have an injury of the spine or spinal cord.[66] Most of these injuries are caused by blunt trauma related to motor vehicle collisions, falls, or athletic injuries.[67-71] Neurologic sequelae can be significant (eg, impaired quality of life and loss of

economic potential). When the injury cannot be prevented, prompt recognition and spinal immobilization may be beneficial. Although the incidence of secondary injury resulting from movement *after* an initial spinal cord injury is unknown, spinal immobilization is still recommended. Research relating spinal immobilization techniques to improved survival or neurologic outcome is needed.

Out-of-hospital and emergency healthcare providers are the first medical professionals to assess and manage spinal injuries. These providers should learn the principles of spinal immobilization. This section discusses the key anatomic features of children affecting management of spinal injuries and the priorities of management.

Anatomic and Physiologic Considerations

Spinal injuries in children often differ from spinal injuries in adults.[72-74] The vertebral column does not begin to assume adult characteristics until approximately 8 to 10 years of age; adult patterns of injury

---

Critical Concepts:
External Signs That Suggest Intra-Abdominal Injury and Risk of Abdominal Hemorrhage

- Abdominal contusion
- Abdominal abrasion
- Lap-belt marks on the abdomen
- Abdominal distension

If external signs of intra-abdominal injury are present and you suspect hemorrhage, additional tests may be useful. Focused abdominal sonography for trauma (FAST), abdominal CT scan, or diagnostic peritoneal lavage (DPL) may help to clarify the diagnosis. (These tests are beyond the scope of the PALS course.)

---

are not fully manifested until after the age of 15 years.[75] Much of the strength of the spinal column in children is derived from cartilage and ligaments. Because the ligaments of children are not as strong as the ligaments of adults, children may sustain damage to ligaments and the spinal cord without damage to the bone (vertebrae). This damage results in the spinal cord injury without radiographic abnormality (SCIWORA) syndrome. The SCIWORA syndrome is often associated with a poor neurologic outcome, a high susceptibility to delayed onset of neurologic deficit, and a high proportion of complete neurologic injuries.[76,77]

In proportion to body size, a child's head is much larger than an adult's head. As a result the fulcrum of movement is higher in the child than the adult.[76] For this reason injuries and fractures at vertebrae C1 to C4 are much more common in children <8 years of age than are injuries of the lower cervical spine, which are seen in adolescents and adults.[68,78]

The pediatric cervical spine has other unique features. For example, the bodies of the vertebrae are wedge shaped, and the vertebrae are cartilaginous rather than bony. The facet is relatively horizontal in orientation, and it becomes more vertical with ossification between 7 and 10 years of age. Paraspinous muscles are undeveloped, and vertebral ligaments and surrounding soft tissues are elastic.[75] These features make the pediatric cervical spine more mobile than the adult cervical spine. They also contribute to spinal cord injuries, particularly during acceleration-deceleration trauma and falls.

If pediatric-sized equipment is unavailable, providers must modify adult-sized equipment to properly immobilize the cervical spine of infants and small children. Extension is the proper position to reduce cervical spine injuries and maintain a patent airway. But this position is difficult to achieve in the young child (<8 years of age) because the head is large and the occiput is prominent. For these reasons the neck may be flexed if the child is placed on a standard backboard. Providers should use a spine board with an occiput cutout (head well) if possible. If the board does not contain an occiput cutout, you can maintain neutral neck extension by placing padding under the child's torso to lift it relative to the child's head.[17,38] The child's neck is in the correct position if the external auditory meatus aligns with the anterior shoulder. This position aligns the cervical spine and avoids anterior displacement and forward flexion.

Rigid infant and pediatric collars may provide better spinal immobilization than foam collars. But a collar alone cannot provide acceptable immobilization. A combination of a rigid collar and supplemental devices, such as a backboard, towels, and tape, provides much better immobilization than a collar alone.[79]

Indications for spinal immobilization rely on a high index of suspicion for injury. Protocols for out-of-hospital clearance of the cervical spine by paramedics were recently developed.[80-83] The following mechanisms of injury and physical findings suggest a possible spine injury. These features indicate the need for spinal immobilization before movement of the patient or radiologic investigation.[37,84-86]

- Mechanism of injury suggestive of spinal cord injury:
  — Multisystem trauma
  — Penetrating trauma to the head, neck, or torso
  — Submersion or diving injuries
  — Fall from height
  — Rapid acceleration-deceleration injury

- Physical findings suggestive of spinal cord injury:
  — Isolated moderate to severe traumatic head injury
  — Altered level of consciousness or intoxication with a possible mechanism of neck injury (head injury

fall, motor vehicle crash, struck pedestrian, etc)
  — Complaints of neck pain or evidence of neck injury after trauma
  — Neurologic abnormalities or subjective complaints of neurologic abnormalities (even if no longer present)

- Characteristics that may complicate diagnosis of spinal cord injuries:
  — Preverbal age or level of development
  — Distraction (ie, painful) injuries

Providers must carefully assess and support the airway with spinal immobilization in all patients. The child's airway can be occluded by the tongue or by neck flexion. Carefully position the infant or young child on the spine board to ensure that the neck remains in a neutral position and the airway is patent; continue to monitor the child during transport. Airway compromise is particularly likely to develop, both during and after immobilization, in children with facial injuries, altered level of consciousness, and neck or torso injuries.

Priorities of Management

Airway maintenance in the injured child with possible spinal injury generally requires two rescuers: one to immobilize the head and neck and one to assess and manage the airway. Rescuers should provide supplemental oxygen, assisted ventilation, and tracheal intubation as needed. Ensure that suction is available at all times.

The goal of spinal immobilization is to maintain alignment of the spine in a neutral position. A neutral position minimizes the risk of further spinal cord injury. Providers must ensure that the spine stays in this neutral position despite the patient's spontaneous attempts to move, maneuvers to control the airway, or transfer of the patient. If minimal gentle movement can return the head and neck to the midline position, the rescuer can generally restore alignment without causing pain or airway obstruction. If a child has a grossly

misaligned cervical spine and a patent airway, use extreme caution; if the airway is patent, it may be unnecessary to return the spine to a neutral position.

If any resistance, pain, impairment of the airway, or neurologic change develops during the attempt, immobilize the child as found. Do not reattempt to align the spine until you evaluate the child's injury. If the child has a grossly misaligned cervical spine and cannot maintain an adequate airway, gently move the cervical spine back toward the neutral position until the airway is opened and maintained.

General Technique of Spinal Immobilization

There is a scientific basis for some but not all of the techniques used for spinal immobilization.[38,79] The techniques outlined here were consolidated from many sources,[84-88] including the medical literature and educational courses offered by subspecialty organizations. Local protocols and procedures may differ, but all should adhere to the basic principles described in this section. If there is a risk of spinal injury, maintain spinal immobilization until appropriate examinations and diagnostic studies can be performed.

Airway Opening and Cervical Spine Immobilization

During initial evaluation and support of the airway, the provider must manually control the cervical spine and open the airway. The combined jaw thrust/spinal stabilization maneuver is a simple modification of the jaw thrust. If two rescuers are present, the first rescuer positions himself/herself at the head of the victim; this rescuer will perform the maneuver. The second rescuer performs bag-mask ventilation or other rescue treatments. If you are a lone rescuer and you think the patient may need rescue breathing and chest compressions, position yourself at the victim's side (see Chapter 3, Figure 25).

To perform this maneuver when you are positioned at the victim's head, grasp the sides of the child's head symmetrically.

Gently rest your palms over the patient's ears and the tips of your ring and small (4th and 5th) fingers on each side of the patient's occiput. Cradle the angles of the patient's mandible with the tips of your index and middle (2nd and 3rd) fingers. Rest your thumbs on the zygomatic arches. Once your hands are in the correct position, apply firm upward pressure with the tips of the index and middle (2nd and 3rd) fingers; this lifts the angle of the mandible anteriorly.

The child is in the position recommended for simultaneous airway opening and cervical spine immobilization when the external auditory meatus aligns with the anterior shoulder. This position aligns the cervical spine and avoids anterior displacement and forward flexion.[17]

To apply the rigid cervical collar, the second rescuer assembles the collar so that the chin piece is properly formed. Holding the collar right side up at the side of the patient's head, the second rescuer slides the flat posterior segment under the back of the neck, tucks the chin piece snugly under the jaw so that it fits tightly against the chin, and tightens and attaches the Velcro strap. The first rescuer should maintain manual immobilization until the child is moved to the spine board. Both rescuers should then assess the patient to determine the need for continued airway opening maneuvers, such as the jaw thrust, or the need for ventilation support.

Immobilizing the Body on a Spine Board

Once rescuers immobilize the cervical spine with a rigid cervical collar and complete the primary survey, they can place the child on a spine board. The standard spine board is often not ideal for immobilization of the small infant or child. Because the child's occiput is relatively large, the head and neck may flex forward and out of the neutral position if you place the child on a flat board.[17,38] When using a standard spine board (with no head well), rescuers generally need to place a ½- to 1-inch layer of towels or sheets on the board under the child's torso (shoulders to buttocks). Placing towels under the torso will position the head and body for alignment of the cervical spine (Figure 5A). If the child is obese, rescuers may need to place towels or sheets under the *occiput* to maintain the cervical spine in a neutral position.

When you strap a small child to a wide board, there will be gaps between the child's body and the site where you secure the straps. If you do not fill these gaps, the child can slide sideways on the board during transport, during transfer, or when you roll the child to the side to clear the airway during vomiting. To reduce or eliminate lateral movement, fill these gaps with rolled towels or blankets (Figure 5B). You may use a rolled towel to immobilize the cervical spine if a cervical collar of appropriate size is unavailable (Figure 5C).

The standard technique used to place the child onto the spine board is the logroll. To logroll the child onto the board, use enough providers to control movement of the torso completely (Figure 6A). At least 2, but preferably 3 or 4, rescuers are needed to move an injured child onto a spine board. The first rescuer controls the head and neck; the second and third rescuers control the body. If present, a fourth rescuer moves the board against the child.

To secure the child to the board, place the straps or cravats over *at least 3* anatomic points: the thighs, pelvis, and shoulders (see Critical Concepts: "Basic Steps of Spinal Immobilization" and Figure 7A and B). To secure the pelvis, place the strap directly over the pelvic girdle. Ensure that there is no pressure on the abdomen; any abdominal pressure or constraint could reduce ventilatory efficiency and increase the potential for vomiting. To secure the shoulders, place the strap over the shoulder girdle, not the lower chest. This position will minimize the risk of respiratory compromise due to immobilization.

Secure the head to the spine board after the body is secured to the board. The rescuer at the head can monitor and support the airway continuously while other rescuers complete spinal immobilization. Use a cervical immobilization device to help secure the head if needed. Alternatively, position rolled towels, rolled blankets, or foam blocks around the head. Do not use sandbags or IV fluid bags to support cervical immobilization and secure the head. These objects can shift during transport or procedures (eg, if you roll the child for airway clearance), moving the head or neck out of alignment.

If there is a risk of spinal injury, maintain spinal immobilization until appropriate examinations and diagnostic studies can be performed. These procedures can usually be done in the ED or the tertiary care center.

Critical Concepts:
Basic Steps of Spinal Immobilization

- Immobilize the cervical spine (manually and then with cervical collar) while providing airway support.

- Place and center the child on a spine board with the neck in neutral alignment.

- Fill any gaps between the child and the edges of the board.

- Secure at least 3 anatomic points to the board:
  - Thighs
  - Pelvis
  - Shoulders

- Secure the child at the feet first and work toward the head. Make sure there is no compromise of oxygenation or ventilation.

- Secure the head last. Make sure there is no compromise of the airway.

FIGURE 5. **A,** If the spine board does not have a head well, place a layer of linens under the child's torso to support alignment of the spine in a neutral position. **B,** Use rolled towels to fill any gaps between the child's body and the site where you secure the straps. **C,** If a rigid cervical collar of appropriate size is unavailable, use a rolled towel to immobilize the cervical spine. (Each victim below has a patent airway and effective ventilation.)

A

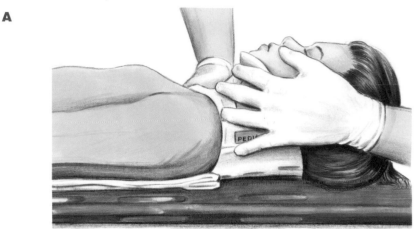

B

C

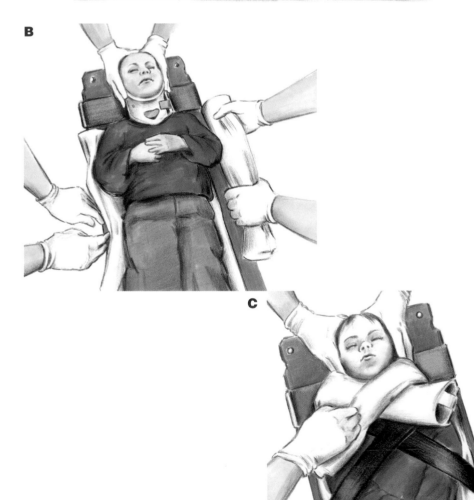

Spinal Immobilization Devices

Cervical Collars

A rigid, properly fitting cervical collar limits flexion and extension of the cervical spine. These collars are an *adjunct* to cervical spine immobilization; they do not fully immobilize the cervical spine when used alone.[79] After you apply the collar, you should continue manual stabilization until the body and head are fully immobilized against the spine board.

If the cervical collar fits correctly, the chin sits snugly in the chin cup. The collar must not force the mandible posteriorly; doing so may compromise the airway. The lower portion of the collar must rest firmly against the chest and clavicles. An improperly fitted cervical collar may place the child at greater risk for spinal injury and may block access to or compromise the airway.

If none of the commercially available collars fits the child, rescuers may immobilize the cervical spine using a rolled towel (Figure 5C).[89] Soft cervical collars (usually made of foam) *cannot* immobilize the cervical spine.

Spine Boards

Spine boards are made of wood, nonporous plastic, or metal. Spine boards for children may contain a head well. Most boards contain cutout handles and tabs for securing the straps.

Long spine boards are "full-length" spine boards. Long spine boards are versatile and widely available. You can secure a patient of any size to a long board. But the child is often much smaller than the long board, so you will need to place additional padding to prevent shifting of the child. This extra padding can block access to the child's extremities or sides.

The short spine board was designed for extrication of occupants of crashed motor vehicles. The short spine board is just as wide as the long board but usually only half the length. The shorter length makes this board better suited for pediatric patients. Because it is as wide as a conventional board, you will still need to use extra padding to secure the child.

FIGURE 6. A, Preparation for placement of child on spine board. The cervical collar is in place, as is a layer of linens that will be under the child's torso. This child has a patent airway and effective ventilation. B, Three rescuers roll the injured child onto her side, supporting the head, neck, torso, and extremities to maintain alignment of the spine. A rescuer will then move the spine board against the child's back. C, Rescuers have logrolled the child onto the spine board. The layer of linen is under the child's torso. Rescuers will now secure the child to the board at a minimum of 3 anatomic points.

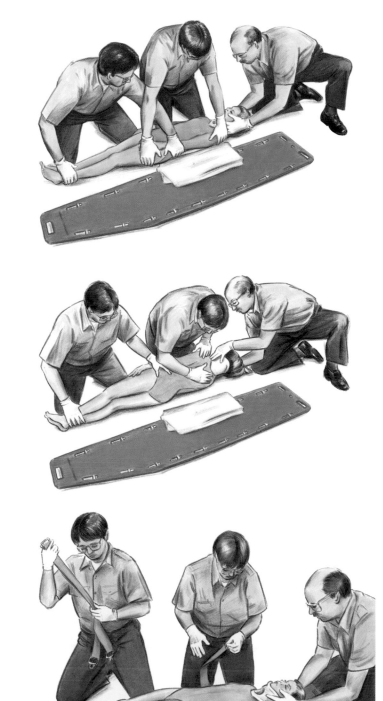

A

B

C

Vacuum Splints and Boards

Several companies produce nylon devices filled with small polystyrene beads. When a vacuum is created inside the nylon bag, the material creates a firm layer that conforms to the shape of the body part it supports, preventing that body part from flexing or moving. These devices can provide both axial stabilization and immobilization if they support the child's head, neck, torso. They are light and portable, making them favorable for use in air transport.

Cost limits the availability of these devices, but their multiple uses may improve cost-effectiveness. Vacuum boards provide immobilization equivalent to that provided by a spine board but with greater comfort.[90-92] A vacuum board also can be applied to the patient faster than a spine board.[92] The main disadvantage of vacuum splints is risk of puncture. If the surface is punctured, the vacuum is lost; the device becomes flexible, so it will no longer immobilize the body part. To prevent this loss of immobilization, providers should place patients with a vacuum splint onto a long spine board during transport.

Infant and Child Safety Seats

Management of the injured child found in a car seat is controversial. There is no information in the peer-reviewed medical literature to evaluate the relative merits of routinely immobilizing the children in the seats for transport or extricating them from the seats. Many EMS jurisdictions routinely use safety seats to transport children; others routinely remove injured children from safety seats before transport. If the integrity of the seat is maintained and the child has no evidence of injury, rescuers can transport the child in the safety seat.

The recommendation to remove a potentially injured patient from a safety seat before transport is based on several concerns. If left in the car seat, the child cannot be fully immobilized while rescuers provide continual assessment, support of airway and breathing, and establishment

FIGURE 7. Spinal immobilization of pediatric trauma victims. **A,** Infant. **B,** Child. Immobilization of an infant's or young child's cervical spine in a neutral position must not compromise the airway, breathing, or circulation. Place straps and immobilizers in a way that allows visual and auscultatory assessment.

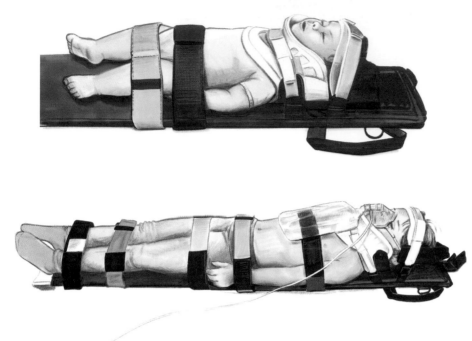

of vascular access if needed. If the child deteriorates during transport, rescuers will have to extricate the child before they can provide support.

Removal of an Infant or Child From a Safety Seat

If an infant or child requires a complete trauma assessment and intervention for airway, breathing, or circulation, rescuers should remove the child from the car safety seat. One rescuer provides cervical immobilization while another rescuer removes the seat restraints.

While the first rescuer maintains cervical immobilization, the second rescuer tips the seat back toward a spine board. The second rescuer then places a pediatric immobilizer, long arm board, or other device behind the infant's head, neck, and back. The second rescuer gently transfers (slides) the child out of the seat in the axial direction and onto the spine board. The spine board should contain a head well or a

layer of blankets or towels to ensure neutral position of the spine.

Immobilization of an Infant or Child in a Safety Seat

If an infant or a toddler has no signs of significant injury and is still restrained in a safety seat, rescuers may immobilize and transport the child in the seat. One rescuer stabilizes the cervical spine by applying manual head and neck immobilization with the car seat in the upright position.

Apply a cervical collar if one of appropriate size is available. Use a rolled towel or small rolled blanket to pad the child's lap and fill any gaps between the child and the seat. Use wide tape to secure the pelvis and upper chest (across the shoulders) to the seat. Place rolled towels on both sides of the head to further stabilize the head, neck, and cervical spine. Apply tape across the forehead and across the cervical collar to further immobilize the child's head and neck.

Risks of Spinal Immobilization

There are risks of spinal immobilization, but they remain largely unstudied in children. One risk is upper airway obstruction due to an incorrectly sized cervical collar; another is adverse neck flexion in infants and young children. Other risks (extracted from limited adult data) are interference with airway access or ventilation, delayed transport or delayed physical examination, pain or pressure sores at bony points of contact (eg, occiput or lumbosacral spine), agitation, and increased intracranial pressure.[93-95]

Unresolved Issues and Research Initiatives

No single method of spinal immobilization works in all circumstances. This chapter summarizes the scientific basis for spinal immobilization techniques in infants and children. It also includes consensus recommendations from pediatric resuscitation and trauma specialists. Some recommendations are based on rational conjecture from adult information. More research is needed to support pediatric spinal immobilization techniques. Research might address when or whether to immobilize a child in a car seat, where and how to secure a car seat in an ambulance, and how to properly logroll an injured child onto a spine board when a minimum number of rescuers is available.

Head Injury

Primary brain injury can include parenchymal damage to the brain, diffuse axonal injury or axonal shearing, and brain swelling. These injuries can cause increased intracranial pressure, which can lead to decreased brain perfusion and brain herniation with cardiorespiratory arrest or brain death. Secondary brain injury, including cerebral hypoxia and hypoperfusion, may contribute to morbidity or mortality. Head injuries that cause signs of brainstem herniation, epidural hematoma, or subdural hematoma may require urgent therapy. These problems are briefly summarized in this section; an extensive discussion is beyond the scope of this textbook.

Herniation Syndromes

Herniation syndromes result from pressure on the brain and brainstem. This pressure causes shifting of the brain or brainstem, cranial nerve dysfunction, and loss of brain or brainstem function. Early and intermediate signs of increased intracranial pressure include headache, vomiting, altered mental status, abnormal respiratory pattern, and stereotypic posturing in response to stimulation. Lateral temporal lobe (uncal) herniation compresses the optic nerve on the side involved, producing unilateral pupil dilation. Untreated uncal herniation can progress and ultimately lead to compression of the midbrain and brainstem.

Brainstem (central) herniation is the compression of the brainstem. This condition causes cranial nerve dysfunction, loss of autonomic nervous system cardiorespiratory control, and ultimately cessation of brain function. Herniation causes an altered level of consciousness. As herniation progresses, irregular respirations, asymmetric and dilated pupils, upward gaze paresis, and hypertonia may develop. Typical late features of brainstem herniation include "Cushing's triad" of bradycardia, hypertension, and irregular or absent respiration (see Critical Concepts: "Signs of Brainstem [Central] Herniation"). These features are caused by severe compression of the brainstem. Complete brainstem herniation through the foramen magnum is associated with cessation of brain perfusion and function (ie, brain death).

Immediate intervention to treat evolving herniation includes support of oxygenation, ventilation, and perfusion. Initial mechanical or manual ventilation of an injured intubated patient should provide 100% oxygen; the typical rate is 20 to 30 breaths/min for infants and 12 to 20 breaths/min for older children. Higher rates or tidal volumes may be needed if intracranial hypertension and evolving

Critical Concepts:
Signs of Brainstem (Central) Herniation

One late warning sign of impending brainstem herniation is altered mental status. This sign may occur with the following signs:

- Asymmetric or fixed dilated pupils
- Bradycardia
- Hypertension
- Irregular respiratory pattern

herniation are present. *Routine* hyperventilation is not recommended for the treatment of increased intracranial pressure. But hyperventilation may be effective in the acute management of impending herniation because it may transiently reduce cerebral blood flow and cerebral blood volume. If intravascular volume and systemic perfusion are stable, consider administration of medications to decrease the volume of water or cerebral spinal fluid in the cranial vault (mannitol 0.5 to 1 g/kg IV or furosemide 1 mg/kg IV). Identify and treat reversible causes of increased intracranial pressure (eg, epidural or subdural hematoma or status epilepticus).

Epidural Hematoma

An epidural hematoma results from laceration or contusion of the blood vessels between the dura mater and skull table. Two common causes of epidural hematoma in children are a tear in the middle meningeal artery after parietal skull fracture and damage to the meningeal or diploic veins in the posterior cranial fossa. Epidural hematomas usually occur in the lateral temporal fossa; increased (blood) density and a biconvex (lens) shape are evident on the CT scan. Older children may present with the classic pattern of a "lucid interval" followed by rapid neurologic deterioration, but this presentation occurs in the minority of children with epidural hematoma. A

good outcome depends on prompt recognition and treatment of the hematoma before secondary brain compression and hypoxic and ischemic injury occur.

Subdural Hematoma

A subdural hematoma usually results from trauma to the cranial vault. Such trauma can cause disruption of a vein or venous sinus beneath the dura. Subdural hematoma is about 5 to 10 times more common than epidural hematoma, especially in infants. Subdural hematomas frequently occur in infants and children with nonaccidental trauma, including shaken impact syndrome. In this syndrome violent shaking produces acceleration-deceleration forces that shear the bridging veins in the subdural space.

Nonspecific symptoms of a subdural hematoma include irritability, headache, vomiting, and low-grade fever. Head circumference may increase in infants with open sutures. Providers may observe lethargy, downward gaze preference (eg, "sunsetting" of the eyes), and retinal hemorrhages. Signs of increased intracranial pressure may develop. A good outcome depends on prompt recognition and treatment. The collected blood should be drained by a trained provider or a neurosurgeon before secondary brain compression and hypoxic and ischemic injury occur.

Burns and Smoke Inhalation

Assessment and management priorities for burn patients are the same as the priorities for other trauma patients. The child with flame burns has a risk of inhalation injury and subsequent upper airway obstruction and respiratory failure. Key features of the scene that suggest a risk of airway injury are an enclosed space, heavy smoke, fumes, steam, hot vapor, chemical hazard, and explosions. Assessment of scene safety, removal from the burning source or burning clothes, and provision of 100% oxygen to treat carbon monoxide exposure are appropriate. Signs of inhalation injury include singed eyebrows or nasal hairs, soot in the nasopharynx or oropharynx, carbonaceous (black) sputum, and stridor. Early tracheal intubation by suitably trained providers is appropriate for patients with suspected upper airway inhalation injury. Hidden internal injuries may result from a fall or blast. More comprehensive materials and instruction are available through the American Burn Association Advanced Burn Life Support Course (see **www.ameriburn.org**).

Patterns of Child Abuse and Self-Destructive Behavior

In 1997 child protective service organizations in the United States reported more than 1 million confirmed victims of child abuse.[96] During evaluation and management of pediatric trauma victims, rescuers should be alert to signs of child abuse and self-destructive behavior (see Critical Concepts: "Behaviors Suggesting Risk of Maltreatment").

Physical findings that suggest child maltreatment include injuries out of proportion to the reported history, bruises of different ages (especially on the ears, neck, back, thighs, genitalia, or buttocks), immersion scald burns that cover the area of a stocking or glove without evidence of splash burns, and human bites.[97] Note that not all unusual injuries are the result of maltreatment. Ask questions in an objective and nonconfrontational manner. Carefully and thoroughly document the child's injuries; also document statements made by the child and caregivers.

The mechanisms for reporting suspected child maltreatment differ by location. Healthcare providers should be familiar with local protocols. Anyone reporting suspected child maltreatment in good faith is safe from civil or criminal liability.

Healthcare providers should carefully evaluate symptoms suggestive of self-destructive behavior (eg, wrist slashing or self-inflicted wounds). Refer children with such symptoms for further evaluation as appropriate.

Critical Concepts:
Behaviors Suggesting Risk of Maltreatment

Child maltreatment includes neglect and abuse, whether emotional, physical, or sexual. Rescuers should suspect physical abuse when the injury is out of proportion to or incompatible with the reported history. The following behaviors may suggest maltreatment:

Child	Caregiver
Avoidance of questions	Apathy, lack of concern
History differs from history reported by caregivers	History incompatible with injury
Inappropriate response to caregiver	Bizarre conduct
Wariness of physical contact	Overreaction to child's actions

Healthcare professionals are ethically and legally obligated to report suspicion of abuse or neglect.

Stabilization and Transport

Stabilization of the trauma victim requires continuous assessment and support of airway, breathing, and circulation with simultaneous spinal immobilization. Communication is an essential part of stabilization and transport of trauma victims. Communication is essential whether transport occurs between the trauma scene and ED, between trauma centers, or between locations in a trauma center. Chapter 9 presents principles of postarrest stabilization and transport.

Decision to Transport

The decision to transport an injured child to a tertiary trauma center is based on the following factors:

1. Access to expertise needed for management of the injury (eg, pediatric trauma surgeon, pediatric surgical subspecialist, or ancillary pediatric services)

2. Access to essential equipment needed for evaluation or treatment of the child

3. Likelihood of clinical deterioration requiring resources unavailable at the current hospital

4. Family preference

Before personnel transport a child, the referring and receiving physicians should communicate as frequently as dictated by changes in the patient's status (see Chapter 9). The physicians should discuss recommendations for management of the patient and mode of transport. Before transport, providers should do the following:

- Secure the patient's airway

- Stabilize the patient's respiratory status

- Secure all intravenous or intraosseous lines

- Assess and document neurologic status

- Stabilize fractures

- Assess and document circulation proximal and distal to each fracture

- Immobilize the child's spine

Transport personnel should bring a complete copy of the medical records and radiographs. The transport vehicle should have a warm or neutral thermal environment depending on the ambient temperature. To improve quality of care, the receiving facility should provide follow-up information to the referring facility after the patient arrives.

Summary Points

Most pediatric trauma-related mortality occurs before admission to the hospital,[98] either in the field or the ED. Prehospital stabilization of the pediatric trauma victim requires immediate treatment of respiratory failure, shock, and life-threatening injuries to ensure effectiveness of ventilation, oxygenation, and perfusion until definitive trauma care is available. Providers must immobilize the spine throughout these procedures to limit injury or reinjury.

The most important skills for support of the pediatric trauma victim are rapid cardiopulmonary assessment, airway support, and the establishment of vascular access. Rapid recognition and treatment of trauma-related injuries (eg, tension or open pneumothorax) can be life-saving. Table 6 presents an approach to the initial evaluation and stabilization of the child with multiple injuries and respiratory failure or shock. This approach is fundamentally the same as the approach for any child with potential respiratory failure or shock with additional caveats for trauma. Early consultation with a surgeon is important when the child has severe, potentially severe, or multisystem trauma. Two preventable causes of death in pediatric trauma victims are inadequate airway management and inadequate volume resuscitation.

Spine injuries are uncommon in children. But these injuries require careful assessment and management. Spinal immobilization in children requires practice and planning. Improper use of equipment may result in further injury to the child; it may also impede resuscitative efforts. To deliver excellent trauma care, providers must recognize the unique anatomic features of children and the limitations and benefits of spinal immobilization equipment.

Case Scenarios

Completion of Introductory Case Scenario

A 7-year-old boy runs into the street. A car traveling at 30 mph (approximately 50 km/h) strikes the child, throwing him approximately 30 feet (10 meters). The child immediately loses consciousness. The child continues to breathe spontaneously, but his breathing is labored. He has an obvious contusion to his forehead and a swollen, deformed left thigh. When EMS arrives the boy is lying prone. He has labored respirations at a rate of 10 breaths/min, a pulse of 160 bpm, and a blood pressure of 90/70 mm Hg. Capillary refill time is >3 seconds in all extremities.

Rescuers apply painful stimuli. The child moans, withdraws from stimuli, and localizes pain. But he does not open his eyes in response to painful stimuli.

Answers to Introductory Questions

■ *How would you approach initial assessment and stabilization of this child?*

TABLE 6. Initial Approach to the Child With Multiple Injuries

1. Notify a *trauma surgeon with pediatric expertise.*

2. Open the airway with a jaw thrust while maintaining cervical spine immobilization.

3. Clear the oropharynx with a rigid suction device if indicated; assess breathing.

4. Administer 100% oxygen by nonrebreathing mask if the child is awake and breathing spontaneously.

5. Ventilate with 100% oxygen using a bag mask if the child has significant respiratory distress or altered mental status. Provide hyperventilation if you suspect increased intracranial pressure with impending brain herniation.

6. Provide advanced airway management with appropriate spinal immobilization if the child has signs of respiratory failure or is unresponsive. Appropriately trained providers may attempt orotracheal intubation; confirm tracheal tube placement by a secondary technique. If the victim is unconscious, consider use of an oropharyngeal airway during bag-mask ventilation or cricoid pressure.

7. While maintaining airway patency and spinal immobilization, assess signs of circulation.

8. Initiate chest compressions and control external bleeding with pressure if indicated.

9. Treat tension pneumothorax or hemothorax if present.

10. Establish vascular access; obtain blood samples for blood type and crossmatch studies.

11. If signs of inadequate perfusion are present, rapidly infuse 20 mL/kg isotonic crystalloid.

12. Immobilize the neck with a semirigid collar or head immobilizer and tape. Immobilize the spine on a spine board.

13. Consider gastric decompression (an orogastric tube is preferable).

14. Infuse a second isotonic crystalloid bolus if signs of shock are present. Consider blood products as necessary for treatment of major hemorrhage.

This child has evidence of multisystem injury. Rescuers should use universal precautions and survey the scene to ensure that it is safe to proceed. They should then assess and support the airway with simultaneous spinal immobilization and assess and support breathing and circulation.

■ *What is your rapid cardiopulmonary assessment?*

This child has signs of respiratory distress with probable respiratory failure and shock. The airway needs support and breathing is labored. Tachycardia and delayed capillary refill suggest compromised circulation. The child has a risk of bleeding from a femur fracture. Potential injuries consistent with this mechanism of injury include pelvic fracture and intra-abdominal injury. The child has an altered mental status, which may be caused by hypoxia, poor perfusion, or brain injury.

■ *What are the 3 most important treatment priorities for this child?*

The first priority of the primary survey (initial assessment or ABCDEs) is support of airway with simultaneous cervical spine immobilization. Rescuers should also assess and support breathing and circulation. The breathing assessment should include evaluation for potential pneumothorax or hemothorax and appropriate treatment. The second priority is establishment of vascular access. Administer an isotonic crystalloid bolus to treat shock. The third priority is rapid communication with and safe transport to the nearest trauma center with pediatric expertise.

Case Scenario 2

A 3-year-old girl is loosely restrained by a lap belt in the middle back seat of a car. The car is hit head on by another vehicle. The child's head strikes the interior of the car. EMS personnel find her still restrained in the car. The child has an obvious scalp laceration and bilateral periorbital hematomas. She is appropriately oriented, but she complains of severe pain in her abdomen and back.

Acceptable Actions

The following actions are acceptable for the out-of-hospital care of children who sustain potential multisystem injuries, including potential head and neck injuries:

■ Use universal precautions.

■ Perform a brief primary survey (initial assessment). Manually immobilize the cervical spine before and during extrication of the child.

■ Assess the child's airway (**A**) while immobilizing the cervical spine in the neutral position. Use the jaw thrust rather than the head tilt–chin lift if you need to open the airway.

■ Assess quantity and quality of respirations (**B**) to determine if respiratory effort is adequate.

■ Assess circulation (**C**), including heart rate and quality of pulse and systemic perfusion.

■ Assess disability (**D**); assess initial neurologic status using the Glasgow Coma Scale and AVPU scale.

■ Fully immobilize the spine with a spine immobilization device.

■ Establish vascular access.

■ Prepare for transport.

■ Communicate with the receiving facility and personnel.

Rationale for Acceptable Actions

■ **A**irway assessment and support with cervical spine immobilization: This child is breathing, oriented, and talking, so you can assume that her airway is patent. The child's complaints and the mechanism of injury suggest spinal injury, so you should immobilize the spine. Using universal precautions, maintain the airway before, during, and after spinal immobilization. Airway maintenance usually requires two rescuers: one to immobilize the head and neck in neutral position and one to assess and manage the airway. In unresponsive patients with potential cervical spine injury, open the airway with a jaw thrust. (The head tilt–chin lift may worsen an existing injury to the cervical spine.) This patient has signs of a patent airway, so she does not need a jaw thrust. Ensure that suctioning equipment is immediately available.

■ **B**reathing assessment and support: Although this child can speak, a more detailed assessment of respiratory status is necessary. Perform a rapid visual inspection, observing chest expansion and chest symmetry. You should look for retractions and use of accessory muscles. Evaluate skin color, and look for external signs of trauma. Auscultate both sides of the chest to evaluate the presence and quality of breath sounds. Administer oxygen. If the child's respiratory rate or effort is inadequate, provide assisted ventilation.

■ **C**irculation assessment and support: In this 3-year-old child, assessment of central pulses (carotid or femoral) and peripheral pulses (radial or dorsalis pedis) is important. Evaluate pulse quality (thready, weak, normal, or bounding) and rate (fast, normal, slow, or absent). Apply direct pressure to sites of active external bleeding.

■ **D**isability assessment: You should perform a rapid neurologic assessment using the Glasgow Coma Scale; also assess pupil size and reactivity. To rapidly assess level of consciousness, use the AVPU scale. Bilateral periorbital hematomas suggest a basilar skull fracture. Use an orogastric tube rather than a nasogastric tube for gastric decompression when you suspect basilar skull fracture. (A nasogastric tube may migrate intracranially if a basilar skull fracture causes a dural tear.)

■ **E**xposure and **E**nvironmental control: Expose the victim and monitor the temperature of the environment. Evaluate the environment for the presence of hazardous materials (eg, leaking gasoline and sparks, which may cause a fire). Provide spinal stabilization and immobilization for transport.

— This 3-year-old child has the potential for spinal cord injury, so rescuers must properly immobilize the child during extrication and throughout transport. Stabilize the cervical spine in the neutral position, but avoid traction on the neck. Apply a properly fitting rigid collar if available.

— The child was restrained by a lap belt only. The mechanism of injury was an acceleration-deceleration event. The child also has back pain. These factors place the child at risk for thoracic and lumbar spine injuries. Rescuers should place this child onto a spine board or other pediatric immobilization device. To maintain the child's neck in neutral position, use a spine board with a head well or place padding on the board to elevate the torso.

Secure the child to the board at a minimum of 3 anatomic points: the thighs, pelvis, and shoulders. Using straps or cravats, secure the child's legs (thighs) and torso (pelvis and shoulders) to the board first; then secure the child's head. You may need to use rolled towels and tape to further immobilize the cervical spine. You may also use rolled towels and tape to immobilize the cervical spine if an appropriately sized rigid cervical collar is unavailable.

Apply minimal pressure to the abdomen; abdominal pressure or constraint could reduce ventilation efficiency and increase the potential for vomiting. Place the shoulder strap over the shoulder girdle, not the lower chest. Placing the straps over the shoulder girdle will minimize the chance that immobilization will cause respiratory compromise.

Unacceptable Actions

- Failing to use universal precautions
- Attempting to extricate the child before you assess and support the airway, breathing, circulation, and disability

- Opening the airway, extricating the child, or transporting the child without proper spinal immobilization
- Using a head tilt–chin lift to open the child's airway

Case Scenario 2 Progression

After you support the airway, immobilize the spine, and extricate the child, you reassess the child's respiratory status. The child has an increased respiratory rate and a distended abdomen; she is less responsive to verbal stimulation. You cannot detect a radial pulse; femoral pulses are weak and rapid. As the child is moved into the ambulance, oxygen is provided. You establish vascular access and infuse a 20 mL/kg bolus of isotonic crystalloid en route to the hospital. You contact the receiving facility and give the patient report. If the patient's clinical condition stabilizes in the ambulance, you can perform a secondary (detailed) survey.

Evaluation at the receiving facility reveals a basilar skull fracture, a perforated jejunum, and a vertebral fracture of the lumbar spine (chance fracture of L3). A standard 3-view cervical spine series shows normal findings.

Case Scenario 3

A 2-year-old boy is playing in his driveway behind a parked car. The driver backs up the car, striking the child. The rear wheel runs over the child, but the driver stops the car before the front wheel reaches the child. The child does not lose consciousness at the scene. His breathing is spontaneous but labored. The child has a "tire tattoo" extending from the right clavicle to the right lower costal margin. The child is brought to the ED by private vehicle without activation of EMS.

You see a toddler in obvious respiratory distress. His respiratory rate is 40 breaths/min and labored with grunting and retractions. You note crepitus on palpation of the right chest with no breath sounds on the right side. Breath sounds are present on the left side. There is no obvious dis-

tention of the neck veins and no obvious deviation of the trachea. The child cries intermittently. He is receiving 100% O_2 by face mask; his oxyhemoglobin saturation by pulse oximeter is 100%. The child's skin is pale and cool to the touch. Capillary refill time is approximately 4 seconds, and heart rate is 160 bpm with palpable central pulses. The child is conscious but listless with his knees drawn to his chest. He intermittently responds to verbal commands.

Acceptable Actions

The following actions are acceptable for evaluation and treatment of this child:

- Use universal precautions.
- Open the child's airway (**A**) using the jaw thrust while immobilizing the cervical spine in the neutral position.
- Provide high-flow oxygen by nonrebreathing mask (**B**).
- Assess breathing and assist with bag-mask ventilation (**B**) if necessary. Decompress the right chest with needle thoracentesis (2nd intercostal space in midclavicular line); insert a thoracostomy tube in the right chest (5th intercostal space anterior to midaxillary line). Monitor oxygen saturation using pulse oximetry.
- Assess circulation (**C**), including heart rate and quality of pulse and systemic perfusion. Establish vascular access and administer fluid boluses as needed.
- Assess disability (**D**) using the GCS and AVPU scale. Perform initial and serial assessments of neurologic status.
- Expose (**E**) the patient to rapidly examine for other life- or limb-threatening injuries. Logroll the patient to examine the thoracic and lumbar spine. Protect the cervical spine with full spine immobilization on a spine board. Control the temperature of the environment and monitor the environment for hazards (**E**).
- Continuously monitor ECG and pulse oximetry.
- Begin the secondary survey (detailed examination). (Detailed presentation

of the full secondary survey is beyond the scope of the PALS course.) Obtain further radiographic studies pending completion of the secondary survey when appropriate. Frequently reassess the child to prevent further injury. Control pain as appropriate.

Rationale for Acceptable Actions

■ **A**irway assessment and support with cervical spine immobilization: This child is responsive and cries intermittently, suggesting a patent airway. The mechanism of injury poses a risk of spinal cord injury, so rescuers must immobilize the spine before further movement or transport. Using universal precautions, continuously assess the airway before, during, and after immobilization; be prepared to support the airway as needed. Airway maintenance usually requires two rescuers, one to immobilize the head and neck in the neutral position and one to assess and manage the airway. In patients with potential cervical spine injury and decreased responsiveness or airway obstruction, open the airway with a jaw thrust. (The head tilt–chin lift may worsen an existing injury to the cervical spine.) Ensure that suction equipment is immediately available.

■ **B**reathing assessment and support: You should perform a detailed assessment of the airway and ventilation. This child has tachypnea, absence of breath sounds on the right, crepitus and contusion of the right chest, and a mechanism of injury suggestive of a right tension pneumothorax. Note that in young children, tracheal deviation and distended neck veins (signs of tension pneumothorax) are not always observed. Tension pneumothorax is a life-threatening complication that requires urgent therapy. The treatment of choice is chest tube thoracostomy or needle thoracentesis followed by chest tube thoracostomy. In this symptomatic child, you should perform chest decompression before you obtain a confirmatory chest x-ray. Monitor the child's oxygenation, per-

fusion, and appearance before, during, and after the procedure. Consider administration of sedation or local anesthetic if the child's condition is stable. After chest decompression, reassess the child's respiratory status, including respiratory rate, effort, chest rise, and use of accessory muscles.

■ **C**irculatory assessment and support: In this 2-year-old child, assess central pulses (carotid or femoral), peripheral pulses (radial or dorsalis pedis), and capillary refill. Assess pulse quality (thready, weak, normal, or bounding) and rate (fast, normal, slow, or absent). Because the child has evidence of chest trauma (an external abrasion extending from the right clavicle to the right lower costal margin), the child is at high risk for blunt injury to the liver. You must monitor the patient's hemodynamic status continuously and look for subtle signs of hemorrhage. Establish reliable vascular access, and administer a 20 mL/kg bolus of isotonic crystalloid. Use of a fluid warmer may be appropriate if you anticipate a need for large-volume fluid resuscitation or blood product transfusion.

■ **D**isability assessment: Perform a rapid neurologic assessment using the GCS; also assess pupil size and response to light. To rapidly assess level of consciousness, use the AVPU scale. Continually reassess and record neurologic function.

■ **E**xposure and **E**nvironmental control: This child has the potential for spinal cord injury and requires spinal immobilization. Stabilize the cervical spine in the neutral position while avoiding traction on the neck. Apply a rigid cervical collar if one of appropriate size is available. Prepare to immobilize the child on a spine board or other pediatric immobilization device. Before you place the child on the spine board, logroll the child to examine the back. Palpate the entire back and look for evidence of injury. Maintain the head and neck in a neutral position. You may use a spine board with a head well or place

padding on the board to elevate the torso. Secure the child to the board at a minimum of 3 anatomic points: the thighs, pelvis, and shoulders. Using straps or cravats, secure the child's legs, pelvis, and torso to the board first; then secure the head (see "General Technique of Spinal Immobilization" earlier in this chapter). Obtain additional information about the patient's history and complete a secondary survey (detailed examination) as soon as feasible. Measure the child's core temperature when you check routine vital signs.

Unacceptable Actions

■ Failing to use universal precautions

■ Failing to immobilize the spine appropriately

■ Failing to identify and treat the tension pneumothorax

■ Delaying intervention to obtain a chest x-ray before definitive management of *symptomatic* tension pneumothorax

■ Relying on signs such as tracheal deviation and distended neck veins for diagnosis of tension pneumothorax in a young child

■ Failing to examine the child for concurrent and significant cerebral, abdominal, and thoracic injuries

Case Scenario 3 Progression

After initial assessment, initiation of supplemental oxygen, and chest decompression, breath sounds are symmetric. The child's respiratory rate is now 30 breaths/min with no grunting or distress. His heart rate is 125 bpm, blood pressure is 94 by palpation, oxygen saturation by pulse oximetry is 96%, depth of respirations has increased, and his color is improving. The child responds to your questions and is now consolable. Findings of a thorough physical examination of the thoracic and lumbar spine are normal. A chest x-ray shows the chest tube in proper position. Cross-table x-rays of the lateral cervical spine and pelvis show no abnormality. A standard 3-view cervical spine series also shows normal results. Results of the secondary

survey (detailed examination), conducted
by a surgeon, are otherwise normal.

Case Scenario 4

EMS is called to the home of an 8-month-old infant. The infant "fell out of bed" 2 days ago; the bed is 2 feet high. When EMS arrives the infant demonstrates minimal respiratory effort; he has slow irregular gasps and an initial heart rate of 80 bpm. Rescuers begin assisted bag-mask ventilation with oxygen and continue ventilation during rapid transport to the ED.

On arrival in the ED, the infant is pale with cool extremities, capillary refill time of 4 seconds, and weak central pulses. His heart rate is 180 bpm. The infant withdraws only in response to painful stimuli. Eye opening occurs only in response to painful stimuli. Pupils are equal and sluggishly reactive bilaterally. You see multiple bruises in various stages of healing over the upper and lower extremities and abdomen. During pauses in assisted ventilation, the infant's spontaneous respiratory pattern is irregular and gasping. You place the child on an ECG monitor and pulse oximeter.

Acceptable Actions

The following immediate actions are acceptable for assessment and treatment of this child:

- Use universal precautions.
- Control the airway with a jaw thrust while immobilizing the cervical spine in the neutral position.
- Provide bag-mask ventilation.
- Assess the quantity and quality of respirations.
- Prepare for tracheal intubation.
- Perform tracheal intubation while immobilizing the cervical spine in the neutral position and applying cricoid pressure. Consider rapid sequence intubation, depending on local protocol, if appropriately trained personnel and equipment are present (see Chapter 14).
- Assess circulation, including heart rate and quality of pulse and systemic perfusion. Establish reliable vascular access,

and administer a 20 mL/kg bolus of isotonic crystalloid.

- Assess initial neurologic status; reassess after initial stabilization of airway, adequate ventilation, and initial fluid bolus.
- Maintain spinal immobilization until you "clear" the cervical spine (ie, rule out fracture and dislocation).
- Expose the child to evaluate bruising and any other signs of injury that might contribute to cardiorespiratory failure.
- Provide support to family and caregivers. Emphasize your role to provide medical care for the child and your responsibility to report the child's injuries to child protective services.

Rationale for Acceptable Actions

- **A**irway assessment and support with cervical spine immobilization: This child is at risk for both head and cervical spine injury. Using universal precautions for exposure to secretions, assess airway patency; remove debris, vomitus, and secretions in the oropharynx to facilitate bag-mask ventilation. While immobilizing the cervical spine in the neutral position, open the airway using the jaw thrust; apply cricoid pressure if the patient is unconscious. Provide assisted bag-mask ventilation if the patient's respiratory rate or effort is inadequate after you open the airway. This patient is at increased risk for aspiration, so you should have suction equipment immediately available.

- **B**reathing assessment and support: The child continues to have poor respiratory effort despite bag-mask ventilation. This poor effort is probably caused by his decreased level of consciousness. To protect the airway and ensure adequate oxygenation and ventilation, prepare for tracheal intubation. Consider rapid sequence intubation if appropriately trained providers and equipment are available. During attempted orotracheal intubation, one provider should immobilize the cervical spine in the neutral position while another provider applies cricoid pressure. Maintain spinal immobilization

until you "clear" the cervical spine (ie, rule out fracture and dislocation).

- **C**irculation assessment and support: This child is pale with cool extremities and weak central pulses. These signs are consistent with shock. Establish reliable vascular access, and infuse an initial bolus of 20 mL/kg warmed isotonic crystalloid.

- **D**isability: Perform a rapid neurologic assessment. Determine and record a GCS score; assess pupil size and response to light. To rapidly assess level of consciousness, use the AVPU scale. The results of this child's examination suggest a traumatic brain injury. The child's level of consciousness and appearance (ie, multiple old bruises) are inconsistent with the history of minor trauma. You should consider nonaccidental trauma as the possible mechanism of injury.

- **E**xposure and **E**nvironmental control: A trained provider should perform a secondary survey (detailed physical examination). This head-to-toe exam reveals additional bruising at the occiput and old scars that look like cigarette burns. Maintain a neutral thermal environment, warm IV fluids before administration, and measure the child's core temperature when you check and record vital signs. Avoid hyperthermia and reduce the child's temperature to normal if it is elevated. Anticipate the need to provide support to the family and caregivers and to involve child protective services.

Unacceptable Actions

- Failing to use universal precautions
- Failing to immobilize the cervical spine in the neutral position during and after the resuscitation until you rule out cervical spine injury
- Failing to recognize respiratory failure or provide assisted ventilation and tracheal intubation
- Failing to establish vascular access and provide fluid resuscitation for this child, who has signs of poor perfusion and shock

- Obtaining x-rays before you complete the initial assessment

- Failing to recognize signs of child abuse (ie, history inconsistent with physical condition of coma with multiple external bruises).

Case Scenario 4 Progression

Providers successfully insert a tracheal tube and confirm its position by exhaled CO_2 detection. The child receives two 20 mL/kg crystalloid boluses. A chest x-ray confirms proper tracheal tube position; multiple rib fractures of various ages with callus formation are visible. There is no evidence of coagulopathy on laboratory studies. A CT scan of the head reveals a large, chronic subdural hematoma requiring neurosurgical consultation. Ophthalmologic examination reveals old and recent bilateral retinal hemorrhages. You notify child protective services; you then provide support to the family while an evaluation is initiated. The child undergoes surgical evacuation of the subdural hematoma, but cerebral edema and increased intracranial pressure later develop. Aggressive management is unsuccessful. The child's condition deteriorates further; he meets criteria for brain death in 48 hours.

Case Scenario 5

A 7-year-old boy is riding unrestrained in the back of a pickup truck. The truck is traveling at low speed. The truck crashes into an oncoming vehicle. The child is thrown from the truck. The child briefly loses consciousness, but he subsequently gets up and walks at the scene. When EMS arrives the boy is crying but awake and alert. He has multiple superficial abrasions, and he complains of abdominal pain. His radial pulse is weak, heart rate is 160 bpm, respiratory rate is 18 breaths/min and unlabored, and blood pressure is 100/65 mm Hg with a capillary refill time of 5 seconds. The nearest hospital is 15 minutes away by ground transport.

Acceptable Actions

The following actions are acceptable for initial assessment and treatment of this child:

- Use universal precautions.

- Assess and support airway patency while immobilizing the cervical spine in the neutral position.

- Assess quantity and quality of respirations; provide oxygen.

- Assess circulation, including heart rate and quality of pulse and systemic circulation. Apply ECG and pulse oximetry monitors.

- Assess initial neurologic status.

- Immobilize the child on a spine board.

- Establish vascular access en route to the hospital, and administer a 20 mL/kg bolus of isotonic crystalloid.

- Communicate with the receiving trauma center.

Rationale for Acceptable Actions

- **Airway assessment and support and cervical spine immobilization:** Although this child has been walking at the scene, the mechanism of injury is an acceleration-deceleration event. The child requires appropriate spinal immobilization. Using universal precautions, one rescuer immobilizes the head and neck in the neutral position while another rescuer assesses the airway and applies an appropriately sized cervical collar. The child has a patent airway and is speaking normally when EMS arrives. But he has a history of loss of consciousness. For this reason providers should continuously monitor his airway and breathing. Assemble suction equipment and ensure that it is ready for use. Immobilize the child on a spine board or other pediatric immobilization device. If necessary, maintain neutral spine position either by using a spine board with a head well or by elevating the torso with padding. Then secure the child's thighs, pelvis, shoulders, and head to the immobilization device.

- **Breathing assessment and support:** The child has no obvious breathing abnormalities, but you must perform a rapid assessment, including chest inspection and bilateral auscultation, to identify any occult injury or abnormality. Oxygen

administration is standard treatment until arrival at a hospital. Administer high-flow oxygen by nonrebreathing mask.

- **Circulation assessment and support:** This child has signs of shock with tachycardia, diminished peripheral pulses, and delayed capillary refill. Compensated shock is present because his systolic blood pressure is adequate (ie, greater than 70 mm Hg + [2 × 7 years] = 84 mm Hg). Assess the quality and rate of radial and carotid pulses. Establish vascular access as soon as possible, but do not delay transport to establish access, especially if transport time is short. Once you establish vascular access, administer a 20 mL/kg bolus of isotonic crystalloid. Apply pressure to sites of external bleeding.

- **D**isability assessment: Perform a rapid neurologic assessment using the GCS; assess pupil size and reaction to light. To rapidly assess level of consciousness, use the AVPU scale. The child has a history of a brief loss of consciousness. The mechanism of injury could have resulted in brain injury, particularly a subdural or epidural hematoma. A hematoma could progress during transport, causing increased intracranial pressure and signs of cerebral herniation. For this reason rescue personnel should frequently reassess and record the child's neurologic status en route to the hospital.

- **E**xposure and **E**nvironmental control: Expose the child to look for additional injuries. Appropriately trained providers should conduct a secondary survey (detailed physical examination) after vascular access is established and treatment of life-threatening injury begins. You note bruises across the upper abdomen and right flank. The abdomen appears full and distended, suggesting the need for prompt surgical evaluation. Measure and control the child's temperature.

Unacceptable Actions

- Failing to use universal precautions

- Failing to assess airway patency and breathing on initial assessment
- Failing to provide oxygen or support airway and breathing as necessary
- Failing to assess circulation and recognize shock
- Failing to assess and reassess the child's neurologic status
- Failing to establish vascular access and administer a bolus of isotonic crystalloid
- Delaying communication with receiving personnel or transport to definitive care

Case Scenario 5 Progression

Rescuers immobilize the child's spine and support airway and breathing. Rescuers then establish IV access and infuse 20 mL/kg isotonic crystalloid. On arrival at the hospital the child responds to verbal stimuli; his GCS score is 14. His pupils are of normal size, and they react briskly to light. The child does not remember the event, and he continues to have abdominal pain. His heart rate is 140 bpm, respirations are unlabored at a rate of 18 breaths/ min with an oxyhemoglobin saturation of 100%, blood pressure is 80/60 mm Hg, and capillary refill time is 5 seconds. Providers start a second bolus of 20 mL/kg isotonic crystalloid and obtain blood samples for a CBC and type and crossmatch studies. A surgical consultant is called.

The child's condition does not change after 3 boluses of crystalloid (60 mL/kg); hemoglobin is 8 g/dL. Providers infuse crossmatched blood. Heart rate improves to 120 bpm; blood pressure, to 100/60 mm Hg; and capillary refill time, to 3 seconds. The child's GCS score is 15, and he is more alert and oriented. A CT scan of the brain shows normal findings. A CT scan of the abdomen and pelvis shows a large, lower pole splenic laceration with a moderate amount of free intra-abdominal fluid. Findings on a standard 3-view cervical spine series are normal. Results of the thoracic and lumbar spine examinations are normal.

Review Questions

1. **A 3-year-old child is an unrestrained back-seat passenger in a low-speed car crash. The child hits her head on the interior of the car. The child is awake and crying at the scene. She has an obvious scalp laceration, bilateral periorbital hematomas, and bleeding from the right nares. Which of the following actions are most appropriate and in the correct order of priority?**

   a. perform immediate tracheal intubation because of the mechanism of injury and manually immobilize the cervical spine

   b. assess airway patency, breathing, circulation, and neurologic function; then immobilize the child on a spine board while applying manual traction to the cervical spine

   c. assess airway patency while manually immobilizing the cervical spine; assess and support breathing, circulation, and neurologic function; and apply pressure to sites of obvious bleeding

   d. apply direct pressure to the nose and scalp; place the child in a recovery position; and assess airway, breathing, and circulation

   The correct answer is c. The first priority of assessment and stabilization is airway assessment and support with cervical spine immobilization.

   Answer a is incorrect because immediate tracheal intubation is not always necessary. Providers should base the decision for advanced airway support on the findings of the ABCDE assessment, not solely on the mechanism of injury.

   Answer b is incorrect because you should not routinely apply traction to the cervical spine.

   Answer d is incorrect because it omits spinal immobilization, which

is part of the primary survey (initial assessment). You should not delay spinal immobilization to complete the primary survey.

2. **A 2-year-old child is playing in his driveway behind a parked car. His mother enters the car without noticing the child. She backs up the car, rolling over the child with the rear wheel. She panics and transports the child to the hospital in the car. On arrival in the ED the child has labored breathing and a "tire tattoo" extending across the right chest. Providers stabilize the cervical spine; the airway is patent. While the child is receiving 100% oxygen by nonrebreathing face mask, his oxyhemoglobin saturation by pulse oximetry is 100%. The child has significant respiratory distress with a respiratory rate of 40 breaths/ min, grunting respirations, and a heart rate of 150 bpm. Heart sounds are present but localized more laterally to the left than normal. The child has crepitus of the right chest wall, no breath sounds over the right chest, but no tracheal deviation or neck vein distention. There are no obvious rib fractures. Which of the following interventions should you perform *first*?**

   a. immediate tracheal intubation without sedation or paralysis

   b. immediate needle decompression of the right chest, with preparation for tracheal intubation if necessary

   c. immediate chest x-ray to determine if a tension pneumothorax is present with preparation for needle decompression of the chest and tracheal intubation if necessary

   d. immediate pericardiocentesis for presumed cardiac tamponade

(Continued on next page)

The correct answer is b. The mechanism of injury places the child at risk for chest injury, and rapid cardiopulmonary assessment reveals respiratory failure and signs consistent with a right tension pneumothorax.

Answer a is incorrect because immediate tracheal intubation may be unnecessary if the tension pneumothorax is rapidly decompressed. In addition, performing tracheal intubation while the patient is awake may be inappropriate under these circumstances.

Answer c is incorrect because providers should not delay needle decompression to obtain chest x-ray. The child's mechanism of injury and clinical signs are consistent with a tension pneumothorax. Tracheal deviation and neck vein distention are *not* always present in children with tension pneumothorax.

Answer d is incorrect. Although cardiac tamponade is a life-threatening potential complication of blunt chest trauma, the patient's symptoms are most consistent with a tension pneumothorax. Providers should not delay decompression.

3. **EMS personnel bring an 8-month-old infant with a history of "rolling out of bed" to the ED. The infant is pale and cool with minimal respiratory effort (apnea). EMS rescuers provide assisted bag-mask ventilation with spinal immobilization. The infant has weak central pulses with a heart rate of 160 bpm. His oxyhemoglobin saturation is 100% while receiving 100% oxygen. He withdraws only in response to painful stimuli. Multiple external bruises in various stages of healing are present over the extremities and abdomen. Which of the following interventions is *not* part of the *primary* survey and support?**

a. assessment and support of airway with simultaneous cervical spine immobilization and assessment of breathing with provision of assisted ventilation if needed

b. assessment and support of circulation, including establishment of vascular access and administration of fluid boluses as needed

c. neurologic assessment with the Glasgow Coma Scale, evaluation of pupil size and response to light, and evaluation of level of consciousness with the AVPU scale

d. CT scan of the abdomen to evaluate for internal bleeding

The correct answer is d. A CT scan of the abdomen to evaluate for internal bleeding may be appropriate, but this test is part of the *secondary survey* (detailed physical exam) and definitive care. Providers should obtain a CT scan after the primary survey.

Answer a is incorrect because assessment and support of airway with simultaneous spinal immobilization are part of the primary survey. Assessment of breathing with support of ventilation if needed is also part of this initial assessment and stabilization.

Answer b is incorrect because assessment and support of circulation, including establishment of vascular access and administration of a fluid bolus, are all part of initial assessment and stabilization.

Answer c is incorrect because a rapid neurologic assessment is part of the initial assessment and stabilization. This assessment is step **D** (Disability) of the ABCDE Approach.

4. **An unrestrained 6-year-old child is riding in the back of a pickup truck. The truck collides head on with another vehicle. The child is ejected from the truck. He briefly loses consciousness, but he later begins to walk at the scene. When EMS arrives the child is complaining of severe abdominal pain. Which of the following is the *first* step you**

should take during your initial assessment and stabilization?

a. if the child requires airway support, you should use a jaw thrust

b. ask the child to lie down on a backboard, perform a head tilt–chin lift to open the airway, assess airway patency, and then immobilize the cervical spine

c. determine the child's Glasgow Coma Scale score and check pupil size and reactivity

d. perform a careful abdominal examination because the child reports pain in his abdomen

The correct answer is a. The mechanism of injury suggests a risk of cervical spine injury. You should immobilize the cervical spine. If the child requires airway support, you should perform the jaw thrust if needed and immobilize the cervical spine.

Answer b is incorrect. If the patient needs airway support, a jaw thrust is preferable to the head tilt–chin lift in injured children.

Answer c is incorrect. Although it is appropriate to apply the Glasgow Coma Scale and to evaluate pupil size and reactivity, these assessments should *follow* assessment and support of airway, breathing, and circulation with cervical spine immobilization. Rapid neurologic assessment is step D (**D**isability) of the ABCDE Approach.

Answer d is incorrect. Providers should assess the abdomen after they perform the primary survey to detect and treat life-threatening injuries.

5. **You have completed initial assessment and stabilization of airway, breathing, and circulation for the 6-year-old child in question 4. The child is breathing spontaneously while receiving 5 L/min oxygen by face mask. You immobilized the cervical spine manually and then with a rigid cervical collar. You and your partner immobilized the child on**

a spine board. You are now transporting the child to a nearby trauma center. During transport the child develops respiratory distress with a respiratory rate of 60 breaths/min, heart rate of 150 bpm, and "seesaw" respiratory pattern of the chest and abdomen. The child has markedly decreased breath sounds over both lung fields with noisy upper airway sounds. Intermittently there are no airway sounds with marked inspiratory respiratory effort. His pulse oximeter shows a falling oxyhemoglobin saturation of 75% and good detection of pulses. He does not respond to verbal commands. Which of the following interventions is *most* appropriate at this time?

a. perform immediate bilateral needle decompression of the chest for suspected bilateral pneumothoraces

b. remove or adjust the cervical collar while maintaining spinal stabilization, perform a jaw thrust to open the airway, suction the oropharynx, and provide assisted bag-mask ventilation if needed

c. increase the flow rate of oxygen from 5 to 10 L/min and ensure that the face mask fits tightly against the face

d. immediately intubate the trachea using a "blind" nasotracheal technique to avoid removal of the cervical spine immobilization device

The correct answer is b. The child has signs and symptoms of an obstructed upper airway: rapid, ineffective respiratory efforts with a "seesaw" pattern of the chest and abdomen; intermittent complete obstruction during inspiration; decreased *bilateral* breath sounds; and noisy upper airway sounds. If obstruction becomes complete, the airway sounds may disappear altogether. The most likely cause of airway obstruction in this child is the cervical immobilization device (improper fit), posterior displacement of the tongue, or secretions in the oropharynx.

Answer a is incorrect because bilateral pneumothoraces are uncommon during spontaneous ventilation. Assessment of airway patency and breathing should precede intervention. The intermittent nature of the distress and noisy airway sounds suggest that intermittent upper airway obstruction is more likely.

Answer c is incorrect. Although it is appropriate to assess the functioning of equipment such as the oxygen delivery device (recall the DOPE mnemonic), tightly applying the face mask will not improve the patient's status. When respiratory distress increases and noisy respirations develop in a child with a cervical collar, providers should first assess airway patency.

Answer d is incorrect. Although preparation for tracheal intubation is appropriate, rescuers should first assess and support airway and breathing. Blind *naso*tracheal intubation is not recommended for trauma victims.

Appendix: Emergency Procedures

Emergency Needle Decompression of Tension Pneumothorax

Needle decompression of a tension pneumothorax may provide temporary relief of respiratory distress. Suitably trained providers can perform this procedure quickly. If a tension pneumothorax is confirmed, the provider should insert the thoracostomy tube *after* initial decompression. The following technique is one of several acceptable techniques for emergency needle decompression.

Equipment

- Gloves, mask, and antiseptic scrub
- Local anesthetic (eg, injectable lidocaine)
- Needle or over-the-needle catheter (18 gauge or larger is preferable)
- 20-mL syringe
- 3-way stopcock (optional)
- Extension tubing with small container of sterile water (optional)

Procedure

1. Use universal precautions and sterile technique.

2. Position the child supine. Restrain the arm on the affected side above the head or out of the way (if appropriate).

3. Locate the 2nd intercostal interspace (between the 2nd and 3rd rib) in the midclavicular line on the side of the suspected pneumothorax. (Alternate site is 5th intercostal space in the anterior axillary line. *Note:* The nipple is usually at the 4th intercostal space.)

4. Clean a wide area around the anticipated site of incision with antiseptic scrub (usually povidone iodine or chlorhexidine). If the patient is responsive, inject a local anesthetic.

5. Using a gloved finger, again locate the 2nd intercostal space, midclavicular line (alternate site: 5th intercostal space, anterior axillary line).

6. Attach the needle to the syringe (3-way stopcock is optional); insert the needle through the skin at a 90° angle just *above* the 3rd rib. (*Note:* The neurovascular bundle lies in a ridge just *below* the rib margin; scraping across the *top* of the rib minimizes the risk of iatrogenic injury.)

7. Advance the needle or catheter while aspirating with the syringe until you aspirate air.

8. Stabilize the needle or catheter and aspirate air. If you are using an over-the-needle system, you can advance the catheter over the needle and remove the sharp needle. Take care to prevent kinking or dislodgment of the catheter.

9. Consider options to maintain decompression of the pneumothorax while you assess the patient's response and prepare to provide definitive treatment (chest tube). Three reasonable options are

   — Leave the needle open to air (equalizing pressure to atmosphere and releasing tension).

   — Aspirate using the 3-way stopcock system.

   — Attach extension tubing, placing the open end into water to let air bubble out through an underwater seal. (This method mimics the underwater seal contained in a pleural evacuation system.)

10. Assign one provider to stabilize the thoracostomy needle or catheter system and ensure that it does not become kinked or dislodged.

11. Reassess breath sounds and patient's response to the procedure.

Emergency Placement of a Thoracostomy Tube for Treatment of Tension or Simple Pneumothorax or Hemothorax

Note: Needle thoracostomy may be accomplished more quickly than chest tube insertion, so needle thoracostomy may precede the use of tube thoracostomy. The following procedure is one of several acceptable approaches for placement of a thoracostomy tube.

Equipment

■ Gloves, mask, antiseptic scrub, and drapes

■ Local anesthetic (eg, injectable lidocaine)

■ Scalpel with blade

■ Curved hemostat or Kelly clamp

■ Chest tube

■ Needle holder

■ Tissue forceps

■ Suture packs (0 or 000 nonabsorbable sutures on a cutting needle)

■ Chest drainage apparatus with underwater seal system

Procedure

1. Use universal precautions and sterile technique.

2. Position the child supine. Restrain the arm on the affected side above the head or out of the way.

3. Locate the 6th rib (generally 2 ribs below the nipple). Follow it laterally to the midaxillary line. You will make the incision and start the subcutaneous "tunnel" at this site.

4. Drape and cleanse a wide area around the anticipated site of tube insertion. Inject a local anesthetic (eg, lidocaine) if the patient is responsive.

5. Select the chest tube. To estimate the appropriate size, use a length-based resuscitation tape or follow these age-based guidelines:

— Newly born: 8F to 12F

— Infant <1 year of age: 14F to 20F

— Children 1 to 8 years of age: 20F to 24F

— Children >8 years and adolescents: 28F to 36F

6. With a gloved finger, again locate the 6th rib (generally 2 ribs below the nipple). Follow it laterally to the midaxillary line. You will make the incision and start the subcutaneous "tunnel" at this site.

7. With a gloved finger, palpate the 5th intercostal space (between the 5th and 6th ribs) in the midaxillary line. The subcutaneous tunnel will end and the chest tube will enter the pleural space at this site.

8. Make a short incision with the scalpel directly over the middle of the rib below the projected entry point (usually the 6th rib). Using the hemostat and your fingers, spread the tissues and loosen the subcutaneous tissue to create a "tunnel" over the rib to the insertion site. The site of insertion will be one interspace above the incision (usually the 5th intercostal space).

9. Apply enough pressure so that the hemostat enters the thoracic cavity directly above the rib. (*Note:* The neurovascular bundle lies in a ridge just *below* each rib; scraping across the *top* of the rib minimizes the risk of iatrogenic injury.) Spread the hemostat to enlarge the entry hole. Mark the entry site with your gloved finger as you remove the hemostat.

10. Grasp the distal tip of the chest tube between the tips of the curved hemostat or clamp. Insert this tube back into the tunnel entry site marked by your gloved finger. When the clamp and chest tube are within the chest cavity, open the hemostat and slide the chest tube forward to ensure

that all of the chest tube holes are within the pleural cavity. (*Note:* Use of trocars is not recommended, especially on the left side, where sharp, rigid trocars may injure vital structures.)

11. Stabilize the tube; take care to prevent kinking or dislodgment of the tube. Assign one provider to stabilize the chest tube and ensure that it does not become kinked or dislodged.

12. Reassess breath sounds and the patient's response to the procedure.

13. Suture the chest tube to the skin.

14. Attach the proximal end of the chest tube to a chest drainage apparatus. Confirm position.

15. Obtain a chest x-ray.

Emergency Pericardiocentesis for Treatment of Pericardial Tamponade

Note: In the uncommon condition of pericardial tamponade with associated shock, pericardiocentesis can be life saving. The technique described below is a simple method of performing pericardiocentesis through a subxiphoid approach. This technique is one of several that are acceptable.

Equipment

■ Gloves, mask, and antiseptic scrub

■ Local anesthetic

■ Spinal needle or over-the-needle catheter long enough to extend from the xiphoid process to the heart (18 gauge or larger is preferable)

■ 20-mL syringe

■ 3-way stopcock (optional)

Procedure

1. Use universal precautions and sterile technique.

2. Position the child supine. Restrain the arms out of the way (if appropriate).

3. Identify landmarks. Cleanse a wide area around the anticipated site of insertion with sterile antiseptic (usually povidone iodine). Inject a local anesthetic if the patient is responsive.

4. Locate the lower margins of the ribs and sternum. Place your finger on the xiphoid process in the midline.

5. Attach the needle to the syringe (3-way stopcock is optional). Insert the needle or over-the-needle catheter at a 45° angle underneath the sternum, just to the left of the xiphoid process; direct the needle or catheter toward the left scapular tip.

6. Aspirate gently with the syringe as you advance the needle.

7. When you aspirate fluid, assess for pulsatile flow and clotting characteristics. In general, blood from the pericardial sac is not pulsatile and will not form a clot; in comparison, blood from the heart chambers may be pulsatile and will usually clot within a few minutes.

8. Secure the needle or catheter manually, and monitor the patient's clinical response to drainage. If an over-the-needle system is used, you can advance the catheter over the needle and remove the sharp needle. Be careful to prevent kinking and dislodgment of the catheter.

9. Monitor for signs of potential complications, including these signs:

— Needle penetration of the pleural space (you will aspirate air)

— Needle penetration of the abdominal or peritoneal cavity (you will aspirate fluid or air)

— Myocardial perforation (you will aspirate blood that clots; the blood may be pulsatile)

10. Consider options to maintain decompression of the tamponade while you assess the patient's response

and plan definitive treatment (pericardial drainage tube or open thoracotomy).

11. Reassess heart and breath sounds and the patient's response to the procedure. The patient will require surgical exploration if pericardiocentesis is successful.

References

1. Committee on Trauma Research (US). Injury in America: A Continuing Public Health Problem. Committee on Trauma Research, Commission on Life Sciences, National Research Council and the Institute of Medicine. Washington, DC: National Academy Press; 1985.

2. *World Health Statistical Annual*, 1994. Geneva, Switzerland: World Health Organization; 1994.

3. Hoyert DL, Kochanek KD, Murphy SL. Deaths: final data for 1997. *Natl Vital Stat Rep.* 1999;47:1-104.

4. National Safety Council. *1999 Injury Facts.* Itasca, Ill: National Safety Council; 1999.

5. Fingerhut LA, Cox CS, Warner M. International comparative analysis of injury mortality. Findings from the ICE on injury statistics. International Collaborative Effort on Injury Statistics. *Adv Data.* 1998:1-20.

6. Guyer B, Ellers B. Childhood injuries in the United States: mortality, morbidity, and cost. *Am J Dis Child.* 1990;144:649-652.

7. From the Centers for Disease Control. Fatal injuries to children—United States, 1986. *JAMA.* 1990;264:952-953.

8. Kraus JF, Fife D, Cox P, Ramstein K, Conroy C. Incidence, severity, and external causes of pediatric brain injury. *Am J Dis Child.* 1986; 140:687-693.

9. Kraus JF, Fife D, Conroy C. Pediatric brain injuries: the nature, clinical course, and early outcomes in a defined United States' population. *Pediatrics.* 1987;79:501-507.

10. Luerssen TG, Klauber MR, Marshall LF. Outcome from head injury related to patient's age: a longitudinal prospective study of adult and pediatric head injury. *J Neurosurg.* 1988; 68:409-416.

11. Tepas JJ III, DiScala C, Ramenofsky ML, Barlow B. Mortality and head injury: the pediatric perspective. *J Pediatr Surg.* 1990; 25:92-95.

12. Rosemurgy AS, Norris PA, Olson SM, Hurst JM, Albrink MH. Prehospital traumatic cardiac arrest: the cost of futility. *J Trauma.* 1993;35: 468-473.

13. Bouillon B, Walther T, Kramer M, Neugebauer E. Trauma and circulatory arrest: 224 preclinical resuscitations in Cologne in 1987-1990 [in German]. *Anaesthesist*. 1994;43:786-790.

14. Hazinski MF, Chahine AA, Holcomb GWI, Morris JAJ. Outcome of cardiovascular collapse in pediatric blunt trauma. *Ann Emerg Med*. 1994;23:1229-1235.

15. Li G, Tang N, DiScala C, Meisel Z, Levick N, Kelen GD. Cardiopulmonary resuscitation in pediatric trauma patients: survival and functional outcome. *J Trauma*. 1999;47:1-7.

16. McKoy C, Bell MJ. Preventable traumatic deaths in children. *J Pediatr Surg*. 1983;18:505-508.

17. Herzenberg JE, Hensinger RN, Dedrick DK, Phillips WA. Emergency transport and positioning of young children who have an injury of the cervical spine: the standard backboard may be hazardous. *J Bone Joint Surg Am*. 1989;71:15-22.

18. Esposito TJ, Sanddal ND, Dean JM, Hansen JD, Reynolds SA, Battan K. Analysis of preventable pediatric trauma deaths and inappropriate trauma care in Montana. *J Trauma*. 1999;47:243-251.

19. Suominen P, Rasanen J, Kivioja A. Efficacy of cardiopulmonary resuscitation in pulseless paediatric trauma patients. *Resuscitation*. 1998;36:9-13.

20. Ramenofsky ML, Luterman A, Quindlen E, Riddick L, Curreri PW. Maximum survival in pediatric trauma: the ideal system. *J Trauma*. 1984;24:818-823.

21. Luterman A, Ramenofsky M, Berryman C, Talley MA, Curreri PW. Evaluation of prehospital emergency medical service (EMS): defining areas for improvement. *J Trauma*. 1983;23:702-707.

22. Dykes EH, Spence LJ, Young JG, Bohn DJ, Filler RM, Wesson DE. Preventable pediatric trauma deaths in a metropolitan region. *J Pediatr Surg*. 1989;24:107-110.

23. Pollack MM, Alexander SR, Clarke N, Ruttimann UE, Tesselaar HM, Bachulis AC. Improved outcomes from tertiary center pediatric intensive care: a statewide comparison of tertiary and nontertiary care facilities. *Crit Care Med*. 1991;19:150-159.

24. Nakayama DK, Copes WS, Sacco W. Differences in trauma care among pediatric and nonpediatric trauma centers. *J Pediatr Surg*. 1992;27:427-431.

25. Cooper A, Barlow B, DiScala C, String D, Ray K, Mottley L. Efficacy of pediatric trauma care: results of a population-based study. *J Pediatr Surg*. 1993;28:299-303.

26. *Advanced Trauma Life Support Course Student Manual*. 6th ed. Chicago, Ill: American College of Surgeons; 1997.

27. Strange GR, ed. *The Pediatric Emergency Medicine Course*. Elk Grove Village, Ill: American Academy of Pediatrics and American College of Emergency Physicians; 1998.

28. Dieckmann RA, Brownstein D, Gausche-Hill M, eds. *Pediatric Education for Prehospital Professionals*. American Academy of Pediatrics. Sudbury, Mass: Jones & Bartlett; 2000.

29. Tepas JJ III, Mollitt DL, Talbert JL, Bryant M. The pediatric trauma score as a predictor of injury severity in the injured child. *J Pediatr Surg*. 1987;22:14-18.

30. Champion HR, Sacco WJ, Copes WS, Gann DS, Gennarelli TA, Flanagan ME. A revision of the Trauma Score. *J Trauma*. 1989;29:623-629.

31. Cooper A, Foltin G, Tunik M. Airway control in the unconscious child victim: description of a new maneuver. *Pediatr Emerg Care*. In press.

32. Pigula FA, Wald SL, Shackford SR, Vane DW. The effect of hypotension and hypoxia on children with severe head injuries. *J Pediatr Surg*. 1993;28:310-314.

33. Copass MK, Oreskovich MR, Bladergroen MR, Carrico CJ. Prehospital cardiopulmonary resuscitation of the critically injured patient. *Am J Surg*. 1984;148:20-26.

34. Durham LAI, Richardson RJ, Wall MJJ, Pepe PE, Mattox KL. Emergency center thoracotomy: impact of prehospital resuscitation. *J Trauma*. 1992;32:775-779.

35. Kloeck WGJ, Kramer EB. Prehospital advanced CPR in the trauma patient. *Trauma Emerg Med*. 1993;10:772-776.

36. Schmidt U, Frame SB, Nerlich ML, Rowe DW, Enderson BL, Maull KI, Tscherne H. On-scene helicopter transport of patients with multiple injuries—comparison of a German and an American system. *J Trauma*. 1992;33:548-553.

37. Curran C, Dietrich AM, Bowman MJ, Ginn-Pease ME, King DR, Kosnik E. Pediatric cervical-spine immobilization: achieving neutral position? *J Trauma*. 1995;39:729-732.

38. Nypaver M, Treloar D. Neutral cervical spine positioning in children. *Ann Emerg Med*. 1994;23:208-211.

39. Teasdale G, Jennett B. Assessment of coma and impaired consciousness: a practical scale. *Lancet*. 1974;2:81-84.

40. Simpson D, Reilly P. Pediatric coma scale [letter]. *Lancet*. 1982;2:450.

41. Yager JY, Johnston B, Seshia SS. Coma scales in pediatric practice. *Am J Dis Child*. 1990;144:1088-1091.

42. Simpson DA, Cockington RA, Hanieh A, Raftos J, Reilly PL. Head injuries in infants and young children: the value of the Paediatric Coma Scale: review of literature and report on a study. *Childs Nerv Syst*. 1991;7:183-190.

43. Boidin MP. Airway patency in the unconscious patient. *Br J Anaesth*. 1985;57:306-310.

44. Safar P, Escarraga LA, Chang F. Upper airway obstruction in the unconscious patient. *J Appl Physiol*. 1959;14:760-764.

45. Muizelaar JP, Marmarou A, Ward JD, Kontos HA, Choi SC, Becker DP, Gruemer H, Young HF. Adverse effects of prolonged hyperventilation in patients with severe head injury: a randomized clinical trial. *J Neurosurg*. 1991;75:731-739.

46. Robertson CS, Valadka AB, Hannay HJ, Contant CF, Gopinath SP, Cormio M, Uzura M, Grossman RG. Prevention of secondary ischemic insults after severe head injury. *Crit Care Med*. 1999;27:2086-2095.

47. Schneider GH, Sarrafzadeh AS, Kiening KL, Bardt TF, Unterberg AW, Lanksch WR. Influence of hyperventilation on brain tissue-PO_2, PCO_2, and pH in patients with intracranial hypertension. *Acta Neurochir Suppl*. 1998;71:62-65.

48. Skippen P, Seear M, Poskitt K, Kestle J, Cochrane D, Annich G, Handel J. Effect of hyperventilation on regional cerebral blood flow in head-injured children. *Crit Care Med*. 1997;25:1402-1409.

49. Fletcher SA, Henderson LT, Miner ME, Jones JM. The successful surgical removal of intracranial nasogastric tubes. *J Trauma*. 1987;27:948-952.

50. Baskaya MK. Inadvertent intracranial placement of a nasogastric tube in patients with head injuries. *Surg Neurol*. 1999;52:426-427.

51. Schwaitzberg SD, Bergman KS, Harris BH. A pediatric trauma model of continuous hemorrhage. *J Pediatr Surg*. 1988;23:605-609.

52. Harte FA, Chalmers PC, Walsh RF, Danker PR, Sheikh FM. Intraosseous fluid administration: a parenteral alternative in pediatric resuscitation. *Anesth Analg*. 1987;66:687-689.

53. Goldstein B, Doody D, Briggs S. Emergency intraosseous infusion in severely burned children. *Pediatr Emerg Care*. 1990;6:195-197.

54. Hodge DD, Delgado-Paredes C, Fleisher G. Intraosseous infusion flow rates in hypovolemic "pediatric" dogs. *Ann Emerg Med*. 1987;16:305-307.

55. Morris RE, Schonfeld N, Haftel AJ. Treatment of hemorrhagic shock with intraosseous administration of crystalloid fluid in the rabbit model. *Ann Emerg Med*. 1987;16:1321-1324.

56. Velasco AL, Delgado-Paredes C, Templeton J, Steigman CK, Templeton JMJ. Intraosseous infusion of fluids in the initial management of hypovolemic shock in young subjects. *J Pediatr Surg.* 1991;26:4-8.

57. Schoffstall JM, Spivey WH, Davidheiser S, Lathers CM. Intraosseous crystalloid and blood infusion in a swine model. *J Trauma.* 1989;29:384-387.

58. Kramer GC, Walsh JC, Hands RD, Perron PR, Gunther RA, Mertens S, Holcroft JW, Blaisdell FW. Resuscitation of hemorrhage with intraosseous infusion of hypertonic saline/dextran. *Braz J Med Biol Res.* 1989; 22:283-286.

59. Halvorsen L, Bay BK, Perron PR, Gunther RA, Holcroft JW, Blaisdell FW, Kramer GC. Evaluation of an intraosseous infusion device for the resuscitation of hypovolemic shock. *J Trauma.* 1990;30:652-658.

60. Guy J, Haley K, Zuspan SJ. Use of intraosseous infusion in the pediatric trauma patient. *J Pediatr Surg.* 1993;28:158-161.

61. Rutledge R, Sheldon GF, Collins ML. Massive transfusion. *Crit Care Clin.* 1986;2:791-805.

62. Niven MJ, Zohar M, Shimoni Z, Glick J. Symptomatic hypocalcemia precipitated by small-volume blood transfusion. *Ann Emerg Med.* 1998;32:498-501.

63. Barlow B, Niemirska M, Gandhi R, Shelton M. Response to injury in children with closed femur fractures. *J Trauma.* 1987;27:429-430.

64. Hannan EL, Farrell LS, Meaker PS, Cooper A. Predicting inpatient mortality for pediatric trauma patients with blunt injuries: a better alternative. *J Pediatr Surg.* 2000;35:155-159.

65. Garcia VF, Gotschall CS, Eichelberger MR, Bowman LM. Rib fractures in children: a marker of severe trauma. *J Trauma.* 1990;30: 695-700.

66. National Pediatric Trauma Registry, April 2000. Boston, Mass: New England Medical Center; 2000.

67. Hadley MN, Zabramski JM, Browner CM, Rekate H, Sonntag VK. Pediatric spinal trauma: review of 122 cases of spinal cord and vertebral column injuries. *J Neurosurg.* 1988; 68:18-24.

68. Osenbach RK, Menezes AH. Pediatric spinal cord and vertebral column injury. *Neurosurgery.* 1992;30:385-390.

69. Orenstein JB, Klein BL, Gotschall CS, Ochsenschlager DW, Klatzko MD, Eichelberger MR. Age and outcome in pediatric cervical spine injury: 11-year experience. *Pediatr Emerg Care.* 1994;10:132-137.

70. Givens TG, Polley KA, Smith GF, Hardin WD Jr. Pediatric cervical spine injury: a three-year experience. *J Trauma.* 1996;41: 310-314.

71. Dietrich AM, Ginn-Pease ME, Bartkowski HM, King DR. Pediatric cervical spine fractures: predominantly subtle presentation. *J Pediatr Surg.* 1991;26:995-999.

72. Medina FA. Neck and spinal cord trauma. In: Barkin RM, ed. *Pediatric Emergency Medicine: Concepts and Clinical Practice.* St Louis, Mo: Mosby Year Book; 1992.

73. Fesmire FM, Luten RC. The pediatric cervical spine: developmental anatomy and clinical aspects. *J Emerg Med.* 1989;7:133-142.

74. Manary MJ, Jaffe DM. Cervical spine injuries in children. *Pediatr Ann.* 1996;25:423-428.

75. Dickman CA, Rekate HL, Sonntag VK, Zabramski JM. Pediatric spinal trauma: vertebral column and spinal cord injuries in children. *Pediatr Neurosci.* 1989;15:237-255.

76. Ruge JR, Sinson GP, McLone DG, Cerullo LJ. Pediatric spinal injury: the very young. *J Neurosurg.* 1988;68:25-30.

77. Pang D, Pollack IF. Spinal cord injury without radiographic abnormality in children—the SCIWORA syndrome. *J Trauma.* 1989; 29:654-664.

78. Hill SA, Miller CA, Kosnik EJ, Hunt WE. Pediatric neck injuries: a clinical study. *J Neurosurg.* 1984;60:700-706.

79. Huerta C, Griffith R, Joyce SM. Cervical spine stabilization in pediatric patients: evaluation of current techniques. *Ann Emerg Med.* 1987;16:1121-1126.

80. Muhr MD, Seabrook DL, Wittwer LK. Paramedic use of a spinal injury clearance algorithm reduces spinal immobilization in the out-of-hospital setting. *Prehosp Emerg Care.* 1999;3:1-6.

81. Domeier RM, Evans RW, Swor RA, Rivera-Rivera EJ, Frederiksen SM. Prospective validation of out-of-hospital spinal clearance criteria: a preliminary report. *Acad Emerg Med.* 1997;4:643-646.

82. Sahni R, Menegazzi JJ, Mosesso VN. Paramedic evaluation of clinical indicators of cervical spinal injury. *Prehosp Emerg Care.* 1997;1:16-18.

83. Brown LH, Gough JE, Simonds WB. Can EMS providers adequately assess trauma patients for cervical spinal injury? *Prehosp Emerg Care.* 1998;2:33-36.

84. *Pediatric Basic Trauma Life Support.* Oakbrook, Ill: BTLS International; 1995.

85. Caroline NL. *Emergency Care in the Streets.* 5th ed. Boston, Mass: Little, Brown; 1995.

86. Sanders MJ, Quick G, Lewis LM, McKenna K, eds. *Mosby's Paramedic Textbook.* Baltimore, Md: Mosby; 1995.

87. *Emergency Care and Transportation of the Sick and Injured.* Rosemont, Ill: American Academy of Orthopedic Surgeons; 1993.

88. De Lorenzo RA. A review of spinal immobilization techniques. *J Emerg Med.* 1996;14: 603-613.

89. Treloar DJ, Nypaver M. Angulation of the pediatric cervical spine with and without cervical collar. *Pediatr Emerg Care.* 1997;13:5-8.

90. Hamilton RS, Pons PT. The efficacy and comfort of full-body vacuum splints for cervical-spine immobilization. *J Emerg Med.* 1996;14: 553-559.

91. Chan D, Goldberg RM, Mason J, Chan L. Backboard versus mattress splint immobilization: a comparison of symptoms generated. *J Emerg Med.* 1996;14:293-298.

92. Johnson DR, Hauswald M, Stockhoff C. Comparison of a vacuum splint device to a rigid backboard for spinal immobilization. *Am J Emerg Med.* 1996;14:369-372.

93. Chan D, Goldberg R, Tascone A, Harmon S, Chan L. The effect of spinal immobilization on healthy volunteers. *Ann Emerg Med.* 1994; 23:48-51.

94. Davies G, Deakin C, Wilson A. The effect of a rigid collar on intracranial pressure. *Injury.* 1996;27:647-649.

95. Raphael JH, Chotai R. Effects of the cervical collar on cerebrospinal fluid pressure. *Anaesthesia.* 1994;49:437-439.

96. Wang CT, Daro D. *Current Trends in Child Maltreatment Reporting and Fatalities: The Results of the 1997 Annual Fifty-State Survey.* Chicago, Ill: National Committee to Prevent Child Maltreatment; 1998.

97. *A Guide to References and Resources in Child Abuse and Neglect.* Elk Grove Village, Ill: American Academy of Pediatrics; 1998.

98. Cooper A, Barlow B, Davidson L, Relethford J, O'Meara J, Mottley L. Epidemiology of pediatric trauma: importance of population-based statistics. *J Pediatr Surg.* 1992;27:149-153.

For Additional Reading

Bickell WH, Wall MJJ, Pepe PE, Martin RR, Ginger VF, Allen MK, Mattox KL. Immediate versus delayed fluid resuscitation for hypotensive patients with penetrating torso injuries. *N Engl J Med.* 1994;331:1105-1109.

Childhood injuries in the United States. Division of Injury Control, Center for Environmental Health and Injury Control, Centers for Disease Control. *Am J Dis Child.* 1990;144:627-646.

Sachdeva RC. Near drowning. *Crit Care Clin.* 1999;15:281-296.

The National Committee for Injury Prevention and Control. Residential injuries. Injury prevention: meeting the challenge. *Am J Prev Med.* 1989; 5(suppl):153-162.

Stiell IG, Hebert PC, Wells GA, Laupacis A, Vandemheen K, Dreyer JF, Eisenhauer MA, Gibson J, Higginson LA, Kirby AS, et al. The Ontario trial of active compression-decompression cardiopulmonary resuscitation for in-hospital and prehospital cardiac arrest. *JAMA*. 1996;275:1417-1423.

Marshall SW, Runyan CW, Bangdiwala SI, Linzer MA, Sacks JJ, Butts JD. Fatal residential fires: who dies and who survives? *JAMA*. 1998;279: 1633-1637.

An Evaluation of Residential Smoke Detector Performance Under Actual Field Conditions. Washington, DC: Federal Emergency Management Agency; 1980.

Pepe PE. Emergency medical services systems and prehospital management of patients requiring critical care. In: Carlson R, Geheb M, eds. *Principles and Practice of Medical Intensive Care.* Philadelphia, Pa: WB Saunders Co; 1992:9-24.

Markenson D, Foltin G, Tunik M, Cooper A, Giordano L, Fitton A, Lanotte T. The Kendrick extrication device used for pediatric spinal immobilization. *Prehosp Emerg Care*. 1999;3:66-69.

Guidelines for cardiopulmonary resuscitation and emergency cardiac care. Emergency Cardiac Care Committee and Subcommittees, American Heart Association. Part VI. Pediatric advanced life support. *JAMA*. 1992;268:2262-2275.

Stylianos S, Jacir NN, Hoffman MA. Optimal intravenous site for volume replacement [abstract]. *J Trauma*. 1992;33:247.

Cooper A, Barlow B, DiScala C, String D. Mortality and truncal injury: the pediatric perspective. *J Pediatr Surg*. 1994;29:33-38.

Garcia V, Eichelberger M, Ziegler M, Templeton JM, Koop CE. Use of military antishock trouser in a child. *J Pediatr Surg*. 1981;16(suppl 1):544-546.

Gaffney FA, Thal ER, Taylor WF, Bastian BC, Weigelt JA, Atkins JM, Blomqvist CG. Hemodynamic effects of Medical Anti-Shock Trousers (MAST garment). *J Trauma*. 1981;21:931-937.

Mackersie RC, Christensen JM, Lewis FR. The prehospital use of external counterpressure: does MAST make a difference? *J Trauma*. 1984;24: 882-888.

Mattox KL, Bickell W, Pepe PE, Burch J, Feliciano D. Prospective MAST study in 911 patients. *J Trauma*. 1989;29:1104-1111.

Kewalramani LS, Kraus JF, Sterling HM. Acute spinal-cord lesions in a pediatric population: epidemiological and clinical features. *Paraplegia*. 1980;18:206-219.

Pang D, Wilberger JEJ. Spinal cord injury without radiographic abnormalities in children. *J Neurosurg*. 1982;57:114-129.

Sneed RC, Stover SL. Undiagnosed spinal cord injuries in brain-injured children. *Am J Dis Child*. 1988;142:965-967.

Bohn D, Armstrong D, Becker L, Humphreys R. Cervical spine injuries in children. *J Trauma*. 1990;30:463-469.

DiScala C, Sege R, Li G, Reece RM. Child abuse and unintentional injuries: a 10-year retrospective. *Arch Pediatr Adolesc Med*. 2000;154.16-22.

Children With Special Healthcare Needs

Introductory Case Scenario

A 16-month-old girl with chronic lung disease, moderate developmental delay, a tracheostomy tube, a cerebral spinal fluid (CSF) shunt, and a gastrostomy tube presents with a 1-day history of fever and mild difficulty breathing. The child typically requires mechanical ventilation on room air while asleep at night and a tracheostomy mist collar with 1 L/min O$_2$ flow while awake during the day.

Yesterday the child developed a cough, and 4 L/min O$_2$ flow was required to maintain an oxyhemoglobin saturation above 90%. The child's illness began with increased secretions in the tracheostomy tube, which necessitated more frequent suctioning.

On examination the child appears alert, but she has labored respirations and mild to moderate intercostal and subcostal retractions. She has bilateral breath sounds, diffuse rales, and an audible wheeze. Her temperature is 39°C (102.2°F), heart rate is 160 bpm, respiratory rate is 40 breaths per minute, blood pressure is 90/60 mm Hg, and capillary refill is <2 seconds.

The pulse oximeter indicates an oxyhemoglobin saturation of 90% with 4 L/min O$_2$ bled into her home ventilator circuit. Large amounts of thick secretions are coming from the child's tracheostomy tube.

- How would you approach initial assessment and stabilization of this child?

- What is your rapid cardiopulmonary assessment?

- What are the most important treatment priorities for this child?

- What assessment steps and treatment priorities are different from those for emergencies in children without special healthcare needs? What assessment steps and treatment priorities are the same as those for children without special healthcare needs?

Learning Objectives

This chapter reviews the assessment, treatment, and priorities of management for children with special healthcare needs. These children typically have a chronic illness and require technologic support or intervention such as a tracheostomy tube, mechanical ventilation, CSF shunt, gastrostomy tube, or long-term central venous catheter.

After completing this chapter the PALS provider should be able to

- Describe the initial approach to assessment and stabilization of a child with special healthcare needs

- Describe how initial assessment steps and treatment priorities are similar to standard PALS evaluation and how they differ for children with special healthcare needs

- Describe the potential complications of equipment that is frequently used in the care of children with a chronic illness

- Recognize common problems (eg, tube displacement, tube obstruction, pneumothorax, equipment or technology failure, and infection) encountered in the care of children with special healthcare needs

- Prioritize assessment and management of life-threatening emergencies in children with special healthcare needs

Introduction

Recent advances in medical science and technology have made it possible for children with complex medical problems and special healthcare needs to live longer lives. Applied technology and knowledge allows children with special healthcare needs (eg, dependence on mechanical ventilation or other technologic support because of severe prematurity, birth defects, or traumatic brain or spinal cord injuries) to receive complicated care at home.

Children with special healthcare needs are those who have or are at risk for chronic physical, developmental, behavioral, or emotional conditions that necessitate use of health and related services of a type or amount not usually required by typically developing children (see Critical Concepts: "Definition of Children With Special Healthcare Needs").[1-3] Approximately 30 000 children in the United States are permanently disabled as a result of serious injuries.[4] An estimated 12 million children in the United States have special healthcare needs,[2] and this number is increasing. These children are frequently encountered by healthcare providers.

Critical Concepts:
Definition of Children With Special Healthcare Needs

Children with special healthcare needs have or are at risk for chronic physical, developmental, behavioral, or emotional conditions that necessitate use of health and related services of a type or amount not usually required by typically developing children.[1-3]

The best source of information about the child with special healthcare needs is the person who cares for the child on a daily basis. Most caregivers and families of children with special healthcare needs complete specialized training and develop expertise in the assessment and management of their child. They are familiar with the management of their child's equipment and problems. In coordination with their child's healthcare team, families are encouraged to develop emergency healthcare plans that list the drugs and devices used in the child's care and recommendations for predetermined interventions to deal with emergencies.[5,6]

The American Academy of Pediatrics (AAP) and the American College of Emergency Physicians (ACEP) created the Emergency Preparedness for Children With Special Health Care Needs Program.[3] This program encourages completion of a standardized Emergency Information Form (EIF) for the child that will be readily accessible in an emergency.[7] This form summarizes the child's medical history and advises how to manage the child's emergency. The form, available at **www.pediatrics.org/cgi/content/full/104/4/e53**, can be kept on the Medic Alert computer database (the child must be registered in the database) so that it can be accessed by medical personnel worldwide.[7]

Emergencies in children with special healthcare needs can be caused by equipment malfunction, drug-related complications, and medical problems. Children

who rely on medical technology or equipment for survival have been called "technology-assisted children" or "technology-dependent children." Their equipment may include a tracheostomy tube, mechanical ventilator (standard or noninvasive bilevel positive airway pressure), long-term central venous catheter, feeding tube, CSF shunt, oxygen, aerosol nebulizer, apnea monitor, pulse oximeter, colostomy tube, pacemaker, splints, crutches, or wheelchair. This equipment may differ in several ways from similar equipment designed for hospital use. Healthcare providers should be able to use the child's equipment and troubleshoot problems related to it.[8-10]

This chapter uses the mnemonic "DOPE" to remind healthcare providers of common causes of deterioration in patients with a tracheal or feeding tube, central venous catheter, CSF shunt, and mechanical ventilator. The DOPE mnemonic reminds providers to look for tube **D**isplacement; tube **O**bstruction; **P**neumothorax, **P**ulmonary thromboembolus, or other complication; and **E**quipment failure (see Critical Concepts: "The DOPE Mnemonic"). Infection should also be ruled out as a cause of deterioration.

Children with a chronic illness often differ from well children of the same age in baseline height and weight, vital signs, and psychosocial development. These factors are important in the assessment of the child and in the identification and management of emergencies. Many children with special healthcare needs are small for age. As a result they may require equipment sizes (eg, tracheal tube) or treatment variables (eg, ventilator tidal volume) that differ from those estimated by age. In addition, baseline vital signs in children with a chronic illness and those who require technologic support may be outside the range of normal for the child's age. Some children with special healthcare needs may have sensory or motor deficits (eg, hearing, vision, or sensation) with normal cognitive function, and others may have cognitive impairment. As a result the child may be unable to communicate.[11]

Critical Concepts:
The DOPE Mnemonic

The DOPE mnemonic may be used to identify common causes of deterioration in the child with an artificial airway (particularly during positive-pressure ventilation) and the child with a central venous catheter. Common causes of emergencies involving a tracheal tube are

Displacement of the tube

Obstruction of the tube

Pneumothorax

Equipment failure

This mnemonic may be modified to identify causes of deterioration in the child with a central venous catheter (Pericardial tamponade is added to the "P" of Pneumothorax), feeding catheter ("P" is changed to Peritonitis or Perforation), or CSF shunt ("P" is changed to Pneumoperitoneum and Peritonitis).

The approach to the child with special healthcare needs should begin with an initial rapid cardiopulmonary assessment (see Critical Concepts: "Initial Approach to the Child With Special Healthcare Needs"). During this assessment the provider should consider the child's baseline vital signs, responsiveness, and developmental level. The provider should also assess the functional status of the equipment used in the child's care (recall the DOPE mnemonic).

This chapter describes the PALS assessment and management priorities for the child with special healthcare needs. It also summarizes signs of equipment malfunction and complications related to technologies commonly used in the care of these children: tracheostomy tubes, chronic central venous catheters, feeding tubes, and CSF shunts.

FIGURE 1. Emergency information form (EIF). Reproduced from American Academy of Pediatrics and American College of Emergency Medicine.[3,7]

Emergency Information Form for Children With Special Needs

Last name:

American College of Emergency Physicians®

American Academy of Pediatrics

Date form completed By Whom	Revised Revised	Initials Initials

Name: Birth date: Nickname:

Home Address:	Home/Work Phone:
Parent/Guardian:	Emergency Contact Names & Relationship:
Signature/Consent*:	
Primary Language:	Phone Number(s):

Physicians:

Primary care physician:	Emergency Phone:
	Fax:
Current Specialty physician: Specialty:	Emergency Phone:
	Fax:
Current Specialty physician: Specialty:	Emergency Phone:
	Fax:
Anticipated Primary ED:	Pharmacy:
Anticipated Tertiary Care Center:	

Diagnoses/Past Procedures/Physical Exam:

1.

Baseline physical findings:

2.

3.

Baseline vital signs:

4.

Synopsis:

Baseline neurological status:

*Consent for release of this form to health care providers.

Diagnoses/Past Procedures/Physical Exam continued:

Medications:

Significant baseline ancillary findings (lab, x-ray, ECG):

1.

2.

3.

4.   Prostheses/Appliances/Advanced Technology Devices:

5.

6.

Management Data:

Allergies: Medications/Foods to be avoided   **and why:**

1.

2.

3.

Procedures to be avoided   **and why:**

1.

2.

3.

Immunizations

Dates						Dates					
DPT						Hep B					
OPV						Varicella					
MMR						TB status					
HIB						Other					

Antibiotic prophylaxis: Indication: Medication and dose:

Common Presenting Problems/Findings With Specific Suggested Managements

Problem   Suggested Diagnostic Studies   Treatment Considerations

Comments on child, family, or other specific medical issues:

Physician/Provider Signature: **Print Name:**

Used with permission from the American Academy of Pediatrics (AAP) and the American College of Emergency Physicians (ACEP). This publication was produced by the AAP and ACEP with funding from the Emergency Medical Services for Children Program, Maternal and Child Health Bureau, Health Resources and Services Administration, US Department of Health and Human Services in collaboration with the National Highway Traffic Safety Administration, US Department of Transportation, Reference No. 99-0649(P).

Tracheostomy Tubes

A tracheostomy is a surgical procedure in which an opening is made through the neck into the trachea. A tube is passed through this opening and into the trachea to provide long-term access to the lower trachea and lungs. Indications for tracheostomy in a child include (1) the need for prolonged ventilatory support, (2) the need to bypass an upper airway obstruction, and (3) the need for removal of secretions when the cough and gag reflexes are ineffective.

Some children who need a tracheostomy tube were born prematurely and subsequently developed bronchopulmonary dysplasia, necessitating prolonged mechanical ventilation. Some children have a congenital or acquired condition requiring establishment of an artificial airway, such as tracheal stenosis, neuromuscular weakness, traumatic brain or spinal cord injury, or lack of airway protective reflexes associated with chronic aspiration.

Tracheostomy tubes come in different sizes (ie, internal diameter, outer diameter, and length), shapes, and brands. Length, cuffs, and cannulas can be standard or custom designed.

Types of Tracheostomy Tubes

Tracheostomy tubes may be plastic or metal, cuffed or uncuffed. Metal tubes have thin walls and do not have a built-in 15-mm tracheal tube connector. All metal tubes have an inner cannula that can be removed for cleaning or if the tube becomes obstructed. Plastic tubes used in pediatric patients usually do not have an inner cannula (see below). Plastic tracheostomy tubes are usually equipped with a 15-mm connector for easy connection to standard oxygen delivery systems, manual resuscitator bags, and ventilation tubing.

There are several different types of tracheostomy tubes. Single-cannula, double-cannula, cuffed, and fenestrated tracheostomy tubes are available (Figure 2). All newborn and most pediatric tubes are single-cannula tubes. A single-cannula tube has no inner cannula, so when this tube is removed, all that is left is the stoma (ie, the skin opening into the trachea).

FIGURE 2. Tracheostomy tubes. **A,** Single-cannula tube without obturator in place. **B,** Single-cannula tube with obturator in place for insertion. **C,** Fenestrated tube. **D,** Cuffed tube on the right (cuff is inflated).

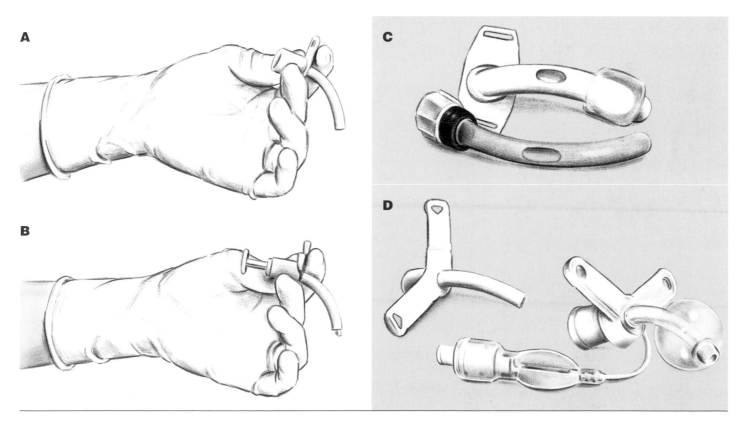

Single-cannula tubes are placed using a solid plastic insert called an obturator, which helps keep the flexible tube from kinking. The obturator must be removed immediately after insertion to avoid obstruction of the airway. If a single-cannula tube becomes occluded and cannot be cleared with suctioning, it must be removed, cleaned, and reinserted or replaced with a clean tube.

Double-cannula tubes have a removable inner cannula that fits inside an outer cannula or sheath. The inner cannula must be in place for manual or mechanical ventilation. The outer cannula remains in the trachea to keep the stoma patent while the inner cannula is removed for cleaning.

Adult tracheostomy tubes and some pediatric tubes have an inflatable cuff. The cuff acts as a seal to eliminate air leaks. Fenestrated tubes are usually used in older children and adults. The fenestrations (openings) in the tube allow air to be directed into the upper airway, which makes speech possible.

Tracheostomy Tube Sizes

The size of the tracheostomy tube is marked on the package and usually on the wings (flanges) of each tube. The size marked on the wings (eg, 00-neonatal or 3.5-pediatric) usually refers to the internal diameter of the tube (see FYI: "Tracheostomy Tube Size"). Tracheostomy tubes are usually labeled as "neonatal," "pediatric," or "adult." One major difference

FYI: Tracheostomy Tube Size

The size marked on the tracheostomy tube refers to the internal diameter of the tube. When changing size or brand, take into account differences in the outer diameter and length of the tubes. You may need to refer to the manufacturer's specifications to select an appropriate tube.

between neonatal, pediatric, and adult tubes of equivalent diameter is the length of the tube.

Tracheostomy Filters, Collars, and Ties

If the child is able to breathe spontaneously through the tracheostomy tube (ie, has periods of spontaneous ventilation when separated from the mechanical ventilator circuit), special attachments to the tracheostomy tube are used during spontaneous ventilation to protect the artificial airway and to humidify inspired air. A tracheostomy "nose" is a filtration device that keeps particulate matter out of the airway and provides humidification. A tracheostomy "collar" is a small mask that fits loosely around the end of the tube to provide humidification with or without oxygen. In older children, adolescents, and adults, valves (eg, Passy-Muir one-way valves) are attached to the outer part of the tube to allow the person to speak. Speech requires use of a fenestrated tube or a small tube with an air leak around it.

Tracheostomy tubes are held in position by ties (usually made of twill tape or Velcro straps). The ties extend from both sides of the tube and are fastened around the neck. The ties must be removed, cut, or detached before the tube can be removed from the trachea. After you cut the ties, grasp the tube and gently withdraw it. Fasten new ties so that only your little finger can pass between the ties and the child's neck. Fastening the ties this way ensures that the ties will hold the tube in place and reduces the risk of tube displacement. The ties should not be so tight that jugular venous return is obstructed.

A pair of scissors and a clean tracheostomy tube prepared with ties should be kept at the bedside of all patients with a tracheostomy tube. A tracheostomy tube one size smaller than normally used should also be available. To facilitate access to the tracheostomy tube, place a rolled sheet or towel under the patient's shoulders so that the head and neck are extended (see next section).

Tracheostomy Emergencies

Children with a tracheostomy tube can become ill for a variety of reasons. They may have underlying pulmonary disease that puts them at risk for respiratory compromise or common infections. These patients will develop typical signs and symptoms of respiratory distress, such as coughing, wheezing, rales, retractions, stridor, nasal flaring, increased respiratory rate, decreased oxygen saturation, cyanosis, increased secretions, and altered level of consciousness. When trying to determine the cause of respiratory distress in these children, consider mechanical obstruction of the tube by increased secretions or a mucous plug. Rule out equipment failure.

When a child with a tracheostomy tube is in respiratory distress, the child's history will help you identify the cause of the problem. If the child has a history of fever and progressive worsening of respiratory status, consider lower airway infection. If the child has a sudden onset of respiratory distress, possibly with increased or thicker secretions in the tracheostomy tube, consider a mucous plug.

A child with a displaced or obstructed tracheostomy tube may have excessive secretions, limited chest wall movement with manual ventilation, increased resistance to ventilation, faint or absent breath sounds bilaterally on auscultation, cyanosis, and accessory muscle use. Exhaled CO_2 monitoring may assist with the assessment for tube displacement; if the tube is displaced out of the trachea, exhaled CO_2 will not be detected.

If you suspect tube obstruction, immediately remove the ventilator and provide manual ventilation. If the bag is difficult to compress, high airflow resistance is likely present. Suction the tracheostomy tube to remove any mucous plugs.

Use the following sequence to evaluate for tube obstruction:

■ Place a rolled towel under the child's shoulders. This position will facilitate access to the tracheostomy tube for evaluation and changing of the tube (Figure 3).

- Consider injecting 1 to 3 mL of normal saline into the tracheostomy tube to dilute secretions.

- Select a suction catheter that will fit through the child's tracheostomy tube. The caregivers may have one with them or may know the correct size. In general use a 6F to 10F catheter. (A length-based resuscitation tape may also be used to estimate the correct size).

- If using wall or portable suction, set the suction to –100 mm Hg or less.

- Preoxygenate, if possible, by administering oxygen at the tracheostoma or by providing manual ventilation before suctioning.

- Insert the suction catheter into the tracheostomy tube and advance the catheter to the tip of the tube. For routine suctioning, determine the distance to the end of the tube and insert the catheter that distance to avoid injuring the tracheal mucosa beyond the tube. If you think an obstruction is located at the end of the tube, pass a catheter beyond the tip of the tube to clear any obstructing secretions. Do not use excessive force to insert the suction catheter.

- Apply suction for a maximum of 10 seconds while withdrawing the catheter. Twist or roll the catheter with your fingers to suction all sides of the tube.

- If there is no improvement in respiratory distress, repeat the procedure or prepare to change the tracheostomy tube.

Caregivers often carry extra tracheostomy tubes with them and know the size, type, and length of the tube. If the caregiver is unavailable, check the wings (flanges) of the tracheostomy tube. If your institution does not stock the patient's brand, then use a tube of similar size. Choose a tube with the same outer diameter as the child's tube or one size smaller. If a tracheostomy tube is unavailable, a standard tracheal tube of equivalent *outer* diameter can be placed through the stoma in an emergency.

Before you insert a clean tracheostomy tube, suction the stoma and trachea with a catheter. Suctioning is particularly important in emergencies because thick secretions may have accumulated in the trachea around the tube. These secretions may be pushed down the trachea by the new tube. If you need to hold the stoma open for suctioning, place two fingers below and on each side of the opening and apply gentle downward, lateral traction. If the patient is not breathing spontaneously, provide bag-mask ventilation through the upper airway until a new cannula is inserted. During bag-mask ventilation, you may need to place a gloved finger over the stoma to prevent air escape and hypoventilation. If total upper airway obstruction is present and the tracheostoma is the only functioning airway, mouth-to-stoma ventilation may be necessary.

Tracheostomy tubes should be changed regularly and whenever there is concern that the tracheostomy tube is obstructed despite suctioning. Recannulation may be difficult during the first week after tracheostomy. When the tracheostoma is new, it is relatively easy to insert a tracheostomy tube into the paratracheal tissues rather than the trachea. Such placement can cause bleeding or a tension pneumothorax. Most surgeons place temporary traction sutures at the lateral margins of the tracheal incision. Gentle lateral traction on these sutures will help open the stoma and facilitate recannulation. Do not use vigorous traction on the sutures. Vigorous traction may damage the trachea or break the sutures. A suction catheter placed through the new tracheostomy tube, through the stoma, and into the trachea should be used to guide the new tube into place. A catheter is much less likely to create a false tract. If one or two attempts to replace the tube fail, the patient should be intubated orally and the tracheostomy tube replaced by the surgeon or someone skilled in airway management.

One procedure for changing the tracheostomy tube is as follows:

- If the existing tube has an inflatable cuff, deflate the cuff by connecting a syringe to the valve on the pilot (cuff inflation indicator) balloon. Aspirate air or water until the balloon collapses. Do not cut the pilot balloon. Cutting the balloon will not reliably deflate the cuff.

- Cut the ties that hold the tracheostomy tube in place. Older children and adolescents may have tubes with Velcro ties that can be detached without cutting.

- If possible, place ties in the flanges of the replacement tube before insertion.

- Remove the obstructed tracheostomy tube.

- Gently insert the replacement tube into the stoma with the curve pointing downward. Never use force to insert

FIGURE 3. Positioning of the child with neck extended for evaluation and changing of the tracheostomy tube.

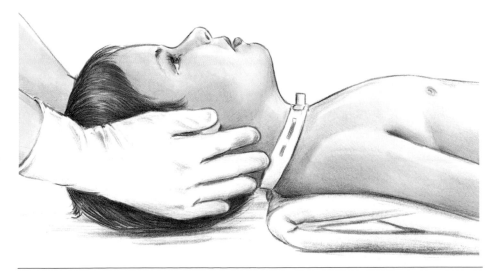

If the tracheostoma is new or small, you can use a suction or feeding catheter as a guide to insert the new tracheostomy tube through the stoma. To prepare for tube replacement, pass a well-lubricated suction catheter through the new tube. Remove the original tube and insert the end of the suction catheter through the stoma and into the trachea. Pass the tracheostomy tube over the catheter into the trachea, using the catheter as a guide. You may use gentle but firm pressure to insert the tube through a tight stoma if a catheter is present. Once the new tube is in place, remove the catheter.

Alternatively, cut the catheter at the end of the suction connector to leave a simple catheter tube. Insert the distal (uncut whistle-tip) end of the suction catheter through the original tracheostomy tube and into the trachea. Hold the catheter in place as a guide and withdraw the original tube from the trachea, pulling it over the cut end of the catheter tubing. Pass the new tracheostomy tube over the cut end of the catheter and along the catheter into the trachea. Then remove the catheter.

A flexible bronchoscope of appropriate size may also be used as a guide. First pass the bronchoscope through a tracheostomy tube and then through the stoma into the trachea. Pass the new tube over the bronchoscope and into the trachea. Remove the bronchoscope.

the tube. It may be helpful to moisten the tube with a sterile, water-soluble lubricant. An obturator should be used with metal tracheostomy tubes (see below). If the tracheostoma is new or small, you may use a catheter to guide the tube into place (see FYI: "Helpful Hint to Place a Tracheostomy Tube").

— During passage of a *plastic* tracheostomy tube into the trachea of a spontaneously breathing child, you should hear air movement through the tube (unless an obturator is used).

— During placement of a *metal* tracheostomy tube, use an obturator. Use of an obturator reduces the risk that the thin-walled, relatively sharp metal tubes will pierce tissue or enter a paratracheal location.

■ If the tube does not easily enter the trachea, withdraw it and attempt to pass a smaller one.

■ If you cannot insert a smaller tracheostomy tube, try to insert a standard tracheal tube of similar size through the stoma. If the tracheal tube has a cuff, once the tube is in place you can inflate the cuff to maintain the position of the tube and to eliminate air leaks around the tube. The advantages of using a tracheal tube in an emergency include the wide range of sizes available and the beveled tip, which facilitates entry through a tight stoma. In addition, condensation from expired air in the tube provides visual reassurance of the continuity of the lumen of the tube with that of the trachea. Typically the tracheal tube must be shortened significantly after its position within the trachea is confirmed.

■ Confirm tracheal tube position by clinical examination and a secondary confirmation technique (exhaled CO_2 detection).

■ If there is no improvement in the patient's condition or if tube placement is unsuccessful, you can usually provide assisted ventilation by covering the stoma and providing manual ventilation through the child's nose and mouth using a bag-mask technique (see FYI: "Upper Airway in Patients With a Tracheostomy Tube").

■ If the child has a double-cannula tracheostomy tube and removal of the inner cannula fails to clear the airway, remove the outer cannula and replace the tracheostomy tube using the procedure described above.

If the tracheostomy tube is inserted correctly, you should feel minimal resistance during insertion. During spontaneous or manual ventilation you should note equal breath sounds and bilateral rise and fall of the chest, and you should detect exhaled CO_2. There should be no bleeding at the site or through the tube and no signs of subcutaneous emphysema (air under the skin).

Many children with artificial airways have chronic lung disease and therefore a low respiratory reserve. Viral infections that produce minor illness in healthy children can be life-threatening in a child with chronic lung disease.

If the child's history and findings of the physical exam suggest infection, the fol-

Most patients with a standard tracheostomy tube have a patent upper airway connected to their trachea. Therefore, bag-mask ventilation and standard tracheal intubation technique (through the mouth) can be used in these patients. In patients with a *tracheal diversion*, the trachea is *separated* from the upper airway and joined directly to the skin at the site of the stoma. These patients no longer have any connection between their upper airway and trachea, so bag-mask ventilation and standard tracheal intubation technique cannot be used.

lowing interventions are indicated: increase the child's inspired oxygen concentration or mechanical ventilatory support, reassess vital signs and oxyhemoglobin saturation, send samples of tracheal secretions for Gram's stain and culture, and consider obtaining a chest radiograph. Depending on the clinical situation and findings of laboratory and radiological studies, therapy could include administration of nebulized β-agonist, racemic epinephrine, inhaled or parenteral steroids, and antibiotics. You should consider transfer of the child and admission to a unit that can manage mechanically ventilated children with a tracheostomy tube.

Home Mechanical Ventilators

Mechanical ventilation may be indicated for chronically ill children with abnormal respiratory drive, severe chronic lung disease, or severe neuromuscular weakness. Some children require continuous mechanical ventilation; others require intermittent support during sleep or acute illness.

Home ventilators may be volume limited or pressure limited (see FYI: "Volume-Limited vs Pressure-Limited Ventilators). All are equipped with alarms. The provider should be familiar with the particular ventilator used.

Ventilator Emergencies

When acute respiratory distress develops in a child who is dependent on a ventilator, it is important to identify and treat reversible causes immediately. Possible reversible causes of acute deterioration in the intubated child receiving mechanical ventilation can be recalled by the DOPE mnemonic:

- **D**isplacement or **D**isconnection of the tube or ventilator circuit
- **O**bstruction of airflow (eg, obstructed ventilator tubing or tracheostomy tube)
- **P**neumothorax or other patient-related condition

FYI: Volume-Limited vs Pressure-Limited Ventilators

Two major types of positive-pressure ventilators are used for home mechanical ventilation, pressure limited and volume limited. The ventilators are distinguished by the mechanism that terminates inspiration. Pressure-limited ventilators deliver a breath over a specified time until a preset pressure limit is reached. The delivered tidal volume may vary from breath to breath depending on the pressure limit, lung compliance, and synchrony between the patient's breaths and ventilator-provided breaths. Volume-limited ventilators deliver a preset tidal volume with each breath, and inspiration is terminated when that volume is reached. With volume-limited ventilation, the peak pressure that develops during inspiration is determined by the child's airway and lung compliance. With either type of ventilator, the effectiveness of ventilation is influenced by airway patency and the presence of any air leak.

Three ventilator *modes* can be used to deliver a desired ventilation rate: synchronized intermittent mechanical ventilation (SIMV), assisted/controlled (AC)

mechanical ventilation, and pressure support (PS) mechanical ventilation.

- In SIMV mode the ventilator ensures delivery of the set number of mechanical breaths, which are coordinated with the patient's respirations. The ventilator does not deliver more than the set number of breaths per minute. Any breaths above the set number are spontaneous breaths of the patient.

- In AC mode the ventilator ensures delivery of the set number of mechanical breaths, which are coordinated with the patient's respiratory effort. In this mode the ventilator will sense any spontaneous breaths above the set number and will provide full support for those breaths as soon as they are sensed.

- In PS mode, which can be combined with either of the above support modes, the ventilator will sense spontaneous breaths and increase airflow to reach a target inspiratory pressure set on the ventilator.

Home ventilators are usually equipped with at least 5 alarms with audible and visual display indicators. The alarms indicate the following problems:

1. *Low pressure or apnea*—may be caused by a loose or disconnected circuit or an air leak in the circuit or at the tracheostoma, resulting in inadequate ventilation.

2. *Low power*—caused by a depleted battery.

3. *High pressure*—can be caused by a plugged or obstructed airway or circuit tubing (eg, due to secretions or water), by coughing, or by bronchospasm.

4. *Setting error*—is caused by ventilator settings outside the capacity of the equipment.

5. *Power switchover*—occurs when the unit switches from alternating-current power to the internal battery.

A full discussion of mechanical ventilators is beyond the scope of this textbook.

- Equipment failure (eg, depleted or disconnected oxygen supply or low battery)

Signs and symptoms of respiratory distress include tachycardia, decreased oxygen saturation, decreased chest expansion, increased exhaled CO_2 values, coarse or decreased breath sounds, increased attempts at spontaneous respiration, intercostal retractions, anxiety, and cyanosis. If a ventilator-dependent child is in respiratory distress and the cause is not easily ascertained and corrected, remove the ventilator and provide assisted manual ventilations.

Although the DOPE mnemonic is used most often to identify causes of acute deterioration in the child who receives positive-pressure ventilation, many of the same complications may cause acute respiratory distress in patients who are supported with negative-pressure ventilators (ie, poncho, shell, vest, or "iron lung") at home.

Continuous Positive Airway Pressure and Bilevel Positive Airway Pressure

Devices that deliver continuous positive airway pressure (CPAP) are used to normalize resting lung volume (functional residual capacity), prevent airway collapse, and improve oxygenation and ventilation in patients who are able to make spontaneous respiratory efforts. During CPAP therapy, a constant positive airway pressure is maintained throughout the respiratory cycle. This support is most often used for patients with restrictive lung disease, tracheomalacia, chronic pulmonary edema, neuromuscular weakness, or obstructive sleep apnea. CPAP is typically delivered by face mask or nasal prongs.

Bilevel positive airway pressure (BiPAP) therapy provides both inspiratory and expiratory positive-pressure ventilatory assistance. When the patient initiates a breath, the device provides the set positive inspiratory pressure to assist ventilation and then maintains the set expiratory positive airway pressure during exhala-

tion. This breathing support augments the patient's spontaneous respiratory efforts, and it has been effective in the treatment of patients with chronic respiratory failure. It is also helpful in the acute transition from invasive to noninvasive respiratory support. BiPAP is delivered through a tight-fitting nasal or facial mask.

Both CPAP and BiPAP use a continuous gas inflow with restriction of outflow to produce the distending airway pressure. If the patient's respiratory function deteriorates during CPAP or BiPAP therapy, healthcare providers should be prepared and suitably trained to initiate more invasive respiratory support. If respiratory distress or inadequate respiratory effort develops, provide assisted manual ventilation with a bag and mask, and invasive airway management may be needed.

Central Venous Catheters

Central venous catheters (CVCs) are used to deliver fluids, parenteral nutrition, medications (eg, antibiotics or chemotherapy), and blood products directly into a central vein and to draw blood samples. A variety of catheters are available for long-term use. The type of catheter to be used is determined by the patient's needs (ie, frequent access for fluid or medication administration or infrequent access for blood sampling, blood component therapy, or medication administration) and the preference of the healthcare team.

Some CVCs exit the skin directly above the vascular access site like a standard IV (Broviac or Hickman catheters). A long-term CVC can be tunneled beneath the subcutaneous tissue of the chest, neck, groin, or arm and inserted into a large central vein. The catheter may have a single, double, or triple lumen. Some catheters have reservoirs that are completely subcutaneous (eg, Port-a-cath or Med-a-port), requiring insertion of a needle through the skin to access the reservoir. External CVCs are typically flushed daily with saline and an anticoagulant

(usually heparin) to prevent blood clots from forming in the catheter. Potential complications of central venous access are infection and bacteremia.

Subcutaneous infusion systems with reservoirs are typically placed in the operating room. The port rests in a subcutaneous pocket in the upper chest, forming a small, palpable bulge under the skin. A flush with anticoagulant (heparin) is needed only once a month or after completion of each access, so there is less risk of infection when the catheter is not in use. Because the catheter is hidden, concerns about altered body image are alleviated, which may be especially important for adolescents. Although the risk of infection is low, these systems are not free of infection risk.

Another type of CVC is a percutaneous intravenous central catheter (PICC). This catheter is typically placed in a peripheral arm (antecubital) vein and threaded into a central (eg, subclavian) vein or the superior vena cava. This catheter is generally used for administration of medications or nutrition temporarily. A PICC may be placed with use of only local anesthesia or sedation.

Central Venous Catheter Emergencies

Emergencies related to CVCs typically result from displacement or disconnection of the catheter, obstruction of the catheter, complications of central venous access, or failure of the device itself. The DOPE mnemonic can be modified to recall common causes of CVC-related emergencies:

- **D**isplacement or **D**isconnection: CVCs can be dislodged, damaged, or disconnected, causing a life-threatening emergency. Children with dislodged or completely withdrawn or separated catheters may present with bleeding. If the catheter is damaged or separated from an external connection, it may be possible to clamp the catheter near the skin entrance site to prevent bleeding. If the catheter is dislodged, apply direct pressure over the site and assess the child's airway, breathing, and circulation to determine if the bleeding has produced cardiorespiratory compromise. Observe for signs and symptoms of shock and treat appropriately (see Chapter 5). The child should be transported to a facility that can definitively treat this problem.

- **O**bstruction: Internal obstruction of the catheter can result from blood clots or the formation of drug or calcium crystals (eg, from parenteral nutrition). Kinking of the catheter at the skin entry site and beneath the skin can also cause obstruction. External obstruction usually results from a blood clot. The most serious risk of clot formation in the CVC is development of an acute pulmonary embolus, which can cause hypoxemia, respiratory distress, or shock (**P**ulmonary embolus is also recalled by the "**P**" of the DOPE mnemonic). If a right-to-left intracardiac shunt is present, a venous clot can potentially flow (embolize) to other areas of the body through the arterial system.

  Signs and symptoms of emboli depend on the organ system affected and include altered mental status, respiratory distress, cyanosis, tachycardia, chest pain, dyspnea, and shock.

  Air embolus is another serious risk for the child with a CVC. Signs and symptoms are the same as for blood clot emboli. Treatment includes clamping the line, placing the child in a supine position with his left side down and head lower than the body, opening the airway, and administering 100% oxygen. Also consider placement of a peripheral IV and administration of IV fluids.

- **P**neumothorax, **P**ericardial tamponade, or **P**ulmonary embolus: Erosion or perforation of the central vein due to the CVC can result in pneumothorax, hemothorax, or even hydrothorax from infusion of the IV fluid. Prompt decompression may be required if these complications produce symptoms. Erosion of the catheter tip through the right

atrium can result in acute pericardial tamponade.

Pulmonary embolus should be considered in all children with an indwelling CVC, particularly older children. A pulmonary embolus may develop if a clot fragment or catheter fragment migrates into the lungs. Signs of pulmonary embolus include hypoxemia despite oxygen administration and adequate ventilation and shortness of breath. A ventilation-perfusion scan or contrast CT scan of the lung will aid diagnosis.

- **E**quipment failure: Leakage at the connections, cracking of the hub, clotting within stopcocks, or damage to the catheter system may cause complications. If there is a question about the functioning of the equipment, remove all interposed equipment and pumps and attempt to manually flush the catheter using a small (1- to 3-mL) syringe. Flushing the catheter often reveals the source of the problem.

If fever develops in a child with a CVC, consider a catheter-related infection. Such infections may be life-threatening, especially in children with a suppressed immune system (eg, due to cancer, chemotherapy, organ transplantation, malnutrition, or HIV infection). These children are at risk for infections, especially bacterial sepsis. A suggested approach to a child with a CVC and a fever is as follows:

1. Assess ABCDEs.

2. Obtain blood samples from the CVC for culture and a complete blood count (some centers also recommend culture of blood from a peripheral site).

3. Administer antibiotics.

If the child does not have a suppressed immune system and appears well, he/she may be discharged with careful follow-up care. If the child is neutropenic, admission to the hospital for IV antibiotics is recommended until the results of blood cultures are known. If the catheter is infected, it will have to be removed.

Feeding Catheters

A feeding catheter is designed to provide total nutrition or to supplement caloric intake in patients who cannot ingest sufficient calories. A feeding catheter can also be used to administer enteral medications. Indications for a feeding catheter include failure to thrive, inability to coordinate swallowing, severe developmental delay or cerebral palsy, coma, burns to the mouth and oropharynx, and short-bowel syndrome.

Types of Feeding Catheters

There are several types of feeding catheters. Some catheters can be passed into the digestive tract through the mouth or nose; others require surgical placement.

Nonsurgical feeding catheters can be left in place for weeks to months and are therefore considered temporary. Nasogastric, nasojejunal, and orogastric tubes are temporary, nonsurgical feeding catheters. Nasogastric tubes are inserted through the nose and end in the stomach. Nasojejunal tubes are inserted through the nose and end in the jejunal portion of the small intestine. These tubes are most frequently used in children who have gastroesophageal reflux and who are at risk for aspiration. Placement in the jejunum is suggested by aspiration of alkalotic fluid (indicating that the tube is no longer in the stomach) and confirmed by x-ray or fluoroscopy. If these tubes are dislodged, replacement at an institution where nasojejunal tubes are routinely inserted is often required.

Orogastric tubes are inserted through the mouth and into the stomach. These feeding tubes are typically placed in young infants or when a tube cannot be placed through the nose (eg, choanal atresia).

Surgically placed feeding catheters include gastrostomy tubes (g-tubes), jejunostomy tubes (j-tubes), and percutaneous endoscopic gastrostomy (PEG) tubes. Jejunostomy tubes are used in children who require specialized nutritional support, including those with gastroesophageal reflux. The tube is surgically placed in the small intestine.

Feeding Catheter Emergencies

Potential causes of emergencies involving complications related to feeding catheters can be recalled using a modification of the DOPE mnemonic:

- **D**isplacement: Feeding catheters can be dislodged, displaced, or damaged. Displacement of a surgically implanted feeding tube is an emergency requiring immediate replacement of the tube. The longer the tube is out, the greater the likelihood that it cannot be replaced easily because the tract between the skin and the gastrointestinal tract narrows quickly. The ostomy can close within several hours. Feeding catheters can be misplaced during initial insertion (eg, into the trachea or esophagus) or displaced after insertion (eg, a nasogastric or orogastric tube can migrate into the jejunum or be pulled into the esophagus). A damaged feeding catheter must be replaced.

- **O**bstruction: Feeding catheters may become obstructed by formula drugs that precipitate or form crystals in the catheter. If the obstruction cannot be cleared with aspiration and gentle irrigation, the feeding catheter should be replaced.

- **P**eritonitis, **P**erforation, or **P**neumoperitoneum: Erosion or perforation of the stomach or intestine due to the feeding catheter can result in pneumoperitoneum and acute peritonitis. Acute perforation may be accompanied by shock and respiratory failure.

- **E**quipment failure: Leakage at the connections, cracking of the hub, and pump failure may cause failure of the feeding tube and feeding system. If you suspect equipment malfunction, remove all interposed equipment and pumps and manually flush the catheter with 5 to 10 mL of air or water. If the catheter flushes easily, the malfunction is likely caused by the infusion pump. If the catheter does not flush easily, the feeding catheter is probably obstructed.

Minor irritation or bleeding at the feeding tube site is not an emergent problem. For bleeding around the site, apply direct pressure. If the site is red, swollen, or discharging pus, evaluate the child for infection and treat on an emergency basis.

Cerebral Spinal Fluid Shunts

CSF shunts are catheters that drain cerebral spinal fluid from the ventricles of the brain to another area of the body where the fluid can be absorbed. CSF shunts frequently drain a lateral ventricle of the brain into a subcutaneous reservoir, which is usually placed under the scalp. This reservoir may contain valves and a pumping mechanism. A conduit from the reservoir is tunneled under the skin to the abdomen (ventriculoperitoneal shunt) or chest (ventriculoatrial or ventriculopleural shunt).

A variety of medical conditions require placement of a CSF shunt. The most common is hydrocephalus, which occurs when the lateral ventricles become dilated with excess CSF. Hydrocephalus results from an imbalance between the production and absorption of CSF. This imbalance results from a block in normal flow of CSF, reduced reabsorption of CSF, or in rare cases, excess production of CSF.

CSF is produced by the choroid plexus in the ventricles, and it circulates through the ventricles and into the subarachnoid space around the brain and spinal cord. Most CSF is reabsorbed by arachnoid villi in the subarachnoid space into the venous channels of the sagittal sinus. If there is a block in the CSF pathway, CSF continues to be produced, but it cannot circulate to be reabsorbed. This form of hydrocephalus is called *obstructive* hydrocephalus. A second form of hydrocephalus, *communicating* hydrocephalus, occurs when the CSF pathway is patent but the CSF is not reabsorbed by the subarachnoid villi. Communicating hydrocephalus

may develop in children with severe head injuries and subarachnoid hemorrhage.

Hydrocephalus can occur without any known cause, or it can be caused by such conditions as a brain tumor, meningitis, trauma, or intraventricular hemorrhage. Congenital hydrocephalus may be caused by fetal infections such as rubella and cytomegalovirus. Hydrocephalus may be associated with congenital abnormalities of the central nervous system. The Arnold-Chiari malformation is often associated with spina bifida (see FYI: "Latex Allergies and Spina Bifida"), meningomyelocele, and hydrocephalus. In Arnold-Chiari malformation central nervous system structures are displaced and block CSF flow, producing obstructive hydrocephalus.

CSF Shunt Emergencies

The most common causes of CSF shunt emergencies are shunt failure (most commonly due to shunt obstruction) and shunt infection. Possible causes of shunt failure emergencies can be recalled using a modification of the DOPE mnemonic:

- **D**isplacement: CSF shunts can be dislodged, damaged, or displaced. If a surgically implanted CSF shunt is dislodged, fractured, or displaced and causes symptoms of increased intracranial pressure, the child requires urgent shunt replacement. When intracranial pressure is elevated, furosemide, acetazolamide (to decrease CSF production), and mannitol may be administered while the operating room is being prepared. If signs of increased intracranial pressure are significant, hyperventilation should be provided to prevent cerebral herniation. If the

FYI: **Latex Allergies and Spina Bifida**

Children with spina bifida are often allergic to latex.[12] Healthcare providers should use nonlatex gloves and supplies when caring for these children.

obstruction in the shunt is *distal* to the reservoir, the shunt reservoir can be tapped and CSF withdrawn to reduce intracranial pressure.

- **O**bstruction: Blood or protein clots can form inside the catheter, leading to catheter obstruction, accumulation of CSF, and increased intracranial pressure. In infants and young children, a *gradual* increase in intracranial volume and pressure may result in expansion of the bones of the skull and separation of the skull sutures. Signs and symptoms of CSF shunt obstruction include headache, irritability, nausea or vomiting, bulging fontanel in infants, change in pupil size, bradycardia, hypertension, ataxia, listlessness, apnea, seizures, and change in mental status. The early signs of CSF obstruction are often nonspecific. Healthcare providers should ensure that the shunt is patent when the child with a CSF shunt presents with vague signs and symptoms.

  Suspected CSF shunt obstruction is an emergency. If shunt failure is documented or strongly suspected, the child should be transported to a facility that can manage this problem. Replacement of the CSF shunt is often indicated.

- **P**eritonitis, **P**erforation, or **P**seudocyst: Erosion or perforation of the stomach or intestines due to the distal CSF shunt catheter can result in symptoms of peritonitis or perforation (ie, pneumoperitoneum and acute abdomen). Acute perforation may be accompanied by the development of shock and respiratory failure.

  A pseudocyst may develop as a complication of CSF catheter insertion. The pseudocyst develops when omentum wraps around the abdominal end of the catheter, creating a sac or cyst into which the CSF flows. When sufficient fluid flows into this sac or closed space, abdominal pain and shunt obstruction can develop.

- **E**quipment failure: Leakage at the connections, cracking of the hub, and fracture of the shunt may cause problems.

If shunt failure or complications produce signs of increased intracranial pressure, consider the following bedside palliative measures pending drainage of CSF:

- Use mechanical advantage: raise the head of the bed 30 degrees.
- Assess and support the child's airway, breathing, and circulation:
  — Support a patent airway.
  — Provide 100% O_2 by face mask.
  — Provide assisted ventilation if necessary.
- Establish vascular access.
- Obtain a CT scan.
- Contact a neurosurgeon as soon as possible.

CSF shunts may also become infected and cause meningitis. Signs and symptoms of a CSF shunt infection include fever, erythema, or tenderness at the shunt site. Children with shunt infections require antibiotic therapy, and they should be transported to a facility capable of providing close observation and definitive care, including replacement of the shunt.

Summary Points

Children with special healthcare needs have chronic illnesses that increase their susceptibility to acute medical problems involving airway, breathing, and circulation. Some of these children have a low respiratory reserve, so a mild illness can cause rapid decompensation. Many children with special healthcare needs have baseline vital signs outside the range of normal for age, so medical personnel must determine the child's baseline condition when performing a rapid cardiopulmonary assessment.

Parents and caregivers are important sources of information for medical personnel. They usually know how to manage the child's problems and equipment. They know the child's baseline vital signs and developmental level. Many children with special healthcare needs carry information cards or medical records containing important information for emergency

providers. To improve access to critical information, you should encourage parents and primary care physicians to enroll children with special healthcare needs in the Emergency Preparedness for Children With Special Health Care Needs Program and to complete an Emergency Information Form.

Use of an organized approach such as the DOPE mnemonic can help you rapidly identify reversible causes of distress in children who rely on technologic support. Whenever the child with an artificial airway deteriorates, particularly during positive-pressure ventilation, tube **D**isplacement or **O**bstruction, **P**neumothorax, and **E**quipment failure should be ruled out or treated immediately. Check the child's oxygen supply, ventilator, and tubing.

Indwelling central venous catheters, feeding catheters, and CSF shunts can become dislodged, obstructed, or infected. Rapid assessment and response to the special healthcare needs of children with these problems can reduce both morbidity and mortality.

Case Scenarios
Completion of Introductory Case Scenario

A 16-month-old girl with chronic lung disease, moderate developmental delay, a tracheostomy tube, a CSF shunt, and a gastrostomy tube presents with a 1-day history of fever and mild difficulty breathing. The child typically requires mechanical ventilation on room air while sleeping at night and a tracheostomy mist collar with 1 L/min O_2 flow while awake during the day. Yesterday the child developed a cough, and 4 L/min O_2 flow was required to maintain an oxyhemoglobin saturation above 90%. The child's illness began with increased secretions in the tracheostomy tube, which necessitated more frequent suctioning.

On examination the child appears alert, but she has labored respirations and mild to moderate intercostal and subcostal retrac-

tions. The child has bilateral breath sounds, diffuse rales, and an audible wheeze. Her temperature is 39°C (102.2°F), heart rate is 160 bpm, respiratory rate is 40 breaths/min, blood pressure is 90/60 mm Hg, and capillary refill is <2 seconds. The pulse oximeter indicates an oxyhemoglobin saturation of 90% with 4 L/min O_2 bled into her home ventilator circuit. Large amounts of thick secretions are coming from the child's tracheostomy tube.

Answers to Introductory Questions

- *How would you approach initial assessment and stabilization of this child?*

This child has chronic special healthcare needs and is dependent on mechanical ventilation. The initial PALS (ABCDE) approach to assessment of airway, breathing, circulation, disability, and exposure is the same for all patients, and this approach should include the rapid cardiopulmonary assessment and the more detailed examination of systems. The child's caregivers can describe baseline activity, responsiveness, vital signs, and appearance to assist in your initial assessment.

- *What is your rapid cardiopulmonary assessment?*

This child demonstrates respiratory distress and potential respiratory failure. Her artificial airway (tracheostomy tube) appears patent, but she is congested with copious secretions. Her breathing appears labored, but it can be maintained with support. This child has an artificial airway and requires mechanical ventilation; these factors introduce the risks of tracheostomy tube obstruction and infection.

- *What are the most important treatment priorities for this child?*

1. Airway and breathing support with evaluation of her tracheostomy tube and mechanical ventilator during completion of the primary survey (ABCDEs)

2. Rapid communication with primary caregivers to compare current condition with baseline condition

3. Consideration of vascular access

4. Evaluation of additional technologies (CSF shunt and gastrostomy tube) for impaired function or infection

- *What assessment steps and treatment priorities are different from those for emergencies in children without special healthcare needs? What assessment steps and treatment priorities are the same as those for children without special healthcare needs?*

The general principles of assessment and management of respiratory distress are identical for children with and children without special healthcare needs. Initial assessment should include a search for common causes of deterioration that require rapid identification and treatment (eg, tube displacement, tube obstruction, pneumothorax, equipment failure, and risk of infection).

Case Scenario 2

An 18-month-old girl with a genetic syndrome presents to the Emergency Department with respiratory distress and fever. She has a tracheostomy tube, gastrostomy tube, and a tunneled central venous catheter (Broviac catheter) for long-term parenteral nutrition supplementation. She requires mechanical ventilation at night, but she typically breathes spontaneously during the day. Today she has needed to remain on the ventilator during the day. When ventilatory support is removed, she immediately becomes hypoxemic and her oxyhemoglobin saturation falls. Her Medic Alert arm bracelet contains a telephone number that can be called for a more detailed medical history. Her Emergency Information Form indicates that she has a 4.5-mm standard Bivona tracheostomy tube and a history of a seizure disorder.

Initial Assessment

This toddler is pale, listless, and cyanotic, with intercostal retractions. Her temperature (rectal) is 39°C (102.2°F), heart rate

is 180 bpm, respiratory rate is 30 breaths/min with the ventilator set at 30 breaths/min, blood pressure is 80/40 mm Hg, and oxyhemoglobin saturation is 88% with her usual O_2 flow of 25% (FiO_2 = 0.25). Coarse breath sounds are heard throughout her chest, but her chest rises bilaterally. Heart sounds are normal, and capillary refill is 3 to 4 seconds. Her extremities are cool, and distal pulses are weak.

What do you conclude from this assessment?

- This child has increased respiratory distress and potential acute respiratory failure. The child is hypoxemic despite adequate oxygen therapy and ventilatory support.

- This child has tachycardia and signs of poor perfusion (capillary refill of 3 to 4 seconds with cool extremities and weak distal pulses). Compensated shock is present because her systolic blood pressure exceeds 72 mm Hg (to estimate the 5th percentile of systolic blood pressure for children 1 to 10 years of age, add 70 mm Hg to twice the child's age in years). In addition, pulse pressure is widened (consider septic shock).

- The child is febrile, so you should search for an infection. A pulmonary infection would not be surprising, but other causes of infection (eg, central venous catheter or gastrostomy tube) should be considered. The presence of signs of shock and a widened pulse pressure make the diagnosis of sepsis likely.

Acceptable Actions

- Position the child's airway by placing a rolled towel under the child's upper back (Figure 3).

- Attach a cardiorespiratory monitor. Consider ECG, pulse oximetry, and exhaled CO_2 monitoring.

- Ask caregivers to describe the child's baseline physical condition and medical history. Ask if the family has any information to add to the Emergency Information Form.

- Increase the concentration of inspired oxygen administered through the tracheostomy tube by the ventilator system.

- Use the DOPE mnemonic (tube **D**isplacement or **O**bstruction, **P**neumothorax, **E**quipment failure) to identify reversible causes of the child's deterioration in respiratory function. Consider increasing the child's mechanical ventilatory support.

- Suction the tracheostomy tube to verify airway patency and to assess the color, odor, consistency, and quantity of secretions.

- Administer a 20 mL/kg bolus of isotonic crystalloid because the child has signs of compromise in peripheral perfusion. Reassess perfusion after the fluid bolus.

- Consider obtaining cultures of blood from the indwelling central venous catheter and a peripheral site, and consider administering broad-spectrum antibiotics.

- Frequently reassess the child's respiratory and circulatory status.

- Consider obtaining a chest radiograph and performing additional diagnostic studies.

- Arrange admission to an appropriate monitored setting and communicate with healthcare providers at the receiving facility.

Rationale for Acceptable Actions

- Positioning the airway may relieve obstruction of the artificial airway if positioning is the cause of the respiratory distress. Placing a rolled towel under the child's upper back will allow the neck to extend slightly so that the tracheostomy tube is accessible. Check for signs of an air leak around the tracheostomy tube because an air leak may cause inadequate ventilation. Cuffed tracheostomy tubes are not often used in infants and young children, so an air leak may develop. An older child or adolescent typically has a cuffed tracheostomy tube. If an air leak is heard upon positioning in an older child, the balloon may have been deflated or the tube may have become dislodged, causing the respiratory distress.

- Continuous monitoring is important in a child with unstable respiratory and cardiovascular status. ECG monitoring can verify that the tachycardia is sinus tachycardia rather than an arrhythmia. Pulse oximetry and exhaled CO_2 monitoring may provide additional information about the adequacy of oxygenation and ventilation.

- Evaluation of vital signs, oxyhemoglobin saturation, and mental status is important. Evaluate $PaCO_2$ to determine the effectiveness of ventilation. Also identify any additional major medical conditions and all medications the child receives.

- Increasing FiO_2 in this child may increase blood oxygen saturation and relieve the distress and cyanosis.

- Increasing the child's mechanical ventilatory support by either bag–tracheostomy tube ventilations or more support by the mechanical ventilator may help improve oxygenation and ventilation.

- This child has signs of compensated shock, including tachycardia, delayed capillary refill, cool extremities, lethargy, and weak distal pulses. So an isotonic crystalloid fluid bolus is indicated.

- Tracheostomy tubes can be obstructed by mucous secretions, exacerbating respiratory distress. Although this child's tachypnea and distress are probably not caused by an obstructed tracheostomy tube, suctioning the tube may facilitate mechanical ventilation if there is any degree of occlusion due to secretions. Suctioning may also help in the assessment of secretions for signs of infection.

- This child has an indwelling central venous catheter and a fever, which suggest infection. Under these circumstances the provider should consider obtaining blood cultures and administering antibiotics.

- This child is at risk for decompensation and requires continued care in a facility equipped to monitor and deal with life-threatening illness.

Unacceptable Actions

The following actions would be inappropriate in this scenario:

- Administering IV fluids or antibiotics before assessing and managing the child's airway and breathing

- Suctioning or changing of the tracheostomy tube before assessment and management of the child's airway, breathing, and circulation

- Failing to obtain critical medical information and history that affect initial emergency assessment and management

Case Scenario Progression

This child's respiratory status improved with increased oxygen administration and increased ventilatory support. Her oxyhemoglobin saturation increased to 99% with an FiO_2 of 0.4. Suctioning revealed no mucous plugs, scant secretions, and no sign of pulmonary infection. The child's heart rate decreased to 140 bpm after two 20 mL/kg boluses of isotonic crystalloid, and her peripheral perfusion improved. Blood cultures indicated the presence of Gram-positive bacteria (Staphylococcus) in the central venous catheter and peripheral blood. The child remained in the hospital for 7 days. She was discharged home on her baseline ventilatory settings to complete her course of antibiotics there.

Review Questions

1. **You are performing an initial evaluation of a 3-year-old child with developmental delay, congenital neuromuscular weakness, and chronic respiratory failure. He has a tracheostomy tube and is dependent on mechanical ventilation. His mother reports that he has been having difficulty breathing and has increased secretions. He is listless, and nasal flaring and grunting are present. His heart rate is 150 bpm, respiratory rate is 80 breaths/min with the ventilator set at 30 breaths/min, and oxyhemoglobin saturation is 82% with his usual O$_2$ flow of 30%. Breath sounds are decreased but present bilaterally, and there is minimal chest movement with respiration. Which of the following is the most appropriate intervention for you to perform first?**

   a. provide 100% oxygen and suction the oropharynx and tracheostomy tube with at least −200 mm Hg suction pressure to remove any tracheal secretions

   b. immediately perform needle decompression on both sides of the chest because the child likely has bilateral pneumothoraces

   c. provide 100% oxygen, attempt manual ventilation through the tracheostomy tube, and assess for displacement or obstruction of the tube

   d. do not touch the tracheostomy tube or mechanical ventilator, and provide 100% blow-by oxygen by face mask over the nose and mouth

   The correct answer is c. The DOPE mnemonic is useful when evaluating respiratory distress or decompensation in any child with an artifical airway, particularly a child with special healthcare needs. During manual ventilation, assess for **D**isplacement or **O**bstruction of the tracheostomy tube, and then assess for **P**neumothorax and **E**quipment failure. The most common causes of distress in children with a tracheostomy tube are tube displacement and obstruction. In this case tube obstruction is the most likely problem because the child has increased secretions, decreased breath sounds, and minimal chest expansion.

   Answer a is incorrect because a suction pressure of −200 mm Hg is excessive for use in children. A suction pressure of −60 to −100 mm Hg is recommended to avoid trauma to the tracheal mucosa.

   Answer b is incorrect because tube obstruction is common in children with a tracheostomy tube. The child has a recent history of increased secretions, and suctioning can be performed rapidly. Bilateral pneumothoraces are uncommon, and needle decompression is not indicated until other causes of decreased breath sounds (tube displacement or obstruction) have been ruled out.

   Answer d is incorrect because this child is in severe respiratory distress and requires intervention. Removal of the mechanical ventilator and provision of assisted ventilation can rule out mechanical ventilator failure as a cause of the distress. Although administration of additional oxygen is not a bad idea, appropriate evaluation of the tracheostomy tube (airway) is the first priority. If the airway is patent, additional oxygen can be administered through the tracheostomy tube.

2. **You are evaluating a child with a tracheostomy tube and respiratory distress. Your assessment reveals an obstructed tube that cannot be cleared with suctioning, so you prepare to replace the tube. The child has a 4.5-mm uncuffed pediatric tracheostomy tube in place. Which of the following statements is most accurate about the tube you may use to replace the obstructed tube?**

   a. neonatal and pediatric tracheostomy tubes are totally interchangeable because they have the same inner diameter and length

   b. if you cannot pass a replacement tracheostomy tube of the same size, you should dilate the stoma starting with a tracheal tube one size larger than the original tracheostomy tube

   c. if you cannot pass the replacement tracheostomy tube, you can attempt to provide bag-mask ventilation using a tightly fitting face mask over the nose and mouth while occluding the leak at the tracheostoma

   d. if the family does not have an extra tracheostomy tube, there is no standard airway support equipment that can be used to support ventilation

   The correct answer is c. A small number of children have total obstruction of the upper airway or laryngotracheal separation. Such children cannot be ventilated by face mask. Alternatively, you may attempt to provide mask ventilation at the tracheostoma by placing a very small (neonatal) mask over the stoma and holding the mask firmly against the neck to prevent any air leak.

   Answer a is incorrect because neonatal and pediatric tracheostomy tubes generally differ in length. Neonatal tracheostomy tubes are much shorter than pediatric tubes of the same diameter.

   Answer b is incorrect. If a tracheostomy tube of the same size does not pass freely, you should attempt to pass a tracheal tube that is *smaller* in diameter than the original tracheostomy tube. Alternatively, a suction catheter may be inserted through the replacement tube and then through the stoma and into the trachea. The new tracheostomy tube is passed over the catheter into proper position.

Answer d is incorrect because standard uncuffed tracheal tubes *can* be used to support ventilation in these children.

3. **A 6-year-old child with acute lymphocytic leukemia presents with fever approximately 1 week after completing a course of maintenance chemotherapy. She has a tunneled central venous catheter in place. Her axillary temperature is 39°C (102.2°F), heart rate is 150 bpm, respiratory rate is 40 breaths/min without distress, and blood pressure is 90/30 mm Hg. Capillary refill is 2 seconds, peripheral pulses are strong, and oxyhemoglobin saturation is 100% on room air. The child is appropriately responsive to all questions. She denies any pain but complains of chills. After evaluation and support of the ABCs, what should be included as part of your routine evaluation and stabilization of this child?**

   a. stat CT scan of the head to rule out meningitis

   b. immediate tracheal intubation

   c. stat echocardiogram to rule out pericardial tamponade

   d. cultures of blood from the central venous line and from a peripheral site

The correct answer is d. This child is at risk for sepsis because she has an indwelling catheter and has just completed a course of chemotherapy that probably produced neutropenia. She has a fever, so infection is likely. Obtaining cultures of blood from her central venous catheter and from a peripheral site is a first step in identifying a source of infection.

Answer a is incorrect because this child has no immediate signs of neurologic infection such as meningitis. In the absence of signs of neurologic infection, you should further evaluate the child and ensure that her cardiorespiratory status is stable before sending her for diagnostic tests that will compromise your ability to monitor and support cardiorespiratory function.

Answer b is incorrect because the child is well oxygenated on room air and is breathing without distress. You should monitor the child's respiratory function closely because it may deteriorate rapidly if sepsis is present or septic shock develops.

Answer c is incorrect because there is no reason to suspect pericardial tamponade. The child has no signs of shock; her pulses are strong, and her capillary refill is brisk.

4. **A 6-year-old child with acute lymphocytic leukemia is admitted with fever and possible sepsis 1 week after chemotherapy. The child has an indwelling central venous catheter. Although the child was in no cardiorespiratory distress on admission, she has become more lethargic while waiting in the Emergency Department for a bed to become available on the pediatric ward. Her heart rate is now 180 bpm, and blood pressure is 70/30 mm Hg. Capillary refill remains brisk (1 second). Axillary temperature is now 40°C (104°F), and respiratory rate remains 40 breaths/min and unlabored. Oxyhemoglobin saturation fell to 91% on room air, so she is receiving 30% oxygen by face mask, which has increased her oxyhemoglobin saturation to 95%. Which of the following interventions does this child require *first*?**

   a. administration of a 20 mL/kg bolus of isotonic crystalloid, followed by reassessment and possibly repeated fluid bolus therapy

   b. immediate tracheal intubation

   c. immediate removal of her central venous catheter

   d. immediate bag-mask ventilation

The correct answer is a. This child has signs of decompensated shock, and she is likely in septic shock. Although her capillary refill is brisk, she is hypotensive and has a widened pulse pressure. In addition, her level of consciousness has deteriorated. Septic shock produces a relative hypovolemia, caused by vasodilation and increased capillary permeability (see Chapter 5, "Shock"). This child requires immediate fluid bolus therapy, and she may require several fluid boluses.

Answer b is incorrect because this child is adequately oxygenated with a relatively small amount of oxygen supplementation. Further attempts at establishment of peripheral vascular access are unlikely to be successful until volume resuscitation is provided.

Answer c is incorrect because the source of the child's fever has not been established. You do not yet know if the child is bacteremic. If the central venous catheter is infected, it will have to be removed, but that decision does not need to be made immediately.

Answer d is incorrect because this child is breathing adequately, is adequately oxygenated, and has no signs of respiratory distress. Note that during volume resuscitation the child may develop pulmonary edema, so you must closely monitor her respiratory function and be prepared to support airway, oxygenation, and ventilation as needed.

References

1. McPherson M, Arango P, Fox H, Lauver C, McManus M, Newacheck PW, Perrin JM, Shonkoff JP, Strickland B. A new definition of children with special health care needs. *Pediatrics*. 1998;102(pt 1):137-140.

2. Newacheck PW, Strickland B, Shonkoff JP, Perrin JM, McPherson M, McManus M, Lauver C, Fox H, Arango P. An epidemiologic profile of children with special health care needs. *Pediatrics*. 1998;102(pt 1):117-123.

3. Emergency preparedness for children with special health care needs. Committee on Pediatric Emergency Medicine, American Academy of Pediatrics. *Pediatrics*. 1999; 104:e53.

4. EMS for children: recommendations for coordinating care for children with special health care needs. Emergency Medical Services for Children, National Task Force on Children With Special Health Care Needs. *Ann Emerg Med*. 1997;30:274-280.

5. Carraccio CL, Dettmer KS, duPont ML, Sacchetti AD. Family member knowledge of children's medical problems: the need for universal application of an emergency data set. *Pediatrics*. 1998;102(pt 1):367-370.

6. Neal W, Kieffer S. Preparing pediatric home care patients for a medical emergency. *Caring*. 1998;17:48-50.

7. American Academy of Pediatrics. Emergency information form. Available at: www. pediatrics.org/cgi/content/full/104/4/e53. Accessed February 18, 2002.

8. American Academy of Pediatrics, Committee on Children With Disabilities. Pediatric services for infants and children with special health care needs. *Pediatrics*. 1993;92:163-165.

9. Foltin G, Tunik M, Cooper A, Markenson D, Treiber M, Phillips R, Karpeles T, Gilbert S. *Teaching Resource for Instructors in Prehospital Pediatrics, Version 2.0. Children With Special Health Care Needs*. New York, NY: Center for Pediatric Medicine; 1998.

10. Diehl B, Dorsey L. High-tech children: interfacing EMS providers with children in the community. *J Emerg Med Serv JEMS*. 1998; 23:78-85.

11. Batshaw M. *Your Child Has a Disability*. Baltimore, Md: Paul H. Publishing; 1991.

12. Bernardini R, Novembre E. Relevance of and risk factors for latex sensitization in patients with spina bifida. *J Urol*. 1998;160:1775-1778.

Toxicology

Introductory Case Scenario

A 16-year-old girl is found lying near the front door of her home when EMS personnel ring the doorbell. The girl called EMS before she collapsed; the mother was asleep and was unaware of any problems until paramedics arrived. The girl is difficult to arouse. An empty bottle of sustained-release 180-mg verapamil tablets is found with a suicide note. EMS personnel provide oxygen, monitor heart rate and rhythm, and rapidly transport the girl to the local medical center. The girl begins to awaken during transport. On arrival in the ED she is awake with a heart rate of 114 bpm, respiratory rate of 28 breaths/min, and blood pressure of 120/60 mm Hg.

■ Does this patient have potential life-threatening toxicity due to ingestion of a calcium channel blocker?

■ Would you use gastric lavage, activated charcoal, or both interventions at this time?

■ What pharmacologic interventions should you prepare to administer in case signs of toxicity develop?

Learning Objectives

After completing this chapter the PALS provider should be able to

■ Identify the clinical signs and symptoms of life-threatening poisoning with cocaine, tricyclic antidepressants, calcium channel blockers (especially sustained-release preparations), β-blockers, and opiates

■ Describe the indications for and limitations of gastrointestinal decontamination in the management of poisonings

■ Recognize the ECG abnormalities and potential life-threatening complications of calcium channel blocker, β-blocker, tricyclic antidepressant, cocaine, and opiate ingestion or exposure

■ Describe the pharmacologic agents and the rationale for interventions used to treat the toxic manifestations of these types of poisoning

Scope of the Problem

Toxic exposures resulting in injury or death are a significant problem for prehospital, Emergency Department, and critical care providers. Exposure to cocaine, tricyclic antidepressants, calcium channel blockers, β-blockers, and opiates may necessitate alterations in resuscitation priorities or approach. Other toxins of concern for children and adolescents are methamphetamines, including MDMA (methylenedioxymethamphetamine or "Ecstasy"), and inhalation of solvents or propellants. Cardiac complications such as tachycardia and hypertension may occur with amphetamine and MDMA overdoses because these drugs produce sympathomimetic effects similar to the effects of cocaine. Sudden cardiac death with ventricular fibrillation (VF) can occur after inhalation of solvents or halogenated hydrocarbon propellants. A comprehensive overview of all types of poisonings including envenomation, toxic inhalation, and biological or chemical exposure is beyond the scope of this chapter.

This chapter addresses the recognition and management of 5 common types of poisoning that require modification in the ALS sequence or priorities.

In 2000 the American Association of Poison Control Centers (AAPCC), using the Toxic Exposure Surveillance System (TESS), reported 2 168 248 cases of human poison exposure.[1] Of these, 1 456 960 (67.2%) poisonings occurred in children 19 years of age or younger. Ingestion was the route of exposure in 76.2% of all cases. A total of 920 fatalities (in *all* age groups) was reported to the AAPCC in 2000. Death due to poisoning is fortunately less common in children than in other age groups. Nevertheless, significant morbidity and life-threatening signs and symptoms occur in children; the TESS reports that 2526 children experienced major effects from poisoning in 2000. The AAPCC defines major patient effects as signs or symptoms that are life-threatening or result in significant residual disability or disfigurement (eg, repeated seizures or status epilepticus, respiratory compromise requiring intubation, ventricular tachycardia with hypotension, esophageal stricture, and disseminated intravascular coagulation). It is likely that the TESS data underestimates the impact of poisoning on both children and adults.

Other sources of data on poisonings are available. For example, the National Center for Health Statistics (NCHS) and National Hospital Ambulatory Medical Care Surveys (NHAMCS) databases contain information on the extent of poisoning injury. The International Classification of Diseases, 9th revision, Clinical Modification (ICD-9-CM), includes a "Supplementary Classification of External Causes of Injury and Poisoning" (ie, E codes). Figure 1 illustrates the burden of poisoning in the United States using data from these sources.

From 1993 to 1996 there were 93 million Emergency Department visits; 1 million of these visits were related to poisoning (ie, classified using E codes). The average annual rate of poisoning-related visits was disproportionately higher among children under 5 years of age (84 visits per 10 000 persons) than among children in older age categories.[2] According to NCHS data, poisoning was the underlying cause of death for 18 549 people in the United States in 1995 alone, and it was the third leading cause of injury-related mortality after motor vehicle traffic injuries and firearm injuries.[3]

Prehospital and Emergency Department providers should consider poisoning as a potential source of life-threatening morbidity. Life-threatening morbidity may manifest as respiratory depression, seizures, hypotension, cardiac arrhythmias, and depressed level of consciousness. Providers caring for children should be aware of these potential complications; rescuers should support the airway, breathing, and circulation of the poisoned child just as they do for any acutely ill or injured child.

Cardiac arrest caused by ingested poisons is uncommon, but it does occur. Ventricular fibrillation, other arrhythmias, and death due to toxic agents such as cocaine ("crack"),[4] ammonium bifluoride,[5,6] calcium channel blockers (amlodipine,[7] nifedipine[8]), β-blockers (acebutolol,[9] propranolol[10]), opiates (methadone[11]), and tricyclic antidepressants in both overdoses (amitriptyline[12]) and normal therapeutic

doses (desipramine, imipramine[13]) have occurred in children. The long-term survival rate among victims of cardiac arrest due to poisoning is good, averaging 24% in 6 studies.

Major obstacles to data gathering and research on poisonings include the relatively low number of life-threatening poisonings and variance in prehospital triage protocols for severe poisonings. In 2000 a Toxicology Working Group and a First Aid Task Force of the AHA Emergency Cardiovascular Care Committee developed evidence- and consensus-based guidelines for treatment of toxicologic emergencies and first aid treatment of poisonings. Providers should apply these guidelines in cases of severe poisoning when the conventional ECC approach to resuscitation is ineffective and poisoning is suspected.[14]

Because research in this area consists primarily of small case series (level of evidence [LOE] 5), animal studies (LOE 6), and case reports, the AHA class of recommendation for most poisoning interventions is Class IIb or Indeterminate. The American College of Emergency Physicians and American Academy of Clinical Toxicology recommend consultation with a medical toxicologist or certified regional poison information center with transfer to a poison treatment center for unusual cases.[15,16]

General Approach to Poisoned Patients

The initial approach in toxicological emergencics follows basic PALS principles: assess and rapidly support the airway, oxygenation, ventilation, and perfusion. The clinician should perform a rapid cardiopulmonary assessment to detect abnormalities in the airway, breathing, and circulation. The patient's history may provide important information if you can obtain it from the patient or parent. A list of drugs and chemicals in the home may offer clues to identify an unknown toxin. The AAPCC reports that analgesics were the most common ingestant and cause of pharmaceutical-

FIGURE 1. Relationship of the number of poison exposures to Emergency Department visits, hospitalizations, and deaths due to poisoning. Sources: Centers for Disease Control and Prevention and National Center for Health Statistics, National Vital Statistics System, 1995; National Hospital Discharge Survey, 1995; National Hospital Ambulatory Medical Care Surveys, 1993-1996; and Toxic Exposure Surveillance System, 1995. Adapted from McCaig LF, Burt CW. Poison-related visits to emergency departments in the United States, 1993-1996. *J Toxicol Clin Toxicol.* 1999;37:817-826.

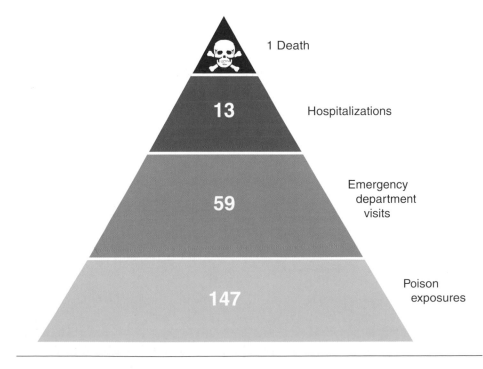

related death in 2000. Knowledge of potential acetaminophen exposure could enable successful antidotal therapy with N-acetylcysteine (Mucomyst) for a toxic exposure that might otherwise remain undetected. If iron pills were in the home, you might need to measure the serum iron level to detect poisoning that might not be detected by a routine comprehensive drug screen. Early discovery of iron ingestion may allow administration of specific antidotal therapy (deferoxamine) before the development of significant toxicity.

Physical findings beyond those detected by the rapid cardiopulmonary assessment may have particular value and diagnostic significance for the patient with a toxic exposure. These physical findings include changes in mental status, seizures, pupil size and response to light, skin temperature and moisture, and presence or absence of bowel sounds. The characteristic clinical manifestations of a specific poisoning or toxin are called a *toxidrome*. For example, dilated pupils, sweaty skin, tachycardia, seizures, and the presence of bowel sounds indicate the possibility of a sympathomimetic overdose, such as that caused by cocaine. On the other hand, a patient with dilated pupils, *dry* skin, tachycardia, seizures, and *no* bowel sounds may have an anticholinergic overdose.

Protection of the airway is extremely important. Many toxins cause respiratory failure by depression of respiratory drive (eg, opiates), hypoperfusion of the central nervous system (CNS), or direct toxic effects on the pulmonary system. Toxins may also affect oxygenation by causing alveolar hypoventilation (eg, opiate intoxication[17]) or direct pulmonary toxicity (eg, tricyclic antidepressants[18]). Table 1 gives examples of these mechanisms and toxic agents that cause decreased oxygenation in poisoned patients. The 5 major toxins addressed in this chapter appear in bold type in the table.

Prehospital providers experienced in tracheal intubation and emergency physicians should consider intubating poisoned patients *earlier* than they would intubate patients with no history of ingestion. Early elective intubation is helpful because poisoned patients are at high risk for progressive or sudden respiratory failure. Subsequent priorities for the support of airway, oxygenation, and ventilation include reversing the effects of the toxin (if possible) and preventing further absorption of the agent. Knowledge of the potential agent or recognition of characteristic clinical signs (toxidromes) for a particular toxin can be key to successful resuscitation.

Poisoned patients may also need anticipatory or emergent tracheal intubation to reduce the risk of aspiration. During initial examination most poisoned patients are still "awake" but confused; they resist manipulation of their airway. If the patient requires intubation, an experienced paramedic or emergency physician may need to induce neuromuscular paralysis to facilitate the procedure. You may be able to effectively support some patients with bag-mask (manual) ventilation. But even this procedure has attendant complications, particularly in the poisoned patient with a full stomach.

When you select agents for sedation and paralysis for tracheal intubation, you must consider the patient's cardiovascular function, pharmacology of the agent, and the possibility of interactions with the toxin (see Chapter 14: "Rapid Sequence Intubation"). For example, organophosphate insecticides can inhibit production of acetylcholinesterase and plasma cholinesterase enzymes. This deficiency prolongs the

TABLE 1. Mechanisms of Decreased Oxygenation in Poisoning

Mechanism	Examples of Toxic Etiology
Alveolar hypoventilation (increased CO_2 with normal $AaDO_2$)	**Opiates**, clonidine, **TCAs**, benzodiazepines, and barbiturates
Ventilation-perfusion mismatch (includes ARDS)	Aspiration of gastric contents, aspiration of hydrocarbons, pulmonary embolism (IV drugs of abuse), and direct pulmonary toxicity with ARDS (eg, **TCAs, calcium channel blockers**)
Shunting	Pneumothorax due to **cocaine**, internal jugular injections ("pocket shots") of **heroin,** and iron intoxication
Diffusion abnormality	Chlorine gas inhalation
Decrease in alveolar oxygen content	Simple asphyxiants: CO_2, methane, inhalants (propane, butane, fluorocarbons), and nitrogen oxides

$AaDO_2$ indicates alveolar-arterial oxygen difference; ARDS, acute respiratory distress syndrome; and TCAs, tricyclic antidepressants.

half-life of succinylcholine, prolonging paralysis. A 1987 case report described persistent paralysis (3 hours, 15 minutes) after administration of succinylcholine to a child with organophosphate poisoning.[19]

Vecuronium and rocuronium (nondepolarizing paralytic agents) are useful for emergency intubation of poisoned patients. These drugs have minimal cardiovascular side effects. Onset of action is short (60 to 90 seconds for rocuronium, slightly longer for vecuronium), and duration of action is relatively brief (30 to 60 minutes for rocuronium, 30 to 90 minutes for vecuronium). Use of sedatives with a brief duration of action will enable you to assess the patient's mental status as soon as possible.

If poisoned patients demonstrate effective spontaneous breathing during prehospital transport and in the ED, it may be prudent to place them on their left side in a recovery position. Some authors recommend the *left* lateral decubitus position to reduce absorption of ingested substances.[20] The lateral decubitus position may also reduce the risk of aspiration.

Gastrointestinal Decontamination

Decontamination of the patient is an issue for both prehospital and Emergency Department personnel. Fresh air and skin decontamination may be of tremendous value in cases of toxic inhalation or skin exposure. Rescuers should be careful to avoid contaminating themselves when treating victims with inhalational or dermal toxic exposure (eg, organophosphate insecticides). You can rinse off most common toxic dermal agents with soap and water. But for some toxins you must follow unique decontamination procedures as advised by "hazmat" (hazardous materials) protocols or consultation with a regional poison center and medical toxicologist.

If the patient can maintain his/her airway and does not require invasive airway procedures, the emergency provider must consider the risks and benefits of administering some form of gastrointestinal decontamination. Most EMS systems follow local protocols for poisoning victims. Paramedics have specific transport and treatment policies and procedures to follow in cases of pediatric injuries, illnesses, and poisonings. EMS personnel typically transport poisoned patients to the nearest Emergency Department. Prehospital personnel or their medical control can obtain valuable information about management of specific exposures and toxicities from their regional poison center. After stabilization it may be beneficial to refer such patients to a center with pediatric expertise.

There have been recent attempts to certify "toxicology treatment centers" where medical toxicologists and specialized equipment and laboratory services can provide diagnostic and treatment services beyond the scope available in most hospitals. Most communities do not have ready access to such a facility. Poisoned *children* with life-threatening complications should ideally receive care at a children's hospital or Emergency Department Approved for Pediatrics (EDAP facility).

Prehospital personnel should not administer anything to the poisoned patient by mouth unless advised by a poison control center or their medical control. Administration of oral fluids for dilution purposes is of no benefit in most poisonings. Prehospital providers should give at-risk patients *nothing per mouth* (maintain "NPO") during transport and observation. This approach will reduce the likelihood of aspiration if mental status deteriorates.

Gastrointestinal decontamination (eg, syrup of ipecac, toxin adsorption by activated charcoal or whole-bowel irrigation) has *not* been shown to change outcome, defined as morbidity, mortality, cost, or length of hospital stay.[21]

Syrup of Ipecac

At this time there is insufficient data to support or exclude administration of syrup of ipecac to induce vomiting in poisoning victims.[22] Because of the potential danger of aspiration and the lack of evidence of benefit, you should not administer ipecac unless specifically directed by a poison control center or other authority (eg, local Emergency Department physician). Ipecac is most effective when it is given within 30 minutes of ingestion. This therapy is appropriate only for ingestion of certain low-risk substances and *only* for victims who are alert and responsive. The decontamination effects of ipecac reported in human studies[22] are not always applicable to poisoned patients because the subjects (volunteers) were given nontoxic drugs. Ipecac is *not* recommended after ingestion of the 5 serious categories of drugs reviewed in this chapter.

Activated Charcoal

Activated charcoal adsorbs numerous compounds, including many drugs, in various degrees.[23] Toxicology experts recently reviewed 115 randomized, controlled trials of activated charcoal conducted in volunteers. Forty-three drugs (including β-blockers and tricyclic antidepressants) were studied in the trials. Activated charcoal reduced the mean bioavailability of the drugs by 69.1% when it was given *within 30 minutes* after drug administration or ingestion.[24] The bioavailability, however, was reduced by only 34.4% when activated charcoal was given 60 minutes or more after drug administration.

Some authors have explored the potential time savings of prehospital administration of activated charcoal.[25,26] If activated charcoal could be provided immediately (within the first 30 minutes) after exposure in the prehospital setting, it would more effectively diminish the amount of toxin absorbed. But activated charcoal can be difficult to administer and unpalatable even under more controlled circumstances. Some clinicians do mix activated charcoal with a sweet drink (eg, chocolate milk) to make it more palatable. Nonetheless most toxicologists and poison centers do not recommend prehospital administration of activated charcoal.

In the Emergency Department activated charcoal may be useful in the treatment of some poisonings. Consider use of activated charcoal if the patient ingested a potentially toxic amount of poison within 1 hour of presentation. There is insufficient data to support or exclude its use more than 1 hour after ingestion.[24] Most children and adolescents present more than an hour after ingestion. A delayed presentation is particularly likely if the patient ingested a sustained-release product (eg, a calcium channel antagonist) because these products often do not produce serious symptoms for several hours.

The optimal dose of activated charcoal has not been established in controlled human trials. The American Academy of Clinical Toxicology and European Association of Poisons Centres and Clinical Toxicologists recommend the following oral doses[24]:

- Children up to 1 year of age: 1 g/kg
- Children 1 to 12 years of age: 25 to 50 g
- Adolescents and adults: 25 to 100 g

Clinicians administering activated charcoal should ensure that the patient has a patent, stable airway. An awake and responsive patient may be able to maintain his/her own airway and protective reflexes. If the patient is obtunded, you should establish a protected airway with tracheal intubation.

Contraindications to the administration of activated charcoal include an unprotected airway and a gastrointestinal tract that is not anatomically intact. You should not administer activated charcoal if it might increase the risk and severity of aspiration (eg, after ingestion of hydrocarbons with high aspiration potential). Although clinicians have used multiple-dose activated charcoal to treat tricyclic antidepressant ingestion for many years, there are potential complications.[27] If the toxic agent slows gastrointestinal motility (eg, tricyclic antidepressants, calcium channel blockers, and opiates), administration of activated charcoal may lead to complications, including regurgitation

and aspiration. Securing the airway with a tracheal tube before administration of activated charcoal reduces the incidence of aspiration,[28] but it does not prevent aspiration.

Gastric Lavage

Although emergency personnel have used gastric lavage for years, there is no convincing evidence that it improves clinical outcome. It may cause significant morbidity, including an increased incidence of aspiration.[29] Gastric lavage may be indicated in patients who ingest life-threatening toxins such as tricyclic antidepressants and present soon after ingestion.

Complications of lavage tube placement include hypoxia,[30] tension pneumothorax and charcoal-containing empyema,[31] and esophageal[32] and gastrointestinal perforation.[33] Lavage tubes inserted to excessive depths may distend the stomach to the confines of the pelvis.[34] A blinded, randomized trial comparing standard external landmark techniques for estimation of tube insertion depth and a patient length-based graphic model found that the graphic method was a more reliable technique for placing tubes in the stomach.[35]

Antidotes

After you apply the basic PALS principles (assessment and support of airway, ventilation, and circulation), you may need to provide antidotal therapy. Use of true antidotes as defined by the International Programme for Chemical Safety (IPCS) is relatively infrequent in pediatric resuscitation. Naloxone is a classic antidote that effectively reverses opiate toxicity. The IPCS classifies naloxone as an A1 agent (A: should be available within 30 minutes or less; 1: effectiveness is well documented).[36,37] The following sections discuss the management of specific poisonings, including the use of specific antidotes where appropriate.

Management of Specific Poisonings

Many ingestions, particularly in adolescents, are mixed exposures ("polypharmacy" overdoses). PALS providers should

be prepared to manage multiple complications of toxic ingestions. A careful history, examination, and drug screens may offer clues to unknown and potential ingestions.

During the Guidelines 2000 Evidence Evaluation Conference, experts reviewed evidence related to the management of 5 types of poisonings. This section includes the recommendations from this conference.

Cocaine

Epidemiology, Pathophysiology, and Clinical Manifestations

Cocaine has complex pharmacologic effects. The route of administration and the form of cocaine affect the onset, duration, and magnitude of these effects.[38] Cocaine is absorbed from all mucous membranes and from the gastrointestinal tract (most common in pediatric unintentional exposure) and genitourinary tract in adults. It is absorbed in the hydrochloride or base form.[39]

Cocaine use may lead to violent fatal injuries in part because of its neurobehavioral effects. In a study of 14 843 adolescents and young adults (age 15 to 44 years) who died of fatal injuries during a 3-year period, 26.7% had the cocaine metabolite benzoylecgonine in their blood or urine; 18.3% had free cocaine. Two thirds of these deaths were due to homicide, suicide, motor vehicle crashes, or falls.[40] In a 20-month prospective, age-matched, controlled study, 34% of adolescent trauma victims tested positive for alcohol or drugs of abuse. The number of positive screens was significantly higher in the trauma group (22 of 65) than the control group (1 of 49) (P <.001). The most commonly detected drugs were alcohol (8), benzodiazepines (8), cocaine (5), and cannabinoids (4).[41]

Children who unintentionally ingest cocaine can present with multiple medical conditions, including altered sensorium, seizures, tachycardia, shock, and cardiovascular compromise. The toxic effects primarily affect the central nervous system, cardiovascular system, and respiratory system in a common 3-phase pattern of early and advanced stimulation and then depression. These phases can occur in rapid succession with death occurring in minutes after a significant overdose. Crack cocaine is considered the most potent and addictive form of the drug; it is also the form that small children may ingest. Ingestion of a small "rock" of crack cocaine by a child may result in toxic manifestations; ingestion of the same amount by an adult is unlikely to produce toxicity.

Cocaine is rapidly metabolized by plasma and hepatic cholinesterases into water-soluble, renally excreted metabolites (mainly benzoylecgonine and ecgonine methyl ester). The parent compound of cocaine has a relatively short half-life. Because cocaine is rapidly metabolized, serum levels are of little use and generally do not correlate with clinical findings.[42] Table 2 summarizes the pharmacokinetics and pharmacodynamics of cocaine hydrochloride.

Cocaine binds to the reuptake pump in presynaptic nerves, blocking the uptake of norepinephrine, dopamine, epinephrine, and serotonin from the synaptic cleft. This action leads to local accumulation of these neurotransmitters (see Figure 2), which produces both peripheral and central nervous system effects depending on which receptors are being activated.

FIGURE 2. Effect of cocaine on presynaptic nerves. Cocaine blocks the uptake of norepinephrine, dopamine, epinephrine, and serotonin from the synaptic cleft. This action leads to local accumulation of these neurotransmitters, which produces adrenergic, dopaminergic, and serotonin effects on the peripheral and central nervous systems. Adapted from Lange RA, Hillis LD. Cardiovascular complications of cocaine use. *N Engl J Med.* 2001;345:351-358.[43]

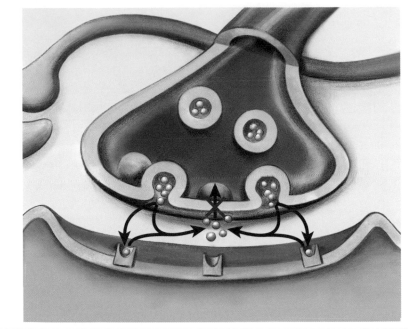

Accumulation of norepinephrine and epinephrine at β-adrenergic receptors results in tachycardia, increased myocardial contractility, tremor, diaphoresis, and mydriasis. The tachycardia increases myocardial oxygen demand while reducing the time for diastolic coronary perfusion.[43] Vasoconstriction and resultant hypertension develop from the accumulation of neurotransmitters at peripheral α-adrenergic receptors. Animal models suggest that vasoconstriction may result from impairment of the peripheral endothelial nitric oxide system.[44] Centrally mediated dopaminergic effects include mood elevation and movement disorders. Centrally mediated stimulation of serotonin (ie, 5-hydroxytryptamine or 5-HT) receptors results in exhilaration, hallucinations, and hyperthermia. Stimulation of peripheral 5-HT receptors results in coronary artery vasospasm.

In adults the most frequent cause of cocaine-induced hospitalization is acute coronary syndrome (ACS) producing chest pain and a variety of cardiac rhythm disturbances.[43,45,46] Although rare in children, cases of acute coronary artery spasm in young people with angiographically normal coronary arteries have been reported in association with ethanol and cocaine abuse.[47] Acute coronary syndrome results from the combined effects of cocaine: stimulation of β-adrenergic myocardial receptors increases myocardial oxygen

TABLE 2. Pharmacokinetics and Pharmacodynamics of Cocaine Hydrochloride

Route	Onset of Symptoms	Peak Effects	Peak Plasma Levels	Duration	Half-Life
Intranasal	5 min	20 min	20-60 min	≥30 min	16-87 min
Intravenous	2 min	5-10 min	3-5 min	30 min	54 min
Oral			50-90 min		48-78 min
Topical to mucous membranes	1 min	5 min	15-120 min	≥30 min	

demand, and the α-adrenergic and 5-HT agonist actions of cocaine cause coronary artery constriction, leading to ischemia. Cocaine also stimulates platelet aggregation and causes an increase in both platelet factor 4 and betathromboglobulin.[48] Cocaine-induced increases in circulating epinephrine may lead to secondary platelet activation.[49] Cocaine blocks reuptake of various amines, and it is a fast (ie, voltage-dependent) sodium channel inhibitor.[38] Sodium channel blockade prolongs propagation of the action potential and thus the QRS interval; it also impairs myocardial contractility.[50,51] Through the combination of adrenergic stimulation and sodium channel blockade, cocaine may cause a variety of tachyarrhythmias, including wide-complex arrhythmias, VT, and VF (see Critical Concepts: "Recognition and Management of Cocaine Toxicity").

Cocaine-induced ACS can lead to myocardial ischemia and subsequent infarction. Cardiovascular complications resulting from cocaine-associated myocardial infarction (CAMI) include ventricular arrhythmias (4% to 17% of patients hospitalized with CAMI), congestive heart failure (5% to 7% with CAMI), and death (<2% with CAMI).[52]

Management

Initial treatment of cocaine toxicity consists of oxygen administration, continuous ECG monitoring, administration of a benzodiazepine (eg, diazepam or lorazepam; Class IIb, LOE 5, 6), and administration of aspirin and heparin (see Critical Concepts: "Recognition and Management of Cocaine Toxicity").[53] You should begin continuous ECG monitoring and monitor for ventricular arrhythmias. A substantial amount of animal data shows that benzodiazepine administration is important for several reasons.[54,55] These drugs have anticonvulsant and CNS-depressant effects. Benzodiazepines reduce heart rate and systemic arterial pressure, and they appear to attenuate the toxic myocardial and CNS effects of cocaine.[43] Phenothiazines and butyrophenones (eg, haloperidol) provide no benefit and may be harmful to patients with cocaine toxidromes.

Critical Concepts:
Recognition and Management of Cocaine Toxicity

Clinical Signs

- **CNS:** Mood elevation, exhilaration, movement disorder, hallucinations, and hyperthermia.
- **CV/ECG:** Acute coronary syndrome (including coronary artery vasoconstriction, myocardial ischemia, and acute chest pain), ventricular tachyarrhythmias, prolonged QRS and QT intervals, impaired myocardial contractility, peripheral vasoconstriction, and hypertension.

Treatment

- Support airway, ventilation, and oxygenation.
- Provide continuous ECG monitoring until stable; treat symptomatic or unstable arrhythmias.
- Administer benzodiazepines.
- Treat acute coronary syndromes with oxygen and nitroglycerin.
- Administer aspirin and heparin.
- Do not administer β-blockers.

If ACS (chest pain with possible myocardial ischemia) develops, administer nitroglycerin (see below). Some experts give aspirin and heparin in an attempt to reverse the platelet-activating effects of cocaine and the biochemical manifestations of a procoagulant state. But this treatment has not been evaluated in clinical trials. For *adult* patients with ACS, the mnemonic "MONA greets all patients" reminds providers to give **M**orphine, **O**xygen, **N**itroglycerin, and **A**spirin. Pediatric patients with cocaine-induced ACS should also receive oxygen, nitroglycerin, and aspirin; you may administer morphine to adolescents with severe chest pain caused by ACS. In patients with cocaine-induced ACS, benzodiazepines are an important addition to this therapy.

Identification of patients with cocaine-induced myocardial infarction is difficult for several reasons. First, the ECG is abnormal in most patients with cocaine-related chest pain (56% to 84%). It is more accurate in *ruling out* an infarction than in confirming one. The sensitivity of ECGs in detecting myocardial infarction is only 36%; specificity is 90% (positive predictive value is 18%; negative predictive value is 96%).[45] This high failure rate is a result of the high rate of repolarization abnormalities in the general population of young adults. These abnormalities complicate ECG interpretation in this age group. Second, rhabdomyolysis causes an increase in the serum creatinine kinase concentration in approximately half of cocaine users who do not have myocardial infarction. If you suspect cocaine-related myocardial infarction, evaluate the serum troponin concentrations. These proteins are a more sensitive indicator of infarction.[43]

β-Adrenergic blockers are recommended for treatment of ACS and myocardial ischemia in adults.[56] But they are *contraindicated* for ACS caused by cocaine intoxication (Class III; LOE 5, 6, 7). In both animals[57] and humans[58,59] the addition of a β-adrenergic blocker results in increased blood pressure and coronary artery constriction. These adverse pharmacologic effects are produced by antagonizing cocaine-induced β-adrenergic receptor stimulation. This β-adrenergic action normally causes vasodilation and counteracts the cocaine-induced increased stimulation of vasoconstricting α-adrenergic receptors. Although labetalol has mixed α- and β-adrenergic blocking actions, the β-adrenergic blocking actions dominate. This agent is not useful in the treatment of cocaine-induced ACS.[60]

Coronary vasospasm may respond to nitroglycerin (Class IIa; LOE 5, 6).[61,62] Intravenous doses of nitroglycerin for children with this condition have not been studied. But the dose used for pulmonary hypertension may be reasonable. Continuous infusions starting at 0.25 to 0.5 µg/kg per minute and titrated up by

1 μg/kg per minute at 20- to 60-minute intervals to desired effect (usual dose 1 to 3 μg/kg per minute; maximum 5 μg/kg per minute) have been recommended for children.[63] To reverse coronary vasoconstriction, you may consider administration of the α-adrenergic blocker phentolamine. But you should administer this drug *after* oxygen, benzodiazepines, and nitroglycerin[53,64] (Class IIb; LOE 5, 6). The optimal dose of phentolamine is unknown. There is a risk of significant hypotension and tachycardia if excessive doses are used. So begin with a small intravenous infusion and titrate doses to effect. You may infuse additional doses if you document ongoing hypertension or evidence of myocardial ischemia. Suggested doses for hypertension in a child are 0.05 to 0.1 mg/kg IM or IV up to a maximum of 2.5 to 5 mg as recommended in adults.[65] You may repeat the dose every 5 to 10 minutes until blood pressure is under control.

Sodium bicarbonate may be useful in the treatment of cocaine toxicity. Because cocaine is a sodium channel blocker, sodium bicarbonate in a dose of 1 to 2 mEq/kg may be effective in the treatment of ventricular arrhythmias. In an experimental model of cocaine-induced ECG changes, anesthetized dogs received cocaine injections and either sodium chloride or sodium bicarbonate. Although sodium chloride did not reverse ECG abnormalities (prolonged PR, corrected QT, and QRS duration), sodium bicarbonate significantly ($P <0.05$) reduced these effects.[51] In one human case series, acidemia appeared to contribute to cocaine toxicity by promoting intraventricular conduction delays (prolonged QRS interval), arrhythmias, and depressed myocardial contractility.[66] Sodium bicarbonate may be clinically useful because it prevents or treats acidosis. Although data from controlled human studies is lacking, theoretical considerations and animal data[67,68] support the use of sodium bicarbonate for ventricular arrhythmias (Class IIb; LOE 5, 6, 7).

The effectiveness of lidocaine in the management of cocaine-induced ACS is questionable. Lidocaine, a local anesthetic that inhibits fast sodium channels, potentiates cocaine toxicity in animals.[69] Cocaine and lidocaine together may have additive effects by depressing γ-aminobutyric acid (GABA) current in CNS neurons, increasing the likelihood of seizure activity.[70] Nevertheless investigators have not documented adverse effects from lidocaine administration, although clinical experience is limited.[71] You may consider lidocaine administration for patients with cocaine-induced myocardial infarction (Class IIb; LOE 5, 6).

Epinephrine may exacerbate cocaine-induced arrhythmias,[72] and it is contraindicated for ventricular arrhythmias (Class III; LOE 6). But if VF or pulseless VT occurs, you may use epinephrine to increase coronary perfusion pressure during CPR (Class Indeterminate).

Animal experiments show that hyperthermia is associated with a significant increase in cocaine toxicity, including seizures.[73] In animals it appears that dopamine DA-1 receptors are involved in cocaine-induced hyperthermia.[74] Some researchers hypothesize that disruption of dopaminergic function is involved in the pathogenesis of cocaine-induced thermoregulatory problems in humans.[75] High ambient temperature has been associated with a significant increase in mortality due to cocaine overdose in humans.[76] For these reasons you should cool children presenting with agitation, delirium, seizures, and elevated body temperature due to unintentional cocaine ingestion.

Cocaine may produce seizures in infants and children after ingestion of the drug itself[77,78] or transmission through breast milk.[79] To manage seizures you should administer a benzodiazepine such as lorazepam; diazepam and midazolam may also be effective. Some pediatric emergency medicine specialists use lorazepam at 0.05 to 0.1 mg/kg (up to 2 mg per dose) and repeat doses as needed. You should monitor patients for respiratory depression after you give benzodiazepines to manage prolonged cocaine-induced seizures.

Flumazenil can unmask seizures; you should *not* use flumazenil to reverse benzodiazepine-induced respiratory depression in patients with cocaine intoxication.

Small children who ingest crack cocaine may present with shock and cardiovascular collapse.[80] Some apparent life-threatening events (ALTEs) may be caused by a number of toxins, including cocaine. In one series of 9 infants with ALTEs, urine drug screens detected cocaine and opiates (codeine, meperidine, and methadone) among other agents.[81] Four of the 9 infants required CPR.

Myocardial infarction in the neonate with a structurally normal heart and coronary arteries is rare, but researchers have reported an association with maternal cocaine abuse.[82] Investigators have statistically correlated maternal use of cocaine with premature rupture of membranes and placental abruption.[83] Infants also may be exposed to cocaine in breast milk[84] or through passive inhalation of vapors from adults smoking crack cocaine.[85] The presence of the cocaine metabolite benzoylecgonine in the urine of infants who are otherwise medically stable may reflect passive inhalation; it does not necessarily indicate poisoning or intentional cocaine administration.[86] This situation raises legitimate concern for the well-being of such infants; 16 infant deaths have been reported to be associated with passive inhalation of crack cocaine smoke.[87] For this reason PALS providers should consider cocaine as an etiologic or contributory factor when assessing, caring for, or attempting resuscitation of infants, children, and adolescents presenting with a wide variety of medical conditions or injuries.

Tricyclic Antidepressants and Other Sodium Channel Blocking Agents

Epidemiology, Pathophysiology, and Clinical Manifestations

Tricyclic (cyclic) antidepressants continue to be a leading cause of morbidity and mortality despite the increasing availability of safer selective serotonin reuptake inhibitors for the treatment of depression. A total of 13 870 ingestions and 111 deaths caused by all cyclic antidepressants were reported to the AAPCC in 2000.[1] Tricyclic antidepressants are currently used to treat depression and a wide variety of disorders in children and adolescents. These other disorders include attention deficit hyperactivity syndrome, migraine headaches, neuropathic pain, cyclic vomiting syndrome, nocturnal enuresis, and sleep disturbances.

Experts are uncertain if these expanding indications for tricyclic antidepressants have magnified the risk of exposure to children. In one recent study both the number of prescriptions for and the number of poisonings due to tricyclic antidepressants increased significantly between two 4-year periods (1988 to 1992 and 1993 to 1997).[88] Most of these ingestions resulted from prescriptions written for extended family members (eg, grandparents). Investigators in England and Wales also reported an increase in the rate of death due to antidepressant poisoning between 1993 and 1997. Those investigators correlated this increased death rate with a more than 3-fold increase in prescriptions for these drugs.[89]

Generally the more high-risk substances there are in a family's environment, the more likely an exposure will occur, assuming all other factors remain unchanged. Clinicians caring for children should be prepared for these poisonings. To reduce the risk of ingestions, physicians caring for children should discuss with caretakers strategies to reduce poisonings such as those due to tricyclic antidepressants.[90]

Other sodium channel blockers include β-adrenergic blockers (particularly propranolol and sotalol), procainamide, quinidine, local anesthetics (eg, lidocaine), carbamazepine, type I_C antiarrhythmics (eg, flecainide and encainide), and cocaine (see above).[50] A common antihistamine, diphenhydramine, can produce prominent sodium channel blocker effects; it causes wide-complex tachyarrhythmias with significant overdoses.[91]

PALS providers who encounter a child with an altered level of consciousness should consider toxin ingestion as a potential cause. For example, doxepin, a cyclic antidepressant, is a component of a topical cream for eczema. An excessive amount could be absorbed if the cream were applied to large areas of a child's skin.[92] A child also could ingest the cream. A caretaker could poison a child but conceal the source of the tricyclic antidepressant (ie, Munchausen syndrome by proxy).[93]

The therapeutic effects of tricyclic antidepressants may take weeks to manifest; toxic effects generally appear within 4 hours of ingestion. The clinical toxicity of these agents results from their 3 major side effects: anticholinergic effects, excessive blockade of norepinephrine reuptake at the postganglionic synapse, and direct sodium channel blockade and quinidine-like effects on the myocardium. Experts have yet to agree on a distinct and well-recognized toxidrome for tricyclic antidepressants. But in general the symptoms consist of **C**oma, **C**onvulsions (seizures), **C**ardiac arrhythmias, and in some cases **A**cidosis. Helpful mnemonics to remember these symptoms are **Three C's, Three C's and an A,** or simply **TCA,** the acronym for tricyclic antidepressant.

Patients may present with symptoms of early CNS stimulation before arrhythmias develop (see Critical Concepts: "Recognition and Management of Tricyclic Antidepressant Toxicity"). These symptoms and signs are likely caused by the anticholinergic effects of the tricyclic antidepressant and include agitation, irritability, confusion, delirium, hallucinations, choreoathetosis, hyperactivity, seizures, and hyperpyrexia.[94] Sinus tachycardia, hypertension, and supraventricular tachycardia may also develop early after ingestion, probably as a result of excessive norepinephrine. These effects are usually short lived, and catecholamine depletion develops because norepinephrine reuptake into neurons is inhibited and the released norepinephrine is metabolized by catechol-*O*-methyltransferase and monoamine oxidase.

The primary toxicity of tricyclic antidepressants results from the inhibition of fast (voltage-dependent) sodium channels in the brain and myocardium. This action is similar to that of other "membrane-stabilizing" agents (also called "quinidine-like" or "local anesthetics").

With serious intoxication, rhythm disturbances result from prolongation of the action potential by inhibition of phase 0 of the action potential. This inhibition causes delayed intraventricular conduction with QRS prolongation (particularly the terminal 40 ms)[95] and a QRS duration ≥100 milliseconds.[96] The presence of these ECG abnormalities may be predictive of seizures and ventricular arrhythmias,[97] but some investigators have not observed this predictive effect.[96,98] Researchers recently reported that an R wave in lead aVR ≥3 mm or an R wave/S wave ratio in lead aVR ≥0.7 is a superior predictor of severe toxicity.[99,100]

Tricyclic antidepressants also inhibit potassium channels, leading to prolongation of the QT interval (see Figure 3). Through blockade of both sodium and potassium channels, high concentrations of tricyclic antidepressants (and other sodium channel blockers) may result in preterminal sinus bradycardia and heart block with junctional or ventricular wide-complex escape beats.[50]

Management

To treat sodium channel blocker toxicity, protect the airway, ensure adequate oxygenation and ventilation, establish continuous ECG monitoring, and treat arrhythmias with sodium bicarbonate (Class IIa; LOE 5, 6, 7). Infuse sodium bicarbonate only after you establish an effective airway and adequate ventilation (see Critical Concepts: "Recognition and Management of Tricyclic Antidepressant Toxicity"). Sodium bicarbonate narrows the QRS complex, shortens the QT interval, and increases myocardial contractility. These actions often suppress ventricular arrhythmias and reverse hypotension.[101,102] Experimental data suggests that the antiarrhythmic effect of sodium

FIGURE 3. Sinus tachycardia with wide QRS complex and prolonged QT interval caused by tricyclic antidepressant overdose.

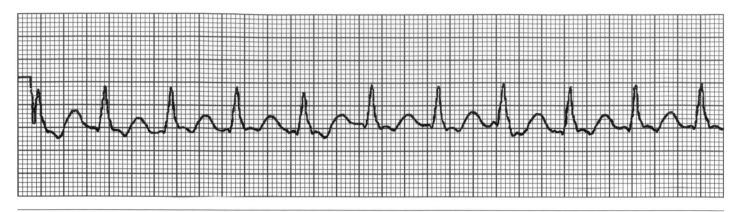

Critical Concepts: Recognition and Management of Tricyclic Antidepressant Toxicity

Clinical Signs

(Remember the mnemonic **Three C's and an A.**)

- **CNS:** Coma, convulsions, agitation, irritability, confusion, delirium, hallucinations, seizures, and hyperpyrexia.

- **CV/ECG:** Cardiac arrhythmias, prolonged action potential, preterminal sinus bradycardia and heart block with junctional or ventricular wide-complex tachycardia or ventricular fibrillation, and possible acidosis and hypotension.

- **Respiratory:** Pulmonary edema, acute lung injury, and possible hypoxemia.

Treatment

- Support airway, ventilation, and oxygenation.

- Provide continuous ECG monitoring until stable. Treat symptomatic or unstable arrhythmias.

- Establish vascular access and treat arrhythmias and shock.

- Administer sodium bicarbonate to treat ventricular arrhythmias. Maintain pH >7.45 (for severe intoxications titrate to keep pH between 7.5 and 7.55).

- If hypotension is present, administer normal saline boluses (10 mL/kg). Monitor for pulmonary edema.

- If hypotension persists, administer a vasopressor.

bicarbonate results from overcoming sodium channel blockade with hypertonic sodium, although the production of alkalosis may be important for some of these agents.[102,103] For example, the percentage of free amitriptyline (potentially available for toxicity) decreases significantly at pH levels achieved by induced alkalosis.[104]

The goal of sodium bicarbonate therapy is to raise the sodium concentration and arterial pH. These increases can be achieved by administering 1 to 2 mEq/kg bolus infusions of sodium bicarbonate until the arterial pH is ≥7.45. After bolus administration sodium bicarbonate may be infused as a solution of 150 mEq $NaHCO_3$ per liter in D_5W titrated to maintain alkalosis. For severe intoxications experts recommend increasing pH to a level between 7.50 and 7.55; higher pH values are not recommended because of the risk of adverse effects.[50,105]

Although hyperventilation-induced alkalosis reportedly improves cardiac conduction,[106] its overall role is unclear.[102] Its benefit may be related to the specific agent ingested.[103] Excessive alkalosis (pH ≥7.6) can develop with combined hyperventilation and intravenous sodium bicarbonate, but the exact causal relationship between arterial pH and any adverse effects remains uncertain.[107] Maintenance of at least normal ventilation is recommended while the pH is raised with sodium bicarbonate administration.

If ventricular arrhythmias do not respond to sodium bicarbonate, you may consider lidocaine. Some investigators argue against use of lidocaine because it is also a sodium channel blocker[69] (Class IIb; LOE 6, 7). Class I_A (quinidine, procainamide) and Class I_C (flecainide, propafenone) antiarrhythmics are contraindicated because they may exacerbate cardiac toxicity (Class III; LOE 6, 8). Class III antiarrhythmics (amiodarone, sotalol) prolong the QT interval; they are also not indicated.[105]

If hypotension is present, administer normal saline boluses (10 mL/kg each) in addition to sodium bicarbonate. Experts recommend more cautious administration of fluid (ie, 10 mL/kg bolus instead of the standard 20 mL/kg bolus) because antidepressants and other sodium channel blocking drugs have myocardial depressant effects. You may repeat this smaller bolus if needed while you carefully monitor the patient's response.

Tricyclic antidepressants block reuptake of norepinephrine at the neuromuscular junction, leading to catecholamine depletion. As a result you may need to administer a vasopressor to maintain adequate vascular tone and blood pressure. Norepinephrine and epinephrine can be effective vasopressors[108]; in an animal model epinephrine and norepinephrine were equally effective, although epinephrine had fewer arrhythmogenic properties.

Anecdotal data supports treatment with norepinephrine rather than dopamine.[109,110] The superiority of norepinephrine over dopamine presumably is due to catecholamine depletion. This catecholamine depletion reduces the hemodynamic effects of dopamine, which partly depend on releasable stores of norepinephrine.[111] Pure β-adrenergic agonists (eg, dobutamine and isoproterenol) are contraindicated because they may worsen hypotension by causing vasodilation.

If vasopressors are insufficient to maintain blood pressure, extracorporeal membrane oxygenation (ECMO) and cardiopulmonary bypass may be effective.[112,113] But these therapies require rapid availability of equipment and trained personnel. Early identification of at-risk patients is important to enable possible referral to a center capable of providing these therapies.

Providers must carefully manage seizures caused by tricyclic antidepressant poisoning in children. Seizures may complicate arrhythmias and cardiac toxicity. In one retrospective study pediatric patients who ingested tricyclic antidepressants and presented with seizures had an increased risk of conduction delays and cardiac arrhythmias.[114]

When considering the differential diagnosis of toxin-induced seizures, remember that tricyclic antidepressants are one of the most common causes. Seizures are more common with amoxapine (a second-generation tricyclic antidepressant) and maprotiline (a tetracyclic antidepressant) than with other tricyclic antidepressants.[115] Authors of a retrospective review of 191

cases of drug-related seizures reported that many were caused by cyclic antidepressants (55 cases, 29%). Other implicated agents were cocaine and other stimulants (55 cases, 29%), diphenhydramine and other antihistamines (14 cases, 7%), theophylline (10 cases, 5%), and isoniazid (10 cases, 5%).[116] The metabolic acidosis associated with seizures may cause hypotension by one or more mechanisms: direct cardiotoxicity, an increase in bioavailability of the tricyclic antidepressant caused by changes in protein binding, or an alteration of the effects of tricyclic antidepressant on cardiac membrane sodium channels.

Initial management of seizures caused by tricyclic antidepressants includes administration of benzodiazepines (eg, lorazepam or diazepam); careful support of the airway, oxygenation, and ventilation; and correction of acid-base disturbances. Because animal studies show increased duration and frequency of ventricular tachycardia after the use of phenytoin for amitriptyline overdose,[117] phenobarbital may be preferable to phenytoin in treating seizures refractory to benzodiazepines.

Tricyclic antidepressant overdose may cause noncardiogenic pulmonary edema and acute lung injury both in humans and in experimental models.[118,119] Children with tricyclic antidepressant overdose may present with depressed level of consciousness, risk of life-threatening arrhythmias, or seizures. The PALS provider should consider early intubation of children and adolescents who have ingested significant amounts of tricyclic antidepressants.

Intubation of at-risk patients may facilitate administration of activated charcoal. Poison centers have traditionally recommended gastric lavage for tricyclic antidepressant overdose, but clear evidence of its efficacy is lacking. If a patient ingests a potentially life-threatening amount of a tricyclic antidepressant and presents within an hour, lavage may be indicated.[29]

If there is no specific history of tricyclic antidepressant exposure but you suspect

an overdose (coma, seizures, and ventricular arrhythmias), you can use a number of bedside rapid urine immunoassays to screen for tricyclic antidepressants.[120] These screening tests are qualitative; you should confirm the results if medically or medicolegally warranted. Some immunoassays may yield false-positive results for tricyclic antidepressants if the patient ingested carbamazepine (a tricyclic structure anticonvulsant).[121] If you care for a patient with coma of unknown origin, you may capitalize on this cross-reactivity by using such an antidepressant screen to reveal carbamazepine overdose.[122] Carbamazepine may also interfere with plasma tricyclic assays.[123]

Blood concentrations of tricyclic antidepressants do not correlate well with clinical toxicity. Providers generally obtain the blood concentration only to confirm an exposure. You should base treatment decisions on clinical and ECG findings.

Calcium Channel Blocker Toxicity

Epidemiology, Pathophysiology, and Clinical Manifestations

The increasing use of calcium channel blockers for the treatment of hypertension and congestive heart failure makes them available for unintentional or intentional overdose. Although most children who unintentionally ingest calcium channel blockers respond to the supportive and specific therapies discussed in this section, some of these therapies have resulted in third-degree atrioventricular (AV) block with cardiac arrest[124] and death.[7,8] In 1999 a total of 8844 exposures to calcium channel blockers were reported to the AAPCC; 2304 of these exposures occurred in children younger than 6 years (26% of reported cases).[12]

Calcium channel blockers are classified into 3 groups on the basis of their relative effects on the myocardium and vascular smooth muscle (Table 3). But in cases of overdose these selective properties are largely inconsequential.[125] All of these agents bind to calcium channels, inhibiting the influx of calcium into cells. The transmembrane and intracellular movement of calcium affects the following:

- Impulse conduction in slow channel-dependent tissue such as the sinoatrial (SA) and AV nodes

- Coupling of myocardial excitation-contraction

- Vascular smooth muscle tone

The life-threatening clinical manifestations of toxicity due to blockade of calcium movement include bradyarrhythmias (due to inhibition of pacemaker cells and AV block) and hypotension (due to vasodilation and impaired cardiac contractility).[125,126] Electrocardiographic changes may include a prolonged PR interval, inverted P waves, AV dissociation, AV block (which may persist for 48 hours or more with amlodipine[127]), moderate ST-segment changes, low-amplitude T waves, sinus arrest, and asystole. Altered mental status (eg, syncope, seizures, and coma) may occur because of cerebral hypoperfusion.

Calcium channel blocker poisoning may affect other organ systems, including the lungs and gastrointestinal tract (see Critical Concepts: "Recognition and Management of Calcium Channel Blocker Toxicity").

These toxicities have implications for providers during advanced life support. For example, pulmonary complications such as cardiogenic or noncardiogenic pulmonary edema[128,129] may necessitate cautious fluid resuscitation and early ventilatory support.

Gastrointestinal hypomotility, ileus,[130] and constipation occur in cases of overdose; these effects may be secondary to the inhibition of gastrointestinal motility hormone release.[131] Patients with calcium channel blocker overdose often have greatly diminished or no bowel sounds. This complication may influence the use of activated charcoal or whole-bowel irrigation.

Generally you should perform careful serial examinations for bowel sounds if you provide any form of gastrointestinal decontamination, particularly if the patient ingested sustained-release products. Some experts advocate whole-bowel irrigation for patients who ingest sustained-release products to prevent further absorption. But no controlled trials have been performed to determine the effect of this intervention after calcium channel blocker overdose. A single published case report describes successful use of whole-bowel irrigation after overdose with a long-acting calcium channel blocker.[132]

Management

The initial approach to therapy for calcium channel blocker overdose is to provide oxygenation and ventilation, continuous ECG monitoring, and frequent clinical assessments. Onset of symptoms may be immediate or delayed for up to 12 to 16 hours, especially with sustained-release preparations.[133] Patients who ingest large amounts of verapamil may initially be conscious; shortly thereafter seizures and respiratory compromise requiring intubation may develop (see Critical Concepts: "Recognition and Management of Calcium Channel Blocker Toxicity").[134]

All patients with a significant overdose require close monitoring of blood pressure and hemodynamic status because severe myocardial dysfunction and hypotension may develop. Consider continuous intra-arterial blood pressure monitoring in symptomatic patients. If hypotension develops in cases of mild intoxication, normal saline bolus administration may restore blood pressure; with more severe intoxication the hypotension may be refractory to fluid administration. To prevent pulmonary edema, limit fluid boluses to 5 to 10 mL/kg and carefully reassess the patient after each bolus.

TABLE 3. Therapeutic Effects of Calcium Channel Blockers by Therapeutic Class

Effect	Phenylalkylamines (eg, verapamil)	Dihydropyridines (eg, nifedipine)	Benzothiazepines (eg, diltiazem)
Net sinus rate	0 to ↓	↑	↓
AV node conduction time	↑↑↑	0	↑↑
Peripheral arteriolar dilation	++	+++	+
Reduced blood pressure	++	+++	+
Myocardial contractility	↓↓↓	↓	↓↓
Cardiac output	0	↑↑	↑
Coronary dilation	++	+++	++

Critical Concepts: Recognition and Management of Calcium Channel Blocker Toxicity

Clinical Signs

- **CNS:** Altered mental status, including syncope, seizures, and coma caused by cerebral hypoperfusion.
- **CV/ECG:** Bradyarrhythmias (caused by inhibition of pacemaker cells and AV dissociation or AV block) and hypotension (caused by vasodilation and impaired myocardial contractility).
- **Pulmonary:** Pulmonary edema.
- **Gastrointestinal:** Ileus.

Treatment

- Support airway, ventilation, and oxygenation.
- Provide continuous ECG monitoring; treat symptomatic or unstable arrhythmias (pacing may be needed to treat bradycardia).
- Establish vascular access; treat shock if present.
  - If hypotension develops, consider normal saline bolus; provide 5 to 10 mL/kg boluses and repeat as needed. Monitor for pulmonary edema.
  - High-dose vasopressor infusion may be needed to treat bradycardia and hypotension.
  - Alternative therapies are calcium chloride, insulin plus glucose (monitor glucose concentration closely), glucagon, cardiac pacing, and extracorporeal membrane oxygenation.

Calcium is often infused to treat calcium channel blocker overdose in an attempt to overcome the channel blockade. But in case reports and one large case series, the effectiveness of this therapy varies (Class IIb; LOE 5, 6, 8).[125,135,136] Calcium chloride is the generally recommended salt because it results in greater elevation of the ionized calcium concentration.[137] The optimal dose of calcium is unclear. You may provide a dose of 20 mg/kg (0.2 mL/kg) of 10% calcium chloride infused over 5 to 10 minutes, followed by infusions of 20 to 50 mg/kg per hour if you observe a beneficial effect. Monitor the patient's serum ionized calcium to prevent toxicity due to hypercalcemia.

High-dose vasopressor therapy (norepinephrine or epinephrine) is reportedly an effective treatment for bradycardia and hypotension associated with severe calcium channel blocker toxicity (Class IIb; LOE 5).[138,139] With this therapy you must carefully monitor the patient and titrate the infusion rate to the desired hemodynamic effect.

Animal data[140,141] and 2 small case series[142,143] suggest that insulin plus glucose may be beneficial in calcium channel blocker toxicity (Class Indeterminate; LOE 5, 6). Precise dosage recommendations are unavailable. You may give a loading dose of glucose (0.5 g/kg) followed by an infusion at 0.5 g/kg per hour. After the glucose bolus an insulin bolus of 0.1 to 0.2 U/kg is suggested, followed by an infusion of 0.1 to 0.2 U/kg per hour. You may titrate infusions up to 0.5 U/kg per hour while monitoring the glucose concentration. Higher doses of glucose may be necessary if these relatively high doses of insulin are used. In general clinicians infuse 3 to 5 g of glucose for each unit of insulin; this regimen has been used safely in adults with acute myocardial infarction to improve cardiac contractility.[144] Insulin infusions of 0.3 U/kg per hour may be sufficient in many cases.

The goal of this therapy is to maintain the glucose concentration between 100 and 200 mg/dL by titrating the rate of glucose administration. Presumably the beneficial effect of combined insulin-glucose therapy results from better myocardial glucose use through activation of pyruvate dehydrogenase, which stimulates production of adenosine triphosphate through aerobic metabolism. In experimental models of verapamil poisoning, insulin administration resulted in increased myocardial uptake of both glucose and lactate and an increase in the myocardial oxygen delivery-to-work ratio.[140] Monitor glucose concentration closely to avoid hypoglycemia, the main adverse effect of this therapy. Insulin and glucose stimulate movement of potassium from the extracellular to the intracellular space; so you must closely monitor the serum potassium concentration. You may need to administer exogenous potassium to prevent or treat hypokalemia.

Laboratory data[145] and recent case reports[127,146] suggest that glucagon may be beneficial in the treatment of myocardial toxicity due to calcium channel blocker overdose. Glucagon treatment causes an increase in the concentration of cyclic adenosine monophosphate (AMP), activation of cyclic AMP-dependent protein kinase, and transient release of intracellular calcium.

Cardiac arrest after calcium channel blocker overdose is more likely with intentional ingestion of a large amount of the drug. If cardiac arrest develops, the patient will require CPR and epinephrine; cardiac pacing and extracorporeal membrane oxygenation may be useful.[147] Pediatric intensive care units have successfully used mechanical cardiopulmonary support (eg, extracorporeal membrane oxygenation, left ventricular assist device, intra-aortic balloon pumping) in the treatment of low cardiac output and cardiac arrest due to several causes.[148] Although the outcome from prolonged cardiac arrest in children is poor, aggressive care may be warranted in cases of calcium channel blocker overdose. Two case reports document recovery after prolonged verapamil-induced pulseless arrest in a young woman[149] and a 15-year-old girl.[150] Possible neuroprotective mechanisms of the calcium channel blocker were implicated.

β-Adrenergic Blocker Toxicity

Epidemiology, Pathophysiology, and Clinical Manifestations

β-Adrenergic antagonists or β-blockers are widely prescribed for a number of medical conditions. These agents are also responsible for a large number of poisonings. Intentional overdose by adolescents and adults may result in severe intoxication. One retrospective review of AAPCC data over an 11-year period (1985 through 1995) revealed 52 156 total β-blocker exposures; overdoses of these agents accounted for 2.5% of all fatalities due to poisons.[10] Investigators in a 6-year prospective cohort study of 280 β-blocker exposures reported to 2 regional poison centers found that propranolol was the most commonly ingested β-blocker (141 of 280 cases); this drug was also most frequently responsible for cardiovascular toxicity.[151] Propranolol, atenolol, or metoprolol was ingested in 87% of all exposures in this cohort.

β-Adrenergic blockers compete with norepinephrine and epinephrine at the β-adrenergic receptor, resulting in bradycardia and decreased cardiac contractility. The clinically important β-adrenergic receptors are divided into 2 subtypes, β_1 and β_2:

- β_1 receptors are located in cardiac, renal, and adipose tissue. These receptors mediate increased rate and force of myocardial contraction, renin release, and lipolysis.

- β_2 receptors are located in the liver and smooth muscle of blood vessels, trachea, bronchi, and gastrointestinal tract. Catecholamine stimulation in the liver results in increased glycogenolysis or gluconeogenesis. Catecholamine stimulation in the smooth muscle of blood vessels results in vasodilation. Such stimulation in the trachea results in tracheal relaxation. Stimulation in the bronchi results in bronchial relaxation, and catecholamine stimulation in the gastrointestinal tract results in decreased gastrointestinal tone or motility.

β-Adrenergic antagonists competitively inhibit the effects of sympathetic neurotransmitters at the receptor site. β-Blockade decreases intracellular cyclic AMP (cAMP), which diminishes the metabolic, chronotropic, and inotropic activities of the heart and other affected organs. Low intracellular cAMP concentration also decreases release of calcium from intracellular stores in the endoplasmic reticulum.[152,153] The result is a decrease in intracellular calcium ion concentration during systole and decreased calcium reuptake during diastole. These decreases depress conduction velocity and contractility, giving rise to bradycardia and conduction disturbances (eg, sinus pauses, prolonged PR interval, various degrees of heart block, intraventricular conduction defects, and prolonged QRS interval).

Arrhythmias including torsades de pointes,[154] ventricular fibrillation, and in rare cases asystole[155] may occur with severe poisoning. Acebutolol, a cardioselective β-blocker with partial agonist and membrane-stabilizing activity, is one of the most toxic β-blockers in overdose. Unlike propranolol, acebutolol may predispose the patient to ventricular repolarization abnormalities that cause ventricular arrhythmias in serious overdose.[9] In severe intoxication some β-adrenergic blockers (eg, propranolol and sotalol) have sodium channel blocking effects, leading to prolongation of the QRS and QT intervals. This effect appears to be due to inhibition of sodium entry through fast inward sodium channels with resultant slowing of phase 0 of the action potential. In one adult case study[156] administration of sodium bicarbonate was effective in the treatment of acebutolol-induced ventricular tachycardia. Hypotension, usually with bradycardia, and various degrees of heart block are common clinical manifestations of β-blocker toxicity (see Critical Concepts: "Recognition and Management of β-Adrenergic Blocker Toxicity").[152]

Altered mental status, including seizures and coma, may develop. Altered mental status is particularly likely with agents that have high lipid solubility (eg, propranolol) because these agents readily cross the blood-brain barrier.[152,157] These CNS effects are separate from the cerebral hypoperfusion that may result from systemic hypotension; they may occur in the absence of clinical signs of cardiac toxicity.[158]

Metabolic disturbances such as hypoglycemia are especially common in children. These disturbances may contribute to diminished level of consciousness. Bronchospasm and increased airway resistance may contribute to airway compromise. The PALS provider should anticipate the possible need for airway support and ventilation in patients who ingest β-blockers.

Management

The initial approach to treatment of β-blocker overdose includes providing adequate oxygenation and ventilation, assessing perfusion, establishing vascular access, and treating shock if present. Continuous ECG monitoring and frequent clinical reassessment are important. To overcome β-adrenergic blockade, epinephrine infusions may be effective,[159] although very high infusion doses may be needed[160] (Class Indeterminate; LOE 5, 6). Other high-dose adrenergic agents (eg, norepinephrine, dobutamine, isoproterenol, and dopamine) have been used successfully.[161-163] Phosphodiesterase inhibitors such as inamrinone (formerly amrinone) have been used successfully in case reports,[164] but neither inamrinone[165] nor milrinone[166] was beneficial in animal models.

Experimental data[145,152] and case reports[159,161] suggest that glucagon may be beneficial in the treatment of β-adrenergic blocker overdose (Class IIb; LOE 5, 6). In adults and adolescents you may infuse 5 to 10 mg of glucagon slowly (over several minutes); follow this dose with an IV infusion of 1 to 5 mg/h. In younger children clinicians have used bolus doses of 0.05 to 0.1 mg/kg up to 1 mg. Note that the diluent supplied by the manufacturer contains phenol. You should not use this diluent with

Critical Concepts: Recognition and Management of β-Adrenergic Blocker Toxicity

Clinical Signs

- **CNS:** Altered mental status, including seizures and coma.
- **CV/ECG:** Bradycardia with prolongation of the QRS and QT intervals and various degrees of heart block, ventricular arrhythmias, decreased cardiac contractility, and hypotension.
- **Respiratory:** Bronchospasm and increased airway resistance.
- **Electrolytes:** Hypoglycemia.

Treatment

- Support airway, ventilation, and oxygenation.

- Provide continuous ECG monitoring; treat symptomatic or unstable arrhythmias.

- Establish vascular access; treat shock if present.
  - Administer epinephrine (very high infusions may be needed).
  - Alternative therapies are glucagon, glucose plus insulin, sodium bicarbonate or calcium (if the patient is unresponsive to glucagon and catecholamines), cardiac pacing, and extracorporeal membrane oxygenation.

---

large bolus doses and subsequent continuous infusions because phenol may cause hypotension, seizures, or arrhythmias.[167] If a dose ≥2 mg is needed, reconstitute the glucagon in sterile water to a final concentration <1 mg/mL.

Glucose plus insulin may be useful. One animal study showed that glucose plus insulin was superior to glucagon (Class Indeterminate; LOE 6) for treatment of β-blocker toxicity.[168] If you observe an intraventricular conduction delay (ie, prolonged QRS interval), you may give sodium bicarbonate (see above).

β-Adrenergic blockade reduces cytoplasmic calcium concentration. Although limited animal data,[169] case reports,[170,171] and a small clinical uncontrolled case series[172] suggest that calcium administration may be beneficial, other clinical reports suggest that it has no effect on bradycardia and hypotension.[162] You may consider calcium administration for patients with β-blocker poisoning unresponsive to glucagon and catecholamines (Class IIb; LOE 5, 6).

Nonpharmacologic therapies such as cardiac pacing[173] and extracorporeal circulation[174] may be successful in β-blocker overdose when other modalities and pharmacologic therapies fail. Children suspected of ingesting massive amounts of β-blockers or manifesting early signs of impending cardiovascular collapse may benefit from transport to a tertiary care pediatric center capable of providing these advanced therapies.

Opioid Toxicity

Epidemiology, Pathophysiology, and Clinical Manifestations

Opiates and related opioids account for a large number of overdose cases reported to poison control centers or presenting to Emergency Departments. A total of 43 500 opioid or opiate exposures were reported to the AAPCC in 2000 (12 227 opioid, 29 418 acetaminophen combined with an opioid, and 1855 heroin).[1] This reporting system may grossly underestimate the total number of opiate and opioid exposures, especially heroin overdoses managed by EMS and Emergency Departments in the United States. Moreover, evidence indicates that opiate exposures and deaths are increasing in some communities in the United States.[3,175] In an 11-year retrospective review

of all deaths from injury and poisoning in the United Kingdom, the largest single category of death due to poisoning was poisoning from opiates and related narcotics.[176]

PALS providers should be prepared to manage toxicity from opiates and opioids after procedural sedation (see Chapter 15) as well as toxicity due to overdoses of these agents. In one large pediatric teaching hospital, 15 cases of respiratory depression (12 of 15 requiring naloxone) were documented in a 3-year surveillance period.[17] Recent reviews of sedation and analgesia for procedures in children highlight the need for providers to be familiar with the sedative agents used and reversal agents such as naloxone.[177]

Narcotic overdose in children may occur from a number of different substances and sources. Morphine, codeine, hydrocodone, oxycodone, hydromorphone, meperidine, pentazocine, and propoxyphene are commonly prescribed narcotic analgesics. Any of these may be ingested by a small child or taken intentionally in a suicide attempt by an adolescent. The synthetic agent oxycodone has recently become a popular recreational drug among adolescents and adults; as a result abuse has increased. Similarly, over-the-counter agents such as dextromethorphan, the D-isomer of the opiate agonist levorphanol, have been abused by adolescents, resulting in overdose deaths.[178] Butorphanol nasal spray may also be abused or accidentally ingested by children.

Methadone is prescribed for pain, but it is more commonly used to prevent withdrawal symptoms in patients recovering from opiate addiction. Because of its widespread use, it may be ingested by children. Methadone intoxication[179] and several methadone-related deaths have occurred in children.[11] Because methadone has a long half-life and active metabolites, the patient with methadone overdose is usually admitted for monitoring and observation. Like opiates, clonidine (a centrally acting imidazoline α_2-receptor agonist) may cause respiratory depression, miosis, and coma. This drug has a prolonged effect, so patients require intensive monitoring.

In children admitted because of coma or respiratory depression of unknown cause, providers should consider the possibility of intentional administration of opiates. These drugs are common in cases of intentional abuse or Munchausen syndrome by proxy.[180] Rapid urine immunoassays may detect opiates, but these tests may produce both false-negative and false-positive results. For example, screening immunoassays often do not detect methadone, but more comprehensive screens do. Gas chromatography/mass spectrophotometry (GC/MS) and high-performance liquid chromatography (HPLC) are more comprehensive but also more expensive.

These tests often do not provide any more clinically useful information than results of limited screening tests coupled with a history and physical exam.[181] Nevertheless, for medicolegal purposes or when child maltreatment is suspected, qualitative screens such as urine immunoassays are insufficient. You should send samples under chain of custody to a reference laboratory for analysis by GC/MS.

Many opiates, most notably codeine, hydrocodone, oxycodone, and propoxyphene, are often formulated in combination with acetaminophen or aspirin. If children present with symptoms or history of overdose with these combination opiates, you should look for additional toxicity from acetaminophen or aspirin. In addition to combination product formulations, some opioids are available in transdermal patch products. Fentanyl patches are formulated to release fentanyl at a rate of 25 to 100 µg/h for adults, but the patches contain very large amounts of the drug (2.5 to 10 *mg* per patch). Ingestion of even a small amount of fentanyl can produce severe toxicity in a child because of the potency of this opioid. The fentanyl on transdermal patches can also be inhaled. In one case severe toxicity developed within seconds after the patient heated a patch and inhaled the vapors.[182]

Heroin may be inhaled, ingested, or injected. Heroin accounts for very few unintentional exposures in children, but it may be abused by adolescents.[183] Heroin overdose is a major problem in most urban Emergency Departments.

Narcotics produce CNS depression and may cause hypoventilation, apnea, and respiratory failure (see Critical Concepts: "Recognition and Management of Opiate or Opioid Toxicity"). Respiration is controlled principally through brain respiratory centers in the medulla with peripheral input from chemoreceptors and other sources. Opioids produce inhibition at the chemoreceptors through mu opioid receptors and in the medulla through mu and delta receptors.

Although a number of neurotransmitters mediate the control of respiration, glutamate and GABA are the major excitatory and inhibitory neurotransmitters, respectively. This mechanism explains the potential for interaction of opioids with benzodiazepines and alcohol: both benzodiazepines and alcohol facilitate the inhibitory effect of GABA, but alcohol also decreases the excitatory effect of glutamate.[184] Children may present with respiratory failure due to ingestion of *only* an opiate or opioid. But adults and adolescents more often mix these agents with alcohol. Noncardiogenic pulmonary edema may occur with heroin overdose; clinical symptoms are usually evident early in the course if it occurs. In one retrospective case series mechanical ventilation was required in only 39% of patients with this complication.[185]

Severe opiate intoxication may cause a number of problems in addition to respiratory compromise. For example, hypotension, bradycardia or tachycardia, arrhythmias, circulatory collapse, and cardiac arrest may occur. Decreased gastrointestinal motility, presumably due to peripheral opioid receptor effects,[186] is common. Delayed gastric emptying may cause "cyclical" coma. That is, the first phase of drug absorption results in a decreased

level of consciousness. This phase is followed by some metabolism of the drug, so the patient begins to awaken. Further (delayed) absorption of the drug may cause another decrease in level of consciousness. It may be prudent to delay administration of activated charcoal during the awake periods because these patients are at risk for further depression in level of consciousness, further respiratory depression, and aspiration. These risks generally preclude administration of activated charcoal unless the airway is protected. Seizures may occur with meperidine,[187,188] further complicating management.

Management

Therapy for opiate or opioid toxicity should begin with assessment and support of the airway, oxygenation, and ventilation. If a rapid cardiopulmonary assessment reveals respiratory failure, provide bag-mask ventilation with oxygen and determine the need for tracheal intubation.

Naloxone is the antidote of choice for treatment of severe opiate or opioid toxicity. You should consider naloxone administration if you identify the opiate toxidrome of coma, depressed respirations, and miosis (pinpoint pupils). In one clinical report the frequency of miosis in relation to the cause of drug-induced coma in children was 88% for narcotics, 72% for phenothiazines, 35% for ethanol, and 31% for barbiturates.[189]

Clinicians have used the opioid receptor antagonist naloxone for more than 20 years. It remains the treatment of choice to reverse narcotic toxicity (Class IIa; LOE 4, 5, 6, 7).[190,191] Although patients generally tolerate naloxone well,[192,193] both animal[194] and clinical data suggest that adverse reactions, including ventricular arrhythmias, acute pulmonary edema,[195] asystole, and seizures, may occur.[196] The opioid and adrenergic systems are interrelated; opioid antagonists stimulate sympathetic nervous system activity.[197] In addition, hypercapnia stimulates the sympathetic nervous system. Animal data

Critical Concepts:
Recognition and Management of Opiate or Opioid Toxicity

Clinical Signs

- **CNS:** CNS depression, hypoventilation, apnea, and cyclical coma.
- **CV/ECG:** Hypotension, bradycardia or tachycardia, arrhythmias, circulatory collapse, and cardiac arrest. Adverse effects may also develop with reversal.
- **Gastrointestinal:** Delayed gastric emptying (may cause cyclical coma).

Treatment

- Support airway, ventilation, and oxygenation.
- Provide continuous ECG monitoring; treat symptomatic or unstable arrhythmias.
- Administer naloxone *after* establishment of effective ventilation. Monitor for adverse effects, including ventricular arrhythmias, pulmonary edema, and seizures.
- Establish vascular access and treat shock if present.

suggests that if ventilation normalizes the partial pressure of arterial CO_2 before naloxone administration, the potential rise in epinephrine concentration and its attendant toxic effects are blunted.[194] For this reason you should establish effective ventilation *before* you administer naloxone (Class IIb; LOE 5, 6).

For treatment of the adverse effects of opiate overdose, the recommended naloxone dose is 0.1 mg/kg IV; you may give up to 2 mg in a single dose.[190] To avoid the sudden hemodynamic effects of opioid reversal, you may give repeated doses of 0.01 to 0.03 mg/kg. Use even lower doses (0.005 to 0.01 mg/kg) to reverse respiratory depression due to therapeutic doses of opiates (see Chapter 15: "Sedation").

To treat respiratory depression in patients with suspected narcotic addiction, many toxicologists use low initial doses of naloxone (eg, 0.01 mg/kg, up to 0.4 mg in a single dose; repeat as needed) to avoid withdrawal symptoms such as vomiting with the attendant risks of aspiration and agitation. The concept of "go low and go slow" may be most appropriate in these patients. After you give the initial doses, you may provide a continuous infusion of naloxone to reverse the toxic effects of opiate poisoning in infants.[198] Continuous naloxone infusion also may be necessary to treat poisoning from certain long-acting opioids such as methadone. You can administer naloxone intramuscularly,[192] subcutaneously,[199] or through the tracheal tube. But use of these routes may delay its onset of action, particularly if perfusion is poor.

Summary Points

- Support of a patent airway and adequate oxygenation, ventilation, and circulation are as necessary for poisoned patients as they are for any patient who requires PALS. Children with overdoses of certain drugs may require modified resuscitation therapies or sequences.
- The rapid cardiopulmonary assessment is a useful tool to assess poisoned patients.
- PALS providers should carefully analyze the ECG for changes that may be caused by tricyclic antidepressants, calcium channel blockers, and β-blockers. Such changes include a widened QRS complex, prolonged corrected QT interval (QT_C), bradycardia, SA and AV nodal conduction delays, VT, VF, and asystole.
- Providers may need to adjust the bolus volume used for fluid resuscitation in children who ingest drugs that affect myocardial contractility or predispose patients to noncardiogenic pulmonary edema. In these patients you may use boluses of 5 to 10 mL/kg or 10 to 20 mL/kg instead of the traditional 20 mL/kg bolus. Reassess the patient carefully between boluses, and repeat the bolus as needed.

- Sudden changes in level of consciousness and respiratory depression may develop in poisoned pediatric patients. For this reason you should support the ABCs and ensure a protected airway before you administer gastrointestinal decontamination. Alert patients may be able to maintain their airway; others will require intubation.
- If you decide to use activated charcoal, administer it early after ingestion; it is most effective within 1 hour of ingestion. Gastric lavage is *not* a routine intervention; its effectiveness is limited in poisoned patients except in patients who present early (usually within 60 minutes or less) after ingestion of a life-threatening toxin. Syrup of ipecac is *not* recommended for any of the 5 types of poisoning discussed in this chapter. Whole-bowel irrigation may be beneficial, but further research is needed.
- Several toxins and drugs (eg, tricyclic antidepressants, β-blockers, and cocaine) have sodium channel blocking effects and effects on cell membrane stability that predispose children to ventricular arrhythmias. These arrhythmias may respond to administration of sodium bicarbonate.
- Specific antidotes that are not used routinely in cardiopulmonary resuscitation may be useful in certain types of drug overdose:
  — Sodium bicarbonate for sodium channel blocking agents, including tricyclic antidepressants and cocaine
  — Calcium chloride for β-adrenergic overdose (more controversial and less uniformly efficacious for calcium channel blockers)
  — Glucose plus insulin or glucagon for calcium channel blocker and β-blocker overdoses
  — Naloxone for opiate intoxication

Case Scenarios

Introductory Case Scenario

A 16-year-old girl is found lying near the front door of her home when EMS personnel ring the doorbell. The girl called EMS before she collapsed; the mother was asleep and was unaware of any problems until paramedics arrived. The girl is difficult to arouse. An empty bottle of sustained-release 180-mg verapamil is found with a suicide note. EMS personnel provide oxygen, monitor heart rate and rhythm, and rapidly transport the girl to the local medical center. The girl begins to awaken during transport. On arrival in the ED she is awake with a heart rate of 114 bpm, respiratory rate of 28 breaths/min, and blood pressure of 120/60 mm Hg.

Introductory Case Scenario Review Questions

■ **Does this patient have potential life-threatening toxicity due to ingestion of a calcium channel blocker?**

Absolutely. The girl is difficult to arouse but then begins to awaken during transport. The drug is a sustained-release drug, so further complications may develop.

■ **Would you use gastric lavage, activated charcoal, or both interventions at this time?**

The time of ingestion is unknown. Gastrointestinal decontamination is unlikely to be effective if ingestion occurred more than 60 minutes ago. Activated charcoal may prevent absorption. Attempts to remove sustained-release products by lavage or whole-bowel irrigation may be warranted, but there is little data from controlled trials to support these interventions. Note that sustained-release calcium channel blockers may slow gastric emptying, which may make gastrointestinal decontamination effective. The slow gastric emptying may, however, increase risk of vomiting and aspiration.

■ **What pharmacologic interventions should you prepare to administer in case signs of toxicity develop?**

The approach to calcium channel blocker toxicity is to support airway, breathing, oxygenation, and perfusion. You should establish vascular access, continuously monitor the ECG, and treat shock if needed. This adolescent may develop bradycardia, decreased cardiac contractility, and hypotension. With severe overdose signs of sodium channel blocking, including prolongation of the QRS and QT intervals and heart block, may develop. This patient may need epinephrine infusions to treat hypotension; glucagon or glucose plus insulin may be effective.

Introductory Case Scenario Rapid Cardiopulmonary Assessment

A rapid cardiopulmonary assessment reveals that the adolescent has a patent airway, RR of 28 breaths/min, good bilateral breath sounds, clear respirations, and normal color. HR is 114 bpm, BP is 120/60 mm Hg, capillary refill is <2 seconds, and peripheral pulses are strong and regular. Pulse oximetry reveals an oxyhemoglobin saturation of 98% on room air. She has a soft, nontender abdomen with no masses but severely diminished to absent bowel sounds. She is alert and talking approximately 1 hour and 15 minutes after ingestion.

Introductory Case Scenario Acceptable Actions and Rationale

■ *Use universal precautions.*

■ *Assess and support the ABCs and provide supplemental oxygen as needed.* Monitoring of respiratory function and cardiac rhythm is particularly important after ingestion of calcium channel blockers.

■ *Place the patient on a cardiac monitor and obtain a 12-lead ECG.* Early ECG changes may be evident before clinical deterioration. Treat symptomatic cardiac arrhythmias.

■ *Obtain a poison exposure history.* Ask about other drugs that may have been ingested. Adolescents often ingest multiple drugs in suicide attempts. When one cardiac drug is in the household, there are often other toxic drugs such as β-blockers and digoxin. Analgesics (eg, acetaminophen and aspirin) are common co-ingestants. Although acetaminophen co-ingestion in this patient is unlikely to result in cardiovascular deterioration, it may produce serious consequences (eg, hepatocellular necrosis and potential hepatic failure) if toxicity is not treated early.

■ *Perform a brief physical exam* to evaluate the patient's cardiopulmonary status; reassess the patient frequently.

■ *Establish IV access.* Obtain blood, urine, or both for drug screens; also obtain blood for evaluation of electrolytes and blood glucose. Many toxins produce metabolic acidosis, hypoglycemia, and other metabolic abnormalities. Drug screens are useful qualitative tools for making a toxicologic diagnosis. But you should confirm the results with more comprehensive tests if medical indications or medicolegal issues arise. Note that drug screens are not standardized; all healthcare providers should know the agents assessed by the drug screen used at their facility. Specific assays for some agents (eg, salicylates and acetaminophen) may be available with established nomograms that correlate acute overdose levels with predicted toxicity. For other agents such as tricyclic antidepressants, cocaine, and calcium channel blockers, specific levels do not correlate well with toxicity, and there are no comparable nomograms to predict outcome.

■ *Contact the regional poison center* for advice about management. Specialized information about toxin exposures and recommended management guidelines are available. Regional poison centers are staffed by certified specialists in poison information and medical toxicologists who can offer consultation and advice on management.

- *Consider gastric lavage or activated charcoal* administration for gastrointestinal decontamination. Ipecac is not very effective for the treatment of calcium channel blocker overdose, particularly more than 30 minutes after ingestion. This intervention may result in seizures or loss of consciousness in patients exposed to certain high-risk substances. Activated charcoal may prevent drug absorption. Attempts to remove sustained-release products by lavage or whole-bowel irrigation may be warranted, but little data from controlled trials is available.

Introductory Case Scenario Unacceptable Actions and Rationale

- *Discharging the patient.* This adolescent's vital signs are relatively normal, and she is alert. But delayed absorption may occur with this sustained-release product. Toxicity may develop over several hours, causing a sudden deterioration in cardiovascular or CNS function.

- *Admitting the patient to a hospital unit with no monitoring.* Conduction delays, bradycardia, or pulseless rhythms may result from ingestion of calcium channel blockers, so monitoring is essential.

Introductory Case Scenario Progression

The ECG shows normal findings at this time. Gastric lavage in the ED removes yellow pill fragments; activated charcoal is administered through an orogastric tube. The patient is admitted to the PICU, and cardiorespiratory monitoring is established. The patient's urine drug screen is positive for verapamil; her blood alcohol level is 37 mg/dL. Eight hours after ingestion her HR falls to the 60s with sinus rhythm and first-degree AV block. Systolic BP is 70 mm Hg.

Introductory Case Scenario Additional Acceptable Actions and Rationale

- *Administer intravenous fluid boluses cautiously.* Fluid bolus administration is appropriate to treat hypotension and

vasodilation, but calcium channel blockers may reduce myocardial contractility and produce cardiogenic or noncardiogenic pulmonary edema (ie, acute respiratory distress syndrome). Closely monitor systemic perfusion, fluid balance, and respiratory function.

- *Consider elective intubation to support ventilation and more safely provide gastrointestinal decontamination.* Patients with severe calcium channel blocker poisoning may develop compromised airway, oxygenation, and ventilation from loss of central control of respirations or direct pulmonary toxicity. This adolescent demonstrates bowel hypomotility, so administration of activated charcoal or whole-bowel irrigation may cause persistent vomiting. These interventions place the patient at risk for aspiration, particularly if the airway is not protected.

- *Administer chronotropic and inotropic adrenergic agents.* Peripheral arteriolar vasodilatation occurs with overdoses of all types of calcium channel blockers, although it is most apparent with nifedipine. Verapamil is a moderate vasodilator. The patient's initial BP of 120/60 mm Hg (note the low diastolic BP and wide pulse pressure) indicated some early vasodilation that has now worsened (systolic BP now 70 mm Hg). You may consider calcium infusion, but this therapy is not uniformly effective.

- *Anticipate the need for cardiac pacing.* Cardiac pacing may be used for calcium channel blocker–induced bradycardia and for β-blocker poisoning.

- *Glucagon* may be effective for calcium channel blocker and β-blocker ingestions, but convincing evidence has not been reported.

Introductory Case Scenario Further Progression and Conclusion

This adolescent receives IV boluses of normal saline, and her hypotension and bradycardia resolve. She vomits activated charcoal with some pills in the emesis. The

medical toxicologist recommends elective tracheal intubation and aggressive whole-bowel irrigation. The patient remains alert, so the physician decides to postpone intubation. Whole-bowel irrigation is started but discontinued because of emesis. Sixteen hours after ingestion the patient's systolic BP falls to 50 mm Hg; her HR is 50 bpm with a wide QRS complex (see Figure 4) and complete heart block. External pacing is unsuccessful. Providers start an epinephrine infusion at 0.1 μg/kg per minute and administer a 500-mg bolus of calcium chloride followed by 1 g of calcium chloride. Providers start dopamine at 15 μg/kg per minute and gradually increase the epinephrine infusion to 0.6 μg/kg per minute. An experienced provider inserts a tracheal tube and verifies its position. Within 30 minutes the adolescent's HR rises to 100 bpm with a BP of 102/50 mm Hg.

Four hours later, despite 40% oxygen administration and mechanical ventilation at a respiratory rate of 20 breaths/min, her SpO_2 drops to 89%. Providers increase the inspired oxygen concentration and provide positive end-expiratory pressure (PEEP) of 6 cm H_2O. Throughout the evening her BP falls frequently, but it responds to increases in epinephrine infusion and glucagon administration. Thirty-six hours after ingestion the patient's blood pressure is stable, and she is weaned from vasopressors and ventilatory support. Gut motility improves.

Case Scenario 2

EMS providers arrive at the home of a 4-year-old, 15-kg boy. The child is unresponsive with minimal to no respiratory effort. The mother called 911 after seeing the child lying supine on the floor, gasping for air. The child was with his mother all morning watching cartoons; he reportedly ate popcorn half an hour before his breathing difficulty developed. Rapid cardiopulmonary assessment reveals cyanosis, a HR of about 64 bpm, and rigid muscle tone. Peripheral pulses are absent and central pulses are weak. Rescuers did not measure BP in the field.

FIGURE 4. ECG effects of slow-release calcium channel blocker overdose in an adolescent. Significant bradycardia with complete heart block and wide QRS complex developed sixteen hours after ingestion.

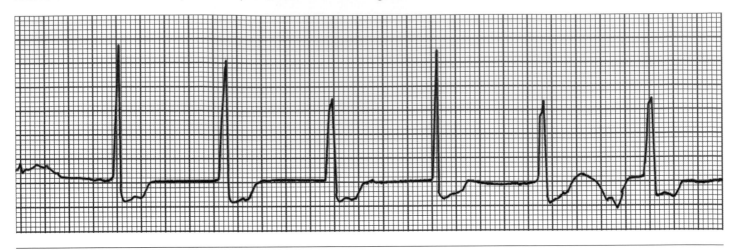

Case Scenario 2 Acceptable Actions and Rationale

■ Use universal precautions.

■ Assess and support the airway and provide bag-mask ventilation with oxygen. This patient requires immediate bag-mask ventilation because he is cyanotic, gasping, and bradycardic. He may progress to full cardiopulmonary arrest if not treated immediately.

■ Perform a brief physical exam while supporting ventilation. Check for possible toxidromes (eg, check pupils for miosis, which would suggest opiate ingestion with apnea and coma).

■ Place the patient on a cardiac monitor and obtain a 12-lead ECG. This patient may have an unknown ingestion. The patient may also be suffering from an arrhythmia that resulted in seizures or cerebral hypoperfusion and respiratory failure.

■ Obtain a focused history targeting possible poisoning. The child's clinical presentation is unusual and is inconsistent with the history. The child may have ingested medications or drugs without the mother's knowledge. Even when the caretaker denies possible ingestion, ask the caretaker to list all drugs available in the home.

■ Establish IV access and obtain blood for a bedside glucose evaluation. Hypoglycemia can cause seizures, unresponsiveness, and respiratory depression in children.

Case Scenario 2 Unacceptable Actions and Rationale

■ *Administering atropine for bradycardia before opening the airway and ventilating the patient.* The bradycardia is caused by hypoxia or heart block.

■ *Failing to check glucose.* The cause of this unconscious child's condition is unclear at this time. Hypoglycemia (one of the **4 H's and 4 T's**) can cause seizure or coma, and it is easy to correct.

Case Scenario 2 Progression

Bag-mask ventilation is difficult because the patient is rigid, but there are no tonic or clonic movements of the extremities. The bedside test reveals a glucose concentration of 154 mg/dL. On arrival at the ED rescuers continue bag-mask ventilation. The child requires insertion of an oral airway and a 2-rescuer ventilation technique. He has thick nasal secretions and a recent history of upper respiratory tract infection. There is no history of fever, head injury, choking, stridor, or ingestion. The child's past medical history reveals no asthma, other pulmonary conditions, *cardiac disorders, or seizures. The child is unresponsive to painful stimuli. No medications or drugs were present at the scene or admitted by the mother. Initial vital signs reveal an HR of 116 bpm and a systolic BP of 76 mm Hg by palpation. There are still no spontaneous respirations. Providers continue 2-rescuer bag-mask ventilation with 100% oxygen to maintain oxygen saturation in the low to mid 90% range. Any attempt to decrease ventilation support results in rapid desaturation. Resistance to hand ventilation is increasing, and episodes of bradycardia occur periodically.*

Case Scenario 2 Additional Acceptable Actions and Rationale

■ *Use universal precautions.*

■ *Perform tracheal intubation.* You must establish an effective and reliable method of ventilation and oxygenation.

■ *Use rapid sequence intubation (RSI) techniques and medications.* Use of RSI sedatives and paralytics will facilitate intubation. Confirm tracheal tube placement. Only experienced providers should perform RSI.

■ *Check pupils for miosis.* This sign may be compatible with an opiate toxidrome (coma, apnea, miosis). If the pupils are pinpoint, use naloxone as an antidote.

Case Scenario 2
Further Progression

An experienced provider administers 0.15 mg of atropine and 15 mg of succinylcholine IV and inserts a 5-mm orotracheal tube. There is no sign of aspiration or foreign-body obstruction, and the epiglottis appears normal on laryngoscopy. Initial blood gas values just before intubation were pH 7.12, PCO_2 54, and PO_2 140 mm Hg (carboxyhemoglobin and methemoglobin were normal). A chest radiograph reveals no pneumonia or foreign body. After securing the airway, providers perform a secondary survey. There is no head trauma or nystagmus, but the pupils are pinpoint (miosis). There is no history of exposure to any medications or drugs, and no pill fragments were removed by gastric aspiration with a nasogastric tube. The patient's core temperature is 35.3°C (95.6°F).

Case Scenario 2
Discussion and Conclusion

The presence of coma, respiratory depression, miosis, bradycardia, hypotension, and hypothermia should lead the provider to consider ingestion of opiates, clonidine, or barbiturates. The provider should also consider CNS anatomic defects or injury such as pontine lesions.

After the patient recovers from succinylcholine, the physician administers 1.5 mg of naloxone twice. Noticeable improvement in responsiveness and spontaneous respirations occurs. Pupils are now 3 mm and reactive. The patient becomes agitated, so midazolam is administered. The physician strongly suspects opiate intoxication and orders a rapid urine immunoassay. The results are negative for drugs of abuse and tricyclic antidepressants. Nevertheless activated charcoal is administered by nasogastric tube after bowel sounds are confirmed and the tracheal tube is secured. A urine sample is sent for a comprehensive screen by GC/MS. The initial results are negative for opiates. A CBC reveals a white blood cell count of $16/200 \text{ mm}^3$ with 19% bands, 67% neutrophils, 8% lymphocytes, 1% variant lymphocyte, and

5% monocytes; hemoglobin is 10.6 g/dL. Ionized calcium is normal (1.21 mmol/L). Serum electrolytes, osmolality, and glucose are normal. A CT scan of the brain shows normal findings.

After naloxone boluses the child demonstrates some respiratory effort; his temperature returns to normal. Repeated blood gas analyses reveal persistent respiratory acidosis (pH 7.10, PCO_2 64.8 mm Hg, PO_2 142 mm Hg), so intermittent mandatory ventilation is provided. PICU providers initiate a continuous infusion of naloxone, which is required for 20 hours after admission. Although the family denied any possibility of ingestion, an uncle was later discovered to be taking methadone for narcotic addiction.

Case Scenario 3

A 14-year-old boy with a history of depression and school-related problems arrives in the ED after telling his parents he took a handful of tricyclic antidepressants 30 minutes ago. On arrival the adolescent is somnolent but arousable and appropriately responsive when stimulated. Vital signs are temperature 38.0°C (100.4°F), RR 10 breaths/min, HR 130 bpm, BP 88/60 mm Hg, and capillary refill time 2 seconds. The patient's skin is dry; his pupils are dilated but reactive.

Case Scenario 3 Acceptable Actions and Rationale

- *Use universal precautions.*
- *Assess and support the ABCs and provide supplemental oxygen.* This patient has signs of decreased responsiveness, hypoventilation, and potential cardiovascular instability.

- *Obtain a 12-lead ECG and provide continuous cardiac monitoring.* Tricyclic antidepressants can delay intraventricular conduction and prolong the QRS interval, particularly the terminal 40 ms (see Figure 3). ECG abnormalities may be predictive of seizures and ventricular arrhythmias. In addition to prolongation of the QRS interval, an R wave in lead aVR ≥3 mm or an R wave/S wave ratio in lead aVR ≥0.7

may be a predictor of serious toxicity. The most common symptomatic arrhythmia associated with tricyclic antidepressant poisoning is a wide-complex tachycardia. More severe intoxication also prolongs the QT interval; high concentrations of tricyclics may result in preterminal sinus bradycardia and heart block with junctional or ventricular wide-complex escape beats. All sodium channel blocking agents prolong the QRS interval and increase the risk of ventricular tachycardia. Many of these agents also inhibit potassium channels, leading to an increased risk of torsades de pointes.

- *Obtain a focused history and perform a rapid cardiopulmonary assessment and targeted physical exam.* This patient has a history and clinical signs (altered mental status, tachycardia, hypotension) consistent with tricyclic antidepressant poisoning. Although peak serum concentrations and drug effects occur within 2 to 8 hours of ingestion, the life-threatening **Three C's** of tricyclic overdose (**C**oma, **C**onvulsions, and **C**ardiac toxicities) can develop rapidly. The **A** of **TCA** overdose (acidosis) may also develop. Most deaths occur within the first several hours of presentation. Your initial approach should focus on the diagnosis, prevention, and treatment of life-threatening complications. For the initial history you should ask about the type and amount of medication taken, time of ingestion, other medications available in the household, past medical history (chronic disease, current medications, recent illnesses), and the possibility of a complicating head injury. The physical exam should assess vital signs, mental status, and cardiopulmonary status. Other portions of the exam can help determine if the patient's presentation is consistent with a particular class of toxins.

- *Establish IV access and obtain blood samples for laboratory studies.* IV access is necessary to treat the patient's hypotension; the adolescent is also at risk for cardiac arrhythmias and seizures.

Determine serum electrolyte and glucose concentrations to identify abnormalities that could exacerbate cardiac dysfunction (eg, hypokalemia, hypocalcemia, or hypomagnesemia). Consider alternative causes of altered mental status (eg, hypoglycemia). Measuring serum osmolality can help identify other possible ingestants by revealing an osmolar gap (ie, the difference between the measured and calculated osmolality). Ingestion of substances like ethanol, methanol, and ethylene glycol can cause a significant osmolar gap. For more information consult a standard toxicology reference. Consider obtaining an initial blood gas analysis to evaluate the effectiveness of ventilation in this drowsy and slowly breathing patient. This patient will probably need alkalinization. You can use the blood gas values as baseline values to measure his response.

■ *Prepare for intubation.* Rationale for immediate intubation: the patient has a low respiratory rate, altered mental status, and hypotension. He is also at risk for prolonged, recalcitrant hemodynamic instability and seizures. Furthermore, adequate ventilation is a necessary prerequisite for sodium bicarbonate therapy.

■ *Obtain a toxicology screen.* Patients who intentionally ingest drugs or medications may not disclose all the agents they took. Some "polypharmacy" ingestions can result in significant comorbidity (eg, acetaminophen). Many toxicologic screens do not detect a number of agents ingested by children, and you may not have time to wait for the results. You should know which medications are detected by the toxicology screen used at your facility and whether tricyclic antidepressants are detected. Detection of tricyclic antidepressants confirms the ingestion, but the level does not reliably indicate severity of toxicity.

■ *Give a fluid bolus.* Initial therapy for hypotension includes administration of a 10 mL/kg bolus of isotonic crystalloid. This patient's hypotension is probably caused by both impaired cardiac contractility and vasodilation, so correction of hypotension will likely necessitate pharmacologic treatment with inotropes. You should administer fluid bolus therapy and carefully monitor the patient for development of pulmonary edema.

■ *Initiate alkalinization.* Infuse sodium bicarbonate if the hypotension does not respond to the initial fluid bolus, the patient's condition deteriorates, or the ECG indicates a high risk of symptomatic tricyclic antidepressant toxicity. After a bolus of 1 to 2 mEq/kg, infuse sodium bicarbonate as a solution of 150 mEq $NaHCO_3$ per liter in D_5W titrated to produce metabolic alkalosis. The initial bolus should raise arterial pH above 7.45. The subsequent infusion should achieve a target pH of 7.50 to 7.55 for severe symptomatic ingestions. If the patient improves after the initial bicarbonate bolus, it is appropriate to infuse sufficient bicarbonate to maintain a pH of 7.45 to 7.50 while monitoring the ECG to ensure that the QRS and corrected QT (QT_C) intervals remain in the normal range. The role of hyperventilation-induced alkalosis is unclear; be aware that sodium bicarbonate can cause paradoxical respiratory acidosis in patients with inadequate or borderline ventilation. You should ventilate intubated patients to at least a normal Pco_2, and you should closely monitor spontaneously ventilating patients for signs of hypoventilation.

■ *Prepare for gastrointestinal decontamination.* Poison control centers and clinical toxicologists are valuable resources for determining the need for gastrointestinal decontamination. This intervention is no longer routinely recommended for several reasons. First, it has limited efficacy with some drugs. Second, many toxins are relatively

benign. Third, it should be performed soon after ingestion. In this case activated charcoal administration is probably warranted because tricyclic antidepressants are highly toxic and the patient presented soon after ingestion. Furthermore, the anticholinergic effect of tricyclic antidepressants delays gastric emptying and increases the amount of drug available for adsorption. If you decide to administer activated charcoal to this patient, perform intubation with a cuffed tracheal tube before administration to decrease the risk of aspiration.

■ *Notify the intensive care unit or appropriate transfer service.* The patient will require close monitoring and possibly invasive support for the next several hours.

Case Scenario 3 Unacceptable Actions and Rationale

■ *Administering syrup of ipecac.* This patient may deteriorate suddenly with seizures, hemodynamic instability, and coma. Ipecac-induced emesis may occur when the patient is unable to protect his airway. This intervention would place him at high risk for aspiration.

■ *Failing to recognize that patients who ingest tricyclic antidepressants may rapidly progress* from being conscious and alert with mild symptoms to manifesting life-threatening toxicity.

■ *Failing to recognize and treat the patient's hypotension; failing to obtain an ECG.*

Case Scenario 3 Progression

Providers take the recommended actions. The ECG reveals a prolonged QRS interval of 140 ms, prolonged QT_C interval of 500 ms, and a tall R wave in lead aVR >3 mm. There are occasional 6-beat runs of ventricular tachycardia, and BP is 70/30 mm Hg. After initial alkalinization with 1 mEq/Kg sodium bicarbonate that is repeated once, BP remains at 80/50 mm Hg with capillary refill of 4 seconds and HR of 70 bpm. The QT_C interval improves to 420 ms, and the QRS interval is 100 ms.

Case Scenario 3 Additional Acceptable Actions and Rationale

■ *Administer a vasopressor.* Tricyclic antidepressants block reuptake of norepinephrine into sympathetic nerves, causing catecholamine depletion. You may need to administer a vasopressor to maintain adequate vascular tone and blood pressure. Use of norepinephrine or epinephrine can be effective. Anecdotal data supports treatment with norepinephrine rather than dopamine.

■ *Consider administering lidocaine.* If ventricular arrhythmias do not respond to sodium bicarbonate, you may administer lidocaine. Some investigators argue against its use because it is a sodium channel blocker. You should generally avoid antiarrhythmics that further prolong the QRS and QT$_C$ intervals (eg, amiodarone, procainamide).

■ *Obtain a blood gas analysis* to confirm sufficient alkalosis. Although the precise degree of alkalosis required to treat tricyclic antidepressant toxicity is unknown, most data suggest a target pH of 7.50 to 7.55 for severe intoxication. A pH >7.55 may produce complications; it is not routinely recommended.

■ Consider preparing for extracorporeal membrane oxygenation (ECMO) or other support of circulation. For high-risk patients who are unresponsive to conventional therapy, consider early transport to a center capable of providing advanced therapies.

Case Scenario 3 Additional Unacceptable Actions

■ *Administering a pure β-adrenergic agonist.* These agents (eg, dobutamine, isoproterenol) may worsen hypotension by causing vasodilation through their action on peripheral β-adrenergic receptors. They are contraindicated.

■ *Administering Class I$_A$ antiarrhythmics other than lidocaine* (eg, quinidine, procainamide) or Class I$_C$ antiarrhythmics (eg, flecainide, propafenone). These drugs are contraindicated because they may exacerbate the cardiac toxicity.

Class III antiarrhythmics (eg, amiodarone, bretylium) prolong the QT interval; they are not routinely indicated, but they have been successful in individual cases.

■ *Administering phenytoin for treatment of cardiac dysfunction.* Phenytoin was previously recommended for ingestion of tricyclic antidepressants. This recommendation was based on case reports and preliminary data suggesting a beneficial effect on cardiac toxicity. But subsequent controlled animal studies failed to confirm a beneficial effect. It is no longer routinely recommended for cardiotoxicity mediated by tricyclic antidepressants. Its role as an anticonvulsant in this setting is unclear.

Case Scenario 4

Paramedics bring a 3-year-old child to the ED. The child was "shaking all over" with both arms and legs "jerking" when found. The mother said the child was "frothing at the mouth" and she could not wake him. When paramedics arrived the child was postictal and unresponsive but breathing. His heart rate was 94 bpm. Paramedics transported the child to the ED.

Case Scenario 4 Acceptable Actions and Rationale

■ *Use universal precautions.*

■ *Place the patient in the recovery position and suction the airway.* This child was described as having copious oral secretions and a seizure. You should establish a patent airway and monitor for additional seizures. Take precautions to prevent aspiration.

■ *Apply high-flow oxygen by face mask.* The patient is unresponsive, and the cause of the event is unknown. Administer oxygen and assess oxygenation by pulse oximetry.

■ *Obtain a focused history.* Ask about the availability of drugs around the house or in the child's environment to try to determine the cause of the seizure.

■ *Perform a brief physical exam and rapid cardiopulmonary assessment.* These assessments may provide clues

about the cause of this seizure. Findings such as dilated pupils (mydriasis), flushed skin versus cool, clammy, pale skin, and absent versus normal bowel sounds may distinguish an anticholinergic toxidrome (mydriasis, flushed skin, absent bowel sounds, tachycardia, central nervous system effects with seizures and coma) from a sympathomimetic toxidrome (mydriasis, pale, cool, clammy skin, tachycardia, seizures, present bowel sounds) due to stimulants such as cocaine.

■ *Establish continuous cardiac monitoring and obtain a 12-lead ECG.* Look for development of toxin-induced arrhythmias.

■ *Perform a bedside glucose test, measure temperature, and establish vascular access.* Drug-induced or metabolic causes of hypoglycemia or high fever may have caused this patient's seizure.

Case Scenario 4 Unacceptable Actions and Rationale

■ *Administering anything by mouth.* You should not give this patient anything by mouth, including syrup of ipecac, even if you suspect ingestion. The patient already manifests adverse pharmacodynamic effects of the toxin. Gastrointestinal decontamination is unlikely to be of any benefit. It may be risky if the patient has another seizure or loses control of his airway and aspirates.

Case Scenario 4 Progression

Your rapid cardiopulmonary assessment reveals a patent airway, RR of 24 breaths/min, HR of 110 bpm, palpable central and distal pulses, but slightly cool, pale skin. Rectal temperature is 97.6°F (36.5°C). Further examination uncovers no trauma to the head, pupils are 4 to 5 mm and reactive to light, there is no odor to the breath, and cardiopulmonary findings are normal. Bowel sounds are present. Bystanders told the paramedics that the child was playing in the backyard of a known crack house. The child's brother said he saw the patient "pick up a rock and eat it." The

patient has no current illness, no symptoms of upper respiratory tract infection,
and no fever. The child has no personal or
family history of seizures. An ECG shows
mild sinus tachycardia but otherwise normal findings. The child begins to awaken
in the ED; he is alert and talking within
an hour.

Case Scenario 4
Additional Acceptable Actions
and Rationale

■ *Obtain laboratory studies to evaluate
the cause of the seizure.* Although many
providers routinely evaluate standard
electrolytes, calcium, magnesium, and
phosphorus, some studies do not support this practice.

■ *Obtain a urine drug screen.* The possibility of cocaine exposure is high.

■ *Administer a benzodiazepine.* These
drugs can attenuate the toxic effects
of cocaine on the heart and central
nervous system.

■ *Consider obtaining a CT or MRI scan
of the brain.* Sympathomimetics such
as cocaine have been associated with
intracerebral hemorrhages and stroke
in children and adults.

Case Scenario 4 Conclusion

*The initial rapid urine immunoassay is
positive for cocaine (metabolites) and
negative for other drugs of abuse and tricyclic antidepressants. Electrolyte, blood
glucose, calcium, magnesium, and phosphorus concentrations are normal. An MRI
scan shows normal findings. You consult
a toxicologist, who recommends sending
urine by chain of custody to a reference
laboratory for GC/MS analysis. This
confirmatory study is important because
of the social history and the possibility of
neglect. The urine screen is negative for
cocaine at the reference laboratory. The
standard level of detection at the laboratory is 300 ng/mL for benzoylecgonine
(cocaine metabolites); anything below that
level is reported as negative. The same
sample is reanalyzed at a forensic toxi-*

*cology laboratory, and the screen detects
benzoylecgonine at 186 ng/mL. You admit
the patient for observation and contact
social services. No other cause of his
seizure was found, and a subsequent
EEG shows normal findings.*

---

1. **You receive a call to evaluate a
toddler who reportedly ingested
a toxic amount of cocaine. You review the complications of cocaine
overdose to anticipate problems
that may develop. Which of the
following is this toddler *not* likely
to develop from cocaine overdose?**

   a. altered sensorium

   b. bradycardia

   c. hypertension

   d. hyperthermia

   The correct answer is b. Bradycardia is unlikely to develop after
cocaine overdose. Cocaine overdose
blocks the reuptake of norepinephrine, dopamine, epinephrine, and
serotonin from the synaptic cleft.
This blockade results in accumulation of norepinephrine and epinephrine at β-adrenergic receptors. The
clinical signs of cocaine overdose
are likely to include adrenergic signs
("fight or flight" response) and possibly signs of acute coronary syndrome. Tachycardia and tachyarrhythmias rather than bradycardia would
be expected.

   Answer a is incorrect because cocaine *can* produce altered sensorium
and even seizures. Cocaine overdose
can produce dopaminergic effects
of mood elevation and movement
disorders. It also can produce serotonin stimulation with possible
exhilaration and hallucinations.

   Answer c is incorrect because hypertension *is* expected with cocaine
overdose. Hypertension results from
accumulation of norepinephrine and
epinephrine at β-adrenergic receptor
sites.

   Answer d is incorrect because
hyperthermia *is* a potential complication of cocaine overdose. Hyperthermia requires aggressive treatment if present. The hyperthermia
results from serotonin stimulation.

Review Questions

2. **You are caring for an adolescent who presents with cocaine-induced myocardial ischemia, tachycardia, and severe hypertension. Which of the following should *not* be part of the care that you provide for him?**

   a. oxygen

   b. benzodiazepine

   c. propranolol

   d. nitroglycerin

   The correct answer is c. Propranolol is *not* part of the treatment for cocaine-induced acute coronary syndromes. β-Blockers are a recommended treatment for myocardial ischemia in adults. But they are contraindicated in patients with cocaine intoxication because they can increase blood pressure and coronary artery constriction.

   Answer a is incorrect because you *should* administer oxygen in the initial treatment of cocaine-induced acute coronary syndromes. Oxygen improves myocardial oxygen delivery. You should also obtain an ECG.

   Answer b is incorrect because benzodiazepine *is* a "first-line" therapy for cocaine overdose. Benzodiazepine is an anticonvulsant and CNS depressant. It may attenuate the toxic effects of cocaine on the myocardium and the central nervous system.

   Answer d is incorrect because nitroglycerin is also a "first-line" treatment for acute coronary syndromes to reverse coronary vasoconstriction.

3. **You are caring for a 15-year-old girl. She was admitted after intentional ingestion of her mother's tricyclic antidepressant. You review the potential complications of TCA overdose to plan this adolescent's care. Which one of the following is *not* a complication of TCA overdose?**

   a. coma

   b. alkalosis

   c. convulsions

   d. cardiac arrhythmias

   The correct answer is b. *Acidemia* is a potential complication of TCA toxicity, but alkalosis is an uncommon complication of TCA overdose. Treatment of TCA overdose requires administration of sodium bicarbonate to induce alkalosis. This therapy will narrow the QRS complex, shorten the QT interval, and increase myocardial contractility. These actions will suppress ventricular arrhythmias and reverse hypotension.

   Answer a is incorrect because coma *is* a potential complication of TCA overdose. To recall the complications of tricyclic antidepressant overdose, use the mnemonic **Three C's and an A** (TCA): Coma, Convulsions (seizures), Cardiac arrhythmias, and at times Acidosis.

   Answer c is incorrect because convulsions are a potential complication of TCA overdose. TCA overdose inhibits fast (voltage-dependent) sodium channels in the brain.

   Answer d is incorrect because TCA overdose *does* inhibit fast sodium channels and potassium channels in the myocardium. This inhibition prolongs the action potential, resulting in delayed conduction with a widened QRS complex and prolonged QT interval; it may also cause sinus bradycardia and heart block with junctional or ventricular wide-complex escape beats.

4. **You initiate continuous ECG monitoring of the adolescent with TCA overdose. A medical student asks which arrhythmias you expect to find. Which one of the following ECG changes is characteristic of severe TCA toxicity?**

   a. a wide QRS complex and prolonged QT_c interval

   b. a narrow QRS complex tachycardia with shortening of the QT_c interval

   c. peaked T waves

   d. supraventricular tachycardia with aberrant conduction

   The correct answer is a. TCA overdose inhibits fast (voltage-dependent) sodium channels in the myocardium and potassium channels. This inhibition prolongs the action potential produced by inhibition of phase 0 of the action potential, resulting in delayed conduction, prolonged QT interval, preterminal sinus bradycardia, and junctional or ventricular wide-complex escape beats.

   Answer b is incorrect because TCA overdose causes *prolongation* of the QT interval and *widening* of the QRS complex.

   Answer c is incorrect because peaked T waves are more common with hyperkalemia than with TCA overdose.

   Answer d is incorrect because tachycardia is less likely than bradycardia with TCA overdose. Ventricular arrhythmias are more common than supraventricular arrhythmias with TCA overdose.

5. **You are listing the priorities of care for the adolescent who ingested the TCA. Symptomatic arrhythmias are beginning to develop. You ensure that her airway is protected and ventilation is adequate, and you initiate continuous ECG monitoring. Which one of the following is the *most* appropriate *initial* therapy for this patient?**

   a. immediate cardioversion for a wide-complex tachycardia even if blood pressure and systemic perfusion are normal

   b. lidocaine administration for a wide-complex tachycardia with palpable pulses and poor perfusion

(Continued on next page)

c. epinephrine administration for a wide-complex tachycardia with weak pulses and poor perfusion

d. sodium bicarbonate administration for a wide-complex tachycardia with palpable pulses and poor perfusion

The correct answer is d. The treatment of choice for symptomatic arrhythmias associated with TCA or sodium channel blocker toxicity includes administration of sodium bicarbonate. The sodium bicarbonate probably overcomes the sodium channel blockade. This therapy will narrow the QRS complex, shorten the QT interval, and increase myocardial contractility.

Answer a is incorrect because cardioversion is not the most appropriate initial therapy. Most patients with TCA overdose have bradycardia and heart block rather than tachycardia.

Answer b is incorrect. Although lidocaine is an optional therapy for the treatment of arrhythmias with this toxidrome, you should consider it only if the patient does not respond to sodium bicarbonate.

Answer c is incorrect. Epinephrine can be an effective treatment for bradycardia and hypotension. But it may be unnecessary if the sodium bicarbonate is effective.

6. **You just evaluated a 12-year-old girl who ingested a large quantity of calcium channel blockers in a suicide attempt. Which of the following abnormalities is *not* likely to be seen with severe calcium channel blocker intoxication?**

a. severe hypotension secondary to vasodilation and diminished cardiac contractility

b. wide-complex tachycardia

c. sinus bradycardia

d. coma or diminished level of consciousness

The correct answer is b. Wide-complex tachycardia is *not* expected after calcium channel blocker overdose. But reflex *sinus* tachycardia may develop in response to nifedipine-induced hypotension. Clinical manifestations of calcium channel blockers include bradyarrhythmias caused by inhibition of pacemaker cells and AV block.

Answer a is incorrect because severe hypotension secondary to vasodilation and diminished cardiac output *is* expected after calcium channel blocker toxicity.

Answer c is incorrect because sinus bradycardia *is* likely to develop after calcium channel blocker overdose.

Answer d is incorrect because coma or diminished level of consciousness *can* be associated with calcium channel blocker toxicity. The toxidrome of calcium channel blocker toxicity may include cerebral hypoperfusion with syncope, seizures, and coma.

7. **You are treating a patient with calcium channel blocker or β-adrenergic blocker toxicity. The patient has cardiac arrhythmias and hypotension with poor systemic perfusion unresponsive to support of airway, oxygenation, and ventilation; volume administration; and vasopressors. You are considering alternative therapies. Which of the following is *not* an appropriate alternative therapy for these types of poisoning?**

a. glucagon administration

b. naloxone administration

c. glucose plus insulin

d. calcium

The correct answer is b. Naloxone has no role in the treatment of β-adrenergic blocker toxicity. Naloxone is appropriate for opioid toxicity.

Answer a is incorrect because glucagon *is* an appropriate alternative therapy for calcium channel blocker or β-adrenergic blocker toxicity.

Answer c is incorrect because glucose plus insulin *is* an appropriate therapy for either β-adrenergic blocker or calcium channel blocker toxicity. In β-adrenergic blocker toxicity glucose plus insulin may be more effective than glucagon. In calcium channel blocker toxicity and β-adrenergic blocker toxicity, glucose plus insulin appears to improve myocardial glucose utilization. It appears to also increase myocardial uptake of glucose and lactate, improving the myocardial oxygen delivery-to-work ratio. You must monitor serum glucose and serum potassium concentrations during this therapy.

Answer d is incorrect because calcium *may* be considered for treatment of either β-adrenergic blocker or calcium channel blocker toxicity. The reports on the effect of calcium in β-adrenergic blocker toxicity are contradictory, but calcium may be considered if glucagon and catecholamines fail.

8. **You are caring for a child with severe narcotic intoxication. Which of the following choices gives the *most* appropriate therapies in appropriate order?**

a. open the airway and support ventilation before you administer naloxone

b. administer epinephrine to reverse bradycardia

c. administer naloxone first; support ventilation if there is no response

d. administer bicarbonate to reverse acidosis

The correct answer is a. For opioid poisoning you should open and protect the airway and support ventilation *before* you administer naloxone. If you provide ventilation to normalize a PaCO₂ *before* you administer naloxone, you will be able to minimize the sudden increase in epinephrine concentration and its potential toxic effects.

Answer b is incorrect because the primary complications of opioid poisoning include hypoventilation, apnea, and respiratory failure. Ventricular arrhythmias may also be present.

Answer c is incorrect because you should provide ventilation to normalize $PaCO_2$ before you administer naloxone.

Answer d is incorrect. If acidosis is present, it is likely to be respiratory acidosis. The buffering action of sodium bicarbonate results in the creation of CO_2. Sodium bicarbonate is likely to make existing hypercarbia worse unless effective ventilation is established.

References

1. Litovitz TL, Klein-Schwartz W, White S, Cobauh DJ, Youniss J, Omslaer JC, Drab A, Benson BE. 2000 Annual report of the American Association of Poison Control Centers Toxic Exposure Surveillance System. *Am J Emerg Med.* 2001;19:337-395.

2. McCaig LF, Burt CW. Poisoning-related visits to emergency departments in the United States, 1993-1996. *J Toxicol Clin Toxicol.* 1999;37:817-826.

3. Fingerhut LA, Cox CS. Poisoning mortality, 1985-1995 [published correction appears in *Public Health Rep.* 1998;113:380]. *Public Health Rep.* 1998;113:218-233.

4. Havlik DM, Nolte KB. Fatal "crack" cocaine ingestion in an infant. *Am J Forensic Med Pathol.* 2000;21:245-248.

5. Klasner AE, Scalzo AJ, Blume C, Johnson P. Ammonium bifluoride causes another pediatric death. *Ann Emerg Med.* 1998;31:525.

6. Klasner AE, Scalzo AJ, Blume C, Johnson P, Thompson MW. Marked hypocalcemia and ventricular fibrillation in two pediatric patients exposed to a fluoride-containing wheel cleaner. *Ann Emerg Med.* 1996;28:713-718.

7. Cosbey SH, Carson DJ. A fatal case of amlodipine poisoning. *J Anal Toxicol.* 1997;21:221-222.

8. Lee DC, Greene T, Dougherty T, Pearigen P. Fatal nifedipine ingestions in children. *J Emerg Med.* 2000;19:359-361.

9. Love JN. Acebutolol overdose resulting in fatalities. *J Emerg Med.* 2000;18:341-344.

10. Love JN, Litovitz TL, Howell JM, Clancy C. Characterization of fatal beta blocker ingestion: a review of the American Association of Poison Control Centers data from 1985 to 1995. *J Toxicol Clin Toxicol.* 1997;35:353-359.

11. Li L, Levine BE, Smialek JE. Fatal methadone poisoning in children: Maryland 1992-1996. *Subst Use Misuse.* 2000;35:1141-1148.

12. Litovitz TL, Klein-Schwartz W, White S, Cobaugh DJ, Youniss J, Drab A, Benson BE. 1999 Annual report of the American Association of Poison Control Centers Toxic Exposure Surveillance System. *Am J Emerg Med.* 2000;18:517-574.

13. Varley CK. Sudden death related to selected tricyclic antidepressants in children: epidemiology, mechanisms and clinical implications. *Paediatr Drugs.* 2001;3:613-627.

14. Albertson TE, Dawson A, de Latorre F, Hoffman RS, Hollander JE, Jaeger A, Kerns WR II. TOX-ACLS: toxicologic-oriented advanced cardiac life support. *Ann Emerg Med.* 2001;37:S78-S90.

15. American College of Emergency Physicians. Poison information and treatment systems. *Ann Emerg Med.* 1996;28:384.

16. American Academy of Clinical Toxicology. Facility assessment guidelines for regional toxicology treatment centers. *J Toxicol Clin Toxicol.* 1993;31:211-217.

17. Gill AM, Cousins A, Nunn AJ, Choonara IA. Opiate-induced respiratory depression in pediatric patients. *Ann Pharmacother.* 1996;30:125-129.

18. Dahlin KL, Lastborn L, Blomgren B, Ryrfeldt A. Acute lung failure induced by tricyclic antidepressants. *Toxicol Appl Pharmacol.* 1997;146:309-316.

19. Selden BS, Curry SC. Prolonged succinylcholine-induced paralysis in organophsophate insecticide poisoning. *Ann Emerg Med.* 1987;16:215-217.

20. Vance MV, Selden BS, Clark RF. Optimal patient position for transport and initial management of toxic ingestions. *Ann Emerg Med.* 1992;21:243-246.

21. Krenzelok E, Vale A. Position statements: gut decontamination. American Academy of Clinical Toxicology; European Association of Poisons Centres and Clinical Toxicologists. *J Toxicol Clin Toxicol.* 1997;35:695-786.

22. Krenzelok EP, McGuigan M, Lheur P. Position statement: ipecac syrup. American Academy of Clinical Toxicology; European Association of Poisons Centres and Clinical Toxicologists. *J Toxicol Clin Toxicol.* 1997;35:699-709.

23. Cooney DO. *Activated Charcoal in Medicinal Applications.* New York, NY: Marcel Dekker; 1995.

24. Chyka PA, Seger D. Position statement: single-dose activated charcoal. American Academy of Clinical Toxicology; European Association of Poisons Centres and Clinical Toxicologists. *J Toxicol Clin Toxicol.* 1997;35:721-741.

25. Wax PM, Cobaugh DJ. Prehospital gastrointestinal decontamination of toxic ingestions: a missed opportunity. *Am J Emerg Med.* 1998;16:114-116.

26. Allison TB, Gough JE, Brown LH, Thomas SH. Potential time savings by prehospital administration of activated charcoal. *Prehosp Emerg Care.* 1997;1:73-75.

27. Mauro LS, Nawarskas JJ, Mauro VF. Misadventures with activated charcoal and recommendations for safe use. *Ann Pharmacother.* 1994;28:915-924.

28. Moll J, Kerns W II, Tomaszewski C, Rose R. Incidence of aspiration pneumonia in intubated patients receiving activated charcoal. *J Emerg Med.* 1999;17:279-283.

29. Vale JA. Position statement: gastric lavage. American Academy of Clinical Toxicology; European Association of Poisons Centres and Clinical Toxicologists. *J Toxicol Clin Toxicol.* 1997;35:711-719.

30. Thompson AM, Robins JB, Prescott LF. Changes in cardiorespiratory function during gastric lavage for drug overdose. *Hum Toxicol.* 1987;6:215-218.

31. Justiniani FR, Hippalgaonkar R, Martinez LO. Charcoal-containing empyema complicating treatment for overdose. *Chest.* 1985; 87:404-405.

32. Askenasi R, Abramowicz M, Jeanmart J, Ansay J, Degaute JP. Esophageal perforation: an unusual complication of gastric lavage. *Ann Emerg Med.* 1984;13:146.

33. Mariani PJ, Pook N. Gastrointestinal tract perforation with charcoal peritoneum complicating orogastric intubation and lavage. *Ann Emerg Med.* 1993;22:606-609.

34. Scalzo AJ, Tominack RL, Thompson MW. Malposition of pediatric gastric lavage tubes demonstrated radiographically. *J Emerg Med.* 1992;10:581-586.

35. Klasner AE, Scalzo AJ, Luke DA. Pediatric orogastric and nasogastric tubes: a new formula evaluated. *Ann Emerg Med.* In press.

36. Jacobsen D, Haines JA. The relative efficacy of antidotes: the IPCS evaluation series. International Programme on Chemical Safety. *Arch Toxicol Suppl.* 1997;19:305-310.

37. Pronczuk de Garbino J, Haines JA, Jacobsen D, Meredith T. Evaluation of antidotes: activities of the International Programme on Chemical Safety. *J Toxicol Clin Toxicol.* 1997;35: 333-343.

38. Bauman JL, Grawe JJ, Winecoff AP, Hariman RJ. Cocaine-related sudden cardiac death: a hypothesis correlating basic science and clinical observations. *J Clin Pharmacol.* 1994;34: 902-911.

39. Goldfrank LR, Hoffman RS. The cardiovascular effects of cocaine. *Ann Emerg Med.* 1991;20:165-175.

40. Marzuk PM, Tardiff K, Leon AC, Hirsch CS, Stajic M, Portera L, Hartwell N, Iqbal MI. Fatal injuries after cocaine use as a leading cause of death among young adults in New York City. *N Engl J Med.* 1995;332:1753-1757.

41. Loiselle JM, Baker MD, Templeton JMJ, Schwartz G, Drott H. Substance abuse in adolescent trauma. *Ann Emerg Med.* 1993; 22:1530-1534.

42. Blaho K, Logan B, Winbery S, Park L, Schwilke E. Blood cocaine and metabolite concentrations, clinical findings, and outcome of patients presenting to an ED. *Am J Emerg Med.* 2000;18:593-598.

43. Lange RA, Hillis LD. Cardiovascular complications of cocaine use. *N Engl J Med.* 2001; 345:351-358.

44. Mo W, Singh AK, Arruda JA, Dunea G. Role of nitric oxide in cocaine-induced acute hypertension. *Am J Hypertens.* 1998;11:708-714.

45. Hollander JE, Hoffman RS, Gennis P, Fairweather P, DiSano MJ, Schumb DA, Feldman JA, Fish SS, Dyer S, Wax P, et al. Prospective multicenter evaluation of cocaine-associated chest pain. Cocaine Associated Chest Pain (COCHPA) Study Group. *Acad Emerg Med.* 1994;1:330-339.

46. Brody SL, Slovis CM, Wrenn KD. Cocaine-related medical problems: consecutive series of 233 patients. *Am J Med.* 1990;88:325-331.

47. Williams JJ, Restieaux NJ, Low CJ. Myocardial infarction in young people with normal coronary arteries. *Heart.* 1998;79:191-194.

48. Heesch CM, Wilhelm CR, Ristich J, Adnane J, Bontempo FA, Wagner WR. Cocaine activates platelets and increases the formation of circulating platelet containing microaggregates in humans. *Heart.* 2000;83:688-695.

49. Karch SB. Cardiac arrest in cocaine users. *Am J Emerg Med.* 1996;14:79-81.

50. Kolecki PF, Curry SC. Poisoning by sodium channel blocking agents. *Crit Care Clin.* 1997; 13:829-848.

51. Parker RB, Perry GY, Horan LG, Flowers NC. Comparative effects of sodium bicarbonate and sodium chloride on reversing cocaine-induced changes in the electrocardiogram. *J Cardiovasc Pharmacol.* 1999;34:864-869.

52. Hollander JE, Hoffman RS, Burstein JL, Shih RD, Thode HCJ. Cocaine-associated myocardial infarction. Mortality and complications. Cocaine-Associated Myocardial Infarction Study Group. *Arch Intern Med.* 1995;155: 1081-1086.

53. Hoffman RS, Hollander JE. Evaluation of patients with chest pain after cocaine use. *Crit Care Clin.* 1997;13:809-828.

54. Derlet RW, Albertson TE. Diazepam in the prevention of seizures and death in cocaine-intoxicated rats. *Ann Emerg Med.* 1989;18: 542-546.

55. Catravas JD, Waters IW, Walz MA, Davis WM. Acute cocaine intoxication in the conscious dog: pathophysiologic profile of acute lethality. *Arch Int Pharmacodyn Ther.* 1978; 235:328-340.

56. Freemantle N, Cleland J, Young P, Mason J, Harrison J. β-Blockade after myocardial infarction: systematic review and meta regression analysis. *BMJ.* 1999;318:1730-1737.

57. Kenny D, Pagel PS, Warltier DC. Attenuation of the systemic and coronary hemodynamic effects of cocaine in conscious dogs: propranolol versus labetalol. *Basic Res Cardiol.* 1992;87:465-477.

58. Sand IC, Brody SL, Wrenn KD, Slovis CM. Experience with esmolol for the treatment of cocaine-associated cardiovascular complications. *Am J Emerg Med.* 1991;9:161-163.

59. Lange RA, Cigarroa RG, Flores ED, McBride W, Kim AS, Wells PJ, Bedotto JB, Danziger RS, Hillis LD. Potentiation of cocaine-induced coronary vasoconstriction by beta-adrenergic blockade. *Ann Intern Med.* 1990;112:897-903.

60. Boehrer JD, Moliterno DJ, Willard JE, Hillis LD, Lange RA. Influence of labetalol on cocaine-induced coronary vasoconstriction in humans. *Am J Med.* 1993;94:608-610.

61. Brogan WC III, Lange RA, Kim AS, Moliterno DJ, Hillis LD. Alleviation of cocaine-induced coronary vasoconstriction by nitroglycerin. *J Am Coll Cardiol.* 1991;18:581-586.

62. Hollander JE, Hoffman RS, Gennis P, Fairweather P, DiSano MJ, Schumb DA, Feldman JA, Fish SS, Dyer S, Wax P, et al. Nitroglycerin in the treatment of cocaine associated chest pain: clinical safety and efficacy. *J Toxicol Clin Toxicol.* 1994;32:243-256.

63. Taketomo CK, Hodding JH, Kraus DM. *Pediatric Drug Handbook.* Hudson, Ohio: Lexi-Corp Inc; 1998.

64. Lange RA, Cigarroa RG, Yancy CWJ, Willard JE, Popma JJ, Sills MN, McBride W, Kim AS, Hillis LD. Cocaine-induced coronary-artery vasoconstriction. *N Engl J Med.* 1989; 321:1557-1562.

65. Benitz WE, Tatro DS. *The Pediatric Drug Handbook.* St Louis, Mo: Mosby-Year Book; 1995.

66. Wang RY. pH-dependent cocaine-induced cardiotoxicity. *Am J Emerg Med.* 1999;17: 364-369.

67. Kerns W II, Garvey L, Owens J. Cocaine-induced wide complex dysrhythmia. *J Emerg Med.* 1997;15:321-329.

68. Beckman KJ, Parker RB, Hariman RJ, Gallastegui JL, Javaid JI, Bauman JL. Hemodynamic and electrophysiological actions of cocaine: effects of sodium bicarbonate as an antidote in dogs. *Circulation.* 1991;83:1799-1807.

69. Derlet RW, Albertson TE, Tharratt RS. Lidocaine potentiation of cocaine toxicity. *Ann Emerg Med.* 1991;20:135-138.

70. Ye JH, Ren J, Krnjevic K, Liu PL, McArdle JJ. Cocaine and lidocaine have additive inhibitory effects on the GABA A current of acutely dissociated hippocampal pyramidal neurons. *Brain Res.* 1999;821:26-32.

71. Shih RD, Hollander JE, Burstein JL, Nelson LS, Hoffman RS, Quick AM. Clinical safety of lidocaine in patients with cocaine-associated myocardial infarction. *Ann Emerg Med.* 1995; 26:702-706.

72. Keller DJ, Todd GL. Acute cardiotoxic effects of cocaine and a hyperadrenergic state in anesthetized dogs. *Int J Cardiol.* 1994;44:19-28.

73. Livezey GT, Sparber SB. Hyperthermia sensitizes rats to cocaine's proconvulsive effects and unmasks EEG evidence of kindling after chronic cocaine. *Pharmacol Biochem Behav.* 1990;37:761-767.

74. Rockhold RW, Carver ES, Ishizuka Y, Hoskins B, Ho IK. Dopamine receptors mediate cocaine-induced temperature responses in spontaneously hypertensive and Wistar-Kyoto rats. *Pharmacol Biochem Behav.* 1991;40:157-162.

75. Ruttenber AJ, Lawler-Heavner J, Yin M, Wetli CV, Hearn WL, Mash DC. Fatal excited delirium following cocaine use: epidemiologic findings provide new evidence for mechanisms of cocaine toxicity. *J Forensic Sci.* 1997;42:25-31.

76. Marzuk PM, Tardiff K, Leon AC, Hirsch CS, Portera L, Iqbal MI, Nock MK, Hartwell N. Ambient temperature and mortality from unintentional cocaine overdose. *JAMA.* 1998;279:1795-1800.

77. Ernst AA, Sanders WM. Unexpected cocaine intoxication presenting as seizures in children. *Ann Emerg Med.* 1989;18:774-777.

78. Conway EEJ, Mezey AP, Powers K. Status epilepticus following the oral ingestion of cocaine in an infant. *Pediatr Emerg Care.* 1990;6:189-190.

79. Chaney NE, Franke J, Wadlington WB. Cocaine convulsions in a breast-feeding baby. *J Pediatr.* 1988;112:134-135.

80. Riggs D, Weibley RE. Acute hemorrhagic diarrhea and cardiovascular collapse in a young child owing to environmentally acquired cocaine. *Pediatr Emerg Care.* 1991;7:154-155.

81. Hickson GB, Altemeier WA, Martin ED, Campbell PW. Parental administration of chemical agents: a cause of apparent life-threatening events. *Pediatrics.* 1989;83:772-776.

82. Bulbul ZR, Rosenthal DN, Kleinman CS. Myocardial infarction in the perinatal period secondary to maternal cocaine abuse: a case report and literature review. *Arch Pediatr Adolesc Med.* 1994;148:1092-1096.

83. Addis A, Moretti ME, Ahmed Syed F, Einarson TR, Koren G. Fetal effects of cocaine: an updated meta-analysis. *Reprod Toxicol.* 2001;15:341-369.

84. Winecker RE, Goldberger BA, Tebbett IR, Behnke M, Eyler FD, Karlix JL, Wobie K, Conlon M, Phillips D, Bertholf RL. Detection of cocaine and its metabolites in breast milk. *J Forensic Sci.* 2001;46:1221-1223.

85. Mott SH, Packer RJ, Soldin SJ. Neurologic manifestations of cocaine exposure in childhood. *Pediatrics.* 1994;93:557-560.

86. Heidemann SM, Goetting MG. Passive inhalation of cocaine by infants. *Henry Ford Hosp Med J.* 1990;38:252-254.

87. Mirchandani HG, Mirchandani IH, Hellman F, English-Rider R, Rosen S, Laposata EA. Passive inhalation of free-base cocaine ('crack') smoke by infants. *Arch Pathol Lab Med.* 1991;115:494-498.

88. Farrar HC, James LP. Characteristics of pediatric admissions for cyclic antidepressant poisoning. *Am J Emerg Med.* 1999;17:495-496.

89. Shah R, Uren Z, Baker A, Majeed A. Deaths from antidepressants in England and Wales 1993-1997: analysis of a new national database. *Psychol Med.* 2001;31:1203-1210.

90. Gerard JM, Klasner AE, Madhok M, Scalzo AJ, Barry RC, Laffey SP. Poison prevention counseling: a comparison between family practitioners and pediatricians. *Arch Pediatr Adolesc Med.* 2000;154:65-70.

91. Mullins ME, Pinnick RV, Terhes JM. Life-threatening diphenhydramine overdose treated with charcoal hemoperfusion and hemodialysis. *Ann Emerg Med.* 1999;33:104-107.

92. Zell-Kanter M, Toerne TS, Spiegel K, Negrusz A. Doxepin toxicity in a child following topical administration. *Ann Pharmacother.* 2000;34:328-329.

93. Mullins ME, Cristofani CB, Warden CR, Cleary JF. Amitriptyline-associated seizures in a toddler with Munchausen-by-proxy. *Pediatr Emerg Care.* 1999;15:202-205.

94. Walsh DM. Cyclic antidepressant overdose in children: a proposed treatment protocol. *Pediatr Emerg Care.* 1986;2:28-35.

95. Wolfe TR, Caravati EM, Rollins DE. Terminal 40-ms frontal plane QRS axis as a marker for tricyclic antidepressant overdose. *Ann Emerg Med.* 1989;18:348-351.

96. Harrigan RA, Brady WJ. ECG abnormalities in tricyclic antidepressant ingestion. *Am J Emerg Med.* 1999;17:387-393.

97. Boehnert MT, Lovejoy FH Jr. Value of the QRS duration versus the serum drug level in predicting seizures and ventricular arrhythmias after an acute overdose of tricyclic antidepressants. *N Engl J Med.* 1985;313:474-479.

98. Foulke GE. Identifying toxicity risk early after antidepressant overdose. *Am J Emerg Med.* 1995;13:123-126.

99. Liebelt EL, Francis PD, Woolf AD. ECG lead aVR versus QRS interval in predicting seizures and arrhythmias in acute tricyclic antidepressant toxicity. *Ann Emerg Med.* 1995;26:195-201.

100. Liebelt EL, Ulrich A, Francis PD, Woolf A. Serial electrocardiogram changes in acute tricyclic antidepressant overdoses. *Crit Care Med.* 1997;25:1721-1726.

101. Hoffman JR, Votey SR, Bayer M, Silver L. Effect of hypertonic sodium bicarbonate in the treatment of moderate-to-severe cyclic antidepressant overdose. *Am J Emerg Med.* 1993;11:336-341.

102. McCabe JL, Cobaugh DJ, Menegazzi JJ, Fata J. Experimental tricyclic antidepressant toxicity: a randomized, controlled comparison of hypertonic saline solution, sodium bicarbonate, and hyperventilation. *Ann Emerg Med.* 1998;32(pt 1):329-333.

103. Bou-Abboud E, Nattel S. Relative role of alkalosis and sodium ions in reversal of class I antiarrhythmic drug-induced sodium channel blockade by sodium bicarbonate. *Circulation.* 1996;94:1954-1961.

104. Levitt MA, Sullivan JB Jr, Owens SM, Burnham L, Finley PR. Amitriptyline plasma protein binding: effect of plasma pH and relevance to clinical overdose. *Am J Emerg Med.* 1986;4:121-125.

105. Liebelt EL. Targeted management strategies for cardiovascular toxicity from tricyclic antidepressant overdose: the pivotal role for alkalinization and sodium loading. *Pediatr Emerg Care.* 1998;14:293-298.

106. Bessen HA, Niemann JT. Improvement of cardiac conduction after hyperventilation in tricyclic antidepressant overdose. *J Toxicol Clin Toxicol.* 1985;23:537-546.

107. Wrenn K, Smith BA, Slovis CM. Profound alkalemia during treatment of tricyclic antidepressant overdose: a potential hazard of combined hyperventilation and intravenous bicarbonate. *Am J Emerg Med.* 1992;10:553-555.

108. Knudsen K, Abrahamsson J. Effects of epinephrine, norepinephrine, magnesium sulfate, and milrinone on survival and the occurrence of arrhythmias in amitriptyline poisoning in the rat. *Crit Care Med.* 1994;22:1851-1855.

109. Teba L, Schiebel F, Dedhia HV, Lazzell VA. Beneficial effect of norepinephrine in the treatment of circulatory shock caused by tricyclic antidepressant overdose. *Am J Emerg Med.* 1988;6:566-568.

110. Tran TP, Panacek EA, Rhee KJ, Foulke GE. Response to dopamine vs norepinephrine in tricyclic antidepressant-induced hypotension. *Acad Emerg Med.* 1997;4:864-868.

111. Zaritsky AL. Catecholamines, inotropic medications, and vasopressor agents. In: Chernow B, ed. *The Pharmacologic Approach to the Critically Ill Patient.* 3rd ed. Baltimore, Md: Williams & Wilkins; 1994:387-404.

112. Williams JM, Hollingshed MJ, Vasilakis A, Morales M, Prescott JE, Graeber GM. Extracorporeal circulation in the management of severe tricyclic antidepressant overdose. *Am J Emerg Med.* 1994;12:456-458.

113. Larkin GL, Graeber GM, Hollingsed MJ. Experimental amitriptyline poisoning: treatment of severe cardiovascular toxicity with cardiopulmonary bypass. *Ann Emerg Med.* 1994;23:480-486.

114. James LP, Kearns GL. Cyclic antidepressant toxicity in children and adolescents. *J Clin Pharmacol.* 1995;35:343-350.

115. Wedin GP, Oderda GM, Klein-Schwartz W, Gorman RL. Relative toxicity of cyclic antidepressants. *Ann Emerg Med.* 1986;15: 797-804.

116. Olson KR, Kearney TE, Dyer JE, Benowitz NL, Blanc PD. Seizures associated with poisoning and drug overdose. *Am J Emerg Med.* 1994;12:392-395.

117. Callaham M, Schumaker H, Pentel P. Phenytoin prophylaxis of cardiotoxicity in experimental amitriptyline poisoning. *J Pharmacol Exp Ther.* 1988;245:216-220.

118. Roy TM, Ossorio MA, Cipolla LM, Fields CL, Snider HL, Anderson WH. Pulmonary complications after tricyclic antidepressant overdose. *Chest.* 1989;96:852-856.

119. Zuckerman GB, Conway EE Jr. Pulmonary complications following tricyclic antidepressant overdose in an adolescent. *Ann Pharmacother.* 1993;27:572-574.

120. Schwartz JG, Hurd IL, Carnahan JJ. Determination of tricyclic antidepressants for ED analysis. *Am J Emerg Med.* 1994;12:513-516.

121. Matos ME, Burns MM, Shannon MW. False-positive tricyclic antidepressant drug screen results leading to the diagnosis of carbamazepine intoxication. *Pediatrics.* 2000;105:E66.

122. Fleischman A, Chiang VW. Carbamazepine overdose recognized by a tricyclic antidepressant assay. *Pediatrics.* 2001;107:176-177.

123. Chattergoon DS, Verjee Z, Anderson M, Johnson D, McGuigan MA, Koren G, Ito S. Carbamazepine interference with an immune assay for tricyclic antidepressants in plasma. *J Toxicol Clin Toxicol.* 1998;36:109-113.

124. Wells TG, Graham CJ, Moss MM, Kearns GL. Nifedipine poisoning in a child. *Pediatrics.* 1990;86:91-94.

125. Ramoska EA, Spiller HA, Winter M, Borys D. A one-year evaluation of calcium channel blocker overdoses: toxicity and treatment. *Ann Emerg Med.* 1993;22:196-200.

126. Moser LR, Smythe MA, Tisdale JE. The use of calcium salts in the prevention and management of verapamil-induced hypotension. *Ann Pharmacother.* 2000;34:622-629.

127. Adams BD, Browne WT. Amlodipine overdose causes prolonged calcium channel blocker toxicity. *Am J Emerg Med.* 1998; 16:527-528.

128. Leesar MA, Martyn R, Talley JD, Frumin H. Noncardiogenic pulmonary edema complicating massive verapamil overdose. *Chest.* 1994;105:606-607.

129. Humbert VH Jr, Munn NJ, Hawkins RF. Noncardiogenic pulmonary edema complicating massive verapamil overdose. *Chest.* 1991;99:258-259.

130. Fauville JP, Hantson P, Honore P, Belpaire F, Rosseel MT, Mahieu P. Severe diltiazem poisoning with intestinal pseudo-obstruction: case report and toxicological data. *J Toxicol Clin Toxicol.* 1995;33:273-277.

131. Ray JM, Squires PE, Meloche RM, Nelson DW, Snutch TP, Buchan AM. L-type calcium channels regulate gastrin release from human antral G cells. *Am J Physiol.* 1997; 273:G281-G288.

132. Stanek EJ, Nelson CE, DeNofrio D. Amlodipine overdose. *Ann Pharmacother.* 1997, 31:853-856.

133. Spiller HA, Meyers A, Ziemba T, Riley M. Delayed onset of cardiac arrhythmias from sustained-release verapamil. *Ann Emerg Med.* 1991;20:201-203.

134. Watling SM, Crain JL, Edwards TD, Stiller RA. Verapamil overdose: case report and review of the literature. *Ann Pharmacother.* 1992;26:1373-1378.

135. Horowitz BZ, Rhee KJ. Massive verapamil ingestion: a report of two cases and a review of the literature. *Am J Emerg Med.* 1989;7: 624-631.

136. Belson MG, Gorman SE, Sullivan K, Geller RJ. Calcium channel blocker ingestions in children. *Am J Emerg Med.* 2000;18:581-586.

137. Broner CW, Stidham GL, Westenkirchner DF, Watson DC. A prospective, randomized, double-blind comparison of calcium chloride and calcium gluconate therapies for hypocalcemia in critically ill children. *J Pediatr.* 1990;117:986-989.

138. Proano L, Chiang WK, Wang RY. Calcium channel blocker overdose. *Am J Emerg Med.* 1995;13:444-450.

139. Oe H, Taniura T, Ohgitani N. A case of severe verapamil overdose. *Jpn Circ J.* 1998;62:72-76.

140. Kline JA, Leonova E, Raymond RM. Beneficial myocardial metabolic effects of insulin during verapamil toxicity in the anesthetized canine. *Crit Care Med.* 1995;23:1251-1263.

141. Kline JA, Tomaszewski CA, Schroeder JD, Raymond RM. Insulin is a superior antidote for cardiovascular toxicity induced by verapamil in the anesthetized canine. *J Pharmacol Exp Ther.* 1993;267:744-750.

142. Boyer EW, Shannon M. Treatment of calcium-channel-blocker intoxication with insulin infusion. *N Engl J Med.* 2001;344: 1721-1722.

143. Yuan TH, Kerns WPI, Tomaszewski CA, Ford MD, Kline JA. Insulin-glucose as adjunctive therapy for severe calcium channel antagonist poisoning. *J Toxicol Clin Toxicol.* 1999;37:463-474.

144. Diaz R, Paolasso EA, Piegas LS, Tajer CD, Moreno MG, Corvalan R, Isea JE, Romero G. Metabolic modulation of acute myocardial infarction. The ECLA (Estudios Cardiologicos Latinoamerica) Collaborative Group. *Circulation.* 1998;98:2227-2234.

145. Zaritsky AL, Horowitz M, Chernow B. Glucagon antagonism of calcium channel blocker-induced myocardial dysfunction. *Crit Care Med.* 1988;16:246-251.

146. Papadopoulos J, O'Neil MG. Utilization of a glucagon infusion in the management of a massive nifedipine overdose. *J Emerg Med.* 2000;18:453-455.

147. Holzer M, Sterz F, Schoerkhuber W, Behringer W, Domanovits H, Weinmar D, Weinstabl C, Stimpfl T. Successful resuscitation of a verapamil-intoxicated patient with percutaneous cardiopulmonary bypass. *Crit Care Med.* 1999;27:2818-2823.

148. Parra DA, Totapally BR, Zahn E, Jacobs J, Aldousany A, Burke RP, Chang AC. Outcome of cardiopulmonary resuscitation in a pediatric cardiac intensive care unit. *Crit Care Med.* 2000;28:3296-3300.

149. Waxman AB, White KP, Trawick DR. Electromechanical dissociation following verapamil and propranolol ingestion: a physiologic profile. *Cardiology.* 1997;99:478-481.

150. Evans JS, Oram MP. Neurological recovery after prolonged verapamil-induced cardiac arrest. *Anaesth Intensive Care.* 1999;27: 653-655.

151. Love JN, Howell JM, Litovitz TL, Klein-Schwartz W. Acute beta blocker overdose: factors associated with the development of cardiovascular morbidity. *J Toxicol Clin Toxicol.* 2000;38:275-281.

152. Kerns W II, Kline J, Ford MD. Beta-blocker and calcium channel blocker toxicity. *Emerg Med Clin North Am.* 1994;12:365-390.

153. Whitehurst VE, Vick JA, Alleva FR, Zhang J, Joseph X, Balazs T. Reversal of propranolol blockade of adrenergic receptors and related toxicity with drugs that increase cyclic AMP. *Proc Soc Exp Biol Med.* 1999;221: 382-385.

154. Assimes TL, Malcolm I. Torsade de pointes with sotalol overdose treated successfully with lidocaine. *Can J Cardiol.* 1998;14:7 53-756.

155. Stinson J, Walsh M, Feely J. Ventricular asystole and overdose with atenolol. *BMJ.* 1992;305:693.

156. Donovan KD, Gerace RV, Dreyer JF. Acebutolol-induced ventricular tachycardia reversed with sodium bicarbonate. *J Toxicol Clin Toxicol*. 1999;37:481-484.

157. Cruickshank JM, Neil-Dwyer G, Cameron MM, McAinsh J. β-Adrenoreceptor-blocking agents and the blood-brain barrier. *Clin Sci*. 1980;59(suppl 6):453s-455s.

158. Lifshitz M, Zucker N, Zalzstein E. Acute dilated cardiomyopathy and central nervous system toxicity following propranolol intoxication. *Pediatr Emerg Care*. 1999;15:262-263.

159. Weinstein RS. Recognition and management of poisoning with β-adrenergic blocking agents. *Ann Emerg Med*. 1984;13:1123-1131.

160. Avery GJ III, Spotnitz HM, Rose EA, Malm JR, Hoffman BF. Pharmacologic antagonism of β-adrenergic blockade in dogs, I: hemodynamic effects of isoproterenol, dopamine, and epinephrine in acute propranolol administration. *J Thorac Cardiovasc Surg*. 1979;77:267-276.

161. Lewis M, Kallenbach J, Germond C, Zaltzman M, Muller F, Steyn J, Zwi S. Survival following massive overdose of adrenergic blocking agents (acebutolol and labetalol). *Eur Heart J*. 1983;4:328-332.

162. Snook CP, Sigvaldason K, Kristinsson J. Severe atenolol and diltiazem overdose. *J Toxicol Clin Toxicol*. 2000;38:661-665.

163. Kalman S, Berg S, Lisander B. Combined overdose with verapamil and atenolol: treatment with high doses of adrenergic agonists. *Acta Anaesthesiol Scand*. 1998;42:379-382.

164. Kollef MH. Labetalol overdose successfully treated with amrinone and α-adrenergic receptor agonists. *Chest*. 1994;105:626-627.

165. Love JN, Leasure JA, Mundt DJ. A comparison of combined amrinone and glucagon therapy to glucagon alone for cardiovascular depression associated with propranolol toxicity in a canine model. *Am J Emerg Med*. 1993;11:360-363.

166. Sato S, Tsuji MH, Okubo N, Nishimoto C, Naito H. Combined use of glucagon and milrinone may not be preferable for severe propranolol poisoning in the canine model. *J Toxicol Clin Toxicol*. 1995;33:337-342.

167. Mofenson HC, Caraccio TR, Laudano J. Glucagon for propranolol overdose [letter]. *JAMA*. 1986;255:2025-2026.

168. Kerns W II, Schroeder D, Williams C, Tomaszewski C, Raymond R. Insulin improves survival in a canine model of acute β-blocker toxicity. *Ann Emerg Med*. 1997;29:748-757.

169. Love JN, Hanfling D, Howell JM. Hemodynamic effects of calcium chloride in a canine model of acute propranolol intoxication. *Ann Emerg Med*. 1996;28:1-6.

170. Brimacombe JR, Scully M, Swainston R. Propranolol overdose—a dramatic response to calcium chloride. *Med J Aust*. 1991;155:267-268.

171. Pertoldi F, D'Orlando L, Mercante WP. Electromechanical dissociation 48 hours after atenolol overdose: usefulness of calcium chloride. *Ann Emerg Med*. 1998;31:777-781.

172. Henry M, Kay MM, Viccellio P. Cardiogenic shock associated with calcium-channel and β blockers: reversal with intravenous calcium chloride. *Am J Emerg Med*. 1985;3:334-336.

173. Kenyon CJ, Aldinger GE, Joshipura P, Zaid GJ. Successful resuscitation using external cardiac pacing in beta adrenergic antagonist-induced bradyasystolic arrest. *Ann Emerg Med*. 1988;17:711-713.

174. McVey FK, Corke CF. Extracorporeal circulation in the management of massive propranolol overdose. *Anaesthesia*. 1991;46:744-746.

175. Unintentional opiate overdose deaths—King County, Washington, 1990-1999. *MMWR Morb Mortal Wkly Rep*. 2000;49:636-640.

176. Roberts I, Barker M, Li L. Analysis of trends in deaths from accidental drug poisoning in teenagers, 1985-95. *BMJ*. 1997;315:289.

177. Krauss B, Green SM. Sedation and analgesia for procedures in children. *N Engl J Med*. 2000;342:938-945.

178. Murray S, Brewerton T. Abuse of over-the-counter dextromethorphan by teenagers. *South Med J*. 1993;86:1151-1153.

179. Brooks DE, Roberge RJ, Spear A. Clinical nuances of pediatric methadone intoxication. *Vet Hum Toxicol*. 1999;41:388-390.

180. McClure RJ, Davis PM, Meadow SR, Sibert JR. Epidemiology of Munchausen syndrome by proxy, non-accidental poisoning, and non-accidental suffocation. *Arch Dis Child*. 1996;75:57-61.

181. Belson MG, Simon HK. Utility of comprehensive toxicologic screens in children. *Am J Emerg Med*. 1999;17:221-224.

182. Marquardt KA, Tharratt RS. Inhalation abuse of fentanyl patch. *J Toxicol Clin Toxicol*. 1994;32:72-75.

183. Remskar M, Noc M, Leskovsek B, Horvat M. Profound circulatory shock following heroin overdose. *Resuscitation*. 1998;38:51-53.

184. White JM, Irvine RJ. Mechanisms of fatal opioid overdose. *Addiction*. 1999;94:961-972.

185. Sporer KA, Dorn E. Heroin-related noncardiogenic pulmonary edema: a case series. *Chest*. 2001;120:1628-1632.

186. Murphy DB, Sutton JA, Prescott LF, Murphy MB. Opioid-induced delay in gastric emptying: a peripheral mechanism in humans. *Anesthesiology*. 1997;87:765-770.

187. Hagmeyer KO, Mauro LS, Mauro VF. Meperidine-related seizures associated with patient-controlled analgesia pumps. *Ann Pharmacother*. 1993;27:29-32.

188. Kyff JV, Rice TL. Meperidine-associated seizures in a child. *Clin Pharm*. 1990;9:337-338.

189. Mitchell AA, Lovejoy FH, Goldman P. Drug ingestions associated with miosis in comatose children. *J Pediatr*. 1976;89:303-305.

190. American Academy of Pediatrics Committee on Drugs. Naloxone dosage and route of administration for infants and children: addendum to emergency drug doses for infants and children. *Pediatrics*. 1990;86:484-485.

191. Kattwinkel J, Niermeyer S, Nadkarni V, Tibballs J, Phillips B, Zideman D, Van Reempts P, Osmond M. An advisory statement from the Pediatric Working Group of the International Liaison Committee on Resuscitation. *Pediatrics*. 1999;103:e56.

192. Sporer KA, Firestone J, Isaacs SM. Out-of-hospital treatment of opioid overdoses in an urban setting. *Acad Emerg Med*. 1996;3:660-667.

193. Yealy DM, Paris PM, Kaplan RM, Heller MB, Marini SE. The safety of prehospital naloxone administration by paramedics. *Ann Emerg Med*. 1990;19:902-905.

194. Mills CA, Flacke JW, Flacke WE, Bloor BC, Liu MD. Narcotic reversal in hypercapnic dogs: comparison of naloxone and nalbuphine. *Can J Anaesth*. 1990;37:238-244.

195. Prough DS, Roy R, Bumgarner J, Shannon G. Acute pulmonary edema in healthy teenagers following conservative doses of intravenous naloxone. *Anesthesiology*. 1984;60:485-486.

196. Osterwalder JJ. Naloxone—for intoxications with intravenous heroin and heroin mixtures—harmless or hazardous? A prospective clinical study. *J Toxicol Clin Toxicol*. 1996;34:409-416.

197. Kienbaum P, Thurauf N, Michel MC, Scherbaum N, Gastpar M, Peters J. Profound increase in epinephrine concentration in plasma and cardiovascular stimulation after mu-opioid receptor blockade in opioid-addicted patients during barbiturate-induced anesthesia for acute detoxification. *Anesthesiology*. 1998;88:1154-1161.

198. Tenenbein M. Continuous naloxone infusion for opiate poisoning in infancy. *J Pediatr*. 1984;105:645-648.

199. Wanger K, Brough L, Macmillan I, Goulding J, MacPhail I, Christenson JM. Intravenous vs subcutaneous naloxone for out-of-hospital management of presumed opioid overdose. *Acad Emerg Med*. 1998;5:293-299.

Neonatal Resuscitation

Introductory Case Scenario

A full-term newborn weighing 3.5 kg is delivered in the Emergency Department. Meconium-stained fluid is present, and the infant is flaccid, apneic, and centrally cyanotic.

- What is the appropriate management of this newly born infant?

- What equipment should be available?

- What is the appropriate size tracheal tube for this newly born infant?

- How does the presence of meconium-stained fluid affect your resuscitation interventions for this newly born infant?

Learning Objectives

After completing this chapter the PALS provider should be able to

- List the questions asked in a targeted history used to prepare for deliveries outside the delivery room

- Describe the key elements of rapid assessment of the newly born infant and the key steps in ongoing evaluation

- Describe the elements of routine care of the healthy term infant

- Differentiate between the initial steps of resuscitation of a newly born infant with clear amniotic fluid and those for an infant with meconium-stained amniotic fluid

- Recognize the importance of establishing adequate ventilation in resuscitation of the newly born infant

- Outline the indications for chest compressions, tracheal intubation, and administration of medication during resuscitation of the newly born infant

Background

Resuscitation in the delivery room is discussed in depth in the Neonatal Resuscitation Program (NRP), a separate course. All personnel who work in the delivery room, mother/baby unit, newborn nursery, and neonatal intensive care should complete the NRP.[1]

This chapter offers a practical approach to resuscitation of the newly born infant in settings other than the delivery room. This approach is based on guidelines established by the American Heart Association in conjunction with the American Academy of Pediatrics and the International Liaison Committee on Resuscitation.[2] Because the guidelines in this chapter are intended for resuscitation of infants *immediately after birth*, they differ in minor ways from the guidelines for resuscitation of infants and children presented in the remainder of this text.

Although the need for resuscitation of the newly born infant often can be predicted, the need may arise suddenly and may occur in locations that do not routinely provide neonatal intensive care. Preparation and training are essential to maximize the outcome of infants born in these locations.

The best resuscitation results are obtained in a well-equipped, well-staffed delivery room. Every reasonable and safe effort should be made to delay birth until the mother can be transported to such a setting. Prehospital delays and stops in the Emergency Department or admitting office are inappropriate.

With adequate anticipation it is possible to optimize any delivery setting with appropriately prepared equipment and trained personnel who are capable of functioning as a team during neonatal resuscitation. At least one person skilled in initiating neonatal resuscitation should be assigned to care for the infant. One additional skilled person capable of performing a complete resuscitation should be immediately available (see Critical Concepts on the next page).

Neonatal Physiology Affecting Resuscitation

Marked changes in the cardiovascular and respiratory systems occur at birth with the transition from fetal to neonatal circulation. After birth the infant's fluid-filled lungs must rapidly fill with air to increase oxygenation and assume the role of ventilation performed before birth by the placenta. For initial lung expansion, fluid-filled alveoli may require higher ventilation pressures than is commonly used in rescue breathing for the older

At least one person skilled in initiating neonatal resuscitation should be on hand to care for the infant. One additional skilled person capable of performing a complete resuscitation should be immediately available.

Neonatal resuscitation can be divided into 4 categories of action:

1. Basic steps, including rapid assessment and initial steps in stabilization

2. Ventilation, including bag-mask or bag-tube ventilation

3. Chest compressions

4. Administration of medications or fluids

infant (see Foundation Facts: "Importance of the Transition to Extrauterine Physiology").[3,4] Before birth only a small fraction of fetal cardiac output passes through the lungs; within seconds after birth the blood vessels in the lungs must relax (dilate) to permit increased blood flow and gas exchange within alveoli filled with air rather than fluid.

Antepartum events that cause asphyxia may preclude a smooth neonatal cardiopulmonary transition. One aim of resuscitation is to reverse asphyxial conditions by restoring and supporting cardiopulmonary function.

The vast majority of term newborns require no resuscitation beyond maintenance of temperature, clearing of the airway, and stimulation of drying. Approximately 5% to 10% of newborns require some degree of active resuscitation at birth.[5] Of the small proportion of newborns who require further intervention, most respond to administration of oxygen and ventilation with bag and mask. Approximately 1%

to 10% of infants born in hospitals are reported to require assisted ventilation.[6]

After drying, stimulation, airway opening, and bag-mask ventilation if needed, subsequent evaluation and interventions are based on assessment of the *Triad of Evaluation*, or 3 clinical characteristics: (1) respirations, (2) heart rate, and (3) color. Most newly born infants require only the basic steps, but for those who require further intervention, the most crucial action is establishment of adequate ventilation.[7] Only a very small percentage will need chest compressions and medications.[8] The inverted pyramid in Figure 1 illustrates the relative frequencies and priorities of neonatal resuscitation.

Some special circumstances, such as the presence of meconium-stained amniotic fluid, may require modification of the resuscitation sequences presented in this chapter. If resuscitative efforts are successful, care of the infant then includes not only supportive care but also ongoing monitoring and appropriate diagnostic evaluation. In certain clinical circumstances, noninitiation or discontinuation of resuscitation in the delivery room may

Physical expansion of the lungs with air and the increase in alveolar oxygen tension mediate a critical decrease in pulmonary vascular resistance and result in an increase in pulmonary blood flow after birth. Failure to normalize pulmonary vascular resistance may result in persistence of right-to-left intracardiac and extracardiac shunts in persistent pulmonary hypertension of the newborn. Inadequate expansion of the alveolar spaces may result in intrapulmonary shunting of blood with resultant hypoxemia. In addition to disordered cardiopulmonary transition, disruption of the fetoplacental circulation (eg, abruptio placentae or placenta previa leading to blood loss from the maternal-fetal unit) also may place the newly born infant at risk for hypovolemia (and need for volume resuscitation) because of acute blood loss.

FIGURE 1. Inverted pyramid illustrates the relative frequencies of interventions for resuscitation of the newly born who does not have meconium-stained amniotic fluid. A majority of infants respond to simple measures.

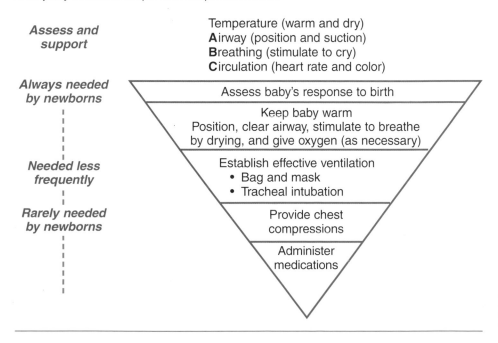

Assess and support
Temperature (warm and dry)
Airway (position and suction)
Breathing (stimulate to cry)
Circulation (heart rate and color)

Always needed by newborns
Assess baby's response to birth

Keep baby warm
Position, clear airway, stimulate to breathe by drying, and give oxygen (as necessary)

Needed less frequently
Establish effective ventilation
• Bag and mask
• Tracheal intubation

Rarely needed by newborns
Provide chest compressions

Administer medications

be appropriate. It is important to document resuscitation interventions and responses in order to understand an individual infant's pathophysiology, to improve resuscitation performance, and to study resuscitation outcomes.[9-11]

Preparation

Appropriate preparation for an anticipated high-risk delivery requires communication between the person(s) caring for the mother and those responsible for resuscitation of the newly born. The person(s) caring for the mother should convey details of antepartum and intrapartum maternal medical conditions and treatment and specific indicators of fetal condition (eg, fetal heart rate monitoring, lung maturity, ultrasonography). A brief targeted history (see Table 1) may help predict newborn distress and the potential need for newborn resuscitation. However, for many infants the need for resuscitation cannot be anticipated.[12] Table 2 lists examples of antepartum and intrapartum factors that place the newly born infant at risk. Several of these conditions have unique implications for resuscitation of the newly born. Prenatal diagnosis and certain features of the perinatal history and clinical course may alert the resuscitation team to these special factors.

The condition of the newly born may also influence priorities of resuscitation. Conditions that may affect opening of the airway, timing of tracheal intubation, and selection and administration of volume expanders are presented in Table 3.

A complete inventory of resuscitation equipment and drugs should be kept in a clean, warm environment wherever deliveries occur. All equipment must be maintained in fully operational condition, and it should be checked on a regular basis. Table 4 lists examples of appropriate neonatal supplies, medications, and equipment. Ideally a radiant warmer should be kept in the Emergency Department; personnel should understand how to use it.

A chart summarizing the sequence of steps in resuscitation and correct medication doses for neonates of various weights is often helpful (Figure 2 and Table 5).

As soon as the need for neonatal resuscitation becomes evident, a prearranged plan should be activated to organize personnel with the necessary skills.

When a newborn is delivered outside the hospital, it may be difficult to maintain the infant's body temperature, airway patency, and vascular access during transport. On arrival in the Emergency Department, it is important to verify tracheal tube placement (or reintubate the trachea) and evaluate the patency and placement of vascular access.

Thus, preparation for resuscitation, stabilization, and advanced life support for the newly born infant in the Emergency Department is identical to that required for any critically ill infant or child.

Universal Precautions

Carefully follow universal precautions in delivery areas, where exposure to blood and body fluids is likely. Treat all fluids from patients as potentially infectious. Wear gloves and other appropriate protective barriers during delivery and when handling newly born infants or contaminated equipment. Do not use techniques involving mouth suction through a tracheal tube.

Resuscitation Procedures

Rapid Assessment

Determination of the need for resuscitative efforts should begin immediately after birth and proceed throughout the resuscitation process. An initial complex of signs (the presence of meconium in the amniotic fluid or on the skin, cry or respirations, muscle tone, color, term or preterm gestation) should be evaluated rapidly and simultaneously by visual inspection. Once intervention begins, the sequence of interventions is determined by the findings of the Triad of Evaluation, which comprises assessment of respirations, heart rate, and color.

Most newly born infants respond to stimulation from the extrauterine environment

TABLE 1. Using a Targeted History to Assess Risk Factors and Need for Resuscitation

Key Question	Example of Risk/Condition	Anticipated Action
How many fetuses?	More than one	Multiple teams
Due date?	Premature	Assisted ventilation
Maternal medications?	Narcotics	Assisted ventilation
Have membranes ruptured? If so, what color is the fluid?	Meconium-stained fluid	Immediate suction; possible tracheal intubation
Bleeding?	Maternal/placental hemorrhage	Vascular access and fluid/blood product administration
Decreased fetal movement or fetal monitoring?	Fetal distress	Assisted ventilation

TABLE 2. Factors Associated With Increased Risk to Newborns

Antepartum Risk Factors	Intrapartum Risk Factors
Maternal diabetes	Emergency cesarean section
Pregnancy-induced hypertension	Forceps or vacuum-assisted delivery
Chronic hypertension	Breech or other abnormal presentation
Chronic maternal illness	Premature labor
Cardiovascular	Precipitous labor
Thyroid	Chorioamnionitis
Neurological	Prolonged rupture of membranes
Pulmonary	(>18 hours before delivery)
Renal	Prolonged labor (>24 hours)
Anemia or isoimmunization	Prolonged second stage of labor
Previous fetal or neonatal death	(>2 hours)
Bleeding in second or third trimester	Fetal bradycardia
Maternal infection	Nonreassuring fetal heart rate patterns
Polyhydramnios	Use of general anesthesia
Oligohydramnios	Uterine tetany
Premature rupture of membranes	Narcotics administered to mother
Post-term gestation	within 4 hours of delivery
Multiple gestation	Meconium-stained amniotic fluid
Size-dates discrepancy	Prolapsed cord
Drug therapy, eg,	Abruptio placentae
Lithium carbonate	Placenta previa
Magnesium	
Adrenergic-blocking drugs	
Maternal substance abuse	
Fetal malformation	
Diminished fetal activity	
No prenatal care	
Age <16 or >35 years	

with strong respiratory efforts, movement of all extremities, improving color (from cyanotic or dusky to pink), and adequate heart rate. Such a vigorous term infant can remain with the mother to receive routine care (warmth, drying, clearing the airway). Determine the need for further assessment and intervention by answering the following rapid assessment questions:

- Is the amniotic fluid clear of meconium?
- Is the baby breathing or crying?
- Is there good muscle tone?
- Is the color pink?
- Is the infant term?

Perform rapid assessment in the first several seconds after an infant is delivered.

If the answer to all of the above questions is "yes," the infant can receive routine care. If the answer to any of these questions is "no," the infant will require further assessment under a radiant warmer and intervention in the form of the initial steps of resuscitation.

Initial Steps

Warmth

All newborns have difficulty tolerating a cold environment.[13] Depressed infants are especially at risk for complications of cold stress, and recovery from acidosis is delayed by hypothermia.[14] Unintended hypothermia is a special problem for the infant born outside the delivery room. Preterm infants cool at a more rapid rate

than full-term newborns when exposed to similar environmental conditions, because the ratio of body surface area to volume is higher in the preterm than in the full-term neonate. For these reasons environmental heat loss should be avoided when caring for preterm infants.[15]

Heat loss may be prevented by (1) placing the infant under a preheated warmer, (2) quickly drying the amniotic fluid from the skin, and (3) removing wet linens from contact with the baby. Radiant warmers are ideal for warming infants, but they may not be readily available in the Emergency Department. Heating lamps become very hot and may be hazardous to both infant and personnel unless precautions are taken to maintain the heating bulb at the recommended distance from the baby. Alternative methods of warming infants include the use of warm blankets or towels, insulating film blankets, infant chemical warming mattresses, and increased ambient temperature. The mother may also help warm the infant by skin-to-skin contact.

Foundation Facts:
Cerebral *Hypothermia* and Avoidance of Perinatal *Hyperthermia*

Preventing heat loss in the newly born infant is vital, especially for preterm infants born outside the delivery room, because cold stress can increase oxygen consumption and impede effective resuscitation.[16,17] Hyperthermia should also be avoided because it is associated with perinatal respiratory depression.[18,19]

Recent studies in animals and humans suggest that selective (cerebral) hypothermia of the asphyxiated infant may protect against brain injury.[20-22] Although this is a promising area of research, routine implementation cannot be recommended until appropriate controlled studies in humans have been performed.

TABLE 3. Conditions That May Affect Resuscitation of the Newly Born Infant

Condition	History/Clinical Signs	Actions
Mechanical blockage of airway		
Meconium or mucus blockage	Meconium-stained amniotic fluid Poor chest wall movement	Intubation for suctioning/ventilation
Choanal atresia	Pink when crying, cyanotic when quiet	Oral airway Tracheal intubation
Pharyngeal airway malformation	Persistent retractions, poor air entry	Prone positioning posterior nasopharyngeal tube
Impaired lung function		
Pneumothorax	Asymmetrical breath sounds Persistent cyanosis/bradycardia	Needle thoracentesis
Pleural effusions/ascites	Diminished air movement Persistent cyanosis/bradycardia	Immediate intubation Needle thoracentesis, paracentesis Possible volume expansion
Congenital diaphragmatic hernia	Asymmetrical breath sounds Persistent cyanosis/bradycardia Scaphoid abdomen	Tracheal intubation Placement of orogastric catheter
Pneumonia/sepsis	Diminished air movement Persistent cyanosis/bradycardia	Tracheal intubation Possible volume expansion
Impaired cardiac function		
Congenital heart disease	Persistent cyanosis/bradycardia	Diagnostic evaluation
Fetal/maternal hemorrhage	Pallor; poor response to resuscitation	Volume expansion, possibly including red blood cells

Critical Concepts:
Integrated Versus Sequential Evaluation

In this chapter evaluation and treatment are presented as a sequential, integrated process. In reality evaluation and intervention are often performed simultaneously. This is particularly true if more than one rescuer is present. Throughout resuscitation the sequence of action is guided by findings from the Triad of Evaluation: assessment of respirations, heart rate, and color. The appropriate response to abnormal findings also depends on how the infant responded to previous resuscitative interventions and the time elapsed since birth.

If initial evaluation indicates that the infant is stable, the dried infant may be placed naked against the mother's chest with blankets placed over both mother and infant. Avoidance of drafts and windows (radiant heat loss) is important for prevention of hypothermia.

Positioning

Place the newly born infant on his/her back or side with the neck in a neutral position. Avoid hyperextension and flexion of the neck, which may produce airway obstruction. To help maintain correct position, place a rolled blanket or towel under the supine infant's back and shoulders, elevating the torso to extend the neck slightly. If copious secretions are present, place the newborn on his/her side with the neck slightly extended to allow secre-

tions to collect in the mouth and cheek rather than in the posterior pharynx.

Clearing the Airway and Treating Meconium

If the amniotic fluid is clear of meconium, clear the airway by suctioning the mouth, then the nose with a bulb syringe or suction catheter (8F to 10F). Negative pressure used to suction should not exceed −100 mm Hg (−136 cm H_2O). Infants who are crying vigorously and have minimal secretions may need only wiping of secretions from the nose and mouth with gauze or a towel. Deep suctioning of the oropharynx may produce a vagal response and cause bradycardia or apnea.[23]

Meconium-stained amniotic fluid is a risk factor for meconium aspiration syndrome.

TABLE 4. Neonatal Resuscitation Supplies and Equipment for the Emergency Department*

Suction equipment
  Bulb syringe
  Mechanical suction and tubing, manometer
  Suction catheters, 5F or 6F, 8F, and 10F or 12F
  8F feeding tube and 20-mL syringe
  Meconium aspirator (for attachment to mechanical suction)

Bag-mask equipment
  Self-inflating or flow-inflating bag with pressure-release valve or pressure manometer (200 to 750 mL); self-inflating bag must have an oxygen reservoir
  Face masks, premature and newborn sizes
  Oxygen with flowmeter (rate up to 10 L/min) and tubing

Intubation equipment
  Laryngoscope with straight blades, No. 0 (preterm) and No. 1 (term)
  Extra bulbs and batteries for laryngoscope
  Tracheal tubes, 2.5, 3.0, 3.5, 4.0 mm
  Stylet (optional)
  Scissors
  Tape or securing device for tracheal tube
  Exhaled CO_2 detector (optional)
  Laryngeal mask airway (optional)

Medications
  Epinephrine 1:10 000
  Isotonic crystalloid
  Naloxone hydrochloride 0.4 mg/mL
  Normal saline for volume expansion
  Sodium bicarbonate 4.2% (5 mEq/10 mL)[†]
  Dextrose 10%
  Normal saline for flushes and sterile water if dilution of bicarbonate or hypertonic glucose solutions is necessary

Miscellaneous
  Gloves and other appropriate personal protection equipment
  Feeding tube, 5F (optional: for administration of tracheal medications)
  Radiant warmer
  Towels and warmed blankets
  Clock (timer optional)
  Stethoscope
  Tape, ½ or ¾ inch
  Syringes, 1, 3, 5, 10, 20, 50 mL
  Needles, 25-, 21-, 18-gauge or puncture device for needleless system
  Alcohol sponges
  Umbilical vessel catheterization supplies:
    Sterile gloves
    Scalpel or scissors
    Umbilical tape
    Umbilical catheters, 3.5F, 5F
    Three-way stopcock
  Cardiac monitor and electrodes (optional)
  Oropharyngeal airways
  Pulse oximeter and probe (optional)

---

*In addition to OB kit.

[†]If the only solution available is 8.4%, it should be diluted 1:1 with sterile water.

This clinical syndrome produces respiratory distress and hypoxemia and is associated with aspiration pneumonia, pneumothorax, and in severe cases, persistent pulmonary hypertension. Meconium aspiration syndrome continues to be a significant cause of morbidity in term infants. Infants who are depressed and delivered through thick meconium are at greatest risk for meconium aspiration syndrome, although a milder form may be observed when the meconium-stained fluid is thin.[24]

If meconium is present in the amniotic fluid, suction the mouth, nose, and posterior pharynx with a large-bore catheter (12F or 14F) or a bulb syringe *after* delivery of the head but *before* delivery of the shoulders.[25,26] Although intrapartum suctioning appears to decrease the risk of meconium-aspiration syndrome, a significant number (20% to 30%) of infants with meconium-stained fluid will have meconium in the trachea *despite* such suctioning and the absence of spontaneous respirations.[24,27] This supports the

Foundation Facts:
Differentiation Between Vigorous and Depressed Infants With Meconium-Stained Amniotic Fluid

Vigorous

Strong respiratory effort

Good muscle tone

Heart rate >100 beats per minute (bpm)

Depressed

Weak or absent respiratory effort

Poor muscle tone, limp

Heart rate <100 bpm

If the newly born infant is depressed and meconium staining of the amniotic fluid is present, delay drying and stimulation and suction the trachea *before* taking other resuscitative steps.[28,29]

FIGURE 2. Overview of resuscitation in the delivery room.

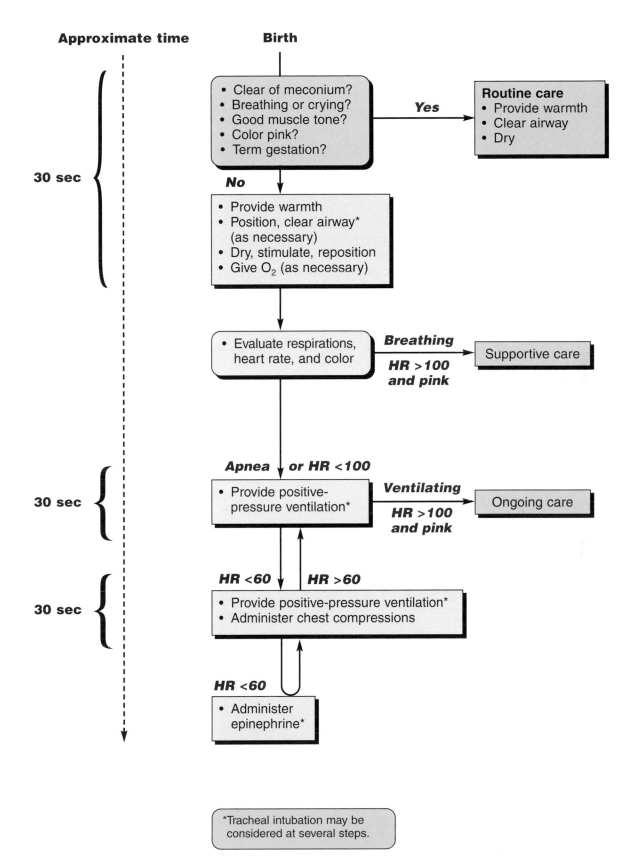

TABLE 5. Medications Used in Resuscitation of the Newborn

Medications	Dose/Route*	Concentration	Wt (kg)	Total volume (mL)	Precautions
Epinephrine	0.01 to 0.03 mg/kg tracheal, IV, or IO	1:10 000	1 2 3 4	0.1-0.3 0.2-0.6 0.3-0.9 0.4-1.2	Give rapidly Repeat every 3 to 5 minutes
Volume expanders **Isotonic crystalloid** **(normal saline** *or* **Ringer's lactate** *or* **blood)**	10 mL/kg IV or IO		1 2 3 4	10 20 30 40	Give over 5 to 10 minutes Reassess after each bolus

Sodium bicarbonate	1 to 2 mEq/kg IV, IO	0.5 mEq/mL (4.2% solution)	1
			2
			3
			4
				2-4
				4-8
				6-12
				8-16
					Give slow push,
					  over at least 2 minutes
					Dilute 8.4% solution 1:1
					  with sterile water
					Give only if infant is
					  effectively ventilated

Naloxone	0.1 mg/kg tracheal, IV, IM, IO, SQ	0.4 mg/mL
		
		1 mg/mL
			1
			2
			3
			4
			1
			2
			3
			4
				0.25
				0.50
				0.75
				1.0
				0.1
				0.2
				0.3
				0.4
					Establish adequate
					  ventilation first
					Give rapidly
					Repeat every 2 to 3 minutes
					  as needed

10% Dextrose	0.2 g/kg IV, IO	0.1 g/mL	1
			2
			3
			4
				2
				4
				6
				8
					Check bedside glucose
					May require dilution from
					  25% or 50% dextrose
					  using sterile water

IV indicates intravenous; IO, intraosseous; IM, intramuscular; and SQ, subcutaneous.

*Note: Tracheal dose may not result in effective plasma concentration of drug, so vascular access should be established as soon as possible. Drugs given tracheally can be diluted to a total volume of 1 mL with normal saline before instillation.

concept of in utero aspiration and the need for tracheal suctioning after delivery in depressed infants.

There is evidence that tracheal suctioning of the vigorous infant with meconium-stained amniotic fluid does not improve outcome and may cause complications.[30,31] After delivery the approach to the infant with meconium-stained amniotic fluid is determined by whether the infant can be described as *vigorous*, with strong respiratory effort, good muscle tone, and a heart rate greater than 100 bpm. If the infant is vigorous, suction the mouth and nose in the same way as for infants with clear fluid.

If the infant is *depressed* (poor respiratory effort, decreased muscle tone, or heart rate less than 100 bpm), delay drying and stimulation and suction the trachea *before* taking other resuscitative steps.[28,30] Place the infant in the prepared warmed environment and perform the following actions immediately:

■ Examine the hypopharynx with a laryngoscope and suction any residual meconium in the hypopharynx.

■ Intubate the trachea and suction the lower airway.

Because meconium may be thick, particulate, and viscous, suction the trachea by

FIGURE 3. One form of adapter (meconium aspirator) is placed between the tracheal tube and the suction tubing. Gloves should be worn.

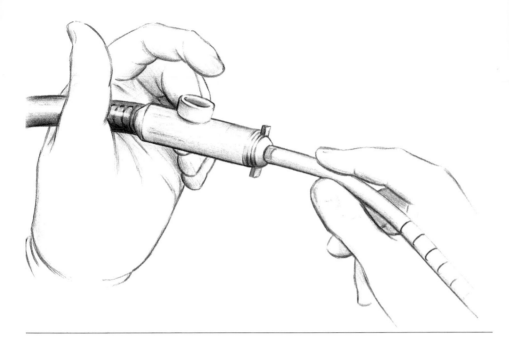

applying suction directly to the tracheal tube as it is withdrawn from the airway (Figure 3). Set mechanical suction no higher than −100 mm Hg. If a significant amount of meconium is obtained, repeat tracheal intubation and suction until little additional meconium is recovered or until the heart rate indicates that resuscitation must proceed without delay. When the infant's heart rate or respiration is severely depressed, it may not be possible to clear the trachea of all meconium before positive-pressure ventilation must be initiated. For infants who develop apnea or respiratory distress, even though they are initially vigorous, provide tracheal suctioning before positive-pressure ventilation. After achieving initial stabilization, place an orogastric tube to empty the newborn's stomach, because swallowed meconium could later be regurgitated and aspirated.

Drying, Stimulation, and Repositioning

Most newborns will begin to breathe effectively in response to mild stimulation, including drying and suctioning. Two additional safe methods of tactile stimulation, slapping or flicking the soles of the feet and rubbing the back, may be used. Avoid more vigorous methods of stimulation. If spontaneous and effective respirations are not established after a few seconds of specific stimulation, positive-pressure ventilation is required. Slow or shallow respirations may be associated with inadequate alveolar ventilation, lung expansion, and pulmonary blood flow, resulting in hypoxemia, hypercarbia, and slowing of the heart rate. Continued stimulation of an obviously depressed, cyanotic, and unresponsive infant increases hypoxemia and delays initiation of ventilation.

Oxygen Administration

If a newly born infant is breathing spontaneously but remains centrally cyanotic, administer 100% free-flow oxygen (see Foundation Facts: "Use of 100% Oxygen"). Ideally oxygen should be warmed and humidified, but this may not be possible in the prehospital or Emergency Department setting. Dry, unheated oxygen may be given for a few minutes during stabilization. Free-flow oxygen may be delivered by a hand cupped over the face and oxygen tubing, a simple face mask held firmly to the infant's face, or a face mask attached to a flow-inflating bag. Self-inflating bags do not reliably deliver free-flow oxygen because they may entrain room air during bag re-expansion between breaths.

Triad of Evaluation

To determine if further resuscitative actions are indicated, evaluate the infant's (1) respiration, (2) heart rate, and (3) color. Monitor this Triad of Evaluation throughout the resuscitation and postresuscitation periods.

Respiration

After initial respiratory efforts the newly born infant should achieve regular respirations that are adequate to improve color and maintain a heart rate greater than 100 bpm. Gasping respirations and apnea after brief stimulation are signs that intervention with positive-pressure ventilation is required.

Heart Rate

Heart rate is a critical determinant of the resuscitation sequence and should be evaluated as soon as respiratory effort has been assessed and appropriate corrective action taken. The heart rate may be evaluated by one of the following methods:

- Palpation of the pulse at the base of the umbilical cord

■ Auscultation of the apical heart sounds with a stethoscope

It may be difficult to palpate the brachial or femoral pulse in the newly born infant.[32] The umbilical pulse is readily accessible in the newly born and permits assessment of heart rate without interruption of positive-pressure ventilation to auscultate the chest. If umbilical pulsations cannot be felt, you will need to auscultate the infant's precordium. A cardiotachometer monitoring system can also be used, but time is required to set up the system, and electrodes may not stick well to the newly born infant's skin until the skin is cleansed. Pulse oximetry also provides an alternative method to monitor heart rate. In an uncompromised newly born infant, the heart rate should be consistently greater than 100 bpm.

Color

Most newly born infants will be centrally cyanotic at birth because normal fetal Po_2 is quite low. With the infant's first breaths, color should rapidly become pink. Central cyanosis is detected by examining the face, trunk, and mucous membranes. Acrocyanosis (blue hands and feet) is common in the first few minutes of life and is not a reliable indicator of hypoxemia.

The Apgar Scoring System

The Apgar scoring system[33] (Table 6) enables rapid evaluation of 5 objective signs (heart rate, respirations, muscle tone, reflex irritability, and color) at 1 and 5 minutes after birth. If the 5-minute Apgar score is less than 7, obtain additional scores every 5 minutes until the score is 7 or greater or for a total of 20 minutes. The Apgar score, however, cannot be used to determine the need for resuscitation. If resuscitative efforts are required, they should be initiated promptly and should not be delayed while the Apgar score is determined.

Ventilation

The key to successful neonatal resuscitation is adequate expansion of the lungs with gas, followed by effective ventilation. The indications for positive-pressure ventilation are

■ Apnea

■ Gasping respirations

■ Heart rate less than 100 bpm

■ Persistent central cyanosis despite administration of 100% oxygen

Effective positive-pressure ventilation with 100% oxygen can usually be accomplished with bag and mask. The self-inflating bag (Figure 4) must be used with an oxygen source and reservoir to deliver a high concentration of oxygen. Many self-inflating bags are equipped with a pressure-release (pop-off) valve that is preset between 30 and 40 cm H_2O. Because the initial inflation of a newborn's lungs may require higher inspiratory pressures, the pop-off valve may prevent effective inflation unless the valve is easily bypassed. The ideal bag volume for neonatal resuscitation is approximately 500 mL (see Foundation Facts: "Small-Volume Manual Resuscitation Bags"); a volume greater than 750 mL makes it difficult to judge the small tidal volumes (6 to 8 mL/kg) administered to neonates and may increase the risk of hyperinflation and potential barotrauma.

The flow-inflating bag (also called an anesthesia bag) inflates only when oxygen enters it from a compressed gas source and a tight seal exists between the mask and face (see Chapter 4, Figure 15). This bag requires a well-modulated flow of gas into the inlet port and correct adjustment of the flow-control valve, which controls the exit of gas not delivered through the

> ## Critical Concepts:
> ### Indications for Positive-Pressure Ventilation
>
> Adequate ventilation is the key to neonatal resuscitation. Indications for positive-pressure ventilation are
>
> ■ Gasping respirations
>
> ■ Apnea
>
> ■ Central cyanosis despite 100% oxygen
>
> ■ Heart rate less than 100 bpm

TABLE 6. The Apgar Scoring System

Sign	0	1	2
Heart rate per minute	Absent	Slow (<100 bpm)	>100 bpm
Respirations	Absent	Slow, irregular	Good, crying
Muscle tone	Limp	Some flexion	Active motion
Reflex irritability (to a catheter in the nares)	No response	Grimace	Cough or sneeze
Color	Blue or pale	Pink body with blue extremities	Completely pink

Apgar V. *Curr Res Anesth Analg.* 1953;32:260.

FIGURE 4. Self-inflating manual resuscitator bag with face mask, with (**A** and **B**) and without (**C** and **D**) oxygen reservoir. **A,** Reexpansion of bag *with* oxygen reservoir. When the rescuer's hand releases the bag, oxygen flows into the bag from the oxygen source and from the reservoir, so the concentration of oxygen in the bag remains 100%. **B,** Compression of bag *with* oxygen reservoir delivers 100% oxygen to the patient (purple arrow). Oxygen continuously flows into the reservoir. **C,** Reexpansion of the bag *without* an oxygen reservoir. When the rescuer's hand releases the bag, oxygen flows into the bag from the oxygen source, but ambient air is also entrained into the bag, so the bag becomes filled with a *mixture* of oxygen and ambient air. **D,** Compression of the bag *without* oxygen reservoir delivers oxygen *mixed* with room air (aqua arrow). Note that with both setups exhaled patient air flows into the atmosphere between the mask and the bag (see gray arrows from mask in **A** and **C**).

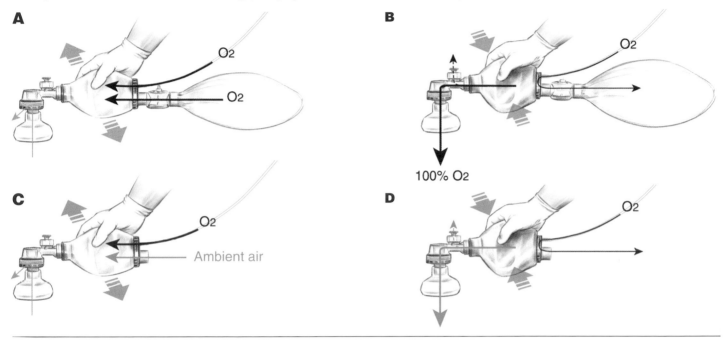

patient outlet. Because a flow-inflating bag can deliver very high pressures, a pressure gauge must be joined to the bag to monitor peak inspiratory pressure. Proper use of a flow-inflating bag requires training and practice, but it can provide a wide range of peak inspiratory pressures and end-expiratory pressures and more reliable delivery of high inspired oxygen concentrations than a self-inflating bag.

Face masks for preterm and term newborns (usually called premature and newborn or neonatal masks) should be available. If the mask is the correct size, it will cover the infant's nose and mouth. The mask should not overlap the eyes or chin because this will prevent creation of a tight seal between the mask and face. Although a tight seal between the mask and face is required to achieve effective ventilation, avoid excessive pressure on the face during bag-mask ventilation. The most effective masks are designed to fit the contours of the newborn's face and

have a cushioned rim and a low volume of dead space (less than 5 mL).

Ventilation of the newly born is provided at a rate of 40 to 60 breaths/min. The tidal volumes required by neonates (especially preterm infants) are smaller than those used for children. To minimize the chance of possible iatrogenic complications (eg, barotrauma), all neonatal ventilation bags should be equipped with a pressure-release valve or manometer to limit inspiratory pressures. The first breaths delivered to an apneic infant may need to be longer (1 to 2 seconds) and use higher inspiratory pressures (30 to 40 cm H_2O) than subsequent breaths. The best indicator of adequate but not excessive tidal volume is gentle rise of the chest wall.

If chest expansion is *inadequate*, identify and treat reversible causes, including an inadequate seal between mask and face, blocked airway, or insufficient inspiratory pressure. Reapplying the mask to the face may correct the problem. A blocked air-

way may be corrected by repositioning the head, suctioning secretions, and ventilating with the mouth slightly open. Finally, if chest expansion remains inadequate, increased inflation pressures may be required.

If adequate ventilation (as indicated by effective chest expansion and improvement in color and heart rate) cannot be achieved by bag and mask, intubation of the trachea for ventilation is required. If bag-mask ventilation is required for more than several minutes or if gastric inflation develops, insert an orogastric tube (8F or 10F), leaving the end open to air. Periodically aspirate the tube with a syringe.

After 30 seconds of adequate ventilation with 100% oxygen, reassess the infant's respirations, heart rate, and color. If spontaneous respirations are present and the heart rate is greater than 100 bpm, positive-pressure ventilation may be gradually discontinued. Gradual reduction in the rate and pressure of assisted ventilation will increase the stimulus for the infant to resume spontaneous breathing. If spontaneous respirations are inadequate, assisted ventilation must continue (see Critical Concepts: "Indications for Positive-Pressure Ventilation"). If the heart rate is less than 60 bpm despite adequate ventilation with

Foundation Facts:
Small-Volume Manual Resuscitation Bags

Although the pressure required to establish air breathing is variable and unpredictable, higher inflation pressures (30 to 40 cm of H_2O or higher) and longer inflation times may be required for delivery of the first several breaths than for subsequent breaths in the newly born. A minimum bag volume of 450 to 500 mL may be necessary to maintain inflation pressure for at least 1 second. Resuscitation bags for neonates should be no larger than 750 mL; larger bag volumes make it difficult to judge delivery of the small tidal volumes (5 to 8 mL/kg) that newly born infants require. If the device contains a pressure-release valve, it should release at approximately 30 to 35 cm H_2O pressure and should have an override feature to permit delivery of higher pressures if necessary to achieve good chest expansion.

Note that the observation that "a minimum bag volume of 450 to 500 mL may be necessary" means that the neonatal recommendations are very close to those used in the PALS guidelines. The PALS guidelines recommend that "resuscitation bags used for ventilation of full-term newly-born infants, infants, and children should have a minimal volume of 450 to 500 mL." It is important to note that the PALS recommendations do *not* encompass the ventilation of *preterm* newborn infants, who will require smaller ventilation volumes than full-term newly born infants.

100% oxygen, continue positive-pressure ventilation and initiate chest compressions.

Prolonged apnea without bradycardia or cyanosis may indicate respiratory depression induced by narcotics administered to the mother within 4 hours of delivery. Administration of naloxone, however, can induce a withdrawal reaction in an infant of a narcotic-addicted mother, so avoid the use of this drug if maternal narcotic addiction is suspected.[34] The dose of naloxone is 0.1 mg/kg (0.1 mL/kg of 1 mg/mL concentration or 0.25 mL/kg of 0.4 mg/mL concentration) administered by intravenous, tracheal, subcutaneous, or intramuscular route. The initial dose may be repeated every 2 to 3 minutes as needed.[35] Because the duration of action of narcotics may exceed that of naloxone, continue to monitor the infant and be prepared to repeat naloxone administration.

Chest Compressions

Asphyxia causes peripheral vasoconstriction, tissue hypoxia, acidosis, poor myocardial contractility, bradycardia, and eventual cardiac arrest. Prompt initiation

of effective ventilation and oxygenation will restore vital signs in the vast majority of newly born infants. Although it has previously been common practice to give compressions if the heart rate is 60 to 80 bpm and not rising, these recommendations have changed to avoid premature focus on chest compressions. Ventilation should be the priority in resuscitation of the newly born. But if a newborn's heart rate is less than 60 bpm despite effective positive-pressure ventilation with 100% oxygen for approximately 30 seconds, you should begin chest compressions.

Two techniques are acceptable for performing chest compressions in the neonate and small infant. In the preferred technique, when 2 or more rescuers (healthcare providers) are present, place both thumbs on the lower third of the sternum, with the fingers encircling the chest and supporting the back (Figure 5).[36,37] Position the thumbs side by side on the sternum just below the nipple line. If the infant is extremely small or the rescuer's thumbs are extremely large, superimpose the thumbs one on top of the other. *Avoid compressing the xiphoid portion of the*

FIGURE 5. Two thumb–encircling hands chest compression technique in infant (2 rescuers).

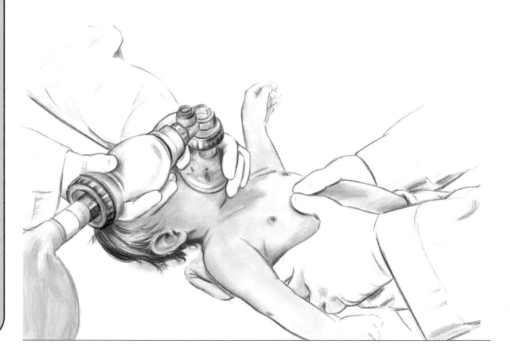

sternum, because such compression may damage the neonate's liver.

If the rescuer's hands are too small to encircle the chest, 2-finger compression may be performed with the ring and middle fingers of one hand on the sternum just below the nipple line. The other hand should support the newborn's back. For more information about this technique of chest compression, see Chapter 3. Compressions should be performed as follows (also see Table 7):

- Compress the sternum approximately one third the anterior-posterior diameter of the chest or to a depth that generates a palpable pulse.

- Provide a smooth (not jerky) compression phase that is slighter shorter than the relaxation phase.

- Do not lift the thumbs or fingers off the sternum during the relaxation phase.

- Deliver compressions at a ratio of 3:1 with interposed ventilations.

- Provide a rate of compressions and ventilations to deliver 120 events per minute (90 compressions and 30 ventilations) or 1 complete cycle of 3 compressions and 1 ventilation every 2 seconds.

- Always accompany compressions with positive-pressure ventilation with 100% oxygen, because ventilation is of primary importance in newborn resuscitation.

- Check the spontaneous pulse rate periodically and discontinue compressions when the heart rate reaches 60 bpm or greater.

Critical Concepts: Confirmation of Tracheal Intubation

After tracheal intubation, confirm proper position of the tracheal tube by

- Observation of symmetric chest movement

- Auscultation of equal and adequate breath sounds in the axillae and absent breath sounds over the stomach

- Improvement in the neonate's color, heart rate, and activity

- Detection of exhaled CO_2. This optional technique is most useful (ie, most sensitive and specific) if there is a perfusing rhythm and the infant weighs more than 2 kg).[38]

Tracheal Intubation

Tracheal intubation is indicated if (1) bag-mask ventilation is ineffective, (2) tracheal suctioning is required in the setting of meconium-stained amniotic fluid, or (3) prolonged positive-pressure ventilation is necessary. Tracheal intubation may also be indicated for delivery of tracheal medications; the tracheal route is generally the most rapidly accessible for administration of epinephrine. If profound bradycardia is present and effective ventilation is achieved with bag and mask, the provider who is inexperienced in neonatal intubation should not delay provision of chest compressions to attempt intubation.

Supplies and equipment for tracheal intubation should be assembled and readily available on the neonatal resuscitation tray. Tubes with a uniform internal diameter are recommended. Most tracheal tubes intended for use in newborns have a black vocal cord line guide near the tip. When this guide is placed at the level of the vocal cords, the tip of the tube is likely to be positioned properly in the trachea, above the carina. Tracheal tube size can be estimated using the infant's weight or gestational age (Table 8). The proper depth of insertion can also be estimated by using the following formula:

Weight in kilograms + 6 cm = Tracheal tube insertion depth at lip in centimeters

After tracheal intubation, verify proper tube position (see Critical Concepts: "Confirmation of Tracheal Intubation"). Once proper tracheal tube position is verified, record the depth of insertion at the lip and secure the tube in position. Obtain a chest x-ray for final confirmation of tracheal tube placement if the tube is to remain in place after resuscitation.

Medications and Fluids

Administration of medications is rarely necessary during resuscitation of the newly born infant.[39] Bradycardia in the newly born infant is usually the result of inadequate ventilation or profound hypoxia; adequate ventilation is the most important step in correcting bradycardia. Medications should be administered if the heart rate remains less than 60 bpm despite adequate ventilation with 100% oxygen and chest compressions.

TABLE 7. Technique of Compressions and Ventilations in the Newly Born

Characteristic of Chest Compressions	Performance in Neonates
Location	Lower one third of the sternum; below an imaginary line between the nipples
Compression-ventilation ratio	3:1
Rate	120 events/min (90 compressions and 30 ventilations per minute)
Depth	One third the anterior-posterior diameter of the chest or to achieve a palpable pulse

TABLE 8. Estimation of Proper Tracheal Tube Size and Depth of Insertion Based on Infant's Gestational Age and Weight

Weight (g)	Gestational Age (wk)	Laryngoscope Blade	Tracheal Tube Size (mm)/ Catheter Size	Depth of Insertion From Upper Lip (cm)
Below 1000	<28	0	2.5/5F	6.5-7.0
1000-2000	28-34	0	3.0/6F	7.0-8.0
2000-3000	34-38	0-1	3.5/8	8.0-9.0
>3000	>38	1	3.5 /8F	>9.0

Foundation Facts:
Technique of Emergency Umbilical Vein Catheterization

Prepare a 3.5F or 5F umbilical catheter with a radiopaque line. Flush the catheter with heparinized saline (0.5 to 1 U/mL) attached to a 3-way stopcock. Prep the umbilical cord and hold it firmly with an encircling tie to prevent bleeding while you cut it with a scalpel blade 1 cm above the skin attachment. The umbilical vein is identified as a thin-walled single vessel distinguishable from the 2 umbilical arteries, which have thicker walls and are often constricted and extend above the cut surface of the cord. The lumen of the vein is usually larger than that of the arteries. Insert the umbilical catheter so that the tip is just below the skin and you can readily aspirate blood. Evacuate any air bubbles to avoid the possible complication of air embolus to the central circulation. Position the umbilical venous catheter just at the point where good blood return is obtained. This should correspond to a depth of insertion of 1 to 4 cm and should avoid advancement of the catheter tip into the portal vein.

Routes of Administration

The tracheal route is generally the most rapidly accessible site for epinephrine administration. Vascular access is necessary, however, if administration of volume expanders or sodium bicarbonate is needed.

Tracheal administration of medications requires prior tracheal intubation. Tracheal intubation is also advisable to secure the airway (if that has not already been done) when chest compressions are being performed. Drugs administered by the tracheal route may be placed directly into the tracheal tube or given through a catheter inserted into the tracheal tube. Adequate drug distribution is promoted if the tracheal drug is followed by a saline flush and positive-pressure ventilations. The drug may be given undiluted and followed by a small volume of normal saline flush (0.5 to 1 mL) or may be diluted to a total volume of 1 mL in normal saline before administration. Administer positive-pressure breaths immediately after drug administration to distribute the drug dose throughout the tracheobronchial tree. Note that this 1-mL dilutional volume of epinephrine is smaller than the dilutional volume recommended for tracheal administration of drugs elsewhere in this text. The smaller volume of administration used in newly born infants reflects differences in size.

The umbilical vein is the most accessible site for vascular access in the newly born because it is easily located and cannulated (see Foundation Facts: "Technique of Emergency Umbilical Vein Catheterization"). However, special training is required to safely perform umbilical vein catheterization and maintain the catheter.

Neonatal liver injury (including hemorrhage) has been linked with the administration of hypertonic and alkaline solution (eg, sodium bicarbonate) into the portal vein, so the tip of the umbilical venous catheter should remain in the distal umbilical vein, away from the portal vein. If the catheter tip remains in the distal umbilical vein, any drugs administered by this route can be diluted by the patient's blood before they reach the liver. The catheter should be removed as soon as possible after resuscitation to minimize the danger of infection or thrombosis.

Vascular access may be obtained by several routes in addition to the umbilical vein. Peripheral veins in the extremities and scalp are difficult to cannulate in neonates during resuscitation, but they may provide adequate venous access even with a 24-gauge catheter. Intraosseous access is not commonly used in newly born infants because of the more readily accessible umbilical vein, the fragility of the infant's small bones, and the small intraosseous space in a premature infant. Intraosseous access can be used as an alternative route for medication and volume administration in the newly born infant if umbilical or other direct venous access is not readily attainable. Insert an 18-gauge needle in the

Foundation Facts:
Epinephrine in the Neonate and the Newly Born

Epinephrine has both α- and β-adrenergic-stimulating properties; in cardiac arrest α-adrenergic-mediated vasoconstriction may be the more important action.[47] Vasoconstriction elevates perfusion pressure during chest compression, enhancing delivery of oxygen to the heart and brain.[41] Epinephrine also enhances the contractile state of the heart, stimulates spontaneous contractions, and increases heart rate.

Critical Concepts:
Medications

Medications are rarely necessary for neonatal resuscitation.

Epinephrine and volume expansion are the most effective neonatal resuscitation medications.

medial aspect of the tibia, just below the tibial tuberosity.[40]

Epinephrine

(See also Chapter 5: "Fluid Therapy and Medications for Shock and Cardiac Arrest.")

The indications for administration of epinephrine are asystole or spontaneous heart rate less than 60 bpm despite adequate ventilation with 100% oxygen and chest compressions (see Foundation Facts: "Epinephrine in the Neonate and the Newly Born"). A dose of 0.01 to 0.03 mg/kg (0.1 to 0.3 mL/kg of 1:10 000 solution) is recommended for IV or tracheal administration. This dose may be repeated every 3 to 5 minutes if required.[41] Some patients who do not respond to standard doses of epinephrine may respond to higher doses.[42,43] The data is inadequate to evaluate the efficacy of high doses of epinephrine in newborns, and the safety of these doses has not been established. High doses of epinephrine may lead to prolonged hypertension,[44,45] which may lead to complications such

as intracranial hemorrhage in preterm infants.[46] If the neonate fails to respond to positive-pressure ventilation with 100% oxygen and a standard dose of epinephrine by the tracheal route, confirm adequate delivery of the dose to the lungs and establish vascular access (IV or intraosseous) to enable administration of epinephrine by the vascular route.[47]

Volume Expanders

Volume expanders are indicated for evidence of acute bleeding from the fetal-maternal unit, including the following signs observed in the newly born: (1) pallor that persists despite oxygenation, (2) faint pulses with a heart rate greater than 100 bpm, and (3) poor response to resuscitation, including effective ventilation.

Administer the volume expander as a bolus over 5 to 10 minutes:

- 10 mL/kg normal saline or Ringer's lactate (albumin is no longer recommended as the first choice for volume expansion—see FYI below).[48]

- 10 mL/kg O-negative blood crossmatched with the mother's blood or "emergency release" uncross-matched

After each volume bolus, re-evaluate the infant with respect to the need for additional boluses. Higher bolus volumes have been recommended for resuscitation of older infants, but volume overload or complications such as intracranial hemorrhage may result from inappropriate intravascular volume expansion in asphyxiated newly born infants as well as in preterm infants.[49,50]

FYI: Glucose Dose

The dose of glucose recommended for neonates during acute resuscitation is 200 mg/kg (2 mL/kg of a $D_{10}W$ solution) as a bolus. In PALS the dose of glucose recommended for infants and children during acute resuscitation is 500 to 1000 mg/kg (volume depends on concentration used). The dose recommended for newly born infants is designed to avoid hyperglycemia, hyperosmolarity, and rebound hypoglycemia because these complications can be particularly problematic in the newly born and premature neonate.

Other Medications

Guide glucose administration by evaluation of bedside blood glucose and avoid hyperglycemia. A dose of 200 mg/kg (2 mL/kg of 10% dextrose) may be given by slow IV push for documented and symptomatic hypoglycemia (see FYI).

There is no evidence that routine administration of sodium bicarbonate, atropine, or calcium is beneficial in the acute phase of neonatal resuscitation at delivery (see Critical Concepts). Do not use sodium bicarbonate during brief resuscitation episodes, although it may be beneficial when other therapies are ineffective and resuscitation is prolonged.[51-55] A dose of 1 to 2 mEq/kg of 0.5 mEq/mL solution may be given by slow IV push (over at least 2 minutes) after adequate ventilation has been established.

FYI: Albumin Volume Resuscitation

Albumin-containing solutions are no longer recommended as the first choice for acute volume expansion because of limited availability, cost, potential risk of infectious disease, and an observed association with increased mortality.[48]

Critical Concepts: Causes of Acute Deterioration During Positive-Pressure Ventilation—the "DOPE" Mnemonic

The mnemonic DOPE may serve as an aid for remembering the causes of deterioration in a patient with a tracheal tube in place:

Displacement of the tracheal tube

Obstruction of the tracheal tube

Pneumothorax

Equipment failure

Stomach inflation with air can impede ventilation. Gastric inflation can be relieved by placement of an orogastric tube and aspiration of stomach contents.

Postresuscitation Care

Three common complications of the post-resuscitation period are tracheal tube migration (including dislodgment), tracheal tube occlusion by mucus or meconium, and pneumothorax. These complications can be recalled using the mnemonic "DOPE" (see Critical Concepts).

Tracheal tube migration can be caused by changes in head position; the tracheal tube is advanced by head/neck flexion and withdrawn by head/neck extension.[56] Tracheal tube malposition or obstruction is suggested by decreased chest wall movement, diminished breath sounds, or the return of bradycardia and decreased arterial oxygen saturation. Unexplained hypercarbia should be assumed to result from tracheal tube obstruction until this complication has been ruled out.

Pneumothorax may complicate positive-pressure ventilation and may be difficult to diagnose by auscultation because breath sounds in the newborn are transmitted from all areas of the lung through the thin chest wall. Pneumothorax should be suspected if a newborn deteriorates after an initial good response to ventilation or fails to respond to resuscitative efforts. Additional signs of pneumothorax include a unilateral decrease in chest expansion, an altered intensity or pitch of breath sounds, and an increased resistance to manual ventilation.

Rule out equipment failure by removing the neonate from the mechanical ventilator and providing manual ventilation. If the equipment is the source of the problem, the infant will improve with hand ventilation. Also consider whether gastric inflation from prolonged bag-mask ventilation might be contributing to reduced effectiveness of ventilation. Gastric inflation may need to be relieved by an orogastric or nasogastric tube and suction.

Once ventilation and heart rate are adequate, additional postresuscitation interventions include

- Provision of a warm environment and frequent assessment of the newborn's temperature

- Monitoring of heart rate, respiratory rate, blood pressure, arterial oxygen saturation, and administered oxygen concentration (as necessary)

- Bedside determination of blood glucose level and treatment of hypoglycemia

- Arterial blood gas determination and correction of documented severe acidosis

- Evaluation of a chest roentgenogram to assess placement of tubes and catheters and lung expansion

- Achievement of vascular access and appropriate fluid therapy

- Treatment of hypotension with volume expanders, inotropic agents, or both; treatment of possible infection or seizures

Communicate with a neonatal ICU and arrange for transport as soon as the need for neonatal resuscitation is evident. Critically ill newborns should ideally be transported by a neonatal transport team specifically trained in the care of sick newborns. Such teams have the expertise and equipment to deliver a high level of neonatal intensive care during transport.

No resuscitation is complete without thorough documentation of actions and notification of the patient's primary care provider. The written record of evaluation and therapy must be sent with the newborn and should include copies of all laboratory results and roentgenograms.

Ethical Issues

In some circumstances noninitiation or discontinuation of resuscitation in the delivery room may be appropriate. These circumstances relate to gestational age, birth weight, known underlying condition, or lack of response to interventions. No single standard can be applied to newly born infants. National and local protocols should dictate the procedures to be followed. Review all such protocols regularly and modify them as necessary.

Noninitiation of Resuscitation

The delivery of extremely immature infants and infants with severe congenital anomalies raises questions about initiation of resuscitation.[57-59] Antenatal information may be incomplete or unreliable. In cases of uncertain gestational age and prognosis, resuscitation options include a trial of therapy and discontinuation of resuscitation after assessment of the infant. In such cases, initiation of resuscitation at delivery does not mandate continued support.

Noninitiation of support and later withdrawal of support are generally considered to be ethically equivalent; the latter approach allows time to gather more complete clinical information and provide counseling to the family. Ongoing evaluation and discussion with the parents and healthcare team should guide continuation versus withdrawal of support. In general there is no advantage to delayed, graded, or partial support. If the infant survives, outcome may be worsened as a result of this approach.

Discontinuation of Resuscitation

It may be appropriate to discontinue resuscitative efforts if resuscitation of an infant with cardiorespiratory arrest does not result in spontaneous circulation (a perfusing rhythm) in 15 minutes. Attempted resuscitation of newly born infants after 10 minutes of asystole is very unlikely to result in survival or survival without severe disability.[60-63] Local discussions should formulate guidelines consistent with local resources and outcome data.

Summary Points

The vast majority of term newborns require only maintenance of temperature, clearing of the airway, and stimulation by drying. At least one person skilled in initiating neonatal resuscitation should be present at every delivery. With adequate anticipation it is possible to optimize the delivery setting with appropriately prepared equipment and trained personnel. Although the need for resuscitation of the newly born infant often can be predicted, such need may arise suddenly and may occur in facilities that do not routinely provide neonatal intensive care. Thus, it is essential that the knowledge and skills required for resuscitation be taught to all providers of neonatal care.

Adequate ventilation is the cornerstone of neonatal resuscitation. Certain special circumstances, such as meconium staining of amniotic fluid, have unique implications for resuscitation of the newly born. Care of the infant after resuscitation includes not only supportive care but also ongoing monitoring and appropriate diagnostic evaluation. It is important to document resuscitation interventions and responses in order to understand an individual infant's pathophysiology, to improve resuscitation performance, and to study resuscitation outcomes.

Case Scenario
Case Scenario 1

A 28-year-old woman is brought into the Emergency Department complaining of severe abdominal pain and vaginal bleeding at 26 weeks of gestation. As she is being moved from the ambulance, her membranes rupture, and the infant is rapidly delivered through bloody amniotic fluid. The female infant is bruised, cyanotic, and flaccid. There are no spontaneous respirations. The infant's appearance is consistent with 26 weeks of gestation.

Note to providers: The presentation of this case scenario is somewhat different from the scenario presentations in other chapters. The "acceptable actions," "unacceptable actions," and rationale are summarized at the end of the scenario presentation.

Initial Assessment

The initial assessment is noted above. The infant is bruised, cyanotic, and flaccid. There are no spontaneous respirations, and the infant appears to be 26 weeks postconceptual age. Although the infant is apparently very ill, it is important to proceed through the initial steps of resuscitation and intervention.

Acceptable Actions

Provide warmth, preferably with a radiant warmer and chemical warming mattress as well as warmed blankets. Position the infant supine with neck slightly extended and clear the airway (mouth, then nose) with a suction catheter. Dry, stimulate, and position the infant as needed. Provide free-flow oxygen in case the infant initiates spontaneous respirations. Call for additional help because intubation and volume administration may be needed to treat an extremely premature infant with evidence of blood loss.

Case Scenario 1 Progression

The infant remains flaccid and apneic despite drying, suctioning, and stimulation by rubbing of the back.

Acceptable Actions

Because the infant failed to respond to brief tactile stimulation with spontaneous respirations, positive-pressure ventilation is necessary. Begin ventilation with a bag and mask. Intubation may be attempted early if bag-mask ventilation is ineffective or if a person skilled in intubation is present. During 30 seconds of positive-pressure ventilation a second person arrives to check the heart rate. After 30 seconds of positive-pressure ventilation, the heart rate will determine the need for chest compressions.

Case Scenario 1 Further Progression

As you continue to provide positive-pressure ventilation with 100% oxygen, a second rescuer attempts to palpate the umbilical cord pulse for 6 seconds. No pulse is detected. When no pulse is palpated at the base of the umbilical cord, the second rescuer listens to the infant's chest with a stethoscope to detect the heartbeat. The heart rate by auscultation is 40 bpm.

Acceptable Actions

A heart rate of less than 60 bpm after 30 seconds of positive-pressure ventilation with 100% oxygen indicates the need for chest compressions. At this stage it is also important to ensure that the airway is clear, that 100% oxygen is being delivered, and that ventilation is adequate. If the infant has not yet been intubated, place a tracheal tube to secure the airway and provide a route for administration of epinephrine if needed. If the heart rate remains less than 60 bpm despite chest compressions and positive-pressure ventilation with a tracheal tube that produce adequate chest wall rise, you must rule out problems and complications. Identify and treat tracheal tube dislodgment or obstruction, pneumothorax, or equipment failure. Also consider myocardial depression from perinatal asphyxia or hypovolemia in this situation. Epinephrine and volume administration may be necessary.

Case Scenario 1 Final Progression and Resolution

Epinephrine 0.3 mL/kg (the infant's estimated weight is 800 g) is given via the tracheal tube. Positive-pressure ventilation and chest compressions are continued for 30 seconds. The heart rate rises to 140 bpm. The infant is transferred to the NICU without incident. Her heart rate is noted to be 180 bpm. Umbilical lines are placed, and the infant is given 8 mL (10 mL/kg) of normal saline for hypotension. Artifical surfactant is administered via the tracheal tube.

The infant must be transferred to an NICU setting for ongoing care. Postresuscitation stabilization should include monitoring of heart rate, respirations, blood pressure, and oxygen saturation, as well as glucose and arterial blood gases. During transport of an infant after resuscitation it will be important to provide thermoregulation and maintenance of a secure airway.

Acceptable Actions

The following actions by the PALS provider are acceptable:

- Performs appropriate assessments throughout resuscitation, focusing on assessment of respirations, heart rate, and color

- Provides a source of supplemental heat during resuscitation of the extremely low-birthweight premature infant

- Performs bag-mask ventilation or immediate intubation for ventilation in a very premature infant who remains apneic after the initial steps

- Listens to the precordium to determine the heart rate when a cord pulse is not detectable

- Initiates chest compressions for a heart rate of less than 60 bpm after 30 seconds of positive-pressure ventilation with 100% oxygen

- Administers epinephrine by the tracheal route for persistent bradycardia (heart rate less than 60 bpm) or asys-

tole despite effective ventilation and chest compressions

Unacceptable Actions

The following actions by the PALS provider are unacceptable:

- Carries out resuscitation of the extremely low-birthweight infant without a source of supplemental heat

- Continues stimulation without positive-pressure ventilation when the infant remains apneic

- Assumes asystole is present before listening to the chest if a cord pulse is not palpable

- Initiates chest compressions *before* adequate ventilation with 100% oxygen

- Performs chest compressions with a heart rate greater than 60 bpm

- Administers epinephrine IM or intra-arterially

Rationale for Acceptable Actions: Ventilation

The key to successful neonatal resuscitation is adequate expansion of the lungs with gas, followed by effective ventilation. *The indications for positive-pressure ventilation include apnea, gasping respirations, a heart rate less than 100 bpm, and central cyanosis unresponsive to 100% oxygen.* Positive-pressure ventilation is provided with 100% oxygen, necessitating a portable oxygen tank in some settings outside the delivery room. Positive-pressure ventilation may be accomplished using either a self-inflating bag with an oxygen reservoir or a flow-inflating bag. Either should be equipped with a method to limit pressure—a pressure-release valve or a manometer. Face masks for both premature and newborn infants should be available; bags for neonatal resuscitation should have a volume of approximately 500 mL.

Ventilation is provided at a rate of 40 to 60 breaths/min. In an apneic infant initial breaths may be provided with longer inspiratory times of 1 to 2 seconds and peak

pressures of 30 to 40 cm H_2O. Subsequent breaths should be given with pressures sufficient to create gentle chest rise. Symmetrical air movement should be audible on auscultation.

Bag-mask manual ventilation of the neonate is perhaps the most crucial skill in resuscitation. The infant who remains thermoneutral and effectively ventilated will rarely need further resuscitation. If continued resuscitation is necessary, it is feasible for a single person to ventilate a neonate for a prolonged period. Unless personnel skilled in neonatal intubation are available, bag-mask ventilation may be the most effective method of supporting ventilation. Placement of an orogastric feeding tube can prevent gastric inflation during prolonged bag-mask ventilation.

After 30 seconds of positive-pressure ventilation, reassess the Triad of Evaluation: respirations, heart rate, and color. Positive-pressure ventilation is gradually discontinued when spontaneous, effective respirations are present, the heart rate is greater than 100 bpm, and the color is pink.

Rationale for Acceptable Actions: Chest Compressions

After 30 seconds of positive-pressure ventilation with 100% oxygen, if the heart rate is less than 60 bpm, administer chest compressions. Table 7 describes the site, compression-ventilation ratio, rate, and depth of chest compressions in the neonate. Compressions may be performed with the 2 thumb-encircling hands technique. Alternatively the 2-finger method may be used for provision of chest compressions and the other hand can support the baby's back.

If an infant requires chest compressions, recruit additional help from pediatric/neonatal specialists. After 30 seconds of chest compressions, check the heart rate again. If the heart rate is greater than 60 bpm, compressions can be discontinued, but positive-pressure ventilation should be continued until the heart rate is greater than 100 bpm, spontaneous respirations have returned, and color is pink.

Rationale for Acceptable Actions: Tracheal Intubation

Tracheal intubation should be considered at several points during resuscitation of a newly born infant. Immediately after birth in the depressed infant with meconium-stained amniotic fluid, tracheal intubation is indicated for tracheal suctioning. Consider intubation early during positive-pressure ventilation in the small preterm infant because tracheal administration of artificial surfactant or prolonged mechanical ventilation may be required. Consider tracheal intubation after several minutes of resuscitation if bag-mask ventilation is inadequate or chest compressions and medications are needed.

Neonatal intubation can be difficult for several reasons. Newly born infants who require intubation may be responsive or even struggling. The laryngeal structures are anteriorly placed and delicate, with less definition than in older infants, and the vocal cord opening is quite small. Secretions tend to be copious immediately after birth, and the newly born infant may rapidly become bradycardic in response to hypoxia and vagal stimulation.

Details of the intubation technique can be found in Chapter 4. Table 8 in this chapter provides information about selection of tracheal tube size and depth of insertion based on estimated gestational age or weight.

Maintenance of a patent airway can be particularly challenging when resuscitation occurs outside the delivery room. During transport the tracheal tube may become displaced or even dislodged. Frequently the tracheal tube moves too deeply and enters the right main bronchus; this results in asymmetrical breath sounds (right greater than left).

Acceptable Actions: Medications

Medications are rarely necessary during newly born resuscitation. Generally an infant who is adequately ventilated and normothermic can reverse asphyxial changes such as bradycardia and acidosis without medications. Hypovolemia, either from acute blood loss or capillary leak, and myocardial dysfunction from severe asphyxial insult may require medication. Table 5 lists dosages and routes of administration.

Acceptable Actions: Stabilization and Transport

After resuscitation outside the delivery room, mother and infant will be transferred to a location for supportive or continuing care. The healthy infant or the infant who has required only the initial steps in resuscitation may be transported with the mother according to local protocols. The infant who has required more extensive resuscitation requires ongoing monitoring with pulse oximetry or cardio-tachometry. The poor adhesive qualities of neonatal skin make it vital to clean the skin before taping tracheal tubes and orogastric tubes or affixing ECG leads. Special care must be taken to maintain the airway during transport. At present there is no scientific information on acceptable general ambulance transport of sick neonates; such situations should be handled according to local operating procedures and availability of specialized neonatal transport.

Review Questions

1. **During resuscitation of the newborn, you repeat the Triad of Evaluation. Which of the following parameters are included in this Triad?**

   a. heart rate, blood pressure, respiration

   b. apnea, pulse rate, grimace

   c. respiration, heart rate, color

   d. Apgar score

   The correct answer is c. The order of the triad indicates the priority of evaluation and interventions: establishment of effective ventilation is the priority for resuscitation of the newly born infant. The Triad of Evaluation should be repeated approximately every 30 seconds to ensure adequate response to interventions and to identify the need to modify support.

   Answer a is incorrect because it lists heart rate before respiration and includes blood pressure instead of color. Blood pressure measurement is not a priority assessment during initial evaluation and resuscitation of the newly born.

   Answer b is incorrect for 2 reasons. First, the evaluation of apnea requires a simple "yes" or "no" answer, whereas the correct evaluation of respiration requires determination of the presence or absence of respiration *and* the effectiveness of any respiratory effort that is present. If respirations are either absent or inadequate, you must support ventilation. Evaluation of respiration also requires clearing of the airway, an assessment that is not covered by assessment for apnea. Finally, a grimace is not a critical assessment parameter.

   Answer d is incorrect because although the Apgar score is important, resuscitation should not be delayed until the score is obtained. If the infant's respiratory effort is inadequate, you must intervene immediately.

2. **Which baby should have tracheal suctioning to reduce the risk of meconium aspiration syndrome?**

   a. vigorous baby with thin meconium-stained amniotic fluid

   b. depressed baby with clear amniotic fluid

   c. vigorous baby with thick meconium-stained amniotic fluid

   d. depressed baby with thick meconium-stained amniotic fluid

   The correct answer is d. You should suction the mouth, nose, and posterior pharynx of all babies with meconium-stained amniotic fluid as soon as the head is delivered but before the shoulders are delivered. This suctioning is recommended whether the meconium is thick or thin. Additional suctioning is determined by whether the infant is vigorous on delivery (see below).

   Answers a and **c** are incorrect because tracheal suctioning is no longer recommended for a vigorous baby whether the meconium is thin or thick. There is evidence that tracheal suctioning of the vigorous infant with meconium-stained amniotic fluid does not improve outcome and may cause complications.[30,31] The infant can be described as "vigorous" if the respiratory effort is strong, muscle tone is good, and heart rate is greater than 100 bpm.

   Answer b is incorrect because if the depressed infant has no meconium in the amniotic fluid, there is no indication for routine suctioning. If there is any concern about airway obstruction caused by secretions, suctioning is required.

3. **You are preparing to assist in stabilization of a newly born. Which of the following interventions will provide the key to successful neonatal resuscitations?**

   a. vascular access

   b. good chest compressions

   c. rapid administration of epinephrine

   d. effective ventilation

   The correct answer is d. Most newly born infants respond to initial measures of warming, drying, suctioning, and stimulation. Bradycardia in the newly born infant is usually the result of inadequate ventilation or profound hypoxia; adequate ventilation is the most important step in correcting bradycardia.

   Answer a is incorrect because vascular access is not often needed during resuscitation. Vascular access will need to be established if the infant requires administration of medications or volume resuscitation. Administration of medications is rarely necessary in resuscitation of the newly born infant.[38] These therapies should be provided only if the infant fails to respond to ventilation and chest compressions.

   Answer b is incorrect because good chest compressions are not the most important intervention during resuscitation of the newly born. Chest compressions are required only if the infant's heart rate remains under 60 bpm after establishment of effective ventilation for 30 seconds or longer.

   Answer c is incorrect because epinephrine administration is indicated only if the newly born fails to respond to establishment of effective ventilation and chest compressions.

References

1. Kattwinkel J, ed. *Textbook of Neonatal Resuscitation*. Elk Grove, Ill: American Academy of Pediatrics and American Heart Association; 2000.

2. American Heart Association in collaboration with International Liaison Committee on Resuscitation. Guidelines 2000 for Cardiopulmonary Resuscitation and Emergency Cardiovascular Care. International Consensus on Science. *Circulation*. 2000;102(suppl 1).

3. Vyas H, Milner AD, Hopkin IE, Boon AW. Physiologic responses to prolonged and slow-rise inflation in the resuscitation of the asphyxiated newborn infant. *J Pediatr*. 1981; 99:635-639.

4. Vyas H, Field D, Milner AD, Hopkin IE. Determinants of the first inspiratory volume and functional residual capacity at birth. *Pediatr Pulmonol*. 1986;2:189-193.

5. Saugstad OD. Practical aspects of resuscitating asphyxiated newborn infants. *Eur J Pediatr*. 1998;157(suppl 1):S11-S15.

6. Palme-Kilander C. Methods of resuscitation in low-Apgar-score newborn infants: a national survey. *Acta Paediatr*. 1992;81:739-744.

7. *The World Health Report: Report of the Director-General*. Geneva, Switzerland: World Health Organization; 1995.

8. Perlman JM, Risser R. Cardiopulmonary resuscitation in the delivery room: associated clinical events. *Arch Pediatr Adolesc Med*. 1995;149:20-25.

9. Cummins RO, Chamberlain DA, Abramson NS, Allen M, Baskett PJ, Becker L, Bossaert L, Delooz HH, Dick WF, Eisenberg MS, et al. Recommended guidelines for uniform reporting of data from out-of-hospital cardiac arrest: the Utstein Style. A statement for health professionals from a task force of the American Heart Association, the European Resuscitation Council, the Heart and Stroke Foundation of Canada, and the Australian Resuscitation Council. *Circulation*. 1991;84: 960-975.

10. Cummins RO, Chamberlain D, Hazinski MF, Nadkarni V, Kloeck W, Kramer E, Becker L, Robertson C, Koster R, Zaritsky A, Bossaert L, Ornato JP, Callanan V, Allen M, Steen P, Connolly B, Sanders A, Idris A, Cobbe S. Recommended guidelines for reviewing, reporting, and conducting research on in-hospital resuscitation: the in-hospital 'Utstein style.' American Heart Association. *Circulation*. 1997;95:2213-2239.

11. Zaritsky A, Nadkarni V, Hazinski MF, Foltin G, Quan L, Wright J, Fiser D, Zideman D, O'Malley P, Chameides L. Recommended guidelines for uniform reporting of pediatric advanced life support: the pediatric Utstein Style. A statement for healthcare professionals from a task force of the American Academy of Pediatrics, the American Heart Association, and the European Resuscitation Council. Writing group. *Circulation*. 1995; 92:2006-2020.

12. Peliowski A, Finer NN. Birth asphyxia in the term infant. In: Sinclair JC, Bracken MB, eds. *Effective Care of the Newborn Infant*. Oxford, UK: Oxford University Press; 1992.

13. Scopes JW, Ahmed I. Range of critical temperatures in sick and premature newborn babies. *Arch Dis Child*. 1966;41:417-419.

14. Adamsons K Jr, Gandy GM, James LS. The influence of thermal factors upon oxygen consumption of the newborn human infant. *J Pediatr*. 1965;66:495-508.

15. Day RL, Caliguiri L, Kamenski C, Ehrlich F. Body temperature and survival of premature infants. *Pediatrics*. 1964;34:171-181.

16. Gandy GM, Adamsons K Jr, Cunningham N, Silverman WA, James LS. Thermal environment and acid-base homeostasis in human infants during the first few hours of life. *J Clin Invest*. 1964;43:751-758.

17. Dahm LS, James LS. Newborn temperature and calculated heat loss in the delivery room. *Pediatrics*. 1972;49:504-513.

18. Perlman JM. Maternal fever and neonatal depression: preliminary observations. *Clin Pediatr*. 1999;38:287-291.

19. Lieberman E, Lang J, Richardson DK, Frigoletto FD, Heffner LJ, Cohen A. Intrapartum maternal fever and neonatal outcome. *Pediatrics*. 2000;105:8-13.

20. Vannucci RC, Perlman JM. Interventions for perinatal hypoxic-ischemic encephalopathy. *Pediatrics*. 1997;100:1004-1014.

21. Edwards AD, Wyatt JS, Thoresen M. Treatment of hypoxic-ischaemic brain damage by moderate hypothermia. *Arch Dis Child Fetal Neonatal Ed*. 1998;78:F85-F88.

22. Gunn AJ, Gluckman PD, Gunn TR. Selective head cooling in newborn infants after perinatal asphyxia: a safety study. *Pediatrics*. 1998; 102:885-892.

23. Cordero L Jr, Hon EH. Neonatal bradycardia following nasopharyngeal stimulation. *J Pediatr*. 1971;78:441-447.

24. Rossi EM, Philipson EH, Williams TG, Kalhan SC. Meconium aspiration syndrome: intrapartum and neonatal attributes. *Am J Obstet Gynecol*. 1989;161:1106-1110.

25. Locus P, Yeomans E, Crosby U. Efficacy of bulb versus DeLee suction at deliveries complicated by meconium stained amniotic fluid. *Am J Perinatol*. 1990;7:87-91.

26. Carson BS, Losey RW, Bowes WA Jr, Simmons MA. Combined obstetric and pediatric approach to prevent meconium aspiration syndrome. *Am J Obstet Gynecol*. 1976; 126:712-715.

27. Falciglia HS. Failure to prevent meconium aspiration syndrome. *Obstet Gynecol*. 1988; 71:349-353.

28. Greenough A. Meconium aspiration syndrome: prevention and treatment. *Early Hum Dev*. 1995;41:183-192.

29. Wiswell TE, Bent RC. Meconium staining and the meconium aspiration syndrome: unresolved issues. *Pediatr Clin North Am*. 1993;40:955-981.

30. Wiswell TE, Gannon CM, Jacob J, Goldsmith L, Szyld E, Weiss K, Schutzman D, Cleary GM, Filipov P, Kurlat I, Caballero CL, Abassi S, Sprague D, Oltorf C, Padula M. Delivery room management of the apparently vigorous meconium-stained neonate: results of the multicenter, international collaborative trial. *Pediatrics*. 2000;105:1-7.

31. Linder N, Aranda JV, Tsur M, Matoth I, Yatsiv I, Mandelberg H, Rottem M, Feigenbaum D, Ezra Y, Tamir I. Need for endotracheal intubation and suction in meconium-stained neonates. *J Pediatr*. 1988;112:613-615.

32. Theophilopoulos DT, Burchfield DJ. Accuracy of different methods for heart rate determination during simulated neonatal resuscitations. *J Perinatol*. 1998;18:65-67.

33. Apgar V. A proposal for a new method of evaluation of the newborn infant. *Curr Res Anesth Analg*. 1953;32.

34. Cloherty JP, Stark AR, eds. *Manual of Neonatal Care: Joint Program in Neonatology, Harvard Medical School*. Boston, Mass: Little, Brown; 1991.

35. American Academy of Pediatrics. Emergency drug doses for infants and children and naloxone use in newborns: clarification. *Pediatrics*. 1989;83:803.

36. Todres ID, Rogers MC. Methods of external cardiac massage in the newborn infant. *J Pediatr*. 1975;86:781-782.

37. David R. Closed chest cardiac massage in the newborn infant. *Pediatrics*. 1988;81:552-554.

38. Repetto JE, Donohue PK, Baker SF, Kelly L, Nogee LM. Use of capnography in the delivery room for assessment of tracheal tube placement. *J Perinatol*. 2001;21:284-287.

39. Burchfield DJ. Medication use in neonatal resuscitation. *Clin Perinatol*. 1999;26:683-691.

40. Ellemunter H, Simma B, Trawoger R, Maurer H. Intraosseous lines in preterm and full term neonates. *Arch Dis Child Fetal Neonatal Ed*. 1999;80:F74-F75.

41. Berkowitz ID, Gervais H, Schleien CL, Koehler RC, Dean JM, Traystman RJ. Epinephrine dosage effects on cerebral and myocardial blood flow in an infant swine model of cardiopulmonary resuscitation. *Anesthesiology*. 1991;75:1041-1050.

42. Goetting MG, Paradis NA. High-dose epinephrine improves outcome from pediatric cardiac arrest. *Ann Emerg Med*. 1991;20:22-26.

43. Paradis NA, Martin GB, Rosenberg J, Rivers EP, Goetting MG, Appleton TJ, Feingold M, Cryer PE, Wortsman J, Nowak RM. The effect of standard- and high-dose epinephrine on coronary perfusion pressure during prolonged cardiopulmonary resuscitation. *JAMA*. 1991;265:1139-1144.

44. Berg RA, Otto CW, Kern KB, Hilwig RW, Sanders AB, Henry CP, Ewy GA. A randomized, blinded trial of high-dose epinephrine versus standard-dose epinephrine in a swine model of pediatric asphyxial cardiac arrest. *Crit Care Med*. 1996;24:1695-1700.

45. Burchfield DJ, Preziosi MP, Lucas VW, Fan J. Effects of graded doses of epinephrine during asphxia-induced bradycardia in newborn lambs. *Resuscitation*. 1993;25:235-244.

46. Pasternak JF, Groothuis DR, Fischer JM, Fischer DP. Regional cerebral blood flow in the beagle puppy model of neonatal intraventricular hemorrhage: studies during systemic hypertension. *Neurology*. 1983;33:559-566.

47. Zaritsky A, Chernow B. Use of catecholamines in pediatrics. *J Pediatr*. 1984;105:341-350.

48. Human albumin administration in critically ill patients: systematic review of randomised controlled trials. Cochrane Injuries Group Albumin Reviewers. *BMJ*. 1998;317:235-240.

49. Usher R, Lind J. Blood volume of the newborn premature infant. *Acta Paediatr Scand*. 1965;54:419-431.

50. Funato M, Tamai H, Noma K, Kurita T, Kajimoto Y, Yoshioka Y, Shimada S. Clinical events in association with timing of intraventricular hemorrhage in preterm infants. *J Pediatr*. 1992;121:614-619.

51. Ostrea EM Jr, Odell GB. The influence of bicarbonate administration on blood pH in a "closed system": clinical implications. *J Pediatr*. 1972;80:671-680.

52. Simmons MA, Adcock EW III, Bard H, Battaglia FC. Hypernatremia and intracranial hemorrhage in neonates. *N Engl J Med*. 1974;291:6 10.

53. Finberg L. The relationship of intravenous infusions and intracranial hemorrhage: a commentary. *J Pediatr*. 1977;91:777-778.

54. Papile LA, Burstein J, Burstein R, Koffler H, Koops B. Relationship of intravenous sodium bicarbonate infusions and cerebral intraventricular hemorrhage. *J Pediatr*. 1978;93:834-836.

55. Graf H, Leach W, Arieff AI. Evidence for a detrimental effect of bicarbonate therapy in hypoxic lactic acidosis. *Science*. 1985;227:754-756.

56. Donn SM, Kuhns LR. Mechanism of endotracheal tube movement with change of head position in the neonate. *Pediatr Radiol*. 1980;9:37-40.

57. Byrne PJ, Tyebkhan JM, Laing LM. Ethical decision-making and neonatal resuscitation. *Semin Perinatol*. 1994;18:36-41.

58. Davies JM, Reynolds BM. The ethics of cardiopulmonary resuscitation, I: background to decision making. *Arch Dis Child*. 1992;67:1498-1501.

59. Landwirth J. Ethical issues in pediatric and neonatal resuscitation. *Ann Emerg Med*. 1993;22:502-507.

60. Davis DJ. How aggressive should delivery room cardiopulmonary resuscitation be for extremely low birth weight neonates? *Pediatrics*. 1993;92:447-450.

61. Jain L, Ferre C, Vidyasagar D, Nath S, Sheftel D. Cardiopulmonary resuscitation of apparently stillborn infants: survival and long-term outcome. *J Pediatr*. 1991;118:778-782.

62. Yeo CL, Tudehope DI. Outcome of resuscitated apparently stillborn infants: a ten year review. *J Paediatr Child Health*. 1994;30:129-133.

63. Casalaz DM, Marlow N, Speidel BD. Outcome of resuscitation following unexpected apparent stillbirth. *Arch Dis Child Fetal Neonatal Ed*. 1998;78:F112-F115.

Rapid Sequence Intubation

Introductory Case Scenario

EMS providers bring a previously healthy 4-year-old, 15-kg child to the Emergency Department. The child was an unrestrained, front-seat passenger in a motor vehicle crash. The vehicle carrying the child was traveling at 30 mph. EMS personnel report that the child was alert and talking coherently at the scene.

On arrival in the ED the child is unresponsive. Respiratory rate is 12 breaths/min with intermittent periods of shallow respirations; breath sounds are clear bilaterally. Oxygen saturation is 100% with 5 L/min supplementary oxygen by face mask. Heart rate is 90 bpm, and blood pressure is 130/84 mm Hg. Central and peripheral pulses are strong, capillary refill is 1 second, and extremities are warm and pink. The child has no purposeful movements; he exhibits flexion posturing in response to painful stimuli. He has no gag reflex, but his pupils are 3 mm and briskly reactive to light. He has a large, soft scalp contusion but no obvious midfacial or mouth injuries. His abdomen is soft and nondistended. There are no gross extremity injuries and no obvious external bleeding.

- What is your assessment of this child's ability to protect and maintain his airway?

- What are the relevant features of the child's initial history and targeted assessment that may affect decisions about rapid sequence intubation (RSI)?

- How would you prepare for tracheal intubation in this child?

- What medications would you give this child for RSI?

- How would you monitor this child after intubation?

Introduction

Rapid sequence intubation uses pharmacologic agents to facilitate emergent tracheal intubation and to reduce the potential adverse effects of intubation. These adverse effects include pain, rise in systemic arterial pressure and intracranial pressure (ICP), airway trauma, regurgitation and aspiration of stomach contents, hypoxemia, arrhythmias, psychological trauma, and death.

Healthcare providers in Emergency Departments and intensive care units use RSI frequently; out-of-hospital providers use this procedure to a lesser extent. Providers who use RSI must have proper training; they should monitor their success rate and the occurrence of complications. Course directors will determine when to include this optional module in their course.

The following recommendations for RSI are based on a review of the literature. The medications discussed are not the only medications you can use, nor are they preferable in all clinical situations. Different centers use different combinations of medications. Inclusion of this information in the PALS course does not represent an endorsement of RSI.

The term *rapid sequence intubation* is preferable to the term *rapid sequence induction*. Rapid sequence *induction* is the technique anesthesiologists use for rapid airway control coincident with the initiation of *anesthesia*. In emergency settings you should view RSI not "as the initiation of anesthesia but rather as the use of deep sedation and paralysis to facilitate . . . tracheal intubation."[1]

RSI Indications and Contraindications

Only properly trained providers who are familiar with the indications and contraindications of RSI should perform this procedure. These providers must be proficient in evaluation and management of the pediatric airway. They must also know the doses, side effects, indications, and contraindications for the medications used during this procedure (ie, sedatives, neuromuscular blockers, and adjunctive agents).

RSI Indications

The indications for RSI are the same as those for tracheal intubation:

- Inadequate central nervous system control of ventilation

- Functional or anatomic airway obstruction

- Loss of protective airway reflexes (cough, gag)

- Excessive work of breathing, which may lead to fatigue and respiratory failure

- Need for high peak inspiratory pressure or positive-end expiratory pressure to maintain effective alveolar gas exchange

- To permit sedation for diagnostic studies while ensuring airway protection and control of ventilation

- Potential occurrence of any of the above if patient transport is needed

RSI Contraindications

The full range of steps and medications of RSI is *not* indicated in patients in cardiac arrest or deeply comatose patients who require immediate intubation. But you may perform some of the steps and use some of the medications for RSI in these patients. Relative contraindications to RSI include

- Provider's concern that attempted intubation or bag-mask ventilation may be unsuccessful

- Significant facial or laryngeal edema, trauma, or distortion

- Spontaneous breathing and adequate ventilation in patients with muscle tone and positioning adequate to maintain the airway (eg, patients with upper airway obstruction or epiglottitis[1])

Steps of RSI

Safe and effective RSI requires you to follow a careful series of steps. You will begin with a review of the patient's history and conclude with postintubation observation, monitoring, and continued sedation. Table 1 lists these steps.

Step 1: Brief Medical History and Focused Physical Assessment

The provider must obtain a concise history before RSI. Use the mnemonic "AMPLE" (**A**llergies, **M**edications, **P**ast history, **L**ast meal, **E**vents leading to the need for intubation) to collect the needed information. This information helps the provider choose the appropriate agents for sedation and paralysis. For example, muscular dystrophy or a previous episode of malignant hyperthermia (**P**) would contraindicate use of

TABLE 1. Steps of Rapid Sequence Intubation

Step 1:	Brief medical history and focused physical assessment
Step 2:	Preparation
	■ Equipment
	■ Personnel
	■ Medications
Step 3:	Monitoring
Step 4:	Preoxygenation
Step 5:	Premedication
Step 6:	Sedation
Step 7:	Cricoid pressure and assisted ventilation (if needed)
Step 8:	Neuromuscular blockade (paralysis)
Step 9:	Tracheal intubation
Step 10:	Postintubation observation and monitoring
Step 11:	Continued sedation and paralysis

succinylcholine. The time since the patient's last meal (**L**) will indicate the risk of regurgitation and aspiration. A common tenet of RSI is to assume that each patient has a full stomach and is at risk for aspiration. The events leading to the patient's need for RSI (**E**) may suggest the potential for complications. Head injury, for example, suggests the potential for increased ICP.

The goal of the focused physical assessment is to determine whether the patient has any anatomic problems that may interfere with successful intubation or mask ventilation once the patient is sedated and paralyzed. You should assess the head, face, eyes, ears, nose, throat, teeth, neck, and cervical spine.

Step 2: Preparation

Assemble all equipment, personnel, and medications, and ensure that they are ready for use.

Equipment. Assemble all equipment needed for tracheal intubation (see Chapter 4). Test the equipment to ensure that it functions properly. Make sure that all equipment is easily accessible.

Personnel. A minimum of 3 providers is recommended:

- A provider experienced in airway management

- A provider to administer medications

- A provider to perform the Sellick maneuver (provide cricoid pressure) throughout the procedure (once the patient becomes sedated or does not have a gag reflex) and to monitor the patient's oxygen saturation, heart rate, and rhythm

Medications. Prepare sedative, paralytic, and adjunctive agents (eg, anticholinergic and analgesic agents). Draw up all drugs and ensure that they are ready for administration.

Step 3: Monitoring

Appropriate monitoring for a child undergoing RSI includes continuous cardiorespiratory monitoring, pulse oximetry, and intermittent blood pressure measurement. One provider should attach monitoring equipment while other members of the team obtain the brief medical history, perform focused anatomic assessment, and prepare equipment and medications. Performing these actions simultaneously will prevent delays in therapy.

Use of an exhaled carbon dioxide detector or other objective method to confirm correct tracheal tube placement is strongly recommended. If available, continuous capnometry monitoring after intubation is ideal; this monitor helps the provider to rapidly detect inadvertent extubation.

Step 4: Preoxygenation

Preoxygenate before administering medication and performing intubation. Preoxygenation maximizes hemoglobin and plasma oxygen saturation and creates an oxygen reservoir in the lungs.[2,3] This reservoir enables a sedated, paralyzed patient to remain well oxygenated and to tolerate the brief period of apnea that occurs during the intubation procedure, postponing the need for bag-mask ventilation. If the patient is breathing spontaneously and ventilating adequately, deliver 100% oxygen through a well-fitted face mask for at least 3 minutes.

During RSI avoid positive-pressure ventilation if possible. Positive-pressure ventilation may cause gastric inflation, increasing the risk of aspiration of stomach contents. Unfortunately the "safe" apnea interval is shorter in children undergoing nonelective tracheal intubation because acute illness, hypoxemia, or other potentially life-threatening conditions may compromise oxygen delivery or increase oxygen demand. Many children requiring urgent tracheal intubation have insufficient respiratory drive, inefficient respiratory mechanics, or an inability to maintain effective ventilation and oxygenation with spontaneous breathing. For these children a variable period of assisted ventilation with supplemental oxygen and bag and mask is desirable to improve the patient's tolerance of tracheal intubation.

Once the patient is adequately sedated, you should apply cricoid pressure (see below) to minimize the risk of aspiration. Apply cricoid pressure *before* initiation of bag-mask ventilation if appropriate, and maintain it until intubation is complete. Administering a paralytic agent as soon as possible after initiation of bag-mask ventilation will facilitate effective ventilation, resulting in less gastric inflation. Placement of a nasogastric tube will aid in stomach decompression. But providers must weigh this benefit against the risk of inducing gagging and emesis and the potential for opening the gastroesophageal sphincter, which increases the risk of gastric reflux.

Step 5: Premedication

Administer adjunctive agents to minimize the potentially dangerous physiologic responses that may occur with laryngoscopy, such as tachycardia, hypertension, increased intracranial and intraocular pressures, and profound vagal stimulation in infants and small children. The clinical status of the patient is the most important consideration for selecting a medication (Table 2). Local custom and availability of medications may also dictate your choice. The following sections describe agents providers typically use for RSI premedication:

- **Anticholinergic agents:** *Atropine* and *glycopyrrolate* minimize the unfavorable responses (bradycardia and asystole) to vagal stimulation that may result from laryngoscopy, hypoxia, or succinylcholine administration. Anticholinergics decrease oral secretions, making it easier to visualize landmarks during intubation. Anticholinergics are indicated for infants less than 1 year of age, children 1 to 5 years of age receiving succinylcholine, and the unusual older child or adolescent who receives a second dose of succinylcholine because of inability to successfully intubate after the initial dose.[1]

  Consider anticholinergics for any child who is bradycardic at the time of intubation. Also consider anticholinergics when you administer ketamine to prevent the increased oral secretions that may occur with succinylcholine administration. The most common side effect of anticholinergics is tachycardia. Because anticholinergics block the bradycardic response to hypoxia, continuous pulse oximetry is strongly recommended.

  — Atropine dose: 0.01 to 0.02 mg/kg IV (minimum 0.1 mg, maximum 1 mg); give 1 to 2 minutes before intubation. You may also combine atropine with succinylcholine for IM administration. The IM dose of atropine is 0.02 mg/kg.

  — Glycopyrrolate dose: 0.005 to 0.01 mg/kg IV (maximum 0.2 mg).

- **ICP protection:** *Lidocaine* reduces the rise in ICP that occurs with laryngoscopy.[4,5] The mechanism by which lidocaine blunts this response is not fully understood. It is likely related to the anesthetic effect of lidocaine on the central nervous system.

  — Lidocaine dose: 1 to 2 mg/kg IV rapid bolus; give 2 to 5 minutes before laryngoscopy.

- **Defasciculation:** Defasciculation is the administration of a small dose of a *nondepolarizing* neuromuscular blocker when succinylcholine (a depolarizing agent) is the chosen paralytic agent. This step inhibits the muscle fasciculations caused by the depolarization of muscle cell membranes that occur with succinylcholine administration. Adverse effects of succinylcholine, such as rhabdomyolysis, myoglobinuria, muscle pain, hyperkalemia, increased ICP, and increased intraocular pressure, are minimized by defasciculation. Consider defasciculation when you give succinylcholine to any child older than 5 years of age. Compared with younger children, children 5 years of age and older have greater muscle mass, which places them at greater risk for complications.[1]

  Providers generally use a low dose of vecuronium or pancuronium. Note that even a low dose of vecuronium or pancuronium may cause partial paralysis in children with presedation compromise of ventilatory efforts. This partial paralysis may necessitate early initiation of bag-mask ventilation and intubation, defeating the purpose of RSI.

  — Recommended defasciculation regimen: 1/10th (10%) of the paralyzing dose of vecuronium or pancuronium (eg, 10% of paralyzing dose of 0.1 mg/kg = 0.01 mg/kg for a vecuronium defasciculation dose); give 1 to 3 minutes *before* succinylcholine.

- **Analgesia:** To reduce or prevent pain, it is desirable to use a rapidly acting, potent analgesic that has little hemodynamic effect. Fentanyl has many of the desired characteristics. But fentanyl may cause rigidity of the chest wall after rapid administration; it may also cause increased ICP. For this reason use fentanyl with caution in children with suspected intracranial hypertension.[6] You

TABLE 2. Pharmacologic Agents Used in Rapid Sequence Intubation for Children

Drug	Dose*	Route	Duration	Side Effects	Comments
CARDIOVASCULAR ADJUNCTS					
Atropine	0.01-0.02 mg/kg (minimum 0.1 mg, maximum 1 mg) (IM dose: 0.02 mg/kg)	IV	>30 min	Paradoxical bradycardia can occur with doses <0.1 mg	Inhibits bradycardic response to hypoxia Dilates but does not "fix" pupil response to light
Glycopyrrolate	0.005-0.01 mg/kg (maximum 0.2 mg)	IV	>30 min	Tachycardia Dry mouth	Inhibits bradycardic response to hypoxia Dilates but does not "fix" pupil response to light
NARCOTIC AGENTS					
Fentanyl citrate (Sublimaze®)	2-4 µg/kg	IV, IM	1-2 hours	Respiratory depression Hypotension GI/GU opioid side effects Chest wall rigidity can occur with high-dose rapid infusions	Less histamine release and associated hypotension than with other opioids May elevate ICP Movement disorders can occur with prolonged use
SEDATIVE-HYPNOTIC AGENTS					
Midazolam (Versed®)	0.1-0.2 mg/kg (maximum 4 mg)	IV, IM	30-60 min	Respiratory depression Hypotension	Potentiates respiratory depressive effects of narcotics and barbiturates No analgesic properties
Diazepam (Valium®)	0.1-0.2 mg/kg (maximum 4 mg)	IV	30-90 min		
Thiopental (Pentothal®)	2-4 mg/kg	IV	5-10 min	Negative inotropic effects Hypotension	Ultrashort-acting barbiturate Decreases cerebral metabolic rate and ICP Potentiates respiratory depressive effects of narcotics and benzodiazepines No analgesic properties
Etomidate	0.2-0.4 mg/kg	IV	10-15 min	Myoclonic activity Cortisol suppression	Ultrashort-acting No analgesic properties Decreases cerebral metabolic rate and ICP Minimal cardiovascular and respiratory depression Contraindicated in patients dependent on endogenous cortisol response

Drug	Dose*	Route	Duration	Side Effects	Comments
ANESTHETIC AGENTS (when used in higher doses)					
Lidocaine	1-2 mg/kg	IV	≈30 min	Myocardial and CNS depression with high doses Seizures can occur with repeated doses	Decreases ICP Hypotension less common
Ketamine (Ketalar®)	1-4 mg/kg	IV, IM	30-60 min	Increased ICP and BP Increased secretions and laryngospasm Hallucinations/ emergence reaction	Dissociative anesthetic agent No to limited respiratory depression Bronchodilator
Propofol (Diprovan®)	2 mg/kg (up to 3 mg/kg in young children)	IV	3-5 min	Hypotension, especially in patients with inadequate intravascular volume Pain on injection	Highly lipid soluble with very short duration of action Less likely than barbiturates to increase airway reactivity
NEUROMUSCULAR BLOCKING AGENTS					
Succinyl-choline (Anectine®)	IV: 1-1.5 mg/kg for children IV: 2 mg/kg for infants IM: double the IV dose	IV, IM	3-5 min	Muscle fasciculations Rise in intracranial, intraocular, intragastric pressure Life-threatening hyperkalemia Hypertension	Depolarizing muscle relaxant Rapid onset and short duration of action Avoid in renal failure, burns, or hyperkalemic states Consider defasciculation with a nondepolarizing agent in children ≥5 years of age Do *not* use for maintenance of paralysis
Vecuronium (Norcuron®)	0.1-0.2 mg/kg	IV, IM	30-90 min	Minimal cardiovascular side effects	Nondepolarizing agent 2- to 3-min onset of action
Rocuronium (Zemuron®)	0.6-1.2 mg/kg	IV	30-60 min	Minimal cardiovascular side effects	Nondepolarizing agent Rapid onset of action equaling that of succinylcholine

BP indicates blood pressure; CNS, central nervous system; GI, gastrointestinal; GU, genitourinary; ICP, intracranial pressure; IM, intramuscular; and IV, intravenous.

*Doses provided are guidelines only. Actual dosing may vary depending on the patient's clinical status.

may use morphine for analgesia, but the associated histamine release may cause hypotension.

— Fentanyl dose in hemodynamically stable patients: 2 to 4 μg/kg slow IV infusion or IM injection; give 1 to 3 minutes before intubation.

Step 6: Sedation

You must appropriately sedate all children undergoing RSI except those who are deeply comatose. Sedation will blunt their awareness during paralysis. Ideal sedatives rapidly induce unconsciousness, have a short duration of action, and have minimal side effects. For sedation during RSI providers commonly use benzodiazepines (eg, midazolam or diazepam), barbiturates (eg, thiopental), the nonbarbiturate sedative-hypnotic etomidate, the general anesthetic propofol, and the dissociative anesthetic ketamine (Table 2).

■ **Barbiturates:** Short-acting barbiturates (eg, thiopental) are sedative-hypnotic agents with a rapid onset of action and short duration of action. They have *no* analgesic properties. The primary benefit of short-acting barbiturates is their cerebroprotective effect: they reduce cerebral metabolic rate and cerebral oxygen demands, and they can reduce ICP. [7] Short-acting barbiturates are frequently the sedatives of choice for patients with head trauma, status epilepticus, or suspected ICP elevation. Disadvantages include myocardial depression and hypotension, so you generally avoid use of barbiturates in patients with hypotension or hypovolemia. Decreasing the rate of administration can reduce these adverse effects; if you do select barbiturates for these patients, decrease the dose by at least half. Other adverse effects include respiratory depression (enhanced by benzodiazepines and narcotics), bronchospasm, cough, laryngospasm, and anaphylaxis. Generally avoid use of barbiturates in children with acute asthma. Barbiturates are contraindicated in patients with porphyria.

— Thiopental dose: 2 to 4 mg/kg IV. Onset of action is 10 to 20 seconds; duration of action is 5 to 10 minutes.

■ **Benzodiazepines:** A number of benzodiazepines are available (eg, midazolam, diazepam, lorazepam). But many providers consider midazolam the sedative of choice for RSI. Midazolam is a water-soluble, rapidly acting sedative with potent amnestic properties. It has a quick onset and short duration of action, making it suitable for RSI. Diazepam has a slightly slower onset of action and a slightly longer duration of action, making it more appropriate for continued sedation *after* intubation. Many providers are more familiar with diazepam than midazolam. Both agents can cause respiratory depression, especially with concomitant use of barbiturates or narcotics. Though less common than with barbiturates, hypotension can occur. For this reason you should give only half the recommended dose for patients who are hemodynamically unstable (ie, hypotensive or hypovolemic). Like barbiturates, the benzodiazepines possess no analgesic properties.

— Midazolam dose: 0.1 to 0.2 mg/kg IV/IM (maximum 4 mg); give 2 to 3 minutes before the paralytic. Onset of action is 1 to 2 minutes; duration of action is 30 to 60 minutes.

— Diazepam dose: 0.1 to 0.2 mg/kg (maximum 4 mg); give 2 to 4 minutes before the paralytic. Onset of action is 2 to 3 minutes; duration of action is 30 to 90 minutes.

■ **Propofol:** Propofol is a sedative-hypnotic capable of producing general anesthesia. Its mechanism of action is not understood. Propofol is nearly insoluble in water. It is administered in a lipid emulsion. The high lipid solubility of propofol leads to rapid transfer across the blood-brain barrier and rapid distribution to organs with high blood flow, similar to the short-acting barbiturates. Its short duration of action after bolus administration is due to rapid redistribution from the brain to other organs and rapid metabolism by both hepatic and extrahepatic mechanisms. Patients recover from propofol-induced sedation more rapidly than from barbiturate-induced sedation. There are 2 significant side effects: hypotension and pain on administration. Approximately 15% of patients with normal blood pressure experience transient hypotension secondary to vasodilation. In patients with hypovolemia or shock, you should probably avoid propofol to limit the risk of severe hypotension. To limit pain on injection, administer 0.5 to 1 mg/kg lidocaine through the IV catheter before or during propofol administration.

— Propofol dose: 2 mg/kg IV; young children may require somewhat larger doses (up to 3 mg/kg).

■ **Dissociative deep sedation:** Ketamine, a phencyclidine derivative, is the only agent capable of producing analgesia, rapid sedation, and amnesia while preserving respiratory drive and airway protective reflexes. Use the lower dosing range for patients with hemodynamic compromise. Ketamine-induced catecholamine release helps maintain blood pressure. It may decrease bronchospasm and improve ventilation in patients with asthma.[8,9] These beneficial effects may not occur in chronically ill patients with catecholamine depletion, however.

Adverse effects include increased systemic, intracranial, and intraocular pressures; hallucinations or emergence reactions; laryngospasm; and excessive airway secretions. Pretreatment with 0.01 mg/kg atropine or 0.005 mg/kg glycopyrrolate will decrease airway secretions. Adding a benzodiazepine may decrease the risk of an emergence reaction.

— Ketamine dose to induce rapid sedation: 1 to 4 mg/kg IV. Onset of action is 1 to 2 minutes; duration of action is 30 to 60 minutes. You may give ketamine by the IM route (dose of 3 to 6 mg/kg), but its onset of action will be slower. Do not routinely use the IM route for ketamine.

■ **Etomidate:** Etomidate is an ultrashort-acting, nonbarbiturate, nonbenzodiazepine sedative-hypnotic agent with no analgesic properties. This drug causes minimal cardiovascular or respiratory depression. Some providers consider etomidate the sedative of choice for patients with multisystem trauma or hypotension.[10,11] Etomidate decreases ICP, cerebral blood flow, and cerebral basal metabolic rate,[12,13] so it is recommended for use in patients with head injury.[11] Etomidate may suppress cortisol production after a single dose in a transient, reversible, and dose-dependent manner.[14,15] A single dose may suppress the cortisol response to adrenocorticotropic hormone for up to 24 hours in critically ill patients.[16] But most children appear to tolerate the drug well.[17] Etomidate may cause myoclonic activity, such as coughing and hiccups, and it may exacerbate focal seizure disorders. Known adrenal insufficiency and a history of focal seizure disorder are relative contraindications to etomidate. The agent is stable in solution at room temperature, and it has a long shelf life. Evidence-based experience with etomidate in children is limited.

— Etomidate dose: 0.2 to 0.4 mg/kg IV infused over 30 to 60 seconds will produce rapid sedation lasting only 10 to 15 minutes.

Step 7: Cricoid Pressure and Assisted Ventilation

If possible avoid positive-pressure ventilation so as to decrease the likelihood of gastric inflation and subsequent reflux and aspiration. If the patient requires bag-mask ventilation, you should perform the Sellick maneuver (ie, application of continuous, steady posterior pressure to the cricoid cartilage) *before* initiation of bag-mask ventilation.[18] Cricoid pressure occludes the esophagus, minimizing entry of air into the stomach. It may improve visualization of the vocal cords because it displaces the larynx posteriorly. See Chapter 4, Figure 13.

Do not apply the Sellick maneuver when the patient is awake and responsive because it can stimulate gagging and regurgitation. During RSI apply cricoid pressure as the patient becomes sedated (ie, as the patient loses consciousness) and *before* initiation of manual ventilation.

Maintain cricoid pressure continuously until the tracheal tube is in place. Because cricoid pressure does not eliminate the possibility of regurgitation, you must have a vacuum source and an adequately sized suction catheter readily available.

Step 8: Neuromuscular Blockade (Paralysis)

Desirable paralytic agents for RSI have a rapid onset and short duration of action with minimal adverse effects (see Table 2). The depolarizing agent succinylcholine is the only agent with rapid onset and short duration. But succinylcholine may produce numerous adverse effects, some potentially fatal. The newer nondepolarizing agents rocuronium and vecuronium have a relatively rapid onset and more benign side effects. For these reasons providers frequently use these agents instead of succinylcholine despite their longer duration of action.

- **Rocuronium:** Rocuronium is an aminosteroid nondepolarizing agent with a rapid onset and intermediate duration of action. Rocuronium has minimal cardiovascular side effects at doses used for RSI.[19] It is safe to use in patients with renal[20] and hepatic failure, but neuromuscular blockade may be prolonged in patients with liver disease.[21,22] Rocuronium comes as a premixed solution, an advantage in urgent situations.

  — Rocuronium dose: 0.6 to 1.2 mg/kg IV. Onset of action is within 60 seconds; duration of action is 30 to 60 minutes.[23-25]

- **Vecuronium:** Vecuronium is the aminosteroid from which rocuronium was developed. It is more potent than rocuronium, so it has a slower onset of action. (The onset of action of neuromuscular blockers is inversely related to potency.) Higher doses produce more rapid onset, but they prolong paralysis. Vecuronium has few side effects; it is safe for patients with renal and hepatic failure.[26] Unlike rocuronium, vecuronium is supplied as a powder that must be reconstituted before administration.

  — Vecuronium dose: 0.1 to 0.2 mg/kg IV will produce acceptable paralysis for intubation in 90 to 120 seconds. Duration of action is 30 to 90 minutes in both adults and children, depending on the dose.[27,28]

- **Succinylcholine:** In the past many providers considered succinylcholine the paralytic of choice for RSI because it is the only agent with both a rapid onset and ultrashort duration of action. It is also the only neuromuscular blocker approved for IM administration. The theoretical advantage of a neuromuscular blocker with an ultrashort duration of action is that if intubation is unsuccessful, the effect of the agent quickly wears off and the patient can resume spontaneous ventilation. Resumption of spontaneous ventilation can minimize the need for bag-mask ventilation with its risks of gastric inflation, vomiting, and aspiration. But children who require RSI often have inadequate spontaneous ventilation for several reasons, including sedative-induced respiratory depression or underlying respiratory failure. In RSI for seriously ill or injured children, the advantage of an ultrashort-acting neuromuscular blocker may be largely negated.

Succinylcholine has numerous contraindications and potential side effects (Table 3), some of which may be fatal (albeit rare). The availability of rapid-acting nondepolarizing agents has limited the indications for succinylcholine. Providers who use succinylcholine must know its potential dangers and contraindications. Providers must carefully weigh the risks and benefits of succinylcholine against the risks and benefits of the nondepolarizing agents. Do not routinely use succinylcholine, but you may still consider it for RSI. Never use succinylcholine to maintain paralysis after intubation.[29-31]

TABLE 3. Succinylcholine: Adverse Effects and Relative Contraindications

Adverse Effects	Relative Contraindications
Muscle fasciculations	Increased intracranial pressure
Muscle pain	Open globe injury
Rhabdomyolysis	Glaucoma
Myoglobinuria	Neuromuscular disorders
Hyperkalemia	History (patient or family) of malignant hyperthermia
Hypertension	
Increased intracranial pressure	History of plasma cholinesterase deficiency
Increased intraocular pressure	Crush injuries
Increased intragastric pressure	Trauma or burns >48 hours after injury
Malignant hyperthermia	Hyperkalemia
Bradycardia, asystole	Renal failure

— Succinylcholine IV dose: 1 to 1.5 mg/kg for children and 2 mg/kg for infants. Onset of action is 30 to 60 seconds; duration of action is 3 to 5 minutes.

— Succinylcholine IM dose: Double the IV dose. Many providers combine succinylcholine with atropine in the same syringe for IM administration. Onset of paralysis adequate for intubation may take 2 to 4 minutes.

Step 9: Tracheal Intubation

The patient is ready for intubation once you ensure adequate preoxygenation, premedication, sedation, and paralysis. Clinical indicators of adequate paralysis include lack of spontaneous movements, respiratory effort, and blink reflex. Jaw relaxation is another indicator of paralysis; you should be able to fully open the patient's mouth without resistance. The goal of RSI is to rapidly obtain definitive airway control while avoiding adverse effects. The provider most experienced in pediatric tracheal intubation should perform or directly supervise this step.

After intubation confirm tracheal tube placement using primary and secondary confirmation techniques (see Chapter 4). After primary and secondary confirmation of correct tube placement, secure the tube. Obtain a chest radiograph when possible.

Step 10: Postintubation Observation and Monitoring

After successful tracheal intubation all patients require close observation and monitoring (see Chapter 4).

Step 11: Continued Sedation and Paralysis

The sedatives and paralytics used for RSI have relatively short durations of action. As a result patients will often need additional medications before or during transport or transfer to an intensive care unit. As paralysis wears off, children may breathe asynchronously with positive-pressure ventilation; some may attempt

to dislodge tubes and monitoring equipment. To correct or avoid these problems, you may administer an additional dose of a neuromuscular blocker and a sedative. Healthcare providers must make every effort to detect loss of sedation in children who remain pharmacologically paralyzed.

This awake but paralyzed state can cause fear, tachycardia, hypertension, and a rise in ICP. You should suspect inadequate sedation in patients with unexplained tachycardia, hypertension, or rise in ICP.

You can use a longer-acting sedative, such as lorazepam (0.05 to 0.1 mg/kg), to provide ongoing sedation and amnesia. You may also give additional doses of midazolam (0.05 to 0.1 mg/kg) or diazepam (0.1 to 0.2 mg/kg). You should remember that hypoxia, inadequate ventilation, tube displacement, tube obstruction, tension pneumothorax, or equipment failure may also cause hypertension and tachycardia.

Recommendations for Specific Clinical Circumstances

Providers must use different combinations of agents for RSI in different clinical circumstances. Figure 1 outlines the technique of RSI and recommended RSI agents for the most common situations encountered in children. Table 4 lists the suggested RSI medications for 4 common clinical conditions. These guidelines are only general guidelines; local customs should dictate protocols and provider training requirements.

Summary Points

■ Rapid sequence intubation is a technique of intubation using sedative, paralytic, and adjunctive agents in a stepwise approach to facilitate tracheal intubation and minimize its adverse effects. The steps are

1. Brief medical history and focused physical assessment

2. Preparation: equipment, personnel, and medications

3. Monitoring

4. Preoxygenation

5. Premedication

6. Sedation

7. Cricoid pressure and assisted ventilation (if needed)

8. Neuromuscular blockade (paralysis)

9. Tracheal intubation

10. Postintubation observation and monitoring

11. Continued sedation and paralysis

■ The choice of medications for RSI depends on the clinical scenario, the patient's history, local customs, and the provider's familiarity with the appropriate agents.

■ Providers should be familiar with the recommended drug regimens for 4 common clinical scenarios:

— Head injury, increased ICP or status epilepticus, with or without hypotension

— Normotensive, euvolemic

— Shock: hypotensive, hypovolemic, or cardiogenic; mild or severe

— Status asthmaticus

Case Scenarios
Introductory Case Scenario

EMS providers bring a previously healthy 4-year-old, 15-kg child to the Emergency Department. The child was an unrestrained, front-seat passenger in a motor vehicle crash. The vehicle carrying the child was traveling at 30 mph. EMS personnel report that the child was alert and talking coherently at the scene.

On arrival in the ED the child is unresponsive. Respiratory rate is 12 breaths/min with intermittent periods of shallow respirations; breath sounds are clear bilaterally. Oxygen saturation is 100% with 5 L/min supplementary oxygen by face mask. Heart rate is 90 bpm, and BP is 130/84 mm Hg. Central and peripheral pulses are strong, capillary refill is 1 second, and extremities are warm and pink.

FIGURE 1. Rapid sequence intubation algorithm.

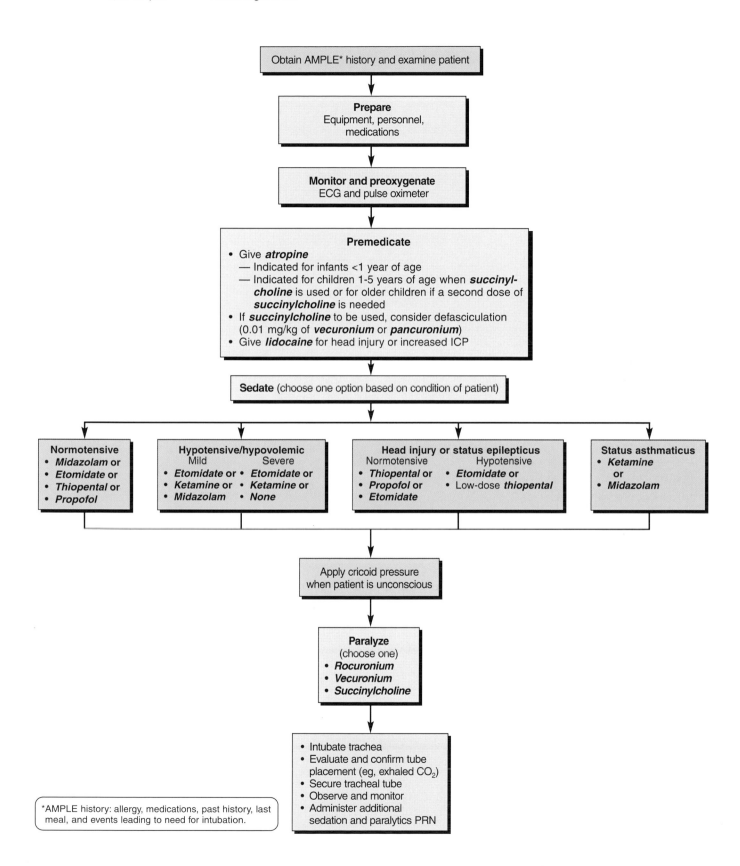

TABLE 4. Recommended Agents for RSI in Common Clinical Conditions

Clinical Scenario		Sedative Agents	Paralytic Agents	Adjunctive Agents
Head injury, increased ICP, status epilepticus	Normotensive	Thiopental, propofol, or etomidate. Midazolam may be used, but it has no specific cerebroprotective effects.	Short-acting NMB*	Lidocaine
	Hypotensive	Etomidate or low-doses of thiopental. Midazolam may be used, but it has no specific cerebroprotective effects.	Short-acting NMB*	Lidocaine
Normotensive, euvolemic		Midazolam, etomidate, propofol, or thiopental.	Short-acting NMB*	
Shock: hypotensive, hypovolemic, cardiogenic	Mild	Etomidate,† ketamine, or low-dose midazolam.	Short-acting NMB*	Atropine‡
	Severe	Etomidate, ketamine, or none.	Short-acting NMB*	Atropine‡
Status asthmaticus		Ketamine or midazolam.	Short-acting NMB*	Atropine

*NMB indicates neuromuscular blocking agent (eg, rocuronium or succinylcholine). Succinylcholine is relatively contraindicated in patients with increased intracranial pressure (ICP).

†Etomidate can suppress corticosteroid production after a single dose. If shock persists, consider adding stress-dose steroids.

‡Atropine is suggested if ketamine is used.

The child has no purposeful movements; he exhibits flexion posturing in response to painful stimuli. He has no gag reflex, but his pupils are 3 mm and briskly reactive to light. He has a large, soft scalp contusion but no obvious midfacial or mouth injuries. His abdomen is soft and nondistended. There are no gross extremity injuries and no obvious external bleeding.

Introductory Case Scenario Self-Evaluation Questions

■ *What is your assessment of this child's ability to protect and maintain his airway?*

This patient has 3 major indications for RSI. First, the patient currently responds to painful stimuli only; he has slow, shallow, intermittent respirations and no gag reflex. These signs indicate that the patient cannot maintain his airway; he needs intervention. Second, the patient's minute ventilation is inadequate with slow and shallow respirations,

so he has potential respiratory failure. The patient has strong pulses, brisk capillary refill, warm extremities, and no hypotension. These signs suggest stable cardiovascular function and systemic perfusion. Third, the patient has a head injury with the potential for increased ICP and delayed cardiovascular deterioration due to occult bleeding.

■ *What are the relevant features of the child's initial history and targeted assessment that may affect decisions about RSI?*

The child has a head injury with possible increased ICP. He responds to painful stimuli. You must assume that the child has a full stomach. RSI is appropriate for this child. If a parent or someone responsible for the child's care is available, begin by obtaining a focused history (use the AMPLE mnemonic). Perform a focused assessment to determine if the patient has any anatomic conditions that will complicate RSI.

The events (**E**) leading to this scenario put the child at risk for significant multisystem injury, including head injury and the potential for cervical spine injury. Rescuers must provide cervical spine immobilization throughout intubation. You must also select drugs appropriate for a child with potential head injury and increased ICP.

The patient has no obvious midface or mouth injuries that would interfere with intubation. The nature of the patient's injury places him at risk for cervical spine trauma. An additional rescuer is needed to maintain alignment of the patient's head and spine in a neutral position throughout the procedure.

■ *How would you prepare for tracheal intubation in this child?*

You should gather appropriate equipment, medications, and personnel. You should also establish monitoring of ECG and oxygenation. Maintaining cervical spine immobilization makes intubation more difficult. The provider most experienced in airway management of patients with potential head and spinal cord injuries should perform intubation.

This patient is breathing spontaneously and has adequate oxyhemoglobin saturation with 5 L/min supplementary oxygen by face mask. You can preoxygenate the patient by delivering 100% oxygen through a tight-fitting mask for 2 to 3 minutes before you initiate paralysis. Preoxygenation will allow the patient to build up an adequate oxygen reserve to tolerate the brief period of apnea between the onset of muscular paralysis and successful intubation.

Avoid manual ventilation if possible; manual ventilation will distend the stomach with air, increasing the risk of regurgitation and aspiration of stomach contents. If the child has specific signs of increased ICP, provide manual ventilation to prevent the development of hypoxia and hypercarbia. Those conditions will contribute to a further increase in ICP. Whenever a patient needs manual ventilation, perform the Sellick maneuver *before* initiation of bag-mask ventilation so as to reduce the risk of regurgitation and aspiration. This child has no gag reflex, so he will tolerate cricoid pressure. Were the child responsive and bag-mask ventilation indicated, you would wait until the child was sedated to perform the Sellick maneuver and then begin positive-pressure ventilation with a bag and mask.

In this scenario immobilization of the cervical spine in a neutral position is necessary *throughout* RSI. Failure to immobilize the cervical spine is unacceptable. Open the airway using the jaw thrust. The head tilt–chin lift is contraindicated.

■ *What medications would you give this child for RSI?*

Once you prepare all equipment and establish monitoring, administer a seda-

tive and then a paralytic. This child has a head injury and possible increased ICP, so you will administer lidocaine at a dose of 1 to 2 mg/kg (15 to 30 mg). Administer lidocaine 2 to 5 minutes before laryngoscopy. Lidocaine will reduce the risk of a further increase in ICP due to laryngoscopy. This child has no external evidence of bleeding; he has normal blood pressure with adequate perfusion. So you have no reason to suspect hypovolemia. Thiopental, propofol, or etomidate (all short-acting agents) are appropriate for sedation. All have cerebroprotective and sedative effects. You may use midazolam for sedation, but it has no cerebroprotective effects.

For paralysis a rapid-onset nondepolarizing neuromuscular blocking agent (eg, rocuronium) is the best choice for this patient with increased ICP. At doses of 0.6 to 1.2 mg/kg, rocuronium has an onset of action comparable to that of succinylcholine. Rocuronium also has more benign side effects.

Ketamine is unacceptable for this patient because this drug may cause increased ICP. Increased ICP is also a relative contraindication to the use of succinylcholine, although this issue is controversial. Defasciculation is not indicated unless succinylcholine is the chosen paralytic.

■ *How would you monitor this child after intubation?*

Immediately after tracheal intubation, you should confirm placement of the tube in the trachea; use both primary and secondary techniques. Monitor the child's heart rate, oxygenation, and exhaled CO_2, preferably continuously. Closely monitor the child's neurologic status.

Because the duration of action of thiopental is only 5 to 10 minutes and the duration of action of rocuronium is 30 to 60 minutes, the patient will most likely awaken from sedation while still

paralyzed. The child may become frightened, which could produce or worsen increased ICP. The stress and fear responses will typically cause the patient's heart rate and blood pressure to rise. For this reason you should administer a longer-acting sedative (eg, lorazepam or midazolam) shortly after intubation. Closely monitor the patient. Signs of inadequate sedation, such as tachycardia or hypertension, could lead to fluctuations in ICP and possibly worse brain injury.

Introductory Case Scenario Progression

Providers apply appropriate monitors and prepare equipment and medications. One provider preoxygenates the patient without manual ventilation. Another provider applies cricoid pressure. You give lidocaine; 1 minute later you give thiopental and rocuronium. After the onset of paralysis an experienced provider performs intubation while another provider immobilizes the cervical spine in a neutral position. You confirm tube position by auscultation over the lateral lung fields and abdomen and by use of a colorimetric exhaled CO_2 detector.

You establish continuous postintubation monitoring. A few minutes later the patient's heart rate is 100 bpm, blood pressure is 102/64 mm Hg, and pupils are equal and reactive to light. Ten minutes after intubation the heart rate rises to 140 bpm and blood pressure rises to 160/88 mm Hg. These signs suggest that sedation has worn off but paralysis continues. You administer a longer-acting sedative (eg, lorazepam), and the patient's heart rate and blood pressure return to normal.

Case Scenario 2

A mother brings her 6-month-old, 5-kg infant to the ED. The mother says the baby has had a runny nose and cough for several days. The infant was feeding well until 1 hour ago, when the mother noticed that the baby was having a hard time breathing. The infant would "stop breathing" between coughing spells, and she was blue around the lips. The mother says the infant has not had fever, vomiting, or diarrhea, and the baby's urine output has been normal.

On arrival in the ED the baby is lethargic and appears ill. Copious, thick secretions are in the baby's nose and mouth. Respiratory rate is 90 breaths/min with shallow breaths. You hear expiratory wheezing and moist inspiratory crackles with poor aeration on auscultation of the lungs. You note significant retractions, nasal flaring, and grunting with each breath. The baby appears cyanotic, and oxygen saturation on room air is only 70%; it increases to 85% with administration of 100% oxygen by face mask. Heart rate is initially 180 bpm and regular, but by the end of your initial assessment it is 90 bpm. Central and distal pulses are strong; blood pressure is 86/54 mm Hg. The baby's mucous membranes are moist, and her diaper is wet.

Acceptable Actions for Case Scenario 2

The following actions are acceptable when performing RSI for this infant:

- Use universal precautions.

- Obtain a brief medical history using the AMPLE mnemonic.

- Perform a rapid cardiopulmonary assessment and brief anatomic assessment. This infant requires urgent support of airway, ventilation, and oxygenation (see below).

- Prepare all needed intubation equipment and medications (sedative, paralytic, and adjunctive agents); have appropriate personnel available.

- Initiate cardiorespiratory and pulse oximetry monitoring.

- Preoxygenate the patient. You will need to provide bag-mask ventilation. You must sedate the patient, perform the Sellick maneuver, and then begin bag-mask ventilation.

- Administer the appropriate adjunctive, sedative (already given), and paralytic agents.

- Perform tracheal intubation and confirm placement of the tube.

- Appropriately observe and monitor the patient after intubation.

- Initiate appropriate treatment for any underlying medical condition (asthma, shock, head trauma, etc).

Case Scenario 2 Initial History and Targeted Assessment

- **Medical history:** Use the AMPLE mnemonic (**A**llergies, **M**edications, **P**ast medical history, **L**ast meal, and **E**vents leading up to the illness) to obtain the relevant history from the infant's mother. Time since the patient's last meal (**L**) will indicate the risk of aspiration. In emergent situations you must assume that all patients have a full stomach and are at risk for aspiration; in this scenario the mother reports that the infant ate well up to an hour ago. The events leading to this scenario (**E**) suggest that the baby had been feeding well and wetting diapers until just recently, so the baby is probably not hypovolemic.

- **Targeted assessment:** This baby has significant secretions in her airway and noisy, obstructed breathing. These symptoms suggest that the airway is not patent, but it is likely maintainable with suctioning. The baby is lethargic with rapid respirations, poor aeration, expiratory wheezing, inspiratory moist crackles, retractions, nasal flaring, and grunting. These are all signs of significant respiratory distress with potential or actual respiratory failure. The wheezing suggests increased airway resistance. The infant will require long expiratory times to avoid air trapping and hyperinflation after intubation.

Rationale for Acceptable Actions for Case Scenario 2

- **Intubation urgency:** This baby requires immediate airway management with

tracheal intubation before respiratory distress and potential respiratory failure lead to full cardiopulmonary arrest. The baby was initially tachycardic, which is appropriate for the level of respiratory distress. But as the baby's distress and hypoxemia worsened, the heart rate dropped to 90 bpm. This heart rate is inappropriately slow for the infant's level of distress; it indicates probable hypoxia and the need for urgent support of airway, ventilation, and oxygenation. Up to this point the baby had strong pulses, appeared well hydrated, and had a wet diaper. These signs suggest that she is euvolemic. Her blood pressure is normal for age.

- **Preparation of equipment, medications, personnel, and monitoring:** This infant has significant airway secretions; suctioning is necessary to maintain a patent airway. The infant has no anatomic features that would make intubation difficult. There is no reason to suspect a head or neck injury, so it is appropriate to open the airway with the head tilt–chin lift. This infant does not require cervical spine immobilization.

Age-based formulas to estimate the appropriate size of tracheal tubes do not apply to infants (less than 1 year of age). You should use the Broselow Resuscitation Tape or a weight- and length-based color coding system to select the correct size of equipment.

- **Patient monitoring:** At a minimum all patients should have continuous cardiorespiratory and pulse oximetry monitoring and frequent blood pressure monitoring. You should use an exhaled CO_2 detector after intubation to confirm tracheal tube placement and effective ventilation. You will note hypercapnia before hypoxia if ventilation is inadequate. To prevent hyperventilation after intubation, continuously monitor exhaled CO_2 once the capnography values are correlated with the infant's arterial P_{CO_2}.

■ **Medication choice and preparation:** This patient is less than 1 year old. She has copious airway secretions, and she has become relatively bradycardic as her respiratory distress has progressed. Atropine is an appropriate adjunctive agent. Providers should routinely give atropine before intubation in patients less than 1 year of age because intubation may induce a strong vagal response in infants and in young children who receive succinylcholine. Succinylcholine (a neuromuscular blocker) enhances cholinergic tone, increasing the risk of bradycardia and asystole. The correct dose of atropine for this infant is 0.1 mg (0.02 mg/kg), the minimum dose. Doses less than 0.1 mg may cause paradoxical bradycardia.

Remember that you will not observe the normal bradycardic response to hypoxia after you administer atropine. For this reason pulse oximetry monitoring of oxyhemoglobin saturation is essential.

Appropriate sedatives for normotensive, euvolemic patients include midazolam, thiopental, propofol, and etomidate. Rocuronium is the paralytic of choice for this patient. Succinylcholine may worsen the infant's bradycardia, although this problem could be corrected with atropine administration. In all infants and most children less than 5 years of age, you should give 0.1 mg of atropine (the minimum dose) 1 to 2 minutes before laryngoscopy. Then give the chosen sedative (midazolam, thiopental, propofol, or etomidate) and neuromuscular blocker (eg, rocuronium) consecutively.

■ **Preoxygenation:** To prevent stomach inflation and subsequent aspiration, you should preoxygenate spontaneously breathing patients by administering high-flow oxygen. But preoxygenation with spontaneous breathing is unfeasible for this infant. The infant has poor aeration with an oxygen saturation of 85% during spontaneous breathing with supplementary oxygen, and she is becoming bradycardic. You must sedate this patient, perform the Sellick maneuver, and provide bag-mask ventilation with 100% oxygen for 2 to 3 minutes before initiating paralysis. This step will build up the infant's oxygen reserve so that she can tolerate the brief period of apnea between the onset of muscular paralysis and successful intubation.

■ **Sellick maneuver:** Apply the Sellick maneuver as the patient becomes sedated and *before* initiation of bag-mask ventilation. Maintain cricoid pressure throughout intubation to avoid aspiration.

■ **Intubation:** The onset of neuromuscular blockade by nondepolarizing agents (eg, rocuronium or vecuronium) typically allows providers to perform intubation about 60 seconds after administration. The loss of spontaneous respirations, lack of movement, and the ability to fully open the patient's mouth without resistance indicate that the patient is ready for intubation. Once intubation is complete, you should confirm tube placement by exhaled CO_2 detection and careful clinical assessment. Carefully secure the tube in place, noting the distance marker at the lip.

■ **Postintubation observation and monitoring:** You must closely monitor the patient after intubation to ensure adequate oxygenation and ventilation, to detect signs of cardiovascular deterioration, and to look for signs of awakening as the effects of the sedative and paralytic wear off. It is appropriate to anticipate the need for prolonged sedation. You may administer a longer-acting sedative once you confirm tracheal tube position and ensure that the patient's condition is stable; you do not need to wait until symptoms of inadequate sedation appear. Thiopental, propofol, and etomidate are short-acting agents; the patient will need supplemental sedation sooner if you use one of these agents instead of midazolam.

Unacceptable Actions for Case Scenario 2

■ Failing to use universal precautions.

■ Failing to obtain a brief medical history. The findings of this assessment may influence which medications you administer during RSI.

■ Failing to perform a rapid cardiopulmonary assessment and brief anatomic assessment. The findings of these assessments may influence which medications you administer during RSI.

■ Failing to emergently address impending respiratory failure.

■ Failing to prepare all necessary equipment. It is unacceptable to find out you don't have the correct size of tracheal tube *after* the patient is paralyzed.

■ Failing to establish adequate monitoring before intubation.

■ Failing to choose appropriate adjunctive, sedative, and paralytic agents; failing to select the correct doses. In this scenario the infant already has copious secretions. So ketamine, which may increase secretions, is not an ideal choice. Succinylcholine increases the risk of worsening bradycardia. Defasciculation is unnecessary for this infant; it is indicated only when succinylcholine is the chosen paralytic. Administering less than 0.1 mg of atropine (the minimum dose) is incorrect. Lidocaine is unnecessary in this scenario because there is no reason to suspect increased ICP.

■ Failing to manually preoxygenate this patient with a bag and mask (administer a sedative, perform the Sellick maneuver when the patient becomes sedated, and begin bag-mask ventilation). Although it is ideal to preoxygenate patients by administering oxygen during spontaneous breathing, in certain cases manual ventilation is the only way to ensure adequate preoxygenation.

■ Failing to monitor the patient before, during, and after intubation. You must monitor the heart rate and clinical appearance during intubation. After intubation confirm correct tracheal tube position by clinical exam and a confirmatory test such as exhaled CO_2 detection. The administered sedative has a shorter duration of action than the paralytic, so this patient will awaken from sedation while still paralyzed. Thus you must monitor for signs of awakening, which indicate the need for more sedation and analgesia.

Case Scenario 2 Progression and Conclusion

Providers apply the appropriate monitors. You give 0.1 mg of atropine as an adjunctive agent; 1 minute later you give midazolam and then rocuronium. As soon as the midazolam takes effect, one provider performs the Sellick maneuver, and you begin bag-mask ventilation. Bag-mask ventilation with 100% oxygen brings the infant's oxygen saturation up to 100% and the heart rate up to 120 bpm. You then successfully intubate the infant. You confirm tube position by primary and secondary techniques, securely tape the tube in place, and record the distance marking at the lip. Providers then safely transport the patient to the PICU.

Case Scenario 3

EMS personnel transport a 16-year-old, 90-kg, muscular male to the ED because of acute onset of severe respiratory distress. The teenager has a history of severe asthma. On arrival of EMS at his home, the patient was sleepy but arousable; he was able to give 1-word responses. On examination the patient had a respiratory rate of 36 breaths/min and diffuse wheezing. Despite treatment with albuterol and oxygen, the patient's condition deteriorated during transport to the ED. EMS personnel established vascular access en route.

On arrival at the ED the teenager is markedly agitated with a look of terror due to lack of air. He is unable to speak and is taking shallow, gasping breaths. You hear minimal air movement. There is severe accessory muscle use with nasal flaring, head bobbing, and shoulder shrugging with each breath. Heart rate is 140 bpm; systolic blood pressure is 130 mm Hg by palpation (the automated BP device does not work). Distal pulses fluctuate with his respiratory cycle, disappearing during inspiration and readily palpable during exhalation. Capillary refill is somewhat sluggish, and extremities are warm. Oxygen saturation on 100% oxygen by face mask averages around 82%, but the monitor is reading only intermittently. The patient's mother tells you the teenager had "a real bad experience" with anesthesia in the past.

Acceptable Actions for Case Scenario 3

The following actions are acceptable when performing RSI for this adolescent:

■ Use universal precautions.

■ Obtain a brief medical history using the AMPLE mnemonic.

■ Perform a rapid cardiopulmonary assessment and brief anatomic assessment. This adolescent requires support of airway, ventilation, and oxygenation (see below).

■ Prepare all needed intubation equipment and medications (sedative, paralytic, and adjunctive agents); have appropriate personnel available.

■ Initiate cardiorespiratory and pulse oximetry monitoring.

■ Preoxygenate the patient. This patient's respiratory efforts are insufficient to maintain oxygenation during spontaneous ventilation. You should sedate the patient, perform the Sellick maneuver when the patient is sedated, and begin bag-mask ventilation.

■ Administer the appropriate adjunctive, sedative (already given), and paralytic agents.

■ Perform tracheal intubation and confirm placement of the tube.

■ Appropriately observe and monitor the patient after intubation.

■ Initiate appropriate treatment for any underlying medical condition (asthma, shock, head trauma, etc).

Case Scenario 3 Initial History and Targeted Assessment

■ **Medical history:** Use the AMPLE mnemonic (**A**llergies, **M**edications, **P**ast medical history, **L**ast meal, and **E**vents leading to status asthmaticus) to obtain the young man's relevant history. This patient previously had "a bad experience" with anesthesia (**P**). This finding suggests plasma cholinesterase deficiency or a risk of malignant hyperthermia. These potential problems contraindicate use of succinylcholine. Time since the patient's last meal (**L**) indicates the risk of aspiration. In emergent situations you must assume that all patients have a full stomach and are at risk for aspiration. The events (**E**) of this scenario suggest a rapid progression of respiratory distress during transport.

■ **Targeted assessment:** This asthmatic patient is lethargic with a relatively slow respiratory rate, minimal aeration, and hypoxia despite administration of high-flow oxygen. His airway appears to be maintainable, but his change in mental status and poor oxygenation are consistent with respiratory failure. He requires urgent tracheal intubation. As expected in a patient with status asthmaticus and respiratory failure, he has marked pulsus paradoxus. Each time he inspires, his hyperinflated lungs compress his heart. This compression impedes venous return and thus cardiac output, so pulse volume declines.

The patient still has fair capillary refill, warm extremities, and normal blood pressure when his pulses are palpable. These signs suggest he is not in decompensated shock. But the potential for worsening cardiovascular status is high because of his respiratory status. You must emergently treat this patient's respiratory failure.

Moreover, the patient is at risk for iatrogenic compromise of cardiac output during positive-pressure ventilation and increased intrathoracic pressure secondary to air trapping. You should consider augmenting his ventricular preload and cardiac output by administering 5 to 10 mL/kg normal saline or lactated Ringer's solution. Such augmentation may be particularly useful immediately after intubation if his perfusion deteriorates.

This patient has no obvious anatomic problems that would interfere with intubation.

Rationale for Acceptable Actions for Case Scenario 3

- **Intubation urgency:** Although this young man's airway appears to be maintainable, his change in mental status and poor oxygenation are consistent with respiratory failure. He requires urgent tracheal intubation.

- **Preparation of equipment, medications, personnel, and monitoring:** It is necessary to prepare all intubation equipment, confirm that it works correctly, and have it readily accessible to the provider performing the procedure. Make sure that tubes 0.5 mm larger and smaller than the estimated size are readily available. Prepare a cuffed tracheal tube for this patient with asthma because he is 16 years old and he is likely to require high airway pressures initially to deliver an adequate tidal volume. A sufficient number of personnel should be available; each provider should have assigned tasks so that all involved know their role in the procedure.

- **Patient monitoring:** At a minimum all patients should have continuous cardiorespiratory and pulse oximetry monitoring and frequent blood pressure monitoring. After intubation you should use an exhaled CO_2 detector to confirm tracheal tube placement and effective ventilation. For this patient the correlation between exhaled CO_2

and arterial pCO_2 is likely to be poor secondary to severe ventilation-perfusion mismatch.

- **Medication choice and preparation:** Ketamine is the sedative of choice for patients with status asthmaticus because it provides dissociative anesthesia, analgesia, and amnesia. Ketamine also has potential bronchodilatory effects. A nondepolarizing neuromuscular blocker (eg, rocuronium) is appropriate. You may consider use of atropine (adjunctive agent) to minimize the secretions that can occur with ketamine administration. Atropine (or other anticholinergics) may also exert a beneficial bronchodilating effect. Once you preoxygenate the patient, administer the appropriate dose of ketamine and rocuronium.

- **Preoxygenation:** This asthmatic patient's spontaneous ventilatory efforts are insufficient for preoxygenation with spontaneous breathing. You will need to provide manual ventilation. To minimize the risk of aspiration associated with manual ventilation, administer a sedative. Then apply cricoid pressure as the patient becomes sedated and *before* initiation of manual ventilation.

- **Sellick maneuver:** Anyone who receives positive-pressure ventilation for RSI needs cricoid pressure. This maneuver reduces the risk of regurgitation and aspiration. You should not apply the Sellick maneuver when the patient is awake and responsive. Apply the Sellick maneuver as the patient becomes sedated but *before* initiation of positive-pressure ventilation. Maintain cricoid pressure throughout intubation.

- **Intubation:** The onset of neuromuscular blockade by nondepolarizing agents (eg, rocuronium or vecuronium) typically allows providers to perform intubation about 60 seconds after administration. The loss of spontaneous respirations, lack of movement, and the ability to fully open the patient's mouth without resistance indicate that the patient is ready for intubation. Once the tube is

in place, confirm its position by exhaled CO_2 detection and careful clinical assessment. Carefully secure the tube in place, noting the distance marker at the lip.

- **Postintubation observation and monitoring:** You must closely monitor the patient after intubation to ensure adequate oxygenation and ventilation, to detect cardiovascular deterioration, and to look for signs of awakening as the effects of the sedative and paralytic wear off. It is appropriate to anticipate the need for prolonged sedation. You may administer a longer-acting sedative once you confirm tube position and ensure that the patient's condition is stable; you do need to wait until symptoms of inadequate sedation appear. Thiopental, propofol, and etomidate are short-acting agents; the patient will need supplemental sedation sooner if you use one of these agents instead of midazolam.

Unacceptable Actions for Case Scenario 3

- Failing to use universal precautions.

- Failing to obtain a brief medical history. This assessment may influence which medications you administer during RSI. Failing to note this patient's previous "bad experience" with anesthesia could lead you to "miss" potential plasma cholinesterase deficiency or risk of malignant hyperthermia. Both of these potential problems are contraindications to succinylcholine administration.

- Failing to perform a rapid cardiopulmonary assessment and brief anatomic assessment; failing to emergently address impending respiratory failure. The findings of these assessments can influence which medications you administer during RSI.

- Failing to provide sedation, cricoid pressure, and bag-mask ventilation. These steps will ensure effective preoxygenation while minimizing the risk of vomiting and aspiration.

- Failing to prepare all necessary equipment. It is unacceptable to find out that you don't have the correct size of tracheal tube available *after* the patient is paralyzed.

- Failing to establish adequate monitoring of the patient before intubation.

- Failing to choose appropriate adjunctive, sedative, and paralytic agents; failing to select the correct doses. Lidocaine is unnecessary in this scenario because there is no reason to suspect increased ICP. Barbiturates, propofol, and benzodiazepines can cause dose-dependent myocardial depression, which can be detrimental in a patient with status asthmaticus. In light of the patient's past experience with anesthesia, succinylcholine is contraindicated. Defasciculation is unnecessary because succinylcholine is contraindicated.

- Failing to monitor the patient before, during, and after intubation. You must monitor heart rate and clinical appearance during intubation. After intubation confirm correct tracheal tube position by clinical examination and a confirmatory test. Because the administered sedative has a shorter duration of action than the paralytic, this patient will awaken from sedation while still paralyzed, so you must monitor for signs of awakening and the need for more sedation and analgesia.

Case Scenario 3 Progression and Conclusion

This patient receives 100% oxygen by non-rebreathing mask while you rapidly prepare the equipment and medications. You administer ketamine and then rocuronium. As soon as the patient is sedated, another provider performs the Sellick maneuver and you provide 100% oxygen with bag and mask. You successfully intubate the patient. You confirm tube position by auscultation over the lateral lung fields and note the absence of breath sounds over the abdomen. Capnography shows low levels of exhaled CO_2 as anticipated. After intubation you initiate additional treatments

with inhaled albuterol and ipratropium bromide and IV corticosteroids. Providers transfer the patient to the ICU.

Case Scenario 4

A 3-year-old girl presents to the ED with a high fever, altered mental status, and a purpuric rash. On examination the child responds appropriately to loud verbal and painful stimuli; she is hypotonic and listless when not stimulated. She is breathing rapidly at a rate of 48 breaths/min with clear breath sounds bilaterally. Rectal temperature is 40°C (104°F), heart rate is 160 bpm, and BP is 62/28 mm Hg. The pulse oximetry monitor detects oxyhemoglobin saturation inconsistently while the child receives supplementary oxygen by face mask. Extremities are cool to the touch with barely palpable distal pulses and weak central pulses. Capillary refill is 7 seconds in a warm room. Extremities are purpuric, and you note scattered petechiae on her trunk. The child has no significant medical history.

Acceptable Actions for Case Scenario 4

The following actions are acceptable when performing RSI for this child:

- Use universal precautions. Also wear a face mask and eye shields because this child probably has meningococcemia.

- Obtain a brief medical history using the AMPLE mnemonic.

- Perform a rapid cardiopulmonary assessment and brief anatomic assessment.

- Prepare all needed intubation equipment; have appropriate personnel available.

- Initiate cardiorespiratory and pulse oximetry monitoring.

- Choose and prepare appropriate sedative, paralytic, and adjunctive agents.

- Preoxygenate the patient.

- Administer the appropriate adjunctive, sedative, and paralytic agents.

- Perform the Sellick maneuver.

- Perform tracheal intubation and confirm placement of the tube.

- Appropriately observe and monitor the patient after intubation.

- Initiate appropriate treatment for any underlying medical condition (asthma, shock, head trauma, etc).

Case Scenario 4 Initial History and Targeted Assessment

- **Medical history:** When the patient's parents or primary caregivers arrive, use the mnemonic AMPLE (**A**llergies, **M**edications, **P**ast medical history, **L**ast meal, and **E**vents leading to intubation) to identify important parts of the patient's medical history and events leading to this illness. This information will help you select appropriate RSI medications; it will also help you determine if there is any problem likely to interfere with intubation and any risk of adverse effects from the medications. In emergent situations you must assume that all patients have a full stomach and are at risk for aspiration. You must have information about the events (**E**) leading to the current medical crisis because they can affect overall management. The events of this scenario suggest meningococcemia, a life-threatening bacterial infection.

- **Targeted assessment:** The patient is responsive to verbal and painful stimuli (AVPU neurologic rating of V and P). She has rapid and shallow respirations, tachycardia, poor perfusion, and hypotension (76 mm Hg is the lower limit of normal systolic blood pressure for a 3-year-old patient). These symptoms indicate that the patient is in decompensated shock and has potential respiratory failure. The patient needs rapid, aggressive treatment. The child's responsiveness to verbal and painful stimuli suggests the need for RSI to minimize further compromise.

This patient has no obvious anatomic problems that would interfere with intubation.

Rationale for Acceptable Actions for Case Scenario 4

- **Intubation urgency:** This patient is in decompensated shock and has potential respiratory failure. Providers must rapidly initiate aggressive treatment.

- **Preparation of equipment, medications, personnel, and monitoring:** It is necessary to prepare all intubation equipment, confirm that it works correctly, and ensure that it is readily accessible to the provider performing the procedure. This patient is in decompensated shock; distal pulsatile flow may be inadequate for pulse oximetry monitoring of oxyhemoglobin saturation. When you prepare the patient for intubation, establish vascular access and administer a rapid isotonic fluid bolus (20 mL/kg) to improve cardiovascular function and systemic perfusion.

  The Broselow Resuscitation Tape may be useful to help select the correct size of tracheal tube. Ensure that tubes 0.5 mm larger and smaller than the estimated size are readily available.

- **Medication choice and preparation:** This patient is in decompensated shock. The only suitable sedatives are ketamine or etomidate, both of which cause little or no cardiovascular depression. Ketamine may actually improve the patient's cardiovascular status because it induces catecholamine release. In this scenario you should use the lower dose range to minimize potential adverse effects. Because this patient is in decompensated shock, it is acceptable to omit the sedative. But once the patient is more hemodynamically stable, administration of a sedative with retrograde amnestic properties is advisable. A non-depolarizing neuromuscular blocker (eg, rocuronium) is the paralytic of choice; succinylcholine is an acceptable alternative.

- **Preoxygenation:** Although this patient is in shock, she has effective spontaneous ventilation and is well saturated with supplemental oxygen. For preoxygenation you can use a tight-fitting mask with 100% oxygen for 2 to 3 minutes before initiating paralysis. Preoxygenation will allow the child to build up an adequate oxygen reserve so that she can tolerate the brief period of apnea between the onset of muscular paralysis and intubation. Avoid manual ventilation: it increases the likelihood of regurgitation and aspiration.

- **Sellick maneuver:** Apply the Sellick maneuver as the patient becomes sedated. To avoid aspiration, maintain cricoid pressure throughout intubation.

- **Intubation:** The loss of spontaneous respirations, lack of movement, and the ability to fully open the patient's mouth without resistance indicate that the patient is ready for intubation. Once the tube is in place, confirm its position by exhaled CO_2 detection and careful clinical assessment. Carefully secure the tube in place, noting the distance marker at the lip.

- **Postintubation observation and monitoring:** Closely monitor the patient after intubation to ensure adequate oxygenation and ventilation, to detect cardiovascular deterioration, and to look for signs of awakening as the effects of the sedative and paralytic wear off. Administer a long-acting sedative before or as soon as signs of inadequate sedation are evident. These signs may include unexplained tachycardia and hypertension. It is appropriate to anticipate the need for prolonged sedation. You may administer a longer-acting sedative once you confirm tube position and ensure that the patient's condition is stable.

Unacceptable Actions for Case Scenario 4

- Failing to use universal precautions, face mask, and eye shields.

- Failing to obtain a brief medical history. The findings of this assessment may influence which medications you administer during RSI.

- Failing to perform a rapid cardiopulmonary assessment and brief anatomic assessment; failing to recognize impending respiratory failure. The findings of these assessments can influence which medications you administer during RSI.

- Failing to prepare all necessary equipment. It is unacceptable to find out you don't have the correct size of tracheal tube available *after* the patient is paralyzed.

- Failing to establish adequate monitoring before intubation.

- Failing to choose appropriate adjunctive, sedative, and paralytic agents; failing to select the correct doses. Lidocaine is unnecessary because there is no reason to suspect increased ICP. Barbiturates, propofol, and benzodiazepines can cause dose-dependent myocardial depression, which can be detrimental to a patient in shock. Defasciculation is not indicated.

- Failing to recognize adequate spontaneous ventilation and providing over-zealous preoxygenation with manual ventilation. This patient appears to be ventilating adequately, but the oxygen saturation is not reliably detected because of the shock. Because her respiratory effort and tidal volume appear to be adequate, it is likely she will be adequately preoxygenated by spontaneous ventilation. You can confirm the adequacy of oxygenation by arterial blood gas analysis. The pulse oximeter will likely begin to work as the rapidly administered fluids restore distal perfusion. The use of manual ventilation could distend the stomach with air, increasing the risk of regurgitation and aspiration.

- Failing to monitor the patient before, during, and after intubation. You should initiate treatment for shock, including volume administration, before you secure the patient's airway. You must also closely monitor the child during intubation and continue shock treatment after the airway is secure. After intubation confirm correct tracheal tube position by clinical assessment and a confirmatory test (eg, exhaled CO_2 detection). Because the administered sedative has a shorter duration of action than the paralytic, this patient will awaken from sedation while still paralyzed. So you must monitor for signs of awakening, which indicate the need for more sedation and analgesia.

Case Scenario 4 Progression and Conclusion

You successfully intubate this patient after she is sedated with etomidate and paralyzed with rocuronium. Another provider applies cricoid pressure as soon as the patient is sedated and maintains it until intubation is complete. You confirm tracheal tube position by primary and secondary techniques (including exhaled CO₂ detection). You started aggressive fluid resuscitation before intubation and continued it after intubation. You administer parenteral antibiotics, and providers transfer the patient to the ICU. Despite maximal therapy the patient dies of multisystem organ failure. Neisseria meningitidis grows from the blood culture within hours of the child's initial presentation.

Case Scenario 5

EMS providers bring an 18-month-old boy to the ED. The toddler is in full cardiac arrest. He was unresponsive when pulled from the family's heated swimming pool. He has remained apneic and pulseless since the event occurred, 20 minutes ago. He is flaccid while receiving bag-mask ventilation and chest compressions. His body temperature is 36.5°C. There is no IV access.

Acceptable Actions for Case Scenario 5

The following actions are acceptable for treatment of this child in cardiopulmonary arrest:

■ Use universal precautions.

■ Perform intubation during resuscitation, but do not use RSI because the child is in cardiopulmonary arrest.

■ Follow PALS protocols for attempted resuscitation from pediatric asystole.

Rationale for Acceptable Actions for Case Scenario 5

■ Providers should follow the pediatric pulseless arrest algorithm in attempts to resuscitate this patient. The likelihood of return of spontaneous circulation with intact neurologic survival in this patient with prolonged normothermic cardiac arrest is poor.

Unacceptable Actions for Case Scenario 5

■ Failing to use universal precautions.

■ Performing RSI. A flaccid, apneic, and pulseless patient does not require sedation or paralysis for intubation. RSI will only delay resuscitative efforts.

1. **A 7-year-old child with a head injury arrives in the ED. The child is combative. He needs to be sedated and intubated for a CT scan evaluation. Which one of the following drugs is *least appropriate* for this child?**

   a. lidocaine

   b. ketamine

   c. propofol

   d. thiopental

   The correct answer is b. Ketamine is thought to increase ICP in patients with head injury. For this reason ketamine is contraindicated in patients with suspected or potentially elevated ICP. Although the validity of this clinical concern has been questioned recently, most airway experts would not recommend using ketamine at this time.

   Answer a is incorrect because lidocaine *is* an appropriate adjunctive drug for RSI in children with head injury and potential increased ICP. Lidocaine may prevent an elevation in ICP during laryngoscopy.

   Answer c is incorrect because propofol *is* an appropriate drug for children with head injury. Propofol is a sedative-hypnotic capable of producing general anesthesia. Its mechanism of action is not understood.

   Answer d is incorrect because barbiturates such as thiopental *are* appropriate for sedation of patients with increased ICP. These drugs may lower ICP, cerebral metabolic rate, and oxygen consumption.

2. **A 10-month-old infant has severe respiratory distress with hypoxemia and mottled skin. The infant is agitated, and his respirations are irregular and inadequate. Despite oxygen administration, the infant continues to deteriorate**

Review Questions

and now requires intubation. You decide to perform RSI, and you must select drugs to use in this patient. Which of the following statements about the drugs you may use during RSI for this patient is *false*?

a. midazolam is an appropriate sedative for this patient

b. succinylcholine is an appropriate depolarizing neuromuscular blocker for this patient

c. atropine is an optional adjunctive agent that can be used to minimize secretions in this patient

d. rocuronium is advantageous for RSI in this patient because it has a rapid onset of action for a nondepolarizing neuromuscular blocker

The correct answer is c. Atropine is an *essential* rather than an *optional* adjunctive agent for infants less than 1 year of age who undergo elective RSI. Atropine can prevent bradycardia and asystole during the procedure. Atropine is recommended for children 1 to 5 years of age if they receive succinylcholine because succinylcholine directly stimulates vagal activity.

Answers a, b, and **d** are incorrect because midazolam, succinylcholine, and rocuronium are appropriate for this patient. All the statements made about these drugs are true.

3. **Listed below are several RSI drugs and potential side effects or limitations to use. Which drug is not associated with the listed side effects or limitations of use?**

a. etomidate: nausea and vomiting

b. propofol: hypotension and rapid termination of effect

c. midazolam: amnesia

d. rocuronium: fasciculations and short duration of action

e. succinylcholine: bradycardia or asystole

The correct answer is d. Rocuronium is a nondepolarizing neuromuscular blocker that does *not* cause fasciculations. This drug has a relatively quick onset of action; it typically produces 30 or more minutes of paralysis.

Answers a, b, c, and **e** are incorrect because these drugs do have the potential side effects or limitations of use listed above.

4. **You are preparing for RSI of a 4-year-old patient with a known history of muscular dystrophy. The child was admitted to the hospital 3 days ago with extensive burns and smoke inhalation caused by a house fire. The child received fluid resuscitation. Systolic blood pressure is 90 mm Hg with adequate systemic perfusion (assessed in nonburned areas). Urine output has been minimal during the last several hours despite effective systemic perfusion. The child has signs of progressive respiratory distress, evidence of pulmonary edema on a chest radiograph, and copious respiratory secretions. In the past hour the child's heart rate began to fall. Which of the following drugs is *inappropriate* for this child during RSI?**

a. succinylcholine

b. rocuronium

c. midazolam

d. atropine

The correct answer is a. Succinylcholine is inappropriate for RSI in this patient for several reasons. First, the child has a known neuromuscular disorder. Second, the child sustained extensive burns more than 48 hours ago, so tissue damage is present. Third, the child may have acute renal failure because urine output has been minimal despite adequate systemic perfusion. These problems are all relative contraindications to use of succinylcholine.

Answer b is incorrect because rocuronium is acceptable for this patient. Rocuronium has minimal or no cardiovascular side effects at doses used for RSI.[19] It is safe to use in patients with renal failure.

Answer c is incorrect because midazolam is often the sedative of choice for RSI. Midazolam is a water-soluble, rapid-acting sedative with potent amnestic properties and minimal cardiovascular effects.

Answer d is incorrect because this child has evidence of bradycardia and copious respiratory secretions. Atropine is not routinely administered to children 1 to 5 years of age. But you should consider it for children with bradycardia or copious secretions.

References

1. Gerardi MJ, Sacchetti AD, Cantor RM, Santamaria JP, Gausche M, Lucid W, Foltin GL. Rapid-sequence intubation of the pediatric patient. Pediatric Emergency Medicine Committee of the American College of Emergency Physicians. *Ann Emerg Med.* 1996;28:55-74.

2. McGowan P, Skinner A. Preoxygenation: the importance of a good face mask seal. *Br J Anaesth.* 1995;75:777-778.

3. Berthoud M, Read DH, Norman J. Pre-oxygenation: how long? *Anaesthesia.* 1983;38: 96-102.

4. Lerman J, Kiskis AA. Lidocaine attenuates the intraocular pressure response to rapid intubation in children. *Can Anaesth Soc J.* 1985;32:339-345.

5. Donegan MF, Bedford RF. Intravenously administered lidocaine prevents intracranial hypertension during endotracheal suctioning. *Anesthesiology.* 1980;52:516-518.

6. Sperry RJ, Bailey PL, Reichman MV, Peterson JC, Petersen PB, Pace NL. Fentanyl and sufentanil increase intracranial pressure in head trauma patients. *Anesthesiology.* 1992; 77:416-420.

7. Walls RM. Rapid-sequence intubation in head trauma. *Ann Emerg Med.* 1993;22:1008-1013.

8. L'Hommedieu CS, Arens JJ. The use of ketamine for the emergency intubation of patients with status asthmaticus. *Ann Emerg Med.* 1987;16:568-571.

9. Sarma VJ. Use of ketamine in acute severe asthma. *Acta Anaesthesiol Scand.* 1992;36: 106-107.

10. Bergen JM, Smith DC. A review of etomidate for rapid sequence intubation in the emergency department. *J Emerg Med.* 1997;15: 221-230.

11. McAllister JD, Gnauck KA. Rapid sequence intubation of the pediatric patient: fundamentals of practice. *Pediatr Clin North Am.* 1999; 46:1249-1284.

12. Hoffman WE, Charbel FT, Ausman JI. Cerebral blood flow and metabolic response to etomidate and ischemia. *Neurol Res.* 1997;19: 41-44.

13. Batjer HH. Cerebral protective effects of etomidate: experimental and clinical aspects. *Cerebrovasc Brain Metab Rev.* 1993;5:17-32.

14. de Jong FH, Mallios C, Jansen C, Scheck PA, Lamberts SW. Etomidate suppresses adrenocortical function by inhibition of 11 beta-hydroxylation. *J Clin Endocrinol Metab.* 1984;59:1143-1147.

15. Wagner RL, White PF. Etomidate inhibits adrenocortical function in surgical patients. *Anesthesiology.* 1984;61:647-651.

16. Absalom A, Pledger D, Kong A. Adrenocortical function in critically ill patients 24 h after a single dose of etomidate. *Anaesthesia.* 1999; 54:861-867.

17. Sokolove PE, Price DD, Okada P. The safety of etomidate for emergency rapid sequence intubation of pediatric patients. *Pediatr Emerg Care.* 2000;16:18-21.

18. Sellick BA. Cricoid pressure to control regurgitation of stomach contents during induction of anaesthesia. *Lancet.* 1961;2:404-406.

19. Maddineni VR, McCoy EP, Mirakur RK, McBride RJ. Onset and duration of action and hemodynamic effects of rocuronium bromide under balanced and volatile anesthesia. *Acta Anaesthesiol Belg.* 1994;45:41-47.

20. Khuenl-Brady KS, Pomaroli A, Puhringer F, Mitterschiffthaler G, Koller J. The use of rocuronium (ORG 9426) in patients with chronic renal failure. *Anaesthesia.* 1993;48: 873-875.

21. Magorian T, Wood P, Caldwell J, Fisher D, Segredo V, Szenohradszky J, Sharma M, Gruenke L, Miller R. The pharmacokinetics and neuromuscular effects of rocuronium bromide in patients with liver disease. *Anesth Analg.* 1995;80:754-759.

22. Khalil M, D'Honneur G, Duvaldestin P, Slavov V, De Hys C, Gomeni R. Pharmacokinetics and pharmacodynamics of rocuronium in patients with cirrhosis. *Anesthesiology.* 1994;80:1241-1247.

23. Fuchs-Buder T, Tassonyi E. Intubating conditions and time course of rocuronium-induced neuromuscular block in children. *Br J Anaesth.* 1996;77:335-338.

24. McDonald PF, Sainsbury DA, Laing RJ. Evaluation of the onset time and intubation conditions of rocuronium bromide in children. *Anaesth Intensive Care.* 1997;25:260-261.

25. Scheiber G, Ribeiro FC, Marichal A, Bredendiek M, Renzing K. Intubating conditions and onset of action after rocuronium, vecuronium, and atracurium in young children. *Anesth Analg.* 1996;83:320-324.

26. Lynam DP, Cronnelly R, Castagnoli KP, Canfell PC, Caldwell J, Arden J, Miller RD. The pharmacodynamics and pharmacokinetics of vecuronium in patients anesthetized with isoflurane with normal renal function or with renal failure. *Anesthesiology.* 1988;69: 227-231.

27. Mirakhur RK, Ferres CJ, Clarke RS, Bali IM, Dundee JW. Clinical evaluation of Org NC 45. *Br J Anaesth.* 1983;55:119-124.

28. Ferres CJ, Crean PM, Mirakhur RK. An evaluation of Org NC 45 (vecuronium) in paediatric anaesthesia. *Anaesthesia.* 1983;38:943-947.

29. Hopkins PM. Use of suxamethonium in children. *Br J Anaesth.* 1995;75:675-677.

30. Morell RC, Berman JM, Royster RI, Petrozza PH, Kelly JS, Colonna DM. Revised label regarding use of succinylcholine in children and adolescents. *Anesthesiology.* 1994;80: 242-245.

31. Badgwell JM, Hall SC, Lockhart C. Revised label regarding use of succinylcholine in children and adolescents [letter]. *Anesthesiology.* 1994;80:243-245.

Sedation Issues for the PALS Provider

Introductory Case Scenario

You are preparing to sedate a 5-year-old girl for bone marrow aspiration. The child has suspected acute lymphoblastic leukemia.

■ What information do you need to develop a safe plan for sedation of this child?

■ Does this patient need sedation, analgesia, or both? What agents can you use to achieve your goals safely?

■ What monitoring does this child require before, during, and after the procedure?

Learning Objectives

After completing this chapter the PALS provider should be able to

■ List the components of a presedation assessment and plan appropriate monitoring of patients undergoing various levels of sedation

■ Explain the difference between sedation and analgesia and choose appropriate medications for specific clinical scenarios

■ Describe the common adverse effects of different sedative and analgesic agents

■ State the appropriate role of benzodiazepine and narcotic reversal agents

Introduction

Ill or injured children frequently require sedation and analgesia. For many years hospitalized young children, especially infants, were inadequately treated for pain and anxiety.[1,2] Recent physiologic observations show that the very young are actually *more* sensitive to pain than adults.[3,4]

Sedation and analgesia are not benign treatments; they can have adverse consequences, especially if used incorrectly. The Joint Commission on Accreditation of Hospital Organizations, American Society of Anesthesiologists, American College of Emergency Physicians, and American Academy of Pediatrics emphasize that sedation should be administered in a safe environment by personnel with appropriate training and credentials.[5-7]

This chapter reviews the drugs, dosages, and techniques you can use to sedate children. In addition, the chapter emphasizes appropriate monitoring during sedation and describes potential complications.

Sedation vs Analgesia

There is a difference between sedation and analgesia. *Sedation reduces the state of awareness.* *Analgesia reduces or eliminates the perception of pain.* Most analgesics have some sedative effects, but many sedatives lack analgesic effects. For example, *benzodiazepines* and *barbiturates* provide sedation only; they have no analgesic effects. Many sedatives produce *amnesia*, the inability to remember.

Critical Concepts:
Definitions of Sedation, Analgesia, and Amnesia

■ *Sedation* reduces the state of awareness; it does *not* relieve pain. Sedation may cause hypnosis (ie, sleep).

■ *Analgesia* reduces or eliminates the perception of pain.

■ *Amnesia* is the inability to remember an event or experience.

Narcotics are primarily analgesics; they typically have little sedative effect unless given in large doses. *Dissociative anesthetic agents* (eg, ketamine) provide both sedation and analgesia.

Types of Sedation

A number of different terms are used to describe the levels of sedation. It is important for providers to understand that sedation is a continuum (see Figure 1). Most sedative agents can induce very deep levels of sedation, sometimes approaching general anesthesia. The level of sedation produced will vary from patient to patient. A dose of sedative that is inadequate to induce any sedation in one patient may render another patient deeply unconscious with the potential for airway compromise.

The American Academy of Pediatrics has defined 3 levels of sedation[5]; the American Society of Anesthesiologists (ASA) has defined 4 levels.[6] More information about these levels is available on the ASA website (**www.asahq.org/Standards/20.htm**). The following sections describe these levels of sedation (see Critical Concepts: "Levels of Sedation").

■ **Minimal sedation (anxiolysis):** A drug-induced state during which patients respond to verbal commands. This level of sedation may impair cognitive function and coordination. Minimal sedation does not affect ventilatory or cardiovascular function.

■ **Moderate sedation/analgesia (formerly called "conscious sedation"):** A drug-induced depression of consciousness during which patients respond purposefully to verbal commands, either alone or with light tactile stimulation. The patient requires no interventions to maintain a patent airway, and spontaneous ventilation is adequate. Cardiovascular function is usually maintained.

■ **Deep sedation/analgesia:** A drug-induced depression of consciousness during which patients cannot be easily aroused but respond purposefully to repeated or painful stimulation. This level of sedation may impair the patient's ability to independently maintain ventilatory function. A patient may require assistance to maintain a patent airway, and spontaneous ventilation may be inadequate. Cardiovascular function is usually maintained.

■ **General anesthesia:** A drug-induced loss of consciousness during which patients cannot be aroused even by painful stimulation. This level of sedation includes general anesthesia and spinal or major regional anesthesia. It does *not* include local anesthesia. General anesthesia frequently impairs the ability to independently maintain ventilatory function. Patients often require assistance to keep their airway patent. Patients may need positive-pressure ventilation because general anesthetics may depress spontaneous ventilation and neuromuscular function. General anesthesia may impair cardiovascular function.

The term *conscious sedation* is no longer used. The American College of Emergency Physicians (ACEP) advocates use of the term *procedural sedation* instead of conscious sedation; the American Society of Anesthesiologists uses *moderate sedation/ analgesia*. Procedural sedation is "a technique of administering sedatives or dissociative agents with or without analgesics to induce a state that allows the patient to tolerate the anxiety and pain of unpleasant procedures while maintaining cardiorespiratory function. Procedural sedation and analgesia is intended to result in a depressed level of consciousness, but one that allows the patient to maintain airway control independently and continuously. Specifically, the drugs, doses, and techniques used are not likely to produce a loss of protective airway reflexes."[7] The ACEP category of procedural sedation could include either moderate or deep sedation and analgesia with preserved airway protective mechanisms and spontaneous ventilation.

Critical Concepts:
Levels of Sedation

■ *Minimal sedation* is generally characterized by a normal response to verbal stimulation with a reduction in anxiety. This level of sedation may impair cognitive function and coordination, but ventilatory and cardiovascular functions remain intact.

■ *Moderate sedation* and *procedural sedation* result in somnolence with a preserved response to verbal stimulation, although the patient may need light tactile stimulation. Airway and protective reflexes remain intact. This level of sedation was formerly called "conscious" sedation because patients remain responsive to stimulation and can protect their airway.

■ *Deep sedation* is characterized by a reduction in consciousness during which patients cannot be easily aroused by verbal and noxious stimuli. Patients respond purposefully to repeated or painful stimulation. Airway and protective reflexes may be preserved or compromised.

■ *General anesthesia* is a state of unconsciousness during which patients are unresponsive to noxious stimuli. Patients typically lose airway protective reflexes. General anesthesia may impair cardiovascular function.

FIGURE 1. Continuum of depths of sedation.

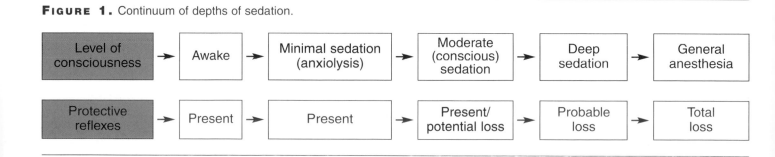

Young children with acute illness or injury are rarely candidates for moderate sedation. Young children cannot cooperate sufficiently for this level of sedation to be adequate during procedures. Moderate sedation, however, may be adequate for radiographic procedures that do not include noxious stimuli. Acutely ill or injured children, especially young children who require a noxious or painful procedure, more often require deep sedation.

Presedation Assessment

The first step in providing safe sedation or analgesia is an adequate presedation assessment. You begin this assessment by obtaining the child's history. To recall the essential components of the history, use the mnemonic AMPLE. Ask the caregiver if the patient has any medication, food, or latex allergies (**A**) or if the patient takes any medications (**M**). Allergies and medications may influence the choice of sedation medications. Also ask about the child's past health history (**P**) because some medi-

cal conditions will affect the approach to sedation. Inquire about previous exposure to and experience with sedatives and anesthetics. This information will help you identify previous problems with these medications and determine the dose required to achieve adequate sedation. Time since the child's last meal (**L**) will indicate the risk of vomiting and aspiration. You must also consider the events (**E**) leading to the need for sedation. For instance, if the patient sustained a wrist fracture in a motor vehicle crash and needs analgesia and sedation for fracture reduction, a complete trauma evaluation is appropriate before sedation. If the patient was burned in a house fire, you should evaluate the airway for inhalation injury before sedation for burn debridement. If a patient being evaluated for hydrocephalus requires sedation for a CT or MRI scan, neurologic evaluation and assessment of airway protective reflexes are necessary before sedation.

In general a patient should not undergo elective sedation for a procedure within 6 hours of eating solid foods or drinking milk. It is often acceptable for the patient to have a small volume of "clear liquids" (eg, soft drinks, transparent fruit juices, and water) within 2 hours of sedation. For breast-feeding infants, a 2- to 4-hour fast is generally sufficient. Protein-containing fluids will increase gastric acid output and delay gastric emptying. You should carefully assess special circumstances that affect gastric motility and aspiration risk; weigh the need for the procedure against the risk of aspiration and its attendant morbidity and mortality.

When a procedure cannot be delayed for the usual time period, some experts advocate use of a histamine type 2 receptor blocker (eg, ranitidine or famotidine) to decrease gastric acidity and volume before administering deep sedation. Prokinetic agents such as metoclopramide have also been used, but there is little data on their efficacy in this application. Table 1 lists the ASA recommendations for fasting before elective procedures.

TABLE 1. ASA Recommendations for Fasting Before Elective Procedures*

Ingested Material	Minimum Fasting Period[†]
Clear liquids[‡]	2 hours
Breast milk	4 hours
Infant formula	6 hours
Nonhuman milk[§]	6 hours
Light meal[‖]	6 hours

*These recommendations apply to healthy patients who are undergoing elective procedures. Complete gastric emptying may require longer than the times indicated.

[†]Fasting periods apply to patients of all ages.

[‡]Examples of clear liquids include water, fruit juices without pulp, carbonated beverages, clear tea, and black coffee.

[§]Nonhuman milk is similar to solids in the time required for gastric emptying. You must consider the amount ingested to determine an appropriate fasting period.

[‖]A light meal typically consists of toast and clear liquids. Fried or fatty foods or meat may prolong gastric emptying time. You must consider both the amount and type of foods ingested to determine an appropriate fasting period.

The presedation physical exam should include evaluation of the ABCs: airway patency and the need for support, breathing pattern and breath sounds, and a cardiovascular exam focused on heart sounds and distal perfusion (see Critical Concepts: "Sedation Checklist"). When you evaluate the airway you should look for characteristics that increase the risk of airway obstruction during the procedure. In particular, you should check for a large tongue, micrognathia (small lower jaw), limited airway opening, severe obesity, excessive secretions, and decreased airway protective reflexes. Carefully evaluate breath sounds and work of breathing to ensure that the patient's respiratory status is not compromised. Document baseline oxygen saturation by pulse oximetry.

Critical Concepts:
AMPLE Presedation History Mnemonic

Always assess the patient before you administer a sedative. This presedation assessment begins with a focused patient history. To reduce the risk of vomiting and aspiration, you should delay elective sedation until the patient is likely to have an empty stomach. Assess individual risk factors for aspiration and weigh these risks against the benefit of sedation and the urgency of the patient's condition.

Allergies

Medications

Past history

Last meal

Events

Critical Concepts: Sedation Checklist

History (Presedation Assessment)

- Allergies (medications, food, latex)

- Medications (current medications, past sedation)

- Past medical history

- Last meal (including times of both solids and liquids)

- Events leading to need for sedation (injuries such as head injury with possible increased intracranial pressure, abdominal injury, or ingestion of other medications)

Vitals Signs and Physiologic Information

- Heart rate

- Respiratory rate

- Blood pressure

- Oxygen saturation by pulse oximetry

- Level of consciousness

Physical Exam

- Upper airway: mouth opening, intra-oral devices (braces, retainers, loose teeth), size of mandible

- Neck flexion: ability to move chin to chest (check for limitation); not applicable to trauma patient with potential cervical spine injury

- Breath sounds

- Heart sounds

- Distal perfusion: distal pulses, skin temperature, capillary refill

Discharge Criteria

(from unit where sedation was administered or from recovery area)

- Airway, vital signs, and pulse oximetry readings are stable and back to baseline

- Patient can follow age-appropriate commands

- Patient is adequately hydrated and can tolerate oral fluids

- Patient is arousable and at baseline level of verbal ability

- Patient can sit unaided (if appropriate for age)

TABLE 2. ASA Classification of Sedation Risk

Class	ASA Score Selection Criterion
I	A healthy patient
II	A patient with mild systemic disease, no functional limitation
III	A patient with severe systemic disease that limits activity but is not incapacitating
IV	A patient with an incapacitating systemic disease that is a constant threat to life
V	A moribund patient not expect to survive 24 hours with or without an operation

For patients in ASA Class III or higher, consider anesthesia consultation.

Assess baseline heart rate, heart sounds, and distal perfusion (skin temperature, color, and capillary refill). Examine other organ systems if the patient's history suggests potential problems. Anesthesiologists often assess sedation risk using the ASA system. This system classifies risk on a scale of I to V (see Table 2). For patients in ASA Class III or higher, consult an airway or sedation specialist before elective sedation. Presedation assessment is summarized in Critical Concepts: "Sedation Checklist."

Monitoring and Training of Personnel

The level of monitoring required during the procedure depends on the anticipated and subsequently observed level of sedation. In all cases a provider trained in sedation practice must be present to observe the patient and document his/her status; this designated provider should *not* perform the procedure. This provider must be able to recognize airway compromise and provide airway and breathing support (open the airway, administer oxygen, and begin noninvasive ventilation) if required.

If possible avoid covering the child's face and chest completely with drapes or equipment during the procedure. You need to be able to observe the color of the mucus membranes and movement of the chest wall continuously. In certain situations (eg, MRI scanning), continuous observation is extremely difficult. In these situations you should use appropriate noninvasive monitoring equipment. Such equipment (ECG, plethysmography, pulse oximetry, and exhaled CO_2) is now available for use in the MRI suite.

When a patient receives light sedation, pulse oximetry monitoring of oxygen saturation is appropriate (see Critical Concepts: "Monitoring During Sedation"). With deeper levels of sedation use full cardiorespiratory monitoring with intermittent blood pressure monitoring. Some centers use capnography (exhaled CO_2) monitoring, especially for patients with artificial airways. Use of this technology, however, has not yet been shown to improve outcome.

Critical Concepts:
Monitoring During Sedation

- For *all sedations:* observation by a designated, trained provider who is *not* performing the procedure

- For *light sedation:* pulse oximetry plus a trained observer

- For *moderate* or *deep sedation*: pulse oximetry, continuous ECG, blood pressure, exhaled CO_2 (recommended but optional), plus a trained observer

You must ensure that appropriate emergency equipment is available to manage sedation-related complications. This equipment includes 100% oxygen with a bag-mask manual resuscitator (including all appropriately sized masks), suction apparatus with a tonsil suction (Yankauer) adapter, airway adjuncts, tracheal tubes, and sedation reversal and cardiac arrest medications. You should also have a length-based resuscitation tape or emergency medication sheet listing doses appropriate for resuscitation.

During sedation providers should record vital signs and oxygen saturation (pulse oximetry). Record these signs at baseline, after each dose of medication, at the end of the procedure, during recovery, and at discharge. When the patient reaches deep sedation, record vital signs, including blood pressure, at least every 5 minutes. Patients with underlying disease or concomitant injuries may require more frequent assessment of vital signs. The recovery period is a high-risk interval; hypoventilation may develop when painful stimuli stop and the patient is still heavily sedated. For this reason the patient needs the same level of monitoring during recovery as during the procedure. "Postsedation Monitoring and Discharge" (later in this chapter) lists typical criteria for scoring sedation recovery. Each institution and locale should develop target recovery criteria pertinent to the scope of practice and patient population.

Sedation Method
Nonpharmacologic Measures

A number of nonpharmacologic adjunctive techniques can decrease anxiety and pain perception in children. These techniques include explanation and preparation before the procedure, distraction, visual imagery, and hypnosis.[8,9] Review of these techniques is beyond the scope of this chapter.

Medications

There are a number of features to consider when selecting a sedative agent. Sedatives can provide 3 distinct effects: sedation, analgesia, or amnesia (see Critical Concepts: "Selecting a Sedative Agent"). Select a sedative to treat anxiety, an analgesic to treat pain, and an amnesic to prevent memory of the procedure. Additional factors to consider are the personnel and equipment available and the drug onset and duration of action. Continuous infusions of sedatives and analgesics are common in monitored and ICU settings; these applications are beyond the scope of this chapter.

- **Topical anesthetics:** Topical anesthetics are useful with both broken and intact skin. Combinations of tetracaine, epinephrine (adrenaline), and cocaine (TAC) have been used extensively in laceration repair. But many institutions have switched to a lidocaine, epinephrine, and tetracaine (LET) solution or gel. This combination is less expensive, and it does not contain a controlled substance.[10] Optimal effect typically occurs in 30 to 45 minutes. For intact skin a mixture of lidocaine and prilocaine (EMLA®) applied for 1 to 2 hours results in a 3- to 5-mm depth of anesthesia.[11] A newer preparation of liposomal 4% lidocaine (ELA-Max®) is often effective within 30 minutes.[12] The time required

FYI: Lidocaine Iontophoresis

You can deliver lidocaine with epinephrine through intact skin by *iontophoresis* (Numby Stuff®). This technique uses an electrical current to drive the drug into the skin. Approximately 10 mm of dermal anesthesia is achieved after 10 to 20 minutes. With shorter delivery times many children report that the tingling induced by the current is uncomfortable.[13]

Critical Concepts: Selecting a Sedative Agent

Sedatives produce 3 distinct effects: sedation, analgesia, or amnesia. Consider these effects when choosing an agent.

Select a sedative to treat anxiety, an analgesic to treat pain, and an amnestic to prevent memory of the procedure.

Medication	Sedation	Analgesia	Amnesia
Barbiturates	+++	−	−
Benzodiazepines	+++	−	+++
Narcotics*	++	+++	−
Ketamine	+++	+++	+
Ketorolac	−	+++	−
Propofol	+++	−	+
Chloral hydrate	++	−	−

*Different narcotics produce different levels of sedation. For example, when given in an equi-analgesic dose, morphine provides deeper sedation than fentanyl.

for its local anesthetic effect precludes its use in urgent situations, but it is practical for elective procedures such as venipuncture or insertion of an intravenous or intra-arterial catheter. You can deliver lidocaine with epinephrine through intact skin using iontophoresis (see FYI: "Lidocaine Iontophoresis").

- **Barbiturates:** Short-acting barbiturates (eg, pentobarbital) are sedative-hypnotic agents. They have a rapid onset of action when given intravenously (1 to 5 minutes) and a short duration of action (15 to 60 minutes). *None has analgesic properties.* A short-acting barbiturate is typically the sedative of choice for patients with head trauma, status epilepticus, or suspected increased intracranial pressure (ICP) because they decrease brain oxygen consumption and ICP. Table 3 lists recommended doses. When given rectally ultrashort-acting barbiturates (eg, thiopental or methohexital) act within 5 to 15 minutes; their effects last 30 to 90 minutes. When given intravenously these agents may rapidly induce general anesthesia. For this reason providers commonly use barbiturates for rapid sequence intubation (see Chapter 14). Providers, however, must use larger doses for rapid sequence intubation than for sedation.

Side effects of barbiturates include dose-dependent myocardial depression and hypotension. You can reduce these adverse effects by decreasing the rate of administration and by providing isotonic crystalloid volume infusion. You should generally avoid use of these drugs in hypotensive or hypovolemic patients. If you use barbiturates in these patients, decrease the dose by at least half. Other adverse effects include respiratory depression (enhanced by benzodiazepines and narcotics), bronchospasm, cough, laryngospasm, and anaphylaxis. You should usually avoid use of barbiturates in children with severe or acute asthma because these drugs stimulate histamine release. Barbiturates are contraindicated in patients with porphyria because they can exacerbate the disease.

- **Benzodiazepines:** Benzodiazepines are sedative-hypnotic agents with potent amnestic effects. When used alone they are very safe because their mechanism of action is to accentuate inhibitory pathways in the brain. When combined with other agents benzodiazepines may have potent sedative effects and may suppress ventilation. Many benzodiazepines are available (eg, midazolam, diazepam, and lorazepam). Midazolam is a frequent choice for moderate or deep sedation (eg, during procedures).

  — Midazolam has a short duration of action (30 to 60 minutes), rapid onset of action, and potent amnestic properties. It is water soluble. You may administer midazolam by the intravenous (IV), intramuscular (IM), intranasal (IN), rectal (PR) or oral (PO) route.

  — Diazepam is fat soluble. It has a slightly slower onset of action but a longer duration of action (30 to 90 minutes). Diazepam often causes pain on injection, and it may irritate the vein.

  — Lorazepam has a sedative effect lasting 2 to 6 hours. You can give lorazepam by the PO, IV, or IM route.

Benzodiazepines can cause respiratory depression, especially with concomitant use of barbiturates or narcotics. Occasionally a paradoxical excitatory reaction occurs (see "Reversal Agents" later in this chapter). Hypotension occurs less frequently with these drugs than with barbiturates. For patients who are hemodynamically unstable (ie, hypotensive or hypovolemic), you should decrease the recommended dose (typically by 50%). Like barbiturates, benzodiazepines possess *no* analgesic properties. Table 3 lists appropriate doses.

- **Narcotics:** Narcotics remain the gold standard for treatment of severe pain.

  — Morphine is a common choice. It has been widely and safely used in infants and children. Pruritus occurs

in some patients. Hemodynamically compromised patients may develop hypotension. Both effects are mediated by histamine release.

— Fentanyl, a synthetic narcotic, also has been widely used in children. It is 50 to 100 times more potent than morphine, and it produces less histamine release. The hemodynamic stability associated with fentanyl and its closely related analogs makes it a preferred agent in cardiovascular surgery. An unusual complication of fentanyl is chest wall rigidity. This complication may occur with large doses (usually >5 µg/kg) given rapidly, especially in infants. You may need to use neuromuscular blockade and tracheal intubation to treat this complication.

— Meperidine has also been used in children. One of its metabolites causes central nervous system excitation and may cause seizures. Use of other narcotics may be preferable.

The most common adverse effects of narcotics are hypoventilation, apnea, and hypotension. The incidence of apnea is higher in very young infants (less than 2 months old) than in older infants and children. To support a patient with apnea or hypoventilation, open the airway as needed, provide assisted ventilation, and give naloxone, a specific narcotic reversal agent (see "Reversal Agents"). Other potential side effects of all narcotics include nausea, vomiting and constipation.

Other Agents

Additional medications include those that may produce amnesia and analgesia, short-acting anesthetics, anti-inflammatory agents, and hypnotics. Some drugs popular several years ago have been replaced by newer agents with better side effect profiles (see FYI: "Meperidine/Promethazine/Chlorpromazine Combination").

TABLE 3. Recommended Doses and Characteristics of Drugs Used for Sedation and Analgesia*

Agent	Dose	Onset of Action	Duration of Action
Benzodiazepines			
Midazolam	IV: 0.05-0.1 mg/kg, maximum single dose 5 mg; may repeat up to maximum total dose 0.4 mg/kg or 10 mg	1-2 minutes	30-60 minutes
	IM: 0.1-0.2 mg/kg	5-15 minutes	30-60 minutes
	IN: 0.2-0.4 mg/kg		
	PR: 0.5-1 mg/kg	5-10 minutes	30-60 minutes
	PO: 0.25-0.5 mg/kg; maximum total dose 20 mg	10 minutes	1-2 hours
Lorazepam	IM, IV: 0.05-0.1 mg/kg, maximum single dose 4 mg	IV: 3-5 minutes	2-6 hours
		IM: 10-20 minutes	2-6 hours
	PO: 0.05-0.1 mg/kg, maximum single dose 2 mg	PO: 60 minutes	2-8 hours
Diazepam	IV: 0.1-0.2 mg/kg	2-3 minutes	30-90 minutes
	PR: 0.3-0.5 mg/kg	5-15 minutes	2-4 hours
Barbiturates			
Pentobarbital	IV: 1-3 mg/kg; may repeat up to 6 mg/kg	1-5 minutes	15-60 minutes
	IM: 2-5 mg/kg	5-15 minutes	2-4 hours
	PO: 2-3 mg/kg	15-60 minutes	2-4 hours
Thiopental	PR: 25 mg/kg	5-15 minutes	60-90 minutes
Methohexital	PR: 20-30 mg/kg	5-15 minutes	30-90 minutes
Narcotics			
Morphine	IV: 0.05-0.1 mg/kg	5-10 minutes	2-4 hours
Fentanyl	IV: 1-4 µg/kg	2-3 minutes	20-60 minutes
Other Agents			
Ketamine	IV: 0.5-2 mg/kg	1-2 minutes	15-60 minutes
	IM: 3-4 mg/kg	3-10 minutes	15-60 minutes
Chloral hydrate	PO, PR: 25-100 mg/kg; maximum 2 g	15-30 minutes	2-3 hours
Ketorolac	IV, IM: 0.5-1 mg/kg	10-15 minutes	3-6 hours
Propofol	IV: 0.5-1 mg/kg; may repeat in 0.5 mg/kg boluses; may give as a titrated continuous infusion of 25-100 µg/kg per minute during the procedure	1-2 minutes	3-5 minutes

IV indicates intravenous; IM, intramuscular; IN, intranasal; PO, by mouth; and PR, by rectum.

*Some of the doses in this table are intentionally *lower* than the doses for rapid sequence intubation (Chapter 14). This table suggests doses for *many* levels of sedation. For rapid sequence intubation, *anesthesia with loss of airway protective mechanisms* is desirable.

This combination has several names: "DPT" (Demerol, Phenergan, Thorazine), "lytic cocktail," and "cath mix." Researchers originally described DPT as a premedication for cardiac catheterization. It is given in variable dose combinations as an IM injection. Problems associated with DPT include prolonged sedation, hypotension, hypoxemia associated with apnea, and even death.[19] Given the alternatives now available, it is best to avoid use of this combined medication.

■ **Dissociative anesthetics (ketamine):** Ketamine is a dissociative anesthetic that produces a cataleptic (ie, trancelike) state in which the eyes remain open with a slow nystagmic gaze. Patients are noncommunicative but they appear awake. Ketamine, a phencyclidine derivative, produces potent analgesia and rapid sedation; it preserves respiratory drive and airway protective reflexes when used in appropriate doses. Ketamine can produce general anesthesia when given in sufficient doses. Its duration of action is variable (15 to 60 minutes). Use the lower dose range for hemodynamically compromised patients.[14,15] Ketamine-induced catecholamine release helps maintain blood pressure. It may decrease or protect against bronchospasm and improve ventilation in asthmatic patients. These beneficial effects may not occur in catecholamine-depleted, chronically ill patients.

Adverse effects of ketamine include increased systemic, intracranial, and intraocular pressures; hallucinogenic emergence reactions (more frequent in adults than children); laryngospasm; and excessive airway secretions. Some experts advocate pretreatment with 0.01 to 0.02 mg/kg atropine or 0.005 to 0.01 mg/kg glycopyrrolate to decrease secretions, but the effectiveness of this approach has not been clearly demonstrated. In one recent review hypersalivation developed despite premedication with atropine in 1.7% of more than 1000 children who received intramuscular ketamine in the Emergency Department.[16] The risk of emergence reactions may be reduced by adding a benzodiazepine to ketamine, but some experts question the need for this measure.[17]

■ **Propofol:** This intravenous anesthetic agent is an increasingly popular choice for deep sedation of children for procedures, but safe use of this drug requires considerable experience. It is short acting, so patients quickly return to their baseline mental status.[18] It closely resembles the short-acting barbiturates in its side effect profile. It may depress cardiac output and cause severe hypotension, particularly in volume-depleted patients. Apnea is also common. Concern for the development of metabolic acidosis in children receiving long duration and high-dose continuous propofol infusions led the FDA to recommend limitation of pediatric use of this drug to short-term and procedural sedation. Like the barbiturates, it has anticonvulsive properties, lacks analgesic activity when used in subanesthetic doses, and lowers ICP. Because of its short duration of action, you must give propofol in frequent boluses or as a continuous infusion.

Propofol is highly fat soluble (it is distributed in a 10% lipid emulsion). High fat solubility leads to rapid passage across the blood-brain barrier. It also leads to a short duration of effect with redistribution from the brain to less well-perfused fat stores.

Patients frequently report pain with IV propofol injection. To reduce this effect, you may inject lidocaine through the IV site before you administer propofol, or you can mix lidocaine with the propofol. Because of the composition of its base solution, propofol is contraindicated in patients with a history of allergy to egg or soybean.

■ **Nonsteroidal anti-inflammatory agents:** Nonsteroidal anti-inflammatory agents (NSAIDs) inhibit prostaglandin metabolism, producing analgesic and antipyretic effects. Ketorolac is a potent nonnarcotic analgesic that is available in an IV formulation for rapid onset of action. Use of this long-acting medication may provide analgesia with little or no sedation. It may allow you to use a lower dose of narcotic to achieve effective pain relief while minimizing adverse effects. The typical dose is 0.5 to 1 mg/kg IV or IM. Like other NSAIDs, this agent may lead to decreased platelet function, gastric ulceration, and gastric bleeding with prolonged use. All NSAIDs can reduce renal blood flow, so they are relatively contraindicated in patients with reduced renal function.

■ **Chloral hydrate:** Chloral hydrate is a hypnotic (sleep-inducing) agent that has been used extensively for sedation of children. Chloral hydrate has no analgesic activity and it has minimal respiratory depressant effect when appropriate doses are used. For these reasons it is a frequent choice for children who require a prolonged diagnostic imaging study (eg, nuclear medicine or MRI scan). It is most useful in children less than 3 years old. In some children chloral hydrate may have a paradoxical excitatory effect. The onset of action is relatively slow and sometimes unreliable. Some children experience prolonged sedation, necessitating prolonged observation and monitoring. Because of these limitations, short-acting barbiturates are often preferable for sedation for radiographic procedures.

■ **Nitrous oxide:** Nitrous oxide is an inhalational anesthetic agent that provides anxiolysis and very mild analgesia. These properties make it useful for short procedures, particularly in the outpatient setting. Providers typically administer a mixture of at least 50% nitrous oxide and 50% oxygen. It is important to combine nitrous oxide with oxygen to avoid delivering a hypoxic gas mixture. Nitrous oxide has been used in prehospital and outpatient settings and the Emergency Department.

Providers frequently use a scavenging device to limit exposure of healthcare personnel. The administration system includes a mask and "demand valve" to enable the patient to control the amount of gas inspired. Because the patient must understand how to control the device, it is most useful in cooperative patients 6 to 8 years of age or older. Side effects include hypoxemia after its discontinuation; all patients should breathe 100% oxygen for 5 minutes after nitrous oxide is discontinued. Nitrous oxide diffuses easily into air-filled cavities, so it is relatively contraindicated in patients with air-leak syndromes (ie, pneumothorax) or closed air spaces (eg, bowel obstruction).

- **Neuroleptics.** Neuroleptics like haloperidol are occasionally used in pediatrics, but they frequently cause dystonic reactions.

- **Continuous infusions of sedatives:** Trained personnel may administer continuous infusions of sedatives and analgesics with appropriate continuous monitoring. Consultation with airway and sedation specialists is advisable for this type of management. Textbooks discussing these topics are available.[20-22] Further discussion is beyond the scope of this chapter.

Reversal Agents

Although you should be familiar with specific reversal agents of narcotics and benzodiazepines to provide safe sedation, you should rarely need to use these agents. If respiratory depression occurs during sedation, you should immediately open and clear the airway. Then provide assisted ventilation and 100% oxygen as needed. Beware of the adverse effects of reversal agents. Weigh the benefit of immediate reversal against provision of respiratory assistance until the adverse effects of the narcotic or benzodiazepine dissipate. If you decide to give a reversal agent, consider the following agents:

- For *narcotic* reversal: naloxone
- For *benzodiazepine* reversal: flumazenil

Note that the half-life of the reversal agent is frequently shorter than the half-life of the sedative agent. Observe for recurrence of sedation after the effects of the reversal agent dissipate.

Naloxone is the prototypical narcotic receptor antagonist. When you suspect that respiratory depression is caused by narcotic effect, use naloxone in small doses (1 to 10 μg/kg). This dose will maintain some analgesia for the underlying pain. Note that this dose is intentionally much lower than the dose recommended for immediate and full reversal of narcotic poisoning (ie, 100 μg/kg or 0.1 mg/kg) in Chapter 12, "Toxicology." If the initial dose is ineffective, repeat titrated doses every 1 to 2 minutes. You may give naloxone by the IV, IM, or tracheal route.

The duration of action of naloxone is usually shorter than that of most narcotics (ie, morphine, fentanyl, and meperidine). As a result you must closely monitor the patient for recurrence of respiratory depression. Use naloxone with caution if the patient is chronically habituated to narcotics: administration can precipitate symptoms of acute withdrawal. In these patients treat hypercarbia by establishing effective ventilation before you administer the naloxone (see FYI: "Potential Adverse Effects of Naloxone").

FYI: Potential Adverse Effects of Naloxone

Naloxone may cause adverse effects. For example, naloxone may cause acute pain in patients receiving analgesics. It can also result in sudden hypertension and acute pulmonary edema. Correction of hypercarbia before administration of naloxone may minimize the risk of this complication. Naloxone has a shorter duration of action than many narcotics, so you may need to give repeated doses of naloxone to treat the narcotic overdose.

FYI: Benzodiazepines and Flumazenil

Some children may have a paradoxical excitatory reaction to benzodiazepine administration. Flumazenil, a benzodiazepine antagonist, can reverse this reaction.[23,24] It also reverses the sedative effects of benzodiazepines.

Flumazenil, a benzodiazepine receptor antagonist, can reverse benzodiazepine-induced respiratory depression and paradoxical excitatory reactions. It is ineffective for narcotic reversal. Providers generally give flumazenil in doses of 0.01 to 0.02 mg/kg; you may repeat these doses every 1 to 2 minutes up to a maximum dose of 1 mg. Like naloxone, flumazenil may have a shorter duration of action than the sedative. The patient will require prolonged observation to ensure that respiratory depression does not recur. Use caution if the patient has a history of seizures because flumazenil may induce seizures (see FYI: "Benzodiazepines and Flumazenil").[23,24]

The role of flumazenil in treatment of patients with drug overdose is controversial and it is rarely used for this indication. Flumazenil may induce seizures, particularly in patients with both tricyclic antidepressant and benzodiazepine overdose. In some patients with cardiorespiratory depression, complete reversal of sedation is undesirable. In most patients you can support ventilation while the respiratory depressant effect of the benzodiazepine dissipates.

Postsedation Monitoring and Discharge

One of the highest-risk periods for sedation-related complications is the recovery phase. For this reason physiologic monitoring

TABLE 4. Sample Recovery Criteria and Scores

Presedation and Postsedation Scoring

Category	Adult/Pediatric Characteristics	Score
Respiration	Able to cough, breathe deeply, or cry	2
	Dyspnea or limited breathing	1
	Apnea or obstructed breathing requiring assistance to maintain airway	0
O₂ Saturation	Able to maintain O$_2$ Sat >90% on room air	2
	Needs O$_2$ supplementation to maintain O$_2$ Sat >90%	1
	O$_2$ Sat <90% with O$_2$ supplementation	0
Circulation	Stable BP within 10% of presedation level	2
	BP within 25% of presedation level	1
	BP >25% higher or lower than presedation level	0
Consciousness	Awake and alert, turns toward voice	2
	Arousable but drifts back to sleep	1
	Unresponsive	0
Pain	No or minimal pain (pain scale 0-2)	2
	Moderate pain (pain scale 3-5)	1
	Significant pain (pain scale ≥6)	0
Activity	Purposeful limb movements	2
	Nonpurposeful movements	1
	No movement	0

Recovery Criteria: Score ≥9 or no less than presedation score

Some patients with an adequate recovery score may not be ready for discharge. If the patient exhibits any of the following signs, notify the physician for intervention or plan of care and approval for discharge:

- Dressing has enlarging area of saturation by blood or other fluid
- Dizzy or lightheaded when supine
- Nausea and vomiting
- Unable to void and uncomfortable

should continue during this period. To be discharged, patients should be arousable, at their baseline level of verbal ability, able to sit unassisted (if appropriate for age), and able to follow age-appropriate commands.[25] Pulse oximeter readings and vital signs should be normal or baseline for that patient. You should document airway patency, protective reflexes, and adequate hydration. Other discharge criteria, such as the ability to tolerate fluids, are site specific. Table 4 lists example recovery criteria and scores.

If the patient received any reversal agents (ie, naloxone or flumazenil), you should observe the patient for at least 2 hours *after* the last dose of the reversal agent. You should instruct patients and caretakers to restrict activities such as walking or crawling alone in the first few hours after sedation. Patients should not participate in high-risk activities such as bicycling, skateboarding, skating, roller-blading, or operating any motorized equipment (car, lawnmower, etc) for at least 6 hours after sedation.

Summary Points

- Safe sedation and analgesia for procedures require careful assessment before administration of any agent. The AMPLE mnemonic is useful to recall the key points of this assessment.

- Patients with significant ongoing medical or surgical issues (ASA class III or above) should receive sedation under the supervision of an anesthesiologist or other expert sedation provider.

- The level of sedation desired (light, moderate, or deep) and achieved determines the intensity of required monitoring. For all levels of sedation a trained provider should be designated to monitor the patient. Monitoring the patient should be this provider's *only* responsibility.

- There is no one correct agent for all scenarios requiring sedation and analgesia. Providers should be familiar with various agents and alternatives and specific reversal agents.

■ Monitoring does not end when the procedure ends. Patients must recover from the effects of the administered medication. You should use predefined criteria to determine the patient's readiness for discharge.

Case Scenarios

Introductory Case Scenario and Review Questions

You need to sedate a 5-year-old girl for bone marrow aspiration. The child has suspected acute lymphoblastic leukemia.

■ *What information do you need to develop a safe plan for sedation of this child?*

You will need to obtain a focused history (use the AMPLE mnemonic) and perform a targeted physical exam.

■ *Does this patient need sedation, analgesia, or both? What agents can you use to achieve your goals safely?*

This patient needs sedation and analgesia because bone marrow aspiration can be very painful. Use the information you obtain during the history and physical assessment to select appropriate medications.

■ *What monitoring does this child require before, during, and after the procedure?*

This patient requires *moderate* or *deep* sedation. Monitoring should include pulse oximetry, continuous ECG, blood pressure, exhaled CO_2 (recommended but optional), plus observation by a trained provider.

Case Scenario 2

A 4-year-old girl is undergoing treatment with IV antibiotics for osteomyelitis. She is scheduled for placement of a peripherally inserted central venous catheter (PICC). You need to sedate her for the procedure.

Case Scenario 2 Initial Assessment

The child is awake and alert with normal respiratory effort. Heart rate is 110 bpm, respiratory rate is 24 breaths/min, temperature is 37°C (98.6°F), and BP is 96/60 mm Hg.

Case Scenario 2 Acceptable Actions

■ Review the patient's history using the AMPLE mnemonic: Allergies, Medications, Past medical history, Last meal, and Events leading to the need for sedation.

■ Obtain baseline vital signs, including oxygen saturation (pulse oximetry). Perform a targeted physical exam including assessment of the airway, breath sounds, heart sounds, and peripheral perfusion.

■ Ensure the availability of 100% oxygen, a bag-mask resuscitator, suction equipment with a Yankauer handle, appropriate monitoring and resuscitation equipment, and personnel capable of providing advanced airway support. Appropriate monitoring for this patient includes pulse oximetry, cardiorespiratory, and noninvasive blood pressure monitoring.

■ Designate a provider who is *not* performing the procedure to monitor the patient.

■ Before the procedure apply a topical lidocaine/prilocaine mixture (EMLA®) or lidocaine cream (ELA-Max®) to the insertion site. You may also apply lidocaine by iontophoresis (Numby Stuff®).

■ Obtain IV access.

■ Select medications. A number of medications are acceptable:

— A short-acting benzodiazepine such as IV midazolam with or without a short-acting narcotic (ie, fentanyl).

— IV or IM ketamine. You may add an anticholinergic agent (ie, atropine or glycopyrrolate) to reduce secretions. Some experts add a small dose of a benzodiazepine to reduce the chance of emergence reactions.

— IV propofol. Use of this anesthetic requires specialized training and close observation to prevent serious hemodynamic and respiratory complications. You may combine propofol with a small dose of a short-acting IV narcotic such as fentanyl.

— Oral, nasal, or rectal medications. You may consider using drugs that can be delivered by these routes if IV access is unavailable.

Case Scenario 2 Rationale for Acceptable Actions

■ Presedation history: Review the patient's history using the AMPLE mnemonic: Allergies, Medications, Past medical history, Last meal, and Events leading to the need for sedation. If the patient's condition is urgent, you must weigh the risk of delaying the procedure to allow gastric emptying against the potential risk of aspiration. Some experts allow 3 to 4 hours for gastric emptying in urgent cases.

■ As part of a targeted physical exam you must determine the patient's weight or length to determine the appropriate medication dosage. Baseline vital signs provide important physiologic information. Airway assessment is important to anticipate difficulties in establishing and maintaining the child's airway or performing tracheal intubation. For example, a child with micrognathia (a small lower jaw) or an obese child has a potentially difficult airway or may develop upper airway obstruction. In some circumstances it is appropriate to arrange for an anesthesiologist or other airway and sedation expert to sedate the child. Many centers assess risk using the ASA classification system (Table 2); an anesthesiologist or other sedation expert should evaluate any patient in ASA class III or higher.

Assessment of breath sounds, heart sounds, and skin perfusion is important to ensure selection of an appropriate sedative medication.

- Topical anesthetics reduce the need for systemic sedation and analgesia. These agents are desirable in elective procedures.

- Establishing IV access is desirable for several reasons. It allows you to titrate doses of sedatives, analgesics, or other medications to effect. Repeated dosing is possible if the procedure lasts longer than anticipated. You can also administer fluids and other medications if necessary during and after the procedure. Alternatives include rectal, oral, nasal, or intramuscular medications.

- This patient is undergoing a painful procedure. The child will require one or more agents to provide sedation and analgesia unless topical anesthesia is used. *Sedation* reduces the state of awareness but does not relieve pain. Sedation may cause hypnosis (ie, sleep). *Analgesia* reduces or eliminates the perception of pain.

Case Scenario 2
Unacceptable Actions

- Failing to perform a presedation assessment including a history (AMPLE assessment) and targeted physical exam.

- Failing to obtain baseline vital signs and apply appropriate monitors, including a pulse oximetry monitor.

- Failing to designate a provider whose *only* responsibility is monitoring the patient. This provider should be skilled in airway management and resuscitation.

- Failing to monitor the patient after the procedure is complete and she returns to her baseline level of consciousness.

Case Scenario 2
Progression and Resolution

The patient's IV line is infiltrated. You give IM ketamine (4 mg/kg of a concentrated solution, 50 or 100 mg/mL), midazolam

(0.1 mg/kg), and atropine (0.01 mg/kg). The child tolerates the procedure well. She is returned to her room after she becomes alert and is cooperative with her parents.

Case Scenario 3

A 1-year-old infant falls from a second floor balcony onto a concrete sidewalk. The infant had a transient loss of consciousness. She also had a brief episode of shaking of all 4 extremities. Her parents said the episode appeared to be a seizure.

Case Scenario 3
Initial Assessment

The infant is awake and screaming. EMS personnel immobilized her cervical spine. Heart rate is 160 bpm, respiratory rate is 40 breaths/min, and BP is 90/60 mm Hg. Breath sounds are equal and adequate bilaterally with good bilateral chest expansion. Heart sounds are normal, and pulses and systemic perfusion are excellent. Pupils are 4 mm and briskly reactive, and the infant opens her eyes in response to voice. The findings of her neurologic exam are otherwise normal. There is a large area of swelling over the right temporoparietal area of her skull. After initial evaluation and stabilization the physician orders a CT scan of the head. The radiologist asks you to sedate the infant because she will not remain still for the exam.

Case Scenario 3
Acceptable Actions

The following actions are acceptable when evaluating a candidate for sedation after a head injury:

- Perform a presedation assessment. Use the AMPLE mnemonic to obtain the infant's history, and perform a targeted physical exam.

- Ensure the availability of oxygen, a manual resuscitator and mask, suction equipment, appropriate monitoring and resuscitation equipment, and personnel capable of providing expert advanced airway support.

- Designate a provider who is *not* performing the procedure to monitor the patient.

- Plan for sedation with a short-acting agent. Common choices are benzodiazepines (midazolam or lorazepam) or ultra-short-acting barbiturates (thiopental or methohexital) given rectally. If the infant requires deeper sedation, consider short-duration deep sedation using IV propofol or higher doses of benzodiazepines, barbiturates, or etomidate. Closely monitor airway protective reflexes and spontaneous breathing.

- Continuously monitor cardiorespiratory function and oxygen saturation, and frequently monitor level of consciousness and blood pressure. If only light sedation is used, you should continue heart rate and pulse oximetry monitoring. You may suspend blood pressure monitoring during the procedure to minimize stimulation of the patient.

- Consider elective rapid sequence intubation and deep sedation with or without brief neuromuscular blockade if the patient has a full stomach or is too unstable for sedation without advanced airway protection.

Case Scenario 3 Rationale
for Acceptable Actions

- Presedation history: The AMPLE mnemonic will provide you with the needed parts of the patient's medical history. See "Case Scenario 2 Rationale for Acceptable Actions" for detailed information. The Events leading to the need for sedation put the child at risk for multisystem injury. The child has head trauma, potential cervical spine injury, and other injuries. All of these injuries may influence the sedation plan.

- Perform a targeted physical exam before sedation as noted in Case Scenario 2. If this patient is hypertensive or bradycardic, had irregular respirations, or becomes unresponsive, you would need to perform rapid sequence intubation instead of sedation because these signs suggest increased ICP.

Assessment of cardiopulmonary status is important because marked tachycardia and prolonged capillary refill suggest hypovolemia due to internal injuries.

- Oxygen (100%) and the equipment to deliver positive-pressure ventilation should always be readily available when you administer sedation. Have a suction apparatus with a tonsil (Yankauer) handle available. Vomiting may occur, and you may need to suction large particulate matter to clear the airway. Equipment appropriate for the patient's size and age and appropriately trained personnel are standard for sedation procedures.

- In this patient vascular access permits titration of small IV doses of medication with rapid onset of action to the level of sedation required for the procedure. If the patient remains combative after more than one dose of medication, ensure that the catheter is patent and the medication is being delivered. If the IV is nonfunctional, consider use of an IM dose of a rapidly acting agent (eg, midazolam) while vascular access is reestablished.

- A trained provider should be designated to monitor the patient. This provider must be immediately available to manage the airway, provide oxygen, suction the airway and manage sedation complications if needed.

- Determine the level of sedation required. Because this infant is undergoing a painless procedure, moderate sedation may be adequate. Titration of a short-acting benzodiazepine (midazolam or lorazepam at a dose of 0.05 to 0.1 mg/kg IV) may be sufficient. Benzodiazepines occasionally cause agitation; use of another class of sedative (eg, barbiturates) may be better in this circumstance. For this reason you should ensure that equipment and personnel appropriate for deep sedation are available. Chloral hydrate is not desirable because it has a slow, variable onset of action and prolonged duration of action. Propofol may be an acceptable choice when providers with proper training and credentials are available. Propofol is short acting and titratable, and it lowers ICP. Because it is short acting, you can perform the neurologic exam soon after the procedure.

- Cardiorespiratory and oxygen saturation monitoring are important for any sedation. Monitoring the level of consciousness is necessary to titrate the dose to the desired effect and to minimize the risk of deeper sedation. In light of the risk of hypotension, blood pressure monitoring is an important component of safe sedation. In certain situations, such as when the patient is only lightly sedated for a painless procedure like a CT scan, inflation of a blood pressure cuff may be sufficient to cause agitation. You must weigh the risk of not monitoring the patient's blood pressure against the risk of inducing a deeper level of sedation.

Case Scenario 3
Unacceptable Actions

- Failing to perform a presedation assessment including a targeted history (AMPLE strategy) and physical exam.

- Failing to have 100% oxygen, a bag-mask resuscitator, functional suction equipment, resuscitation equipment, and appropriately trained personnel available.

- Failing to have a designated, trained provider whose *only* responsibility is to monitor the patient.

- Using an agent that may increase ICP or risk of seizure (eg, ketamine).

- Using a long-acting agent for this short procedure. A long-acting agent will prevent thorough neurologic assessment for a prolonged period.

- Giving narcotics for sedation for a painless procedure. To achieve adequate sedation with narcotics alone, you may need to give large doses. Large doses of narcotics may result in respiratory depression.

- Failing to monitor heart rate, respiratory rate, blood pressure, and oxygen saturation. Monitoring these vital signs greatly reduces the likelihood of an adverse event from sedation.

Case Scenario 4

A previously healthy 5-year-old boy was a restrained passenger in a high-speed motor vehicle crash. The child is awake and alert; he has an obvious deformity of his left thigh. The trauma team has evaluated him. His only identifiable injury is a midshaft fracture of the left femur, which is now immobilized in an air splint.

Case Scenario 4
Initial Assessment

The child is awake and moaning in pain. Heart rate is 120 bpm, respiratory rate is 20 breaths/min, and BP is 100/60 mm Hg. Oxygen saturation is 98% on room air. The child can wiggle his toes; his dorsalis pedis and posterior tibial artery pulses are readily palpable. He says he can feel light touch on the top, bottom, and sides of his left foot. The right leg is normal. The child moans continuously, and he identifies his leg as the source of pain. An IV line of normal saline was established at the scene and is running at a maintenance rate.

Case Scenario 4
Acceptable Actions

- Ensure appropriate immobilization of the injured leg.

- Obtain an AMPLE history, perform a physical exam, and rule out other traumatic injuries (eg, abdominal injury and hemorrhage or head injury).

- Measure the child's length or weight, and ensure that appropriate resuscitation equipment and reversal medications are available.

- Administer an IV dose of analgesic (usually a narcotic).

- Maintain cardiorespiratory and oxygen saturation monitoring while treating the pain.

- Assess hemodynamic status before and after you administer a narcotic.

Case Scenario 4 Rationale for Acceptable Actions

- Immobilization is the first step in reducing fracture-related pain. Providers frequently use pediatric traction splints until more sufficient stabilization can be achieved. Minimize movement of the patient during diagnostic studies, offer reassurance, and allow the parents or guardian to provide ongoing support.

- After you assess the child's neurologic function, intravenous doses of narcotics are the treatment of choice for treatment of acute, severe pain. You can give morphine at a dose of 0.05 to 0.1 mg/kg up to a maximum of 2 to 3 mg. If the child does not respond to this dose, you can repeat it in 5 to 10 minutes. Remember that increasing the cumulative dose increases the risk of adverse reactions. Common side effects include nausea and vomiting. Morphine is generally preferable to meperidine, but morphine does cause histamine release. In some patients a transient erythematous rash may develop and blood pressure may fall. Although shorter-acting narcotics such as fentanyl can be used, this child may need analgesics for many hours or days, so use of a longer-acting agent is more appropriate.

- Cardiorespiratory and oxygen saturation monitoring are appropriate because this patient is at risk for multisystem injury. Not all injuries may be apparent at initial presentation. The child's femur fracture places him at risk for hemorrhage, hypovolemia, and development of a fat embolism.

Case Scenario 4 Unacceptable Actions

- Failing to obtain an AMPLE history before administering the narcotic.

- Failing to prepare resuscitation equipment and medications, including reversal agents, or failing to gather trained resuscitation personnel before administering the narcotic.

- Failing to immobilize the extremity appropriately. Immobilization greatly reduces pain; it may decrease blood loss and the potential for nerve and vascular injury.

- Giving an IM dose of analgesic in this patient, who has a significant injury and a functional IV line.

- Giving only a sedative with no analgesic activity (eg, a benzodiazepine like midazolam or lorazepam). You may consider combining sedatives with analgesics if anxiety or discomfort persists after adequate analgesia (eg, because of muscle spasm). Likewise, chloral hydrate would not be a good choice because it lacks analgesic activity.

Case Scenario 4 Progression

After receiving morphine 0.1 mg/kg slow IV, the child is much more comfortable. Over the next 30 minutes his heart rate rises to 135 bpm, but he appears comfortable and denies significant pain. He responds appropriately and follows verbal commands; the findings of his neurologic assessment remain normal. He has good distal pulses in all extremities, and capillary refill is <2 seconds. An orthopedist evaluates the child and recommends traction. Placing the child in the skin traction device will be quite painful until traction is applied. The child needs to be relatively cooperative for the procedure, so the orthopedist requests your assistance.

Case Scenario 4 Additional Acceptable Actions

- Give a 20 mL/kg bolus of isotonic crystalloid solution such as normal saline or lactated Ringer's.

- Send blood to the laboratory for cross-matching.

- Choose a sedative to be given in combination with the previously administered narcotic, or choose an agent with both sedative and analgesic properties (eg, ketamine).

- Monitor the patient during and after the procedure.

Case Scenario 4 Rationale for Additional Acceptable Actions

- The presence of tachycardia despite successful pain relief may indicate the development of hypovolemia. You should administer a fluid bolus and monitor the child closely for other signs of occult injury. Recognition of hypovolemia is important when planning a sedative regimen.

- Although this child demonstrates no specific signs of hypovolemia, he is at risk for hemorrhage. You should send a blood specimen for cross-matching. Worsening hemodynamic status may necessitate blood transfusion if shock develops and signs of compensated shock persist despite 2 boluses of crystalloid. The child may require urgent blood administration if decompensated shock develops despite the first fluid bolus.

- There are many appropriate choices for sedatives in this scenario:

  — Any benzodiazepine could be used. The benzodiazepines also offer amnestic properties, which may be beneficial.

    • Midazolam (0.05 to 0.1 mg/kg IV) has a short duration of action. This characteristic allows assessment of neurologic function when the drug effect disappears.

    • Lorazepam (0.05 to 0.1 mg/kg) has a longer duration of action. You can give this drug every 4 to 6 hours.

    • Diazepam is acceptable, but it has active metabolites that persist for several days.

  — Propofol is another alternative, but it may be less desirable. Propofol tends to cause hypotension, especially in the face of potential hypovolemia.

  — Ketamine (1 to 2 mg IV) may be useful in this scenario. At doses for sedation and analgesia, airway reflexes usually remain intact.

Providers frequently combine ketamine with an anticholinergic to minimize increased secretions or with a small dose of a benzodiazepine to decrease the risk of emergence reactions.

■ If pain increases with the procedure, you should give another dose of analgesic.

Case Scenario 4 Additional Unacceptable Actions

■ Failing to recognize the increasing tachycardia as a possible sign of compensated shock and failing to treat the underlying hypovolemic shock appropriately.

■ Giving a fluid bolus with dextrose-containing IV fluids in the absence of suspected or proven hypoglycemia.

■ Failing to monitor the patient adequately until he returns to his previous level of consciousness.

Case Scenario 4 Further Progression

You administer a bolus of normal saline and IV midazolam. The orthopedist applies the traction apparatus, and you transfer the patient to an inpatient unit. At the time of transfer the child's heart rate is 100 bpm, respiratory rate is 25 breath/min, and BP is 98/60 mm Hg.

On the ward, ECG and pulse oximetry monitoring are discontinued. About 1 hour later you receive an urgent call to evaluate the child in his room. His parents say the child was crying and in pain. The nurse gave him another dose of morphine. The child is floppy, cyanotic, and unresponsive with a respiratory rate of 8 breaths/min, heart rate of 100 bpm, and capillary refill of 4 seconds. Distal pulses are strong and palpable. He moans only slightly in response to a sternal rub, and his pupils are 2 mm bilaterally.

Case Scenario 4 Additional Acceptable Actions

■ Immediately open the airway and administer supplemental oxygen. If cyanosis does not rapidly improve,

begin manual ventilation with 100% FiO$_2$ while another provider applies cricoid pressure.

■ While providing assisted ventilation, administer a small dose of naloxone intravenously (1 to 10 µg/kg or 0.001 to 0.01 mg/kg). Follow it with a normal saline flush (5 to 10 mL) and observe for effect. If respiratory efforts do not improve within 1 to 2 minutes, repeat this dose of naloxone and the saline flush.

■ Begin both cardiorespiratory and oxygen saturation monitoring.

■ Check the patient's responsiveness, blood pressure, and perfusion after airway support.

■ If the child does not respond to naloxone, perform intubation with positive-pressure ventilation.

■ Turn the patient to the recovery position (left lateral decubitus) if adequate spontaneous breathing resumes.

■ Monitor the patient for recurrence of respiratory depression.

Case Scenario 4 Rationale for Additional Acceptable Actions

■ The patient has clinical evidence of significant hypoxemia associated with hypoventilation. You should immediately provide airway support plus 100% oxygen. If the patient's respiratory effort is insufficient to improve his oxygenation, you should open his airway and provide positive-pressure ventilation. The most likely cause of this child's deterioration is hypoventilation. Hypoventilation may develop after cessation of painful stimuli in a heavily sedated patient. In this case an additional dose of narcotic was given after splinting and traction reduced the pain.

■ Naloxone is a specific narcotic antagonist. Because this patient had significant pain, complete reversal of the narcotic effect is undesirable. Administering a small dose of naloxone (1 to 10 µg/kg or 0.001 to 0.01 mg/kg) frequently

reverses the respiratory depression while maintaining the analgesic effect. If this dose is inadequate, you can repeat the dose every few minutes and titrate it to effect. When you administer small doses of naloxone you must be sure to flush it to ensure that it reaches the central circulation.

■ Cardiorespiratory and oxygen saturation monitoring are necessary to assess the adequacy of interventions and to monitor for recurrence.

■ Because of its histamine-releasing effect, morphine may cause hypotension. Blood pressure assessment is essential.

■ If the child's hypoventilation persists after several doses of naloxone, you must provide ongoing positive-pressure ventilation. Tracheal intubation is the best means of providing airway access for prolonged support.

■ Because naloxone has a shorter duration of action than morphine, you must monitor the patient for recurrence of respiratory depression. You should transfer the patient to a unit where continuous cardiorespiratory and oxygen saturation monitoring are possible and trained personnel are immediately available.

Case Scenario 4 Additional Unacceptable Actions

■ Obtaining a blood gas analysis or chest x-ray before attempting to improve oxygenation.

■ Failing to recognize the respiratory depression as a complication of analgesia and failing to institute appropriate treatment.

■ Administering flumazenil. Although the patient received midazolam in the Emergency Department, he was monitored there until he returned to his baseline level of consciousness. Because of its short duration of action, the more recent dose of IV morphine, and the symptoms of narcotic overdose (small pupils, hypoventilation), the narcotic is the most likely source of respiratory depression.

- Failing to institute appropriate monitoring and failing to continue this monitoring. This child requires continuous monitoring because of the risk of recurrence of respiratory depression.

- Failing to observe the patient in an appropriate setting where trained personnel are immediately available to intervene if respiratory depression recurs. Unrecognized and untreated respiratory depression can progress to respiratory arrest with subsequent cardiopulmonary arrest.

Review Questions

1. **You need to sedate a child for a procedure. You do not yet know about the child or the specific procedure. Which of the following should be part of all presedation assessments?**

   a. complete blood count

   b. 12-lead ECG

   c. chest x-ray

   d. oxygen saturation by pulse oximetry

   The correct answer is d. You should monitor oxygen saturation by pulse oximetry before, during, and immediately after all sedation procedures. Monitor oxygen saturation regardless of the level of sedation.

   Answer a is incorrect because you do not need to obtain a complete blood count for every presedation assessment. You will evaluate medications and past medical history before sedation. This information will help you determine the need for a complete blood count.

   Answer b is incorrect because you do not need to obtain a 12-lead ECG for presedation assessment for all patients. You will evaluate heart rate and heart sounds before sedation.

   Answer c is incorrect because you do not need to obtain a chest x-ray for presedation assessment for all patients. You will evaluate the upper airway and breath sounds before sedation.

2. **You are gathering equipment to sedate a child for a painful procedure. Which of the following equipment or personnel is *essential* for this sedation?**

   a. one provider assigned to both assist in the procedure and monitor the patient

   b. capnograph (exhaled CO_2 monitor)

   c. appropriately sized tracheal tubes

   d. soft, flexible suction catheters in sizes 6F and 8F

   The correct answer is c. You will be providing deep sedation for the child. You should have appropriately sized tracheal tubes readily available in case the child needs intubation.

   Answer a is incorrect because one provider must monitor the child throughout the procedure. That provider should have no responsibilities for assisting with the procedure.

   Answer b is incorrect. Experts recommend capnography during sedation, but it is not essential.

   Answer d is incorrect because small catheters (6F and 8F) will not enable you to clear the child's airway of vomitus and particulate matter. You will need a Yankauer adapter and large-bore suction catheters for that purpose.

3. **You cared for a child with acute lymphoblastic leukemia who was sedated for bone marrow aspiration. The child is now awake, and her mother asks when she can take her daughter home. Which of the following criteria should the patient meet before discharge after recovery from sedation?**

   a. ability to ambulate unassisted

   b. ability to follow age-appropriate commands

   c. 1 hour has passed since any reversal agent (eg, naloxone) was given

   d. ability to tolerate solids without vomiting

   The correct answer is b. The child should be responsive (for age) and alert before discharge.

   Answer a is incorrect. Discharge criteria require the child to be able to sit unaided, not walk unaided.

Answer **c** is incorrect. If the child received any reversal agent, you should observe the child for at least 2 hours after administration of the agent. The half-life of narcotics and benzodiazepines typically exceeds the half-life of reversal agents. The effects of the reversal agent may dissipate after 1 to 2 hours, but respiratory depression may still develop.

Answer **d** is incorrect because the child must be able to tolerate clear liquids but not solids.

4. **You must sedate a child for a painful procedure. The child has a possible closed head injury. Which of the following medications should you *avoid* in patients with increased intracranial pressure?**

   a. thiopental

   b. midazolam

   c. ketamine

   d. pentobarbital

The correct answer is c. Ketamine may produce increased systemic, intracranial, and intraocular pressures. You should not use ketamine in patients with the potential for development of increased ICP.

Answers a and **d** are incorrect. A barbiturate is often the sedative of choice for a patient with increased ICP provided the patient has no hypotension. Barbiturates lower ICP and decrease brain oxygen consumption. But they can produce dose-dependent myocardial depression and hypotension.

Answer b is incorrect because you may use midazolam for patients with increased ICP. This drug has a very short duration of action, so it will not prolong the time to neurologic examination.

5. **A 5-year-old boy is sedated for bone marrow aspiration. After the child receives midazolam and fentanyl, gurgling respirations develop and oxygen saturation falls to 83%. Which of the following is the *most* appropriate *initial* intervention?**

   a. open the airway and provide suction

   b. perform tracheal intubation using rapid sequence intubation

   c. administer IV naloxone

   d. administer IV flumazenil

The correct answer is a. The gurgling respirations indicate airway obstruction due to secretions; the child's oxygen saturation may improve after suctioning. You should also administer oxygen. Be prepared to provide bag-mask ventilation with oxygen if the child's oxygen saturation does not improve.

Answer b is incorrect because it is not yet clear that the child needs tracheal intubation. Begin with suctioning and oxygen administration; then provide bag-mask ventilation.

Answers c and **d** are incorrect because it is not clear that the child needs a reversal agent. You should first assess the degree of respiratory depression that is present (if any), support airway and ventilation if needed, and then determine the need for a reversal agent.

References

1. Burokas L. Factors affecting nurses' decisions to medicate pediatric patients after surgery. *Heart Lung.* 1985;14:185-191.

2. Eland JM, Anderson JE. The experience of pain in children. In: Jacox AK, ed. *Pain: A Sourcebook for Nurses and Other Health Professionals.* Boston: Little, Brown; 1977.

3. Anand KJ, Hickey PR. Halothane-morphine compared with high-dose sufentanil for anesthesia and postoperative analgesia in neonatal cardiac surgery. *N Engl J Med.* 1992;326:1-9.

4. Anand KJ. Physiology of pain in infants and children. *Ann Nestle.* 1999;57:1-12.

5. American Academy of Pediatrics Committee on Drugs. Guidelines for monitoring and management of pediatric patients during and after sedation for diagnostic and therapeutic procedures. *Pediatrics.* 1992;89:1110-1115.

6. Practice guidelines for sedation and analgesia by non-anesthesiologists: a report by the American Society of Anesthesiologists Task Force on Sedation and Analgesia by Non-Anesthesiologists. *Anesthesiology.* 1996;84:459-471.

7. American College of Emergency Physicians. Clinical policy for procedural sedation and analgesia in the emergency department. *Ann Emerg Med.* 1998;31:663-677.

8. Kissoon N, McGrath PA, Glebe D. Children's understanding of the need for painful procedures in the emergency department modifies their response to pain. *Pediatr Emerg Care.* 1989;5:284.

9. Wain HJ, Amen DG. Emergency room use of hypnosis. *Gen Hosp Psychiatry.* 1986;8:19-22.

10. Ernst AA, Marvez E, Nick TG, Chin E, Wood E, Gonzaba WT. Lidocaine adrenaline tetracaine gel versus tetracaine adrenaline cocaine gel for topical anesthesia in linear scalp and facial lacerations in children aged 5 to 17 years. *Pediatrics.* 1995;95:255-258.

11. Hallen B, Olsson GL, Uppfeldt A. Pain-free venepuncture: effect of timing of application of local anaesthetic cream. *Anaesthesia.* 1984;39:969-972.

12. Bucalo BD, Mirikitani EJ, Moy RL. Comparison of skin anesthetic effect of liposomal lidocaine, nonliposomal lidocaine, and EMLA using 30-minute application time. *Dermatol Surg.* 1998;24:537-541.

13. Irsfeld S, Klement W, Lipfert P. Dermal anaesthesia: comparison of EMLA cream with iontophoretic local anaesthesia. *Br J Anaesth.* 1993;71:375-378.

14. L'Hommedieu CS, Arens JJ. The use of ketamine for the emergency intubation of patients with status asthmaticus. *Ann Emerg Med.* 1987;16:568-571.

15. Sarma VJ. Use of ketamine in acute severe asthma. *Acta Anaesthesiol Scand.* 1992;36: 106-107.

16. Green SM, Rothrock SG, Lynch EL, Ho M, Harris T, Hestdalen R, Hopkins GA, Garrett W, Westcott K. Intramuscular ketamine for pediatric sedation in the emergency department: safety profile in 1,022 cases. *Ann Emerg Med.* 1998;31:688-697.

17. Sherwin TS, Green SM, Khan A, Chapman DS, Dannenberg B. Does adjunctive midazolam reduce recovery agitation after ketamine sedation for pediatric procedures? A randomized, double-blind, placebo-controlled trial. *Ann Emerg Med.* 2000;35:229-238.

18. Hertzog JH, Campbell JK, Dalton HJ, Hauser GJ. Propofol anesthesia for invasive procedures in ambulatory and hospitalized children: experience in the pediatric intensive care unit. *Pediatrics.* 1999;103:E30.

19. American Academy of Pediatrics Committee on Drugs. Reappraisal of lytic cocktail/ demerol, phenergan, and thorazine (DPT) for the sedation of children. *Pediatrics.* 1995;95:598-602.

20. Yaster M, Krane EJ, Kaplan RF, Cote CJ, Lappe DG. Pediatric *Pain Management and Sedation Handbook.* St Louis: Mosby; 1997.

21. Krauss B, Brustowicz RM. *Pediatric Procedural Sedation and Analgesia.* Philadelphia: Lippincott Williams & Wilkins; 1999.

22. Deshpande JK, Tobias JD. *The Pediatric Pain Handbook.* St Louis: Mosby; 1996.

23. Kankaria A, Lewis JH, Ginsberg G, Gallagher J, al-Kawas FH, Nguyen CC, Fleischer DE, Benjamin SB. Flumazenil reversal of psychomotor impairment due to midazolam or diazepam for conscious sedation for upper endoscopy. *Gastrointest Endosc.* 1996;44:416-421.

24. Fulton SA, Mullen KD. Completion of upper endoscopic procedures despite paradoxical reaction to midazolam: a role for flumazenil? *Am J Gastroenterol.* 2000;95:809-811.

25. Krauss B, Green SM. Sedation and analgesia for procedures in children. *N Engl J Med.* 2000;342:938-945.

Coping With Death and Dying

Introductory Case Scenario

A 2-year-old girl is found face down in a backyard swimming pool during the summer. The child is unresponsive when pulled from the water. An adult neighbor starts CPR. When the EMS team arrives, the child is apneic and pulseless with no movement, cough, or response. Her ECG shows asystole. The child remains pulseless after initial ALS, including tracheal intubation and intraosseous administration of epinephrine. EMS personnel provide ventilation and chest compressions during transport. The child's distraught mother follows the ambulance to the ED and accompanies the child to the door of the treatment room. Despite ongoing resuscitative efforts, the child remains in asystole.

- Is this child likely to respond to resuscitative efforts?

- What message about the child's prognosis should be communicated to the healthcare team at this time? What message should be communicated to the mother?

- Should the mother be asked to leave the treatment room?

Learning Objectives

After completing this chapter the PALS provider should be able to

- Discuss the outcome of cardiopulmonary arrest in children

- Understand the issues involved with family presence during pediatric emergencies

- Avoid actions and phrases that may upset or offend bereaved family members or colleagues

- List actions healthcare providers can take to help families, themselves, and their colleagues cope with a child's emergency or death

The main objectives of pediatric advanced life support are (1) to detect and treat prearrest conditions to prevent cardiopulmonary arrest and (2) to resuscitate and preserve young lives. Many children who require resuscitation for cardiopulmonary arrest do not survive; those who do survive often have a poor neurologic outcome.[1-3] Healthcare providers involved in pediatric resuscitation must be prepared for the death of many of their patients. All healthcare providers who care for dying children are also responsible for supporting the child's family members. Surviving family members may be emotionally devastated. But families can benefit from skilled, sensitive support from healthcare providers.[4] Your behavior at this critical time can have a positive or negative effect on the family's adaptation to the loss of their child.[5,6]

The death of a pediatric patient can have a profound effect on healthcare providers.[7]

Providers cite the death of a child as one of the most powerful sources of discomfort.[7-9] Childhood death frequently triggers staff requests for critical incident debriefing. Some healthcare providers leave the profession because of the emotional stress experienced after failure of resuscitative efforts.[10-12] Thus it is important for both surviving family members and healthcare providers that interactions during ALS be as constructive and supportive as possible.[10,13]

This chapter describes the role of the healthcare provider in grief support during attempted resuscitation and after pronouncement of death. The chapter identifies common needs of surviving family members and healthcare providers and describes how to address those needs. Long-term grief support and therapy for complicated or pathological grief behaviors are beyond the scope of this text.

General Principles

There is little published data-driven information to help healthcare providers develop skills to support surviving family members after the death of a child.[14] Healthcare provider training typically emphasizes scientific information and life-saving medical techniques; little time is devoted to development of communication skills for use with grieving parents and siblings.[4] In fact, emotional support practices are often ignored in healthcare provider education.[15,16] But resources are available.

For example, you can order or download the *Bereavement Practice Guidelines* from the website of the EMS-C Resource Center **www.ems-c.org/cfusion/Publication: Detail.cfm?id=000822.**

No single "formula" can be applied to acute grief support. Some surviving family members report that the healthcare provider's approach made no difference in their experience or actually made it worse.[11,15,17] Some families report that elaborate and rigid protocols appeared to replace the empathetic, individualized communication the bereaved really needed.[18] Pathological grief reactions by family members are rare in the healthcare environment.[19] Most survivors and family members report that they want only empathy and truthfulness from healthcare providers.[18]

The healthcare professional should ensure that family members receive support during the time of the child's death to help them understand and feel more comfortable with their grief.[4] Colleagues or support personnel experienced in bereavement counseling, such as social workers, clergy, or even volunteers, are often available to help.

Needs of Surviving Family Members
Emotional Support

Family members require emotional support. They need the following:

- *Immediate communication and support.* Family members need information as soon as they arrive. This information helps them begin to understand the child's medical status and treatment and deal with the shock of the child's injury or illness.[4]

- *Privacy.* If at all possible find a private place for family members where they will be free to express their grief, talk, and comfort one another. Ideally this place should be near a bathroom; it should contain facial tissue, drinking water, and a telephone.

- *Consistent staff members serving as parental liaisons.* Continuity of care

and communication with a small number of healthcare providers will be less stressful for the family than having to relate to a large number of strangers.

- *Acknowledgment.* Family members need you to acknowledge their loss without "apologizing" for the care you have given. As obvious as it may seem, it is helpful to simply express sympathy.

- *Availability.* Do not abandon family members. Maintain contact, but allow the family to be alone if they request it.

- *Listening.* Listening is probably the most important intervention you can offer. Parents often need to reminisce about their child. Some parents may share feelings of helplessness and begin to explore the question "Why?" Often you don't have to *say* anything; parents may need you simply to *listen*. It is far better to offer respectful silence than to make an awkward comment.

- *Empathy.* Communicate feelings of caring and concern with both words and body language. Do not lose your professional demeanor. Grieving survivors do not expect you to feel as bad as they feel. Acknowledge the pain they are experiencing. Convey that the child's death is not just a routine part of your day.

- *Respect.* Grant permission and provide assistance for family members to cope with their grief in a way that will comfort them. For example, parents may want to hold the child's body (or not) or to observe cultural rituals or practices.[20,21] Recognize that there are cultural differences in the way families grieve and outwardly demonstrate their grief.

Help With Cognitive Tasks

Many family members enter a state of crisis when forced to deal with the imminent or actual death of a child. They may need help with a variety of practical tasks, including the following:

- *Planning.* Help family members identify tasks that need to be completed soon (eg, inform siblings or relatives of the death or contact a funeral home).

- *Prioritizing.* Be prepared to help surviving family members prioritize additional tasks. Families dealing with a crisis may be unable to separate high-priority from low-priority activities.

- *Guidance.* Anticipate and explain common stresses the family will encounter and tasks they must confront. For example, family members, particularly young parents, may be unaware of procedures for postmortem organ recovery, death scene investigation, autopsy, organ tissue recovery, and funeral arrangements. If you are unsure of the sequence of upcoming events, simply say you will seek the information they need. Ask if there are siblings, family members, and caregivers greatly affected by this death, and discuss how they can be supported.[22,23]

- *Information.* Answer questions simply and honestly. When family members repeatedly ask questions about the child's illness, injury, medical treatment, resuscitation, and death, they are attempting to understand and accept the crisis that has just occurred. They often seek reassurance that the dying child did not experience pain or that the child was aware that family members were present. Published resources are available. ADM Publishing produces the *National Directory of Bereavement Support Groups and Services*.[23] This directory includes 24-hour hotline numbers. The directory is also available online: **www. admpublishing.com/page585444.htm.** You may want to recommend books and pamphlets for surviving family members who have concerns about reactions of spouses, siblings, grandparents, and childcare workers.[23] Grief counselors and support groups can also provide information and guidance.

Factors That Prevent Providers From Meeting Family Needs

Meeting the needs of surviving family members requires empathy and communication skills. It may be difficult for healthcare providers to meet the needs of family members when the providers themselves have an emotional response to the child's death. Normal reactions such as withdrawal, irritability, or inattention can reduce the provider's capacity to communicate and express empathy.[6,13] Some surviving family members report feeling ignored or blamed. Comments that appear to minimize the loss, such as "You should be glad you have another child" or "Try to be strong for the rest of your family," are not helpful. Avoid making such comments.

The most common cause of negative interactions with family members is defensive reactions from healthcare providers.[24] Your actions and conversations should be driven by the needs of the surviving *family members*, not by *your* needs. Unfortunately the healthcare provider often perceives a "failed" resuscitation attempt (ie, death) as a personal and professional failure; such perceptions lead to feelings of guilt or remorse even if the medical care was perfect. As a result the healthcare provider may look for acceptance and support *from* the family rather than for a way to provide support *to* the family. To avoid negative interactions with family members, you must be aware of your coping reactions, and you must recognize and change defensive behaviors.

Needs of Healthcare Providers

Healthcare providers often experience emotional reactions similar to those of family members. Healthcare providers require support when an attempted resuscitation ends in the death of a child.[6,25] Healthcare providers have emotional, physical, and cognitive needs:

- *Emotional needs.* Providers may experience such emotions as sadness, anger, anxiety, irritability, and exhaustion. Numbness, or a lack of visible reaction, is normal. Providers may wish to talk about the experience with a colleague. Some call home just to hear a

---

FYI: Responsibility vs Obligation to Support the Family

The professional's role is to ensure that the family receives support during their loss. But this responsibility does not impose an obligation that each provider personally provide that support. A healthcare provider struggling with his/her own reaction may find it helpful to withdraw from a personally stressful situation if other professionals can support the family. The provider who tries to suppress emotions may relate awkwardly to the family.

---

familiar voice. Many providers wish to be alone; others want only to get busy with something else.

- *Physical needs.* Healthcare providers may have trouble eating, sleeping, or focusing on detailed tasks. They may become forgetful. They may need a brief respite from their normal duties to deal with their feelings. Relief from normal duties may also prevent errors.

- *Cognitive needs.* Most healthcare providers need reassurance that they did all that was possible. Often a brief constructive review of the resuscitation can reinforce the feeling that everything possible was done for the child. Address any significant mistakes when the resuscitation team is rested and everyone can review the events objectively (typically several days after the event).

The Transition From Life Support to Grief Support

Healthcare providers must quickly shift from intense attempts to preserve life to support of family members and staff who must cope with the child's death. Emotions often must be suppressed during a resuscitation attempt to avoid distraction. In contrast, communication with family members requires empathy and is often emotionally charged. Most providers find this abrupt shift in approach difficult to make.[17] It is unrealistic, and in fact counterproductive, to expect healthcare providers to give acute grief support without addressing their own reactions and needs (see FYI: "Responsibility vs Obligation to Support the Family").[6,13]

How Providers Perceive Their Role

A healthcare provider's perceptions of his/her role during a resuscitation attempt affects the provider's reactions to a failed resuscitation attempt. If you believe your role is to "cure" or "save" all children, then any death is a failure.[24,26] If you feel a sense of failure, you may demonstrate *defensive* rather than *supportive* interactions with surviving family members. Try to set realistic goals for your own performance. You often cannot control a patient's outcome, but you can control your own performance.[14] Realistic professional goals you might set include

- To prevent cardiopulmonary arrest, when possible, through early detection and appropriate management of respiratory failure and shock

- To provide appropriate resuscitative efforts for every infant and child

- To use your best effort and skills *whether or not they change the outcome*

Managing the Emotional Needs of Survivors and Providers

Healthcare providers must be aware of their reactions and defenses. This awareness will help them gain insight into their responses and greater sensitivity to the effects of their responses on family members. For example,

- A healthcare provider who is shocked and numb after a failed resuscitation attempt may prefer to avoid all contact with surviving family members. This avoidance may be interpreted by distraught family members as aloofness or lack of concern. If the healthcare provider can maintain contact with family members and offer even a brief empathetic remark, the perception of aloofness may be avoided.

- A healthcare provider who maintains a calm demeanor and presents information to the family in a "matter of fact" way may send the message that the child's death was a matter of routine. Surviving family members do not perceive their loss as routine. It is possible to reflect the experience of the grieving person without *feeling* it personally.

- Family members will usually resent any attempt to minimize their loss by emphasizing hope for the future (eg, suggesting that they "look for the silver lining in a black cloud"). Such observations may be made by the surviving family members.

Maintaining Composure

Most healthcare providers agree that they should maintain composure when supporting grieving family members. There is little guidance about the range of feelings that is acceptable for a provider to express, and opinions vary.[27] Bereaved survivors more often express dissatisfaction about providers who appear unemotional than about providers who are too emotional. Within reasonable limits, it is appropriate to shed tears and express grief; family members frequently appreciate such expressions. But the healthcare provider should avoid role reversal. Family members should not have to stop grieving to support the provider.

The healthcare provider's obligation is to provide support that is empathetic and "in tune" with the temperament of the family. But the support should also be in tune with *the provider's* temperament. The provider is not obligated to show

any prescribed level of emotion or to be disingenuous.

Strong emotional reactions to the death of a child are normal. You should expect such reactions. There will be times when you need to acknowledge that your own emotions are interfering with your ability to support the family. If that happens, there are ways to maintain or regain your composure. For example,

- Mentally focus on the mechanics of CPR or ALS during the resuscitation attempt. Avoid dwelling on the "life or death" implications of the protocols.

- After the resuscitation attempt, take a break from the stress. Spend a few minutes in the staff locker room, the medication room, or an empty office. When you have more time, walk to the hospital cafeteria, lobby, or even around the building.

- Define a specific, active role for yourself in grief support for survivors (eg, offer to find a phone or refreshments for the family). Your emotional response may be exaggerated if you feel helpless. Engaging in even a small but helpful task can help you regain composure.

- Acknowledge how difficult it is to maintain composure in these situations.

Priorities for Family Support
Communication With Family Members

The sudden death of a family member is often the worst experience a family will ever endure. Carefully plan the words you will use to tell the family about the child's imminent or actual death. A careful choice of words will help prevent misunderstanding.

When you are reporting the child's death to the family, it is important to be specific.[11,13,14,16,28] Say "death," "died," or "dying." Avoid vague expressions such as "passed on" or "expired."

The following principles may be useful when you talk to family members about the attempted resuscitation or death of a child. Modify these principles according to the situation; combine them with suggestions from other available resources as appropriate.

- *Introduce yourself and identify caregivers who should receive the information.* Information about the child's attempted resuscitation and death is personal and confidential. Caregivers who have both legal and emotional ties to the child should hear the news first. *They* should decide who is present for the discussion. Begin the interaction by introducing yourself. If several family members are present, be sure you know their names and their relationship to the child.

- *Use the child's name.* Avoid referring to the child by impersonal terms such as "the patient" or "your child." Use of the child's name will help the parents feel that you took a "personal" interest in their child.

- *Provide the appropriate environment and support personnel to deliver the news.* Find a private setting with appropriate seating, facial tissues, water, and a telephone. Identify a support person who can remain with the family after the news is delivered. Whenever possible sit with the family. When you stand it appears that you are not prepared to spend much time with the family.

- *Speak directly and simply.* Even sophisticated, medically oriented family members and caregivers require simple explanations during a crisis. If you have to ask family members to make decisions or provide informed consent for procedures after only a brief interaction, give them the simplest explanation of the relevant issues. Family members overwhelmed with emotion are more likely to understand small, concrete bits of information that are reinforced several times. At the end of the conversation, reinforce the important points again.

- *Give information in increments.* During attempted resuscitation it is usually easier for the family to deal with several small pieces of information every few minutes than with a single announcement of death. It is often helpful to initially introduce possible outcomes and describe the intensity of treatment efforts under way. Subsequently you can relate the decreasing prospects for a good outcome. It is important for all involved to know that everything possible is being done. Some providers advocate this incremental approach even when surviving family members arrive late to the resuscitation, sometimes continuing life support efforts until the family has received more than one progress report.[14]

- *Pause to allow time for the reactions and questions of family members.* Communication is only as good as what is *heard* and *understood* by the listener. Pause after you present critical information. To assess understanding you can ask, "This is a lot to take in all at once. Can you tell me what you understand so far?" Often after a brief pause a family member will respond with an answer or another question. It is important for surviving family members to know that information is available whenever they ask for it. They should know they do not need to grasp all the details at one time.

- *Expect the unexpected.* Family members may cope with crisis by denial, withdrawal, anger, intellectualizing, or emotional outburst. Some family members show no visible reaction at all, making it difficult to determine their needs.

- *Anticipate common questions.* Surviving family members often ask the same questions: What did the child experience? Was he/she in pain? Did the child know what was happening? Should I have done something differently? Was everything possible done? Give simple, truthful, and empathetic responses.

- *Consider providing written reinforcement of key points.* It may be helpful for you to write down the child's diagnosis, the name of the attending physician, and contact numbers for the family to call if they have questions after they leave.

- *Ensure that someone is available to remain with the family, if appropriate, after the "bad news" is delivered.* You cannot abandon family members in crisis, but you should respect their desire to be alone at times.

Your most important communication tool is your ability to be a good listener, offering a silent presence and conveying empathy. Your silence allows the bereaved the opportunity to ask questions and direct the conversation to meet their needs. "Reflective" listening, a simple reiteration of what family members said, can help them feel that their feelings have been acknowledged. Family members often react negatively to memorized "protocols" or "prepared statements."

You can support family members even after they leave the hospital. Many Emergency Departments and ICUs have programs to provide follow-up contacts (calls or letters) a month or more after the death of a child. If your hospital has such a program, you should tell the family so they are not surprised when they are contacted by a nurse or social worker.

Assessment of Initial Family Reactions

Most acute grief reactions are "normal." Denial of the death is not unusual. This response temporarily shields the person from the full weight of the tragedy. You should not "attack" denial; instead, gently and truthfully reinforce reality over time. Some survivors may have a "fight-or-flight" response; they may exhibit combative behavior or even leave the scene. Visual and auditory hallucinations occasionally occur. These hallucinations are also considered normal,[29] but they can be disturbing to other family members.

Any family member demonstrating a grief reaction requires support in the days after the child's death. Usually these behaviors are short-lived and the family member can be redirected with a calm and honest approach. Routine administration of sedatives to surviving family members is *not* recommended; sedatives may impair memory or comprehension of events.

Acute depression and questioning the value of one's own life are normal grief reactions. But occasionally a grief reaction becomes maladaptive or unsafe. People with such reactions require professional intervention and support. A person who expresses suicidal ideation or plans may need evaluation by a psychiatrist or other mental health professional. Family members who exhibit reactions that may result in harm to themselves or others, or family members with preexisting psychiatric disorders, may also need evaluation and support from mental health professionals.

Chronic medical conditions such as asthma, seizures, and cardiovascular disease are often exacerbated during grief. Exacerbation may result from a stress response, lack of sleep, irregular schedule, unpredictable diet, or failure to take medications. You should ensure that family members have appropriate medications and food. Encourage family members to sleep (or at least rest) at regular intervals. Refer family members to appropriate providers for treatment of exacerbations of medical conditions.

Issues Before Death

Family Presence During Attempted Resuscitation

According to surveys in the United States and the United Kingdom, most family members would like to be present during the attempted resuscitation of a loved one.[30-35] Parents and caregivers of chronically ill children are often knowledgeable about and comfortable with medical equipment and emergency procedures. Family members with no medical background report that being at the side of a loved one and saying goodbye during the final moments of life are extremely comforting.[30-38] Parents or family members often do not ask if they can be present. Healthcare providers should offer the opportunity whenever possible.[30,37,39,40]

Family members present during resuscitation attempts report that their presence helped them adjust to the death of their loved one[31-33]; most indicate they would ask to be present again.[31] One small but detailed prospective, randomized, controlled trial compared the functioning of family members who witnessed attempted resuscitation with the functioning of family members not offered the option. Researchers found a trend toward less anxiety and depression and more constructive grief behavior among family members who were present during the attempted resuscitation.[34]

In out-of-hospital emergencies, family members are typically present during the attempted resuscitation of a loved one. But out-of-hospital providers may be too busy caring for the patient to offer undivided attention to the emotional needs of family members. Brief explanations and the opportunity to remain with the loved one can be comforting to family members. Some EMS systems provide follow-up visits to family members after unsuccessful resuscitation attempts; these visits can be helpful in clarifying information, answering questions, and assessing the family's need for additional support.

Some medical and nursing personnel resist the presence of family members at in-hospital resuscitation attempts, concerned it will violate the patient's privacy or distract the medical team. But surveys of healthcare providers confirm that family members are not disruptive; the presence of family members also helps the staff to view the patient as more human.[37,41] In one study the small number of patients who were successfully resuscitated all expressed satisfaction that family members were present; patients also reported that the presence of family comforted them.[34]

A successful and supportive family member experience requires planning. The hospital should develop a protocol to prepare family members for the resuscitation attempt and to support them during and immediately after the experience; this protocol should indicate each team member's responsibilities.[40,41] One such protocol, adapted from recommendations of the Association for Care of Children's Health,[40] is available on the Parkland Hospital website: **www3. utsouthwestern.edu/parkland/fp/fp.htm** and in the *American Journal of Nursing*.[41]

A facilitator should be available to prepare the family for the sights and sounds they may notice during the attempted resuscitation. This facilitator should remain with the family to answer their questions and provide comfort. The facilitator will leave the medical team free to focus on the attempted resuscitation. Resuscitation team members should be aware that family members will be near the bedside.

During some attempted resuscitations it may be unfeasible for family members to remain at the patient's side. For example, if multiple resuscitations are being conducted by a small number of healthcare providers, there may be no one to support family members and answer their questions. In some EDs or trauma rooms there is insufficient space for the family to be at the bedside during a sterile procedure, particularly if the procedure involves surgical exploration for bleeding or open-chest massage. Nonetheless, family members appreciate the opportunity to be nearby, to whisper in the child's ear (from the head of the bed), or to stand at the door to the room even if they cannot be at the child's side.

The decision to offer family members the opportunity to be present during resuscitation should be a team decision. The time to develop the protocol for family presence and address the concerns of medical and nursing staff is *before* a resuscitation attempt.

Organ Donation

Organ donation may play a powerful role in bereavement for some families.[42] Although the search for meaning in a child's death occurs much later in the grief process, some parents find comfort by donating organs that can save the life of another child. It may be difficult for healthcare providers to broach the subject of organ donation in the midst of a crisis. But you must not overlook this vital and important issue. Most researchers suggest that you separate discussions about the child and the child's prognosis from discussions about organ donation. Otherwise family members may think the child's prognosis or your resuscitative efforts are linked to donation of the child's organs (ie, that you are saying, "if you will donate the child's organs, we will stop trying to save him/her"). Give the family time to absorb the information about the child's prognosis before you mention organ donation.

You can help parents make a decision by providing them with information about the positive aspects of organ donation and the logistics of how it is done.[43] Organ donation coordinators are usually happy to talk with the family and answer questions if the family needs specific information you cannot provide. The process of organ donation will not delay typical funeral arrangements. Although organ donation is allowed by most coroners and medical examiners, even in the case of a suspected homicide, you should contact your local coroner or medical examiner to verify his/her cooperation.

Support of Surviving Family Members

Surviving family members may be unable to articulate their needs. Almost all parents have experienced the death of a family member (eg, parent or grandparent) or friend. But most parents of young children have not been the principal "manager" of postmortem care and bereavement for a close family member. You can play a key role in helping family members cope with the child's death if you help them identify the things that will comfort them and then help them gain that comfort.

Procedures and checklists have been developed to organize support efforts for grieving family members.[44] These checklists remind healthcare providers of useful steps to take and decisions the family may need to make. The checklists are not appropriate for all people in all situations.

Family members will probably need to notify relatives and friends. It may be helpful for the family to appoint one "spokesperson" to act as the contact person for relatives and friends.

Spirituality

Healthcare providers should encourage surviving family members to express their spirituality in a way that will provide comfort.[45,46] Providers can be reflective listeners during prayers even if they have no particular knowledge of the family's religious beliefs or spirituality. If you are uncomfortable providing this support, ask the family if they would like you to call someone who shares their beliefs (eg, a priest, minister, or rabbi).

In your attempts to be supportive, do not refer to the child's death as "God's will." That statement is common but presumptuous; it should be left to the family members to make if they believe it is true.

Cultural Sensitivity

Healthcare providers should treat all patients and family members as unique with a unique culture. You should ask family members about their practices and beliefs; do not assume that their practices and beliefs are the same as yours or predictable and consistent because of their name, clothing, or declared religion. A variety of publications describe grief in specific cultural groups.[21,47-49] Use these guides with care; there is individual variation within any culture.

Local Resources

To find local resources, contact a tertiary pediatric center, the state sudden infant death syndrome program, a local hospice, or the division of maternal and child nursing of your local health department. National and local resources are listed in several guides.[23] Articles describing work with the dying and the bereaved are available in every professional area.[50-52] Some professional societies issue statements of suggested practice. These statements may be helpful in applying principles for specific settings and roles.

Summary Points

- The main objectives of pediatric advanced life support are

  — To prevent cardiopulmonary arrest through detection and treatment of respiratory failure and shock

  — To develop the skills to resuscitate and preserve young lives

- When cardiopulmonary arrest develops and resuscitation attempts are unsuccessful, PALS providers must support grieving family members.

- The most important skill for the healthcare provider at the time of a child's death is the ability to communicate in a clear, truthful, and empathetic manner.

- Providers should modify the suggested approaches to supporting the family according to the individual locale, family, and providers.

Case Scenario
Introductory Case Scenario

A 2-year-old girl is found face down in a backyard swimming pool during the summer. The child is unresponsive when pulled from the water. An adult neighbor starts CPR. When the EMS team arrives, the child is apneic and pulseless with no movement, cough, or response. Her ECG shows asystole. The child remains pulseless after initial ALS, including tracheal intubation and intraosseous administration of epinephrine. EMS personnel provide ventilation and chest compressions during transport. The child's distraught mother follows the ambulance to the ED and accompanies the child to the door of the treatment room. Despite ongoing resuscitative efforts, the child remains in asystole.

Answers to Introductory Questions

- ***Is this child likely to respond to resuscitative efforts?***

  This child is unlikely to respond to resuscitative efforts. The child received basic and advanced life support, yet she remains in pulseless arrest on arrival in the ED. Successful resuscitation after prolonged submersion has been documented in only very small children submerged in very cold (icy) water. The child in this scenario was submerged during the summer. Healthcare providers should search for and treat any reversible causes of persistent asystole, but this child's prognosis is poor.

- ***What message about the child's prognosis should be communicated to the healthcare team at this time? What message should be communicated to the mother?***

  The team and the mother should be aware that the child likely suffered a severe hypoxic insult that may have caused irreversible damage to her brain and other organs. Aggressive resuscitation will be attempted. The fact that the child's heart rate and cardiac function have not returned is very worrisome and suggests that the child may not survive.

- ***Should the mother be asked to leave the treatment room?***

  If a staff member is available to serve as facilitator for the mother and to remain with her at all times, the mother should be asked if she would like to stay. The mother should be prepared for the sights and sounds of the resuscitation attempt. The facilitator should make it clear that the mother can ask questions or leave at any time.

Initial Cardiopulmonary Assessment

- *Airway:* The child is orally intubated. Verify that the tube is in the trachea using primary and secondary techniques. Note that exhaled CO_2 may be minimal in the presence of cardiopulmonary arrest despite correct placement of the tube in the trachea.

- *Breathing:* The child is easily ventilated with 100% O_2; bilateral, equal breath sounds are present.

- *Circulation:* The ECG monitor documents asystole; there are no palpable pulses and no apical pulse. The child's skin is cold despite a warm ambient temperature; her core body temperature is 97°F (36.1°C).

Acceptable Actions

- Ensure that a staff member remains with the mother. This person should keep the mother informed of resuscitative efforts and the child's lack of response to these efforts.

- Provide support and immediate communication. Give the mother the option of going to a private waiting room or remaining with her daughter during the resuscitative effort.

- Describe the resuscitation process (chest compressions, bag-mask ventilation, and administration of drugs) and the intensity of these efforts.

- Begin to introduce possible outcomes (poor prognosis).

- Ask the mother if there is someone you can call for her.

Rationale for Acceptable Actions

- An unsuccessful resuscitation attempt creates difficult emotional issues for parents and healthcare providers. A supportive staff member can facilitate communication with the family and help prepare them for the child's death.

- A single provider interacting with the family improves continuity of information. One provider who interacts with the family throughout the resuscitation attempt can better assess their needs.

- The mother will have questions about the resuscitation effort. It is helpful for her to know that "everything possible" is being done.

- The mother should be gradually prepared for a poor outcome.

- The arrival of a relative, friend, or someone who shares her spiritual beliefs (eg, priest or rabbi) may comfort the mother.

Unacceptable Actions

- Abandoning the mother or other family members in the waiting room without news

- Creating false hope

- Describing the resuscitation process with complex terminology

- Implying that the child's submersion was the mother's "fault"

Case Scenario Progression

The providers continue to check for reversible causes of arrest (the 4 H's and 4 T's). Tube position in the trachea is reconfirmed. The mother says the child was not seen for 30 minutes before she was found in the pool; the mother called EMS as soon as the child was discovered. EMS personnel arrived 5 minutes after the call. BLS and ALS were provided for 12 minutes before the child arrived at the ED. Chest compressions and ventilations continue, and the bedside nurse prepares to administer a third IV dose of epinephrine. The child remains in asystole; her extremities are cool and her skin is mottled. The mother holds the child's hand and tells the child she is loved. The mother is not interfering with any resuscitative efforts. She asks that someone call her best friend.

Acceptable Actions

- Allow the mother to remain at the child's side. A facilitator should be present to answer questions and support the mother.

- Tell the mother that the child has not responded to maximal resuscitative efforts and that additional efforts are unlikely to succeed.

- Ensure that the mother's friend is called, and keep the mother informed about the success of that contact. Determine if the child's father lives nearby and if he has any legal or emotional role in the child's life.

Rationale for Acceptable Actions

- If family members are not interfering with the child's care and are able to be present without causing harm to themselves (eg, passing out and falling), it is acceptable to let them stay. Family members say it is comforting to stay at the child's side. Being present at the child's side may help the mother grasp the reality of the child's sudden, unexpected death, and she will see that everything possible was done. It will also allow the mother the opportunity to say goodbye to her daughter.

- Parenting is an active role. Allowing the mother to fulfill this role in the last few moments of her child's life may provide comfort.

- Preparing the mother incrementally for the child's death gives her time to understand all that has happened.

- The mother may be comforted by the arrival of her friend. The father may need to be contacted and informed of the child's serious condition.

Unacceptable Actions

- Failing to consider the mother's need to be with her child or dismissing it out of hand

- Failing to prepare the mother for the death of her daughter

Case Scenario Progression

It has now been 20 minutes since the toddler arrived in asystole. The physician leading the resuscitative effort gently touches the mother's shoulder and says there is nothing further to be tried. He tells her that resuscitative efforts were unsuccessful for 12 minutes before hospital arrival and 20 minutes after arrival. The physician tells the mother that resuscitative efforts will stop within the next few minutes, and he asks if she has any questions that she would like answered before that happens. The mother indicates she has no questions. The physician asks if the mother would like to be at the child's side when resuscitative efforts stop. The mother says, "Yes." Healthcare providers stop chest compressions and ventilations, and the attending physician pronounces the child dead. The mother kisses her daughter and tells the child goodbye. The mother then tells the physician that she is ready to talk with him.

Acceptable Actions

■ The facilitator and the physician walk with the mother to the waiting room. The facilitator remains with the mother while the physician briefly explains what has happened to the child since her arrival at the hospital, including the effects of submersion and the attempted resuscitation. The physician tells the mother that the child's oxygen deprivation was so severe that the child's heart and brain could not recover.

■ Use the word *death* rather than a euphemism (eg, *expired* or *passed away*). Avoid medical jargon.

■ Ideally this communication occurs in a quiet, private place away from the child's bedside. Seating should be provided for all involved in the discussion.

■ Sit with the mother during the discussion. You may not need to say anything, but be sure the mother knows you are listening.

■ Explain the local requirements for disposition of the child's body. Also explain any legal or investigative requirements (eg, mandatory autopsy, police interviews, or organ recovery issues).

■ Offer to help the mother find the information she needs to make any necessary arrangements.

■ Determine if the child's father is available and how to contact him (if not already done).

Rationale for Acceptable Actions

■ Conversations about the child's death should take place where the mother can grieve freely but privately.

■ Incremental, progressively more serious reports every few minutes during the resuscitation attempt appear to be more helpful than a sudden announcement of death without warning.

■ The facilitator should be present when the attending physician talks to the mother. If available, a social worker or spiritual support person may also be helpful.

■ It is important to provide information to help the mother begin to make plans about funeral arrangements and contacting relatives.

Unacceptable Actions

■ Providing false hope or not keeping the mother updated.

■ Holding these conversations at the child's bedside or the hallway (unless it is the mother's preference).

■ Saying "I know how you feel." Everyone grieves differently.

■ Making comments that minimize the mother's loss, such as, "You can have other children."

■ Informing the mother of the child's death and then abruptly leaving her alone, abandoning the mother to deal with disposition of the body, or leaving the mother to get home by herself.

Review Questions

1. You are assisting with the attempted resuscitation of a child. The boy suffered blunt trauma in a school bus crash. He was in pulseless (cardiopulmonary) arrest when EMS personnel arrived at the scene. Despite aggressive BLS and ALS during transport and in the ED, the child remains in asystole with no apparent reversible causes. His family arrives and asks to see the child to say goodbye. Which of the following is likely to be the *most effective* therapy you can provide for this child and family at this time?

a. Review the 4 H's and 4 T's one more time to identify any reversible causes of arrest

b. Administer at least 2 more doses of high-dose epinephrine

c. Prepare the family and arrange for them to be present during the remaining moments of the child's attempted resuscitation

d. Obtain a CT scan of the head and an ultrasound scan of the abdomen to identify occult bleeding

The correct answer is c. Survival after out-of-hospital cardiopulmonary arrest due to blunt trauma is unlikely. This child has not responded to a trial of BLS and ALS, and there are no reversible causes of arrest. This family has requested the opportunity to say goodbye to the child. At this time the greatest potential for healing you can offer will be to the family.

Answers a, b, and **d** are incorrect. These therapies are unlikely to be effective if the child has not yet responded (see Chapter 10 for more information).

2. You have been asked to sit with a mother and father immediately after the death of their daughter, Amy. The parents were with Amy when she died. They are now in the family room, awaiting the arrival of relatives. After you introduce yourself, which of the following comments is most appropriate?

a. "I am very sorry about the death of your daughter, Amy."

b. "I know just how you feel, and I feel terrible."

c. "You should know how upset the entire staff is. It is very hard for us to lose a patient."

d. "This is God's will."

The correct answer is a. The most appropriate comment you can make is a simple and honest expression of sympathy. It is important to call the child by name.

Answer b is incorrect. Unless you have experienced the death of a daughter under identical circumstances, it is unlikely that you know how the parents feel. This comment focuses on your feelings rather than the parents' feelings.

Answer c is incorrect for several reasons. First, it focuses on the needs of the staff instead of the needs of the family. Second, it suggests that the loss of the staff is somehow equivalent to the loss of the family. Third, it sounds defensive.

Answer d is incorrect because you do not know the family's religious orientation and you are presuming to know what their god thinks. It is inappropriate.

3. You are comforting family members after the unexpected death of a child. Several of them express their grief. Which of the following statements would be most worrisome to you?

a. "This is the saddest day of my life."

b. "This is my fault. I left her at home with a baby-sitter so I could go back to work."

c. "I don't want to live without her. Life is not worth living. I have been saving some sleeping pills, but I didn't take them for her sake. Now I can join her in heaven."

d. "How will I ever find the energy to do anything for the rest of the family?"

The correct answer is c. These comments are specific statements about self-harm (suicide). The statements mention an intent and a realistic mechanism to carry out the intent. You should refer this person to a provider who specializes in mental health.

Answer a is incorrect because the statement is a normal response to the unexpected death of a child.

Answer b is incorrect because it is a natural response to the unexpected death of a child. Parents or those who normally care for the child often assume blame for the child's illness or injury.

Answer d is incorrect because fatigue and depression are normal responses to the death of a child.

References

1. Young KD, Seidel JS. Pediatric cardiopulmonary resuscitation: a collective review. *Ann Emerg Med.* 1999;33:195-205.

2. Kuisma M, Suominen P, Korpela R. Paediatric out-of-hospital cardiac arrests: epidemiology and outcome. *Resuscitation.* 1995;30:141-150.

3. Torres A, Pickert CB, Firestone J, Walker WM, Fiser DH. Long-term functional outcome of inpatient pediatric cardiopulmonary resuscitation. *Pediatr Emerg Care.* 1997;13:369-373.

4. Lipton H, Coleman M. *Bereavement Practice Guidelines for Health Care Professionals in the Emergency Department.* Washington, DC: Emergency Medical Services for Children National Resource Center; 1999. Available at: www.ems-c.org/cfusion/PublicationDetail.cfm?id=000822. Accessed February 22, 2002.

5. Frader J, Sargent J. Sudden or catastrophic illness: family considerations. In: Fleisher R, Ludwig S, eds. *Textbook of Pediatric Emergency Medicine.* 3rd ed. Baltimore, Md: Williams & Wilkins; 1993:1164-1173.

6. Linton JC, Kommor MJ, Webb CH. Helping the helpers: the development of a critical incident stress management team through university/community cooperation. *Ann Emerg Med.* 1993;22:663-668.

7. Vachon MLS, Pakes E. Staff stress in the care of the critically ill and dying child. In: Wass H, Corr CA, eds. *Childhood and Death.* New York, NY: Hemisphere Publishing; 1984:151-182.

8. Price DM, Murphy PA. Emotional depletion in critical care staff. *J Neurosurg Nurs.* 1985;17:114-118.

9. Ahrens WR, Hart RG. Emergency physicians' experience with pediatric death. *Am J Emerg Med.* 1997;15:642-643.

10. Death of a child in the emergency department. American Academy of Pediatrics Committee on Pediatric Emergency Medicine. *Pediatrics.* 1994;93:861-862.

11. Neidig JR, Dalgas-Pelish P. Parental grieving and perceptions regarding health care professionals' interventions. *Issues Compr Pediatr Nurs.* 1991;14:179-191.

12. Watson P, Feld A. Factors in stress and burnout among paediatric nurses in a general hospital. *Nurs Prax N Z.* 1996;11:38-46.

13. Buckman R. *How to Break Bad News: A Guide for Health Care Professionals' Interventions.* Baltimore, Md: The Johns Hopkins University Press; 1992.

14. Ahrens W, Hart R, Maruyama N. Pediatric death: managing the aftermath in the emergency department. *J Emerg Med.* 1997;15:601-603.

15. Segal S, Fletcher M, Meekison WG. Survey of bereaved parents. *CMAJ.* 1986;134:38-42.

16. Harper MB, Wisian NB. Care of bereaved parents: a study of patient satisfaction. *J Reprod Med.* 1994;39:80-86.

17. Schmidt TA, Tolle SW. Emergency physicians' responses to families following patient death. *Ann Emerg Med.* 1990;19:125-128.

18. Leon IG. Perinatal loss: a critique of current hospital practices. *Clin Pediatr (Phila).* 1992;31:366-374.

19. Paterson GW. Managing grief and bereavement. *Prim Care.* 1987;14:403-415.

20. Yoder L. Comfort and consolation: a nursing perspective on parental bereavement. *Pediatr Nurs.* 1994;20:473-477.

21. Culturally effective pediatric care: education and training issues. American Academy of Pediatrics Committee on Pediatric Workforce. *Pediatrics.* 1999;103:167-170.

22. Corr CA, Corr DM, eds. *Handbook of Childhood Death and Bereavement.* New York: Springer; 1996.

23. Wong MM, ed. *The National Directory of Bereavement Support Groups and Services.* Forest Hills, NY: ADM Publishing; 1998. Available at: www.admpublishing.com/page585444.htm. Accessed February 22, 2002.

24. Holman EA. Death and the health professional: organization and defense in health care. *Death Stud.* 1990;14:13-24.

25. Neimeyer GJ, Behnke M, Reiss J. Constructs and coping: physicians' responses to patient death. *Death Educ.* 1983;7:245-264.

26. Ross DD, O'Mara A, Pickens N, Keay T, Timmel D, Alexander C, Hawtin C, O'Brien W, Schnaper N. Hospice and palliative care education in medical school: a module on the role of the physician in end-of-life care. *J Cancer Educ.* 1997;12:152-156.

27. Wagner RE, Hexel M, Bauer WW, Kropiunigg U. Crying in hospitals: a survey of doctors', nurses' and medical students' experience and attitudes. *Med J Aust.* 1997;166:13-16.

28. Iserson KV. *Grave Words: Notifying Survivors About Sudden, Unexpected Deaths.* Tucson, Ariz: Galen Press Ltd; 1999.

29. Horowitz MJ, Siegel B, Holen A, Bonanno GA, Milbrath C, Stinson CH. Diagnostic criteria for complicated grief disorder. *Am J Psychiatry.* 1997;154:904-910.

30. Meyers TA, Eichhorn DJ, Guzzetta CE. Do families want to be present during CPR? A retrospective survey. *J Emerg Nurs.* 1998;24:400-405.

31. Doyle CJ, Post H, Burney RE, Maino J, Keefe M, Rhee KJ. Family participation during resuscitation: an option. *Ann Emerg Med.* 1987;16:673-675.

32. Hanson C, Strawser D. Family presence during cardiopulmonary resuscitation: Foote Hospital emergency department's nine-year perspective. *J Emerg Nurs.* 1992;18:104-106.

33. Barratt F, Wallis DN. Relatives in the resuscitation room: their point of view. *J Accid Emerg Med.* 1998;15:109-111.

34. Robinson SM, Mackenzie-Ross S, Campbell Hewson GL, Egleston CV, Prevost AT. Psychological effect of witnessed resuscitation on bereaved relatives. *Lancet.* 1998;352:614-617.

35. Boie ET, Moore GP, Brummett C, Nelson DR. Do parents want to be present during invasive procedures performed on their children in the emergency department? A survey of 400 parents. *Ann Emerg Med.* 1999;34:70-74.

36. Adams S, Whitlock M, Higgs R, Bloomfield P, Baskett PJ. Should relatives be allowed to watch resuscitation? *BMJ.* 1994;308:1687-1692.

37. Boyd R. Witnessed resuscitation by relatives. *Resuscitation.* 2000;43:171-176.

38. Hampe SO. Needs of the grieving spouse in a hospital setting. *Nurs Res.* 1975;24:113-120.

39. Offord RJ. Should relatives of patients with cardiac arrest be invited to be present during cardiopulmonary resuscitation? *Intensive Crit Care Nurs.* 1998;14:288-293.

40. Shaner K, Eckle N. Implementing a program to support the option of family presence during resuscitation. *Assoc Care Child Health Advocate.* 1997;3:3-7.

41. Meyers TA, Eichhorn DJ, Guzzetta CE, Clark AP, Klein JD, Taliaferro E, Calvin A. Family presence during invasive procedures and resuscitation: the experience of family members, nurses and physicians. *Am J Nurs.* 2000;100:32-43. Protocol available at: www3.utsouthwestern.edu/parkland/fp/fp.htm. Accessed February 22, 2002.

42. Nesbit MJ, Hill MN, Peterson N. A comprehensive pediatric bereavement program: the patterns of your life. *Crit Care Nurs Q.* 1997;20:48-62.

43. Hohenhaus S, Phillippi R. Death of a child. *Emergency Medical Services for Children Pediatric Emergency Care Course.* Washington, DC: Emergency Medical Services for Children National Resource Center; 2000:1-18.

44. Smith TL, Walz BJ, Smith RL. A death education curriculum for emergency physicians, paramedics, and other emergency personnel. *Prehosp Emerg Care.* 1999;3:37-41.

45. Balk DE. Bereavement and spiritual change. *Death Stud.* 1999;23:485-493.

46. Mayer J. Wholly responsible for a part, or partly responsible for a whole? The concept of spiritual care in nursing. *Second Opin.* 1992;17:26-55.

47. Lipson JG, Dibble SL, Minarik PA, eds. *Culture and Nursing Care: A Pocket Guide.* San Francisco, CA: UCSF Nursing Press; 1996.

48. Irish DP, Lundquist KF, Nelsen VJ, eds. *Ethnic Variations in Dying, Death and Grief: Diversity in Universality.* Washington, DC: Taylor & Francis; 1993.

49. National Center for Cultural Competency, 1-880-788-2066. http://gucdc.georgetown.edu/nccc/cultural.html. Accessed February 22, 2002.

50. Andrew CM. Optimizing the human experience: nursing the families of people who die in intensive care. *Intensive Crit Care Nurs.* 1998;14:59-65.

51. Olsen JC, Buenefe ML, Falco WD. Death in the emergency department. *Ann Emerg Med.* 1998;31:758-765.

52. Lynch D. Dealing with pediatric death and dying: a prehospital caregiver's perspective. *Issues Compr Pediatr Nurs.* 1989;12:333-338.

53. Eichhorn DJ, Meyers TA, Mitchell TG, Guzzetta CE. Opening the doors: family presence during resuscitation. *J Cardiovasc Nurs.* 1996;10:59-70.

54. Wolfelt A. Reconciliation needs of the mourner: reworking a critical concept in caring for the bereaved. *Thanatos.* 1988;13:6-10.

55. Rando T. *Parental Loss of a Child.* Champaign, Ill: Research Press; 1986.

56. Woolley MM. The death of a child: the parent's perspective and advice. *J Pediatr Surg.* 1997;32:73-74.

Ethical and Legal Aspects of CPR in Children

Introductory Case Scenario

A 2-year-old child is found in the family swimming pool. Bystanders call EMS and provide CPR at the scene until EMS personnel arrive. On initial assessment the child appears lifeless and does not respond to basic and advanced life support interventions. The child is transported to the Emergency Department; CPR efforts continue, and epinephrine is administered en route.

On arrival in the ED the child is in cardiac arrest, but after several doses of epinephrine there is a return of spontaneous circulation, and the child is subsequently admitted to the pediatric ICU. Over the next 2 days the child remains hemodynamically unstable, and there is no evidence of return of brain function. Several discussions are held with the family about the next appropriate interventions for the child.

■ Should EMS personnel discontinue CPR at the scene if the parents ask them to do so?

■ Would it be appropriate for the ED physician to discontinue support after the child arrives in the ED?

■ Is discontinuation of technological support, such as removal of the tracheal tube, ethically or morally different from withholding initiation of that support?

■ In the PICU the child's parents want everything done, but the attending physician realizes that the child's outcome

is poor. In the event of sudden cardiac arrest, is a physician order for a "slow code" legally and ethically appropriate?

■ Death by neurologic criteria ("brain death") is documented using an accepted methodology. Is it necessary to obtain parental consent to discontinue mechanical ventilation and other support of the child?

Learning Objectives

After completing this chapter the PALS provider should be able to

■ Understand the legal and ethical implications of caring for a patient who is a child

■ Understand the relationship between parent, child, and healthcare provider in reaching decisions on limiting therapy or not attempting resuscitation

■ State the essential elements of medical malpractice

■ State the general principles for writing "do not attempt resuscitation" (DNAR) orders

■ Understand the special legal and ethical implications of prehospital resuscitation of a child

■ Describe the criteria for determination of brain death in infants and children and the responsibilities of the healthcare provider in that circumstance

Introduction

The technique of external chest compression to attempt resuscitation was introduced 4 decades ago.[1] Since that time CPR has gained acceptance as an effective emergency technique that can save lives and can be mastered by healthcare professionals and laypersons alike. CPR has become a standard treatment modality with attendant legal and ethical implications.

The long-term goals of both CPR and advanced life support are the same as those for other medical interventions—to preserve life, restore health, relieve suffering, and limit disability. CPR tries to reverse clinical death, but this outcome is achieved in a minority of patients. CPR attempts may conflict with the wishes of the patient or family, and the attempt to restore life may result in suffering and disability. Decisions about the use of CPR, particularly in the prehospital setting, may be complicated by the need for rescuers to decide within seconds to attempt resuscitation when they may be unaware of the wishes of the patient and family.

The search for principles to guide the conduct of potential rescuers in sudden death situations is part of the larger, continuing exploration of the impact of modern medical technology on the traditional patient-provider relationship. The evolving position of children in our society, their legal standing, and the legal predicates of the special relationships among provider, parent, and child in the pediatric healthcare setting are additional considerations in the care of infants, children, and adolescents.

This chapter presents some of the general principles underlying the ethical and legal rights of pediatric patients and the responsibilities of healthcare providers and hospitals and how those principles relate specifically to resuscitation attempts and pediatric advanced life support. Aspects of ethical and legal issues unique to the care of children are highlighted.

The Child as Patient

The subspecialty discipline of pediatrics requires an appreciation of the physical, physiologic, and psychosocial development of children. Practitioners and hospitals that provide care for children should be aware of the unique legal issues related to children, particularly those involving surrogate decision makers and emancipated minors.

The Patient-Physician Relationship
Ethical Principles

Throughout much of medical history physicians have been guided by principles derived from the Hippocratic oath. The dominant Hippocratic theme instructs physicians to use their knowledge and skills for the benefit of patients and to protect patients from harm. Contemporary writers have noted the absence of an explicit *patient* role in decision making in the Hippocratic oath and have questioned whether this paternalistic stance is appropriate in an era in which highly invasive technology may blur the borders between "benefit" and "harm."[2]

The modern view frames the patient-physician relationship as a collaborative process in which the physician contributes medical knowledge, skill, and judgment and the patient contributes a personal valuation of the potential benefits and risks inherent in the proposed treatment, thus incorporating important moral principles of patient autonomy and right to self-determination.

The broad principles of *beneficence, non-maleficence, autonomy, and justice* appear to be accepted across most cultures (see Critical Concepts: "Principles of Ethics"). The relative importance of these principles, however, varies among countries and cultures. In the United States the emphasis is on patient autonomy. In Europe there is often more reliance on the autonomy of healthcare providers, who are assigned an ethical duty to make informed decisions about their patients. In some cultures concern for the community outweighs the autonomy and needs of the individual.

Issues of patient autonomy, shared decision making, and the dilemma of balancing benefit and harm are particularly germane to CPR and the appropriate use of life-support technology. These issues are further complicated in cases involving minors because such cases may challenge highly valued traditions of family privacy and parental authority.

At times conflicts of interest may lead parents to make decisions that are not in the best interest of the child. If patients, surrogates, or parents cannot agree with the physician on a course of action, outside consultation should be obtained. When this occurs, the physician may seek the assistance of another consultant, the patient's

Critical Concepts:
Principles of Ethics

The following ethical principles guide decision making:

- Beneficence (benefit to the child)
- Nonmaleficence (do no harm)
- Autonomy (right of self-determination)
- Justice (social and community rights)

Note that when ethical principles conflict, autonomy is often given the greatest emphasis.

primary care physician, the hospital ethics committee, or as a last resort, a governmental child protection agency. When children with chronic and potentially life-threatening conditions are living in foster care under state jurisdiction, ambiguities about the scope of decision-making authority vested in custodial guardians, especially decisions about CPR and prolonged life support, must be resolved.

Legal Principles

Physicians generally enter into a legal relationship with a patient by 2 routes. Typically the physician agrees in advance to provide a specific course of treatment in exchange for compensation. Less typical, but more applicable in an acute resuscitation context, are the legal obligations that arise when a physician renders care without prior agreement. Once a physician or other person performs an act that may be construed as rendering care, a legal *duty* generally follows to meet some "reasonable standard" (discussed more fully below) in the performance of that act and to continue the effort.[3]

Once treatment is undertaken either in the hospital or in the prehospital setting, the provider may not unilaterally terminate the legal relationship unless care is no longer needed, the patient agrees to the termination, or appropriate procedures for the transfer of care have been carried out.[4]

Informed Consent

Central to the patient-physician relationship is the notion of "consent," a traditional moral and legal concept that has evolved into a complex codification of patients' rights of self-determination. At first glance these considerations may seem irrelevant in emergency care situations, in which consent to treatment is usually implied.[5] But providers must be familiar with this issue, particularly in light of the increasing use of advance patient directives prescribing preferred treatment in the event of cardiac arrest, the rising number of competent patients refusing consent for life support, and the frequency with which third parties serve as proxy decision makers for patients who are incompetent.

In his classic assertion that every person of sound mind and mature age has the right to determine what shall happen to his or her own body,[6] Cardozo defined patients' rights to grant *permission* for treatment. He asserted that unless this permission is provided, a physician may be guilty of committing an assault. Modern court decisions and state statutes have shaped this concept into the doctrine of "informed consent," which requires much more than mere acquiescence.

The essential operational elements of informed consent involve a careful assessment of the patient's decision-making capacity, a judgment as to the "voluntariness" of the decision, and a determination of the nature and extent of the information to be disclosed (see Critical Concepts: "Informed Consent"). The patient's decision-making capacity is reflected in his/her ability to comprehend, communicate, and appreciate the consequences of the available choices. "Voluntariness" refers to the absence of internal or extrinsic pressures that may coercively restrict patient options.[7]

Considerable controversy and legal variability surround the required content of the information disclosure. Truly informed decisions require that patients (or a surrogate decision maker) receive and understand accurate information about their condition and prognosis, the nature of the proposed intervention, the alternatives, and the risks and benefits. Traditionally and in many locales, prevailing practice patterns have been accepted as the reference standard for required disclosure.

The modern view enhances patient autonomy by often rejecting this professional standard in favor of a lay, objective, "reasonable person" standard that requires physicians to disclose those material facts concerning treatment alternatives and risks that a reasonable person would need to make an informed decision.[8]

The law recognizes several exceptions to the informed consent doctrine that may apply in cases involving CPR and life support. Most significant, in emergencies

Critical Concepts:
Informed Consent

The following operational elements are essential for informed consent:

- Assessment of the patient's decision-making capacity
- Judgment of "voluntariness" of the decision (absence of coercion)
- Extent and accuracy of disclosure of risks and benefits

Local community rules and standards determine whether the standard is a "prevailing professional practice" model or "reasonable layperson" model.

involving the risk of serious injury or death, consent may be implied if the need for treatment is immediate or the patient has lost the capacity to make decisions. If there is strong reason to believe that the disclosure involved may cause serious psychological harm, physicians may rely on "therapeutic privilege" and be excused for failing to obtain informed consent.[9] States vary considerably with respect to their statutory or common-law definition of informed consent.[10]

Although the need to obtain informed consent is generally recognized in conducting clinical research, attempting to conduct research on potentially life-sustaining or life-saving therapies in acutely ill patients introduces complex issues. Clearly there are circumstances when it is not feasible to obtain prospective or proxy consent for enrollment in an emergency research protocol, but vulnerable patients requiring resuscitation or urgent interventions must be protected.

In these circumstances patients are vulnerable not only to research risks but also to being denied potentially beneficial therapy when there is no known effective treatment for their life-threatening condition. When the need to rapidly apply an

investigational therapy precludes prospective consent for participation in emergency research, specific criteria should be met.[11,12] Elimination of the requirement for informed consent is appropriate only if it is highly likely that patients would want to participate in the research study if they were capable of providing consent and could express themselves.

The Parent-Child-Professional Triad
The Rights of Parents and Children

Decisions about the provision of life-sustaining therapies to critically ill infants and children should be individualized and based on careful discussion and consideration of what is in the best interest of the patient and family.[13] An increased potential for conflict is introduced into the patient-professional relationship when the patient is a minor under parental guardianship. Parental decision making on behalf of children, particularly in the area of life support, can provoke questions about the rights of parents versus the rights of children, the rights of parents versus the duty of the pediatric healthcare professional, and the interests of the decision makers versus those of the state and community.

As a rule, the law protects the natural rights of parents to raise children free from unwarranted interference, presuming that parents will act in the best interests of their children (see FYI: "Protection of Parents and Legal Custodians").[14] Accordingly, parents are allowed considerable latitude in making medical decisions on behalf of their children even if the choices may not concur with the physician's recommendation.[15,16] These rights are conditional on parental fulfillment of the duty to provide necessary care for minor children. If parents fail to provide their children with at least a minimum standard of medical care, the government may assert its legal interest in protecting the welfare of children by invoking child protection statutes to override parental wishes. Courts regularly uphold such interventions when the parents' refusal to provide care may be life-threatening even if the parents' decision is genuinely motivated by strong family convictions.[17]

When the consequences for the child are grave but not life-threatening, however, courts have varied in their willingness to intervene legally, reflecting the continuing struggle to balance the rights of individual children and family privacy.[18] Thus courts have overruled parental refusal to consent when cosmetic surgery is recommended for a severely deformed child[19] but have upheld parental objections to a spinal fusion that would correct the child's paralytic scoliosis.[15]

The courts have been inconsistent in decisions about medically inappropriate parental decisions in which the treatment chosen is predictably ineffective but not immediately life-threatening. In one case the court ordered conventional chemotherapy for a child with leukemia over the objections of the parents, who preferred metabolic and laetrile treatment.[20] Conversely, another court upheld a parental decision to treat the child with laetrile, reasoning that the parents fulfilled the legal requirement of providing the minimum treatment necessary by showing that some medical opinion exists supporting the use of laetrile.[21] Many child-protection statutes include exemptions for parents who seek nontraditional forms of treatment based on religious convictions, although the American Academy of Pediatrics has urged states to repeal such provisions.[22]

FYI: Protection of Parents and Legal Custodians

Parents and legal custodians acting in the best interest of their minor child and providing at least a minimum standard of medical care are generally protected from community legal reproach.

"Baby Doe" Cases

The widely publicized "Baby Doe" cases of the early 1980s involved decisions by parents and physicians to withhold life-sustaining treatment from severely handicapped or critically ill newborn infants. In these situations the general ethical and legal concepts of physician-patient relationships, informed consent, rights of the incompetent, and conflict between the family and the state are at issue.

The President's Commission for the Study of Ethical Problems in Medicine and Biomedical and Behavioral Research identified significant problems in the decision-making process concerning neonates and offered an approach to a "best interest" analysis, in which ethics committees were asked for advice in ambiguous cases.[23] Congress established controversial guidelines suggesting that treatment may be withheld from neonates under the following conditions:

- The infant is chronically and irreversibly comatose.
- Treatment would merely prolong dying or would not be effective in ameliorating or correcting all of the infant's life-threatening conditions.
- Treatment would be virtually futile in terms of survival and therefore inhumane.

The Department of Health and Human Services interpreted these provisions narrowly to specifically exclude any consideration of the potential "quality of life" of the affected infant.[24] Although many neonatologists believe that these guidelines have led to excessive treatment of hopelessly ill infants,[25] other neonatologists report that the guidelines have not affected practice patterns.[26]

Difficult decisions about initiating CPR may arise unexpectedly in the delivery room with the birth of a very premature, critically ill neonate or a baby with multiple congenital malformations. Many hospitals follow a policy of initiating resuscitation attempts in the delivery room

Critical Concepts: Ethics Committees

Ethics committees may help resolve difficult ethical dilemmas. The following key questions are often addressed by ethics committees:

- Is the nature of the illness chronic and irreversible?
- Will the treatment offered prolong the dying process without altering the ultimate outcome?
- Is the treatment futile?

for all viable neonates pending a thorough assessment and review of therapeutic options. In most cases a well-documented review of the clinical data supported by appropriate clinical consultation and discussions with the family will result in a clear consensus about the appropriateness of continued life-support measures based on the child's best interest.

Ethical dilemmas remain, however, in those complex cases in which the decision makers must balance the benefits of prolonging life through the use of multiple invasive medical and surgical procedures against the continuing burden on the child and family. Consultation with hospital ethics committees (see Critical Concepts: "Ethics Committees") can provide a method to ensure careful consideration of the clinical and ethical issues in such cases.[23,27]

Consent by Minors

Historically the right of self-determination in the United States is recognized at the legal age of maturity, which is defined as 18 years. Many legislatures and courts have expanded the rights of minors to consent to medical treatment, although great variability in this approach exists from state to state. Depending on state law, a child may acquire status as an "emancipated minor" entitled to treatment as an adult through marriage, judicial decree, military service,

Emancipated minors with decision-making capability are defined by each community. The following factors are often considered:

■ Marriage

■ Judicial decree

■ Military service

■ Parental consent

■ Financial independence

■ Motherhood

The consent given by a minor is valid if the minor is considered capable of comprehending the clinical consequences of the therapeutic options being offered.

parental consent, failure of the parents to meet legal responsibilities, living apart from and being financially independent of parents, and (in some circumstances) motherhood (see FYI: "Emancipated Minor Status"). In addition, statutory "mature minor" rules uphold the validity of consent given by minors if the treatment is appropriate and the minor is considered capable of comprehending the clinical consequences of the therapeutic options.[28]

In many communities statutes permit minors to consent to treatment for specified conditions, such as venereal disease and substance abuse. A "variable competence" approach to minors' consent, which considers developmental aspects of cognitive and psychosocial maturation, may be used.[29] As a child's powers to interpret and integrate life experiences evolve from a characteristically concrete, shortsighted perspective to an appreciation of abstract, future-oriented concepts, a concomitant expansion of decisional rights involving increasingly complex and risky alternatives may follow.

Healthcare providers have been encouraged to obtain "assent" for some treatments from children as young as 7 years and, in the interest of promoting children's rights, to consider persistent expressions of dissent by young children.[30]

Courts have recognized the rights of minors approaching the age of 18 years to participate in decision making, including choices involving life-and-death consequences.[31,32]

Essential Elements of Medical Malpractice
General Considerations

Medical malpractice actions are based on allegations of negligent conduct by the healthcare provider. To prevail, the plaintiff must prove that the healthcare provider failed in his/her *duty* to provide the patient with the degree of knowledge, skill, and care usually exercised by a reasonable and prudent healthcare provider under similar circumstances, given the prevailing state of medical knowledge and available resources,[33] and that the *alleged injury* was *caused* by that failure. Each emphasized element of this definition must be supported separately by sufficient evidence to make the allegation more likely to be accurate than not. Poor results, complications of treatment, and errors in judgment are not necessarily evidence of malpractice.[33]

The provider's legal duty toward the patient begins with a mutual agreement to provide care for compensation or exists with any act that may represent an undertaking to provide care. To prevail in a malpractice action, the patient must prove that the provider breached that duty by failing to provide care or by providing care that did not meet an acceptable standard. In addition, the patient must have suffered an injury.

Therefore, even if evidence demonstrates that the care provided was substandard, a claim of medical malpractice will fail if the patient escaped injury. Finally, the plaintiff must prove that the provider's failure to provide care of an acceptable standard caused the patient's injury. Although these general elements apply to medical malpractice cases, specific criteria may vary considerably from state to state.

Standards of Care
General Standards

The *standard of care* by which the provider's conduct will be measured is key to the finding of medical malpractice. Healthcare providers are required to exercise the degree of care and skill expected of a reasonably competent practitioner of the same class, acting in the same or similar circumstances. Courts vary, however, on the geographic limits from which the comparison practitioner may be drawn. The traditional "strict locality rule," which limited the comparison standard to the same geographic area as the defendant provider, has been abandoned in most courts in favor of a regional or national standard.[34]

Recognizing the effects of widespread improvement in the standard of medical care, greater access to information and facilities, and standardized training programs for medical specialists, many courts prefer to use nationally accepted standards of care. This wider geographic standard greatly expands the range of medical expert opinions available to parties in malpractice litigation.

Medical malpractice cases concerning CPR primarily involve in-hospital cases in which the risk of cardiac arrest could be anticipated. Successful action against laypersons attempting out-of-hospital CPR is uncommon.[35]

Standards and Guidelines for CPR

As noted above, successful medical malpractice litigation is often determined by comparing the defendant's actions with a reference standard of care. A person at the scene of a cardiac arrest may be bound by a duty to provide care based on a previous or existing relationship with the patient or by employment in an organized EMS system. The standard of care by which the rescuer's conduct in initiating, performing, or terminating CPR may be measured takes into account the type of rescuer, the level of expertise that he/she may have or is expected to have, and the nature of the emergency. Whether a person trained in CPR may be legally held to the AHA ECC guidelines is unclear. Some courts regard the ECC guidelines as a national standard of care.[35,36] However, adaptation and interpretation of the ECC guidelines to meet unique community and individual needs is expected and encouraged.

Failure to Obtain Consent

Negligence in malpractice cases may be based on uninformed consent. In most cases the plaintiff must prove that the provider failed to disclose the material facts that a reasonable person would require to make an informed decision, that the patient's injury was caused by the provider's act (for which the patient granted uninformed permission), and that a reasonable person would have withheld consent had the material facts been fully disclosed.[8] These elements may vary according to the laws of individual states.

Consent for CPR may be implied in cases of cardiac arrest, as it is in any emergency in which circumstances preclude an opportunity for prior discussion with the patient or decision maker. However, problems may arise in emergency situations in which documents on the victim's person or statements by family members purport to represent the victim's intended refusal of CPR. Authorities encourage the exercise of medical judgment in such cases.[5,37] It is extremely difficult to validate such information in an emergency setting, so the practice of initiating resuscitative efforts is generally accepted with the understanding that CPR may be discontinued based on subsequent authentication of the patient's previously expressed wishes or advance directives.

Hospital Liability

The healthcare professional who provides CPR often functions as part of an organization. Emergency Department staff, hospital-based resuscitation teams, hospital medical staff, trained technicians in an EMS system, firefighters, and police deal with complex issues of accountability and legal liability.

A hospital may be held liable not only for the organized services it provides but also for the individual acts of its employees. A hospital that represents itself as operating an Emergency Department has a duty to accept and treat all patients coming through its doors and to provide a properly equipped facility.[38] A hospital has a duty to maintain sufficient personnel properly trained in CPR, to provide appropriate equipment for CPR, to implement an emergency response system within the hospital, and to monitor CPR performance. In many jurisdictions this legal duty of hospitals to ensure organization of CPR services and competence of their cardiac arrest teams has deprived hospital-based personnel of the limited legal immunity available to out-of-hospital rescuers.[39]

In recent years courts have expanded the notion of hospital liability beyond responsibility for the facility to include the duty to ensure that competent medical care is provided to each patient.[40,41] By this doctrine a hospital is considered an entity composed of both administrative and medical staff (paid and volunteer), each sharing joint responsibility for the development of standards and monitoring the quality of patient care.

With the validation and publication of national (and even international) guidelines for pediatric CPR, the courts will likely recognize a hospital's corporate liability for provision of appropriate CPR services to infants and children, including provision of trained personnel, proper equipment, an organized system for response to pediatric cardiopulmonary arrests, and continuous monitoring of resuscitation performance.

Vicarious Liability

Customary CPR practices include prompt designation of a leader from among the responders to a cardiac arrest. This raises questions about the potential special liability of the leader for the actions of others. Similar issues may arise in connection with the role of hospital-based medical personnel directing care via telecommunications with EMS personnel in the field.

The traditional legal view applied the "captain of the ship doctrine" to such cases so that a leader would be held vicariously liable for the conduct of others in the group, depending on his/her level of control or right of control of group member actions. The modern legal trend, generally articulated with reference to surgical teams, recognizes the distinct areas of expertise contributed by each member and tends to hold each to a standard of his/her class and ultimately his/her employer rather than to shift liability to the team leader.[42]

Duty to Rescue
Ethical and Legal Aspects of Duty to Rescue

The AHA stresses the crucial role the first responder plays in initiating CPR before an organized resuscitation team arrives.[43,44] Under the generally accepted moral principles of beneficence and nonmaleficence, the fundamental proscription against actively harming others is complemented by an affirmative duty to benefit others when in a position to do so.[45] Traditional American law, however, does not enforce this moral obligation. Precedents in case law distinguish between an *affirmative act* that may give rise to liability in rescue situations if it is performed *inappropriately* and *failure to act,* which however ignoble, may be above legal reproach.[3,46] This distinction may result in a moral paradox in which a person making a well-intentioned but incompetent attempt to rescue another is held legally liable, whereas failure to act may not produce legal consequences.

Certain preexisting relationships may create a legal duty to rescue in emergency situations. These duties may stem from implied contracts, as in the case of Emergency Department staff, police, lifeguards, or emergency medical technicians (EMTs). Special relationships, such as parent-child, captain-passenger, and employer-employee, may carry a general legal duty to rescue if the effort can be made without endangering the rescuer.[47]

When not functioning in an official, obligatory capacity, healthcare providers are subject to similar disparate moral and legal standards. Although the moral obligation of providers to assist in emergencies is asserted in the professional code of ethics,[48] no legal duty to act has been imposed on healthcare providers simply because they are providers.[49]

Despite reluctance to assign legal liability for failure to act, courts have ruled that once steps are initiated and termination would place the victim in a worse position or compromise the likelihood of assistance from others, the potential rescuer incurs a legal duty to perform appropriately. This element of the law of rescue, coupled with the dramatic growth in medical malpractice litigation, created well-grounded fears that healthcare professionals would hesitate to offer assistance, and this fear ultimately led to "Good Samaritan" statutes in all states.

Good Samaritan Status

Good Samaritan statutory language generally identifies a protected class, usually focusing on protection of healthcare professionals, to encourage a response by trained persons. Some state statutes protect any person offering emergency assistance. As a general rule, limited legal immunity is granted only to persons rendering aid without compensation or attempts to collect compensation. Many state statutes, however, protect trained professionals in the course of their official duties.

There is considerable variability in the scope of Good Samaritan limited immunity granted by statute. Common to all is the requirement that the rescuer show "good faith" that the situation called for the immediate action undertaken. Most statutes confer limited legal immunity, which typically provides limited immunity for rescue attempts unless the actions were grossly negligent (conduct that would be considered reckless, offensive, and shocking to most people).

The rescue settings covered by Good Samaritan statutes also vary. In some states only actions at the site of the emergency are covered; other states include events during transport to a medical facility.[50] Some states extend limited immunity to persons responding to an emergency within a hospital if they have no preexisting duty to offer assistance. In contrast, other states have denied protection to these same persons, reasoning that members of a hospital staff are presumed to have sufficient expertise in emergency medical care.[50]

Traditional legal concepts hold persons offering assistance in an emergency to a "reasonable care" standard, taking into account all of the circumstances surrounding the incident and the rescuer's level of skill. Thus common law formula considers the existence of an emergency in determining what degree of care is reasonable.[51]

First responders should not be dissuaded by fear of possible litigation from making reasonable attempts at CPR, regardless of their level of experience or training. Whether under Good Samaritan statutes or traditional principles of common law, CPR attempts in emergencies are likely to be viewed as reasonable even when provided by an inadequately trained rescuer as long as there is a good-faith belief that the possible benefits of the attempt outweigh the risk of the rescuer's incompetence.[52]

Decisions to Initiate and Terminate CPR

First responders at the scene of a cardiac arrest are encouraged to initiate full CPR measures unless advance directives are immediately available, clear, and substantiated. Because there are no widely accepted criteria for immediate determination of death, most rescuers responding to the scene of a cardiac arrest will initiate resuscitation attempts.[53,54] The *ECC Guidelines 2000*[55] recommend that all patients in cardiac arrest receive resuscitation unless

- The patient has a valid DNAR order
- The patient has signs of irreversible death: rigor mortis, decapitation, or dependent lividity

- No physiologic benefit can be expected because the patient's vital functions have deteriorated despite maximum therapy for specific conditions such as progressive septic or cardiogenic shock
- Attempts to perform CPR would place the rescuer at risk of physical injury

Unreliable or unverifiable information about the patient's prior illness or wishes previously expressed by the patient against CPR should not influence medical judgment in prehospital emergencies. Several states have established protocols to allow EMS providers to accept DNAR orders in the prehospital setting.[56] The use of DNAR orders for children in the prehospital setting are controversial and vary from state to state.

In a hospital setting some children may have preexisting DNAR orders (see below). If it is determined that these orders are valid, CPR should not be initiated or may be discontinued. From both an ethical and legal standpoint, discontinuing or withholding CPR under such circumstances is permissible.[55,57,58]

In the hospital setting a physician is the professional who makes a decision to terminate CPR based on a perceived inability to resuscitate because this decision is equivalent to determining death. Nonphysicians are required to continue CPR to the limits of their physical endurance or until the care of the victim is transferred to another qualified, responsible person.

Once CPR is initiated in the prehospital setting, healthcare providers are required to continue CPR as necessary until the victim is transferred to the care of other properly trained personnel or until death by cardiovascular criteria (defined by cardiovascular unresponsiveness to acceptable resuscitative techniques) is determined.[53-55] An increasing number of states are exploring ways to authorize nonphysician emergency medical personnel to withhold or discontinue resuscitative efforts based on criteria for poor survival or recognition of a patient's request not to be resuscitated (see "Emergency Medical Services" below).[55-57]

Although specific features of the patient, arrest, EMS system, and duration of resuscitation may have prognostic importance, no single factor alone or in combination is clearly predictive of outcome.[55,58] The most consistent factor associated with poor outcome is duration of resuscitative efforts.[59-63] The chance of discharge from the hospital alive and neurologically intact diminishes as resuscitation time increases.[64-67]

The results of available scientific studies have shown that in the absence of mitigating factors, prolonged resuscitative efforts for children with pulseless arrest will probably not be successful.[55,58] If a child fails to respond to at least 2 doses of epinephrine with a return of spontaneous circulation, the child is unlikely to survive.[58,62,68] In the absence of VF or VT, history of a toxic drug exposure, metabolic abnormality, or a primary hypothermic insult, resuscitative efforts may be discontinued if there is no return of spontaneous circulation despite ALS interventions. In general, resuscitative efforts may be discontinued if spontaneous circulation has not returned after 30 minutes. Mitigating factors, such as profound prearrest hypothermia (eg, submersion in icy water) or young age, should be considered when determining if resuscitative efforts should be extended (see Critical Concepts: "Termination of Resuscitative Efforts"). If return of spontaneous circulation of any duration occurs at any time during the resuscitative effort, it may be appropriate to consider extending the resuscitative effort.

For the newly born infant, discontinuation of resuscitative efforts may be appropriate if spontaneous circulation has not returned after 15 minutes (see "The Delivery Room").

DNAR Orders

In marked contrast to earlier times, when most people died at home in the comfort of familiar surroundings, an estimated 80% of all deaths now occur in hospitals.[23]

It is not surprising that a large proportion of hospitalized patients die after one or more attempts at CPR.[69] Recognizing that attempts at resuscitation may not always promote patient well-being, the National Conference Steering Committee stated, "The purpose of cardiopulmonary resuscitation is the prevention of sudden, unexpected death." DNAR orders may be written for children when (1) in the judgment of the treating physician, an attempt to resuscitate the child would be futile, or (2) the parent or surrogate expresses his/her preference that CPR be withheld in the event the child suffers a cardiac arrest, provided this is in accordance with the child's best interests (see FYI. "DNAR vs DNR Terminology").[70]

CPR may not be indicated when death is expected and prolonged cardiac arrest would render resuscitative efforts virtually futile.[71] In fact, attempted resuscitation in these circumstances may violate a patient's right to die with dignity. Contraindications to CPR must be noted in the patient's chart by the attending physician.[70,71]

DNAR orders and chart notes document decisions to forgo attempted resuscitation of hospitalized patients when CPR is not indicated. Decisions to limit resuscitative efforts must be clearly communicated to all healthcare professionals involved in the patient's care. It is also important to note that DNAR orders carry no inherent implications for limiting other forms of treatment. DNAR orders should be reviewed before surgery by the anesthesiologist, attending surgeon, and patient or surrogate to determine their applicability in the operating room and immediate postoperative recovery period.

Under certain circumstances DNAR orders may apply to prehospital care of terminally ill patients when appropriate documentation is provided to the local EMS service.[72,73] Some state laws and regulations, however, prevent prehospital personnel from honoring a hospital DNAR order for a child.

Critical Concepts:
Termination of Resuscitative Efforts

No single factor is predictive of the outcome of attempted resuscitation in all cases. Patient factors, arrest factors, EMS system factors, and duration of the resuscitation attempt all have prognostic importance. *Duration of the resuscitation attempt* is the most consistent factor associated with poor outcome. The patient's chance of being discharged from the hospital alive and neurologically intact diminishes as the duration of attempted (unsuccessful) resuscitation increases. If asystole persists despite provision of effective BLS and ALS and treatment for immediately reversible causes or mitigating factors (eg, the 4 H's and 4 T's), the prognosis for the child's intact neurologic recovery is dismal, and prolonged attempts are not recommended. Effective BLS and ALS include effective compressions, ventilation, oxygenation, establishment of vascular access, appropriate medications, and defibrillation if needed.

Competent Patients

Consistent with the principle of self-determination, a competent patient's right to refuse CPR is virtually absolute.[74,75] Courts have limited the right of a competent patient to refuse lifesaving treatment in only a few narrowly defined circumstances, such as protection of dependent children.[76]

In everyday legal contexts, such as assignment of property rights, the definition of "competence" is straightforward. Determination of competence in terms of decision-making capacity in the healthcare process is considerably more complex yet critical to an analysis of resuscitation decisions. Patients may have decision-making capacity for some medical alternatives but not others.

FYI: DNAR vs DNR Terminology

DNAR (do not *attempt* resuscitation) terminology is replacing DNR (do not resuscitate) terminology to reflect more accurately that resuscitation should not be *attempted*. This acknowledges the fact that even if resuscitation is attempted, it may not be effective. DNR implies that resuscitation would be effective but is not being performed.

The degree to which pain, drugs, or mental state may temporarily or permanently affect a patient's decision-making capacity also must be assessed.[77,78] Under the consent doctrine, once competence is established, the patient has the right to refuse treatment, including lifesaving measures, even if the decision seems foolish or irrational to others.

Unfortunately studies suggest wide disparities in physician practices with respect to discussions of resuscitation with competent patients.[79,80] Legal considerations aside, communication among practitioners, patients, and families on the subject of resuscitation appears to be influenced by the social and ethical values held by staff members and by differing views concerning the propriety of including competent patients in such discussions.[81-86]

Minors may express the wish to have life support withheld.[31] Caregivers may underestimate the capacity of some adolescent patients to deal with the concepts of death, terminal illness, and the consequences of their decisions.[30,87] In several recent cases courts have authorized caregivers to recognize decisions by older adolescents to withhold resuscitation attempts.[32,88] When there is disagreement between parents and the adolescent patient, the courts decide the cases individually.

Incompetent Patients

It may be difficult to promote the autonomy of hopelessly ill and incompetent patients.[89]

Some general recommendations, however, have emerged from a review of court rulings.

The American Medical Association has stated that physicians have no obligation to provide futile or useless treatment. Thus, DNAR orders are often appropriate for patients who are irreversibly and terminally ill when resuscitation would merely prolong the dying process.[90] There is considerable controversy, however, about the meaning of the term *futile* and its implications for unilateral decision making by physicians.[91] The *ECC Guidelines 2000*[55] state that medical treatment is futile if its purpose cannot be achieved. An intervention that cannot increase length or quality of life is futile. In resuscitation a qualitative definition of futility includes a low chance of survival and low quality of life if resuscitation is successful.

Thus, decisions to stop or withhold CPR may be appropriate when survival is not expected. The guidelines caution against unilateral decision making by physicians when value judgments are made about important goals of therapy from the patient's point of view.[55] Nevertheless, healthcare providers must recognize the subjective value judgments inherent in terms such as *hopeless, irreversible,* and *terminal*; open discussion among participants in the decision should be encouraged.[92]

Court decisions have emphasized the same right of self-determination for incompetent patients that is granted to competent patients.[93] Therefore, surrogate decision makers who are engaged in decisions about life-sustaining treatment (including CPR) for incompetent patients are required to ascertain and represent (to the extent possible) the wishes expressed by the patient while the patient was still competent (eg, "substituted judgment"). In other words, the surrogate decision maker attempts to reach the decision that the incapacitated person would make if he/she were able. Previous statements or indirect evidence of the patient's views regarding life-sustaining treatment or resuscitation

provide legal ground for substituted judgment by the surrogate decision maker.[94] If it is impossible to ascertain the patient's prior wishes or if the patient was never competent, as in the case of a minor, physicians and surrogate decision makers may make the decision based on their assessment of the patient's "best interests."[94]

Designations of treatment as "ordinary" or "extraordinary" have been used to distinguish obligatory from optional care (see FYI: "*Ordinary* vs *Extraordinary*"). Recent cases recognize the ambiguity of those terms and suggest that analysis should be shifted from the type of treatment to the condition of the *patient,* highlighting the potential benefit to the patient and the burden of the proposed treatment.[95] CPR, for example, might be considered disproportionately burdensome if it offers no reasonable possibility of benefit beyond very short-term survival.

Because it is difficult to know the previous wishes of minors, parental decisions to withhold CPR or other life-sustaining treatment from children are measured by the "best interest" test (see Critical Concepts: "Best Interest"). Nevertheless, surrogate decision makers are expected to exercise their judgment as to the child's best interest from the point of view of the child—what the child might choose if he/she were competent.[96] The conflicts that may arise between legitimate parental rights of family privacy and the state's interest in protecting the welfare of children will center on whether life-sustaining treatment serves the best interest of an individual child. When decisions must

FYI: Ordinary vs Extraordinary

The terms *ordinary* versus *extraordinary* were previously used to differentiate obligatory versus optional care. More recent terminology emphasizes care that provides "potential benefit" that exceeds "potential burden."

be made on behalf of never-competent patients, some urge that the autonomy of the family unit be upheld by deference to a guardian's or family's reasonable interpretation of a patient's best interest from the perspective of their own beliefs and values.[97]

Policies and Guidelines

Most hospitals have adopted formal policies governing in-patient DNAR orders. These policies are designed to ensure the protection of patients' rights in circumstances in which the healthcare provider must act rapidly with limited personal knowledge of the patient. Explicit DNAR policies encourage prior deliberation, ensure adherence to informed consent requirements, and promote the assignment of decision-making responsibilities to appropriate persons. Such policies should include the following:

- Requirements that DNAR orders be written by an attending physician (rather than a physician-in-training) on the order sheet, accompanied by progress notes that explain the rationale for the decision and identify the participants in the decision-making process

- Recommended interval for renewal or review of the orders

- Guidelines enumerating the circumstances in which judicial review is required[80,98]

DNAR orders refer exclusively to the initiation of resuscitative measures in the event of cardiac or respiratory arrest. These orders do not affect administration of other diagnostic and therapeutic interventions.

Physicians may write orders for "partial codes," which limit the extent of resuscitation offered a patient.[99] Although these are rationalized as serving the patient's presumed best interest, partial code orders may create ethical and legal problems if they are not carefully considered and written. At some institutions DNAR policies and forms provide an opportunity to list specific associated life-support interventions that may or may not be incorporated into the limitation-of-treatment plan

> ### Critical Concepts:
> #### "Best Interest"
>
> Surrogate decision makers are expected to exercise their judgment as to the child's best interest from the point of view of the child—what the child might choose if he/she were competent.

during the *prearrest* phase. It is never appropriate, however, to write orders to perform a "slow code" designed to give the illusion of attempting effective CPR.

Ethics Committees

Legal scholars, professional organizations, and government agencies have recommended that hospitals establish ethics committees to encourage systematic and disciplined approaches to ethical medical decision making. The major functions envisioned for ethics committees are education, consultation, development of hospital policies and guidelines, and case review.

Experience to date suggests that a multidisciplinary ethics committee serves as an effective institutional resource, particularly in cases in which ambiguity, a breakdown in communications, disagreement, or an apparent conflict of interest has complicated life-and-death decisions for incompetent patients. Creation of a forum for discussion of ethical dilemmas, review of policies and guidelines related to medical ethics issues, and nonbinding case consultation may enhance the protection of patients' rights with little need for recourse to judicial intervention.[100]

A major impetus for the development of hospital-based ethics committees was the controversy surrounding the care of critically ill or seriously handicapped neonates in the early 1980s. Some hospitals still have infant care review committees or subcommittees, although many have shifted these responsibilities to hospital ethics committees. These ethics committees are playing an increasing role in life-support decisions.[101,102]

Emergency Medical Services

The establishment of EMS systems has significantly enhanced delivery of emergency care to out-of-hospital cardiac arrest victims. These complex, integrated systems of care are charged with multidimensional responsibilities, including appropriate maintenance of equipment, delineation of standards of care at various levels of training, on-site decisions to initiate or terminate CPR, shared clinical and legal responsibility between the EMT and central medical control, and application of immunity statutes to professional EMTs. All of these areas are subjects of potential litigation.

Specially trained technicians (EMTs, paramedics) working within such systems will generally be held to a standard of care commensurate with their level of training or certification. Most states require paramedics to pass a national course reflecting criteria established by a national accreditation task force. Because EMTs engage in a quasimedical practice outside the hospital, their scope of practice relies on standing order protocols and offline medical direction.[103]

System organization varies widely between communities. In some EMS systems healthcare providers are authorized to terminate resuscitation attempts outside the hospital. In others healthcare responders are required to initiate resuscitation attempts in virtually all instances without determining the patient's viability[104] and to resolve any doubts as to patient viability in favor of the patient. In these systems CPR may be terminated only by order of a physician.[105,106] The *ECC Guidelines 2000* encourage the development of policies to enable termination of resuscitation in the field when appropriate.[55]

As a rule, prehospital healthcare providers may not disregard or countermand an order given by a physician.[107] Conflicts may arise at the scene when trained first responders and a physician who may be less skilled in prehospital emergency care respond to a cardiac arrest. Most EMS systems have specific policies dealing with this issue. The procedure used varies widely from system to system.

When prehospital arrest occurs in a patient without a properly executed DNAR order, EMS providers are generally obligated to attempt resuscitation. Conflicts may also arise for the EMS provider when the patient had a DNAR order in the hospital but is now at home. Unfortunately physicians often fail to provide a DNAR order when a patient leaves the hospital and returns home. In addition, some states do not recognize written DNAR orders for children in the out-of-hospital setting. When EMS personnel determine that resuscitation must be attempted, they should communicate this information to the family sensitively but emphatically. Families should be counseled that more definitive direction regarding ongoing care and further resuscitation attempts can be established when the patient reaches the hospital.

Emergency Department personnel can discontinue treatment initiated by EMS providers in the prehospital setting if there is valid, after-the-fact evidence that this treatment is inappropriate. For example, if the child's attending physician is contacted and confirms that the family does not wish to have resuscitation provided, the resuscitation attempts should be discontinued. Discontinuation of treatment may include removal of the tracheal tube, intravenous access lines, and medication. There is international ethical agreement that withholding resuscitative efforts at the initial collapse is ethically and morally equivalent to withdrawing resuscitative efforts at the terminal event.[55]

Death by Neurologic Criteria (Brain Death)

It is possible to support cardiorespiratory function mechanically in patients with minimal or no brain function and no possibility for recovery. These technologic developments blur the borders between life and death and challenge traditional

> ## Critical Concepts:
> ### Cardiovascular and Neurologic Criteria for Pronouncement of Death
>
> Death may be declared by either cardiovascular or neurologic criteria. Neurologic criteria (brain death) require irreversible cessation of all functions of the brain and brainstem.

legal, cultural, and religious concepts of death. They also highlight the need for a reliable policy for determination of death when cardiorespiratory activity is maintained through technology (see Critical Concepts: "Cardiovascular and Neurologic Criteria for Pronouncement of Death").[108,109]

Neurologic criteria for brain death determination have become well established as a legal standard of death in the United States. Brain death statutes generally conform to the Model Uniform Determination of Death Act[110] and state that a person is legally dead when (1) irreversible cessation of circulation and respiratory function or (2) irreversible cessation of all functions of the entire brain, including the brainstem, has been determined according to accepted medical standards.[110]

Unique modifications to the definition may be found in some locales. For instance, one locale includes a controversial "conscience clause" that provides that in situations in which the physician is aware that the patient's or family's religious convictions would be violated by a declaration of brain death, only cardiorespiratory death criteria may be applied.[111]

The diagnosis of death by neurologic criteria in children (brain death) may be difficult and may not be well understood by clinicians.[112] Specific criteria for brain death developed for adults have not been validated for children. Authoritative statements that may serve as useful working

guidelines have been issued for adults and children of various age groups.[113,114] The use of brain death guidelines for children in the ICU setting has been inconsistent.[115] Diagnosis of death based on neurologic criteria should be made with particular caution in circumstances in which neurologic function may be altered by hypothermia or the use of neuromuscular blocking agents or barbiturates, or when the cause of the brain insult is unknown.[116,117]

Cardiopulmonary support systems may be withdrawn from brain-dead patients without judicial review or fear of legal repercussions. In homicide cases courts have consistently rejected the alleged assailant's defense that the discontinuation of cardiorespiratory support of the brain-dead victim caused death.[118] Similarly courts have authorized the discontinuation of cardiorespiratory support systems for brain-dead victims of child abuse without affecting the criminal charges against the alleged abuser.[119]

Extraordinary situations have occurred in which CPR or mechanical cardiorespiratory support of brain-dead pregnant women was continued for the protection of a viable fetus.[120-122] Rapid advances in perinatology have brought into focus the potential conflicts between maternal and fetal rights. These conflicts of interest are expected to occasionally include the pregnant woman's right to refuse life-sustaining treatment.[123]

Advance Directives

In the United States the Patient Self-Determination Act of 1990 requires hospitals and other healthcare facilities and agencies that participate in Medicare and Medicaid to establish written policies and procedures to inform all adult patients of their right to prescribe binding limits to CPR and life-sustaining measures in the event of future decisional incapacity.[124] An *advance directive* is any expression of a person's thoughts, wishes, or preferences for his/her end-of-life care; advance directives may provide surrogate decision makers with important evidence of an incompetent patient's wishes even in states that do not have living will statutes (see Foundation Facts: "Definition of Advance Directive").[90] The Patient Self-Determination Act was revised in 1991 to require hospitals and healthcare agencies to establish written policies and procedures to inform all adult patients of their right to make decisions concerning medical care, including the right to accept or refuse medical or surgical treatment and the right to formulate an advance directive.[125]

It is now accepted that competent adult patients have the right to decide their treatment with a living will. The usefulness of a living will, however, may be limited by the inability of the patient to foresee all possible situations that may arise. The addition of a durable healthcare power of attorney gives the appointed person the ability to make decisions based on the patient's beliefs.[126]

The application of advance directives in pediatric practice is difficult. Issues of consent by minors and determination of competence must be considered. Despite these limitations, the use of advance directives in pediatric patients is increasing.[127]

The Delivery Room

The standard of care in the delivery room has improved dramatically in recent years. Professional organizations such as the

American Academy of Pediatrics and the American Heart Association have promulgated national guidelines and educational programs for the organization of skilled personnel and equipment to ensure delivery of acceptable resuscitation services to high-risk neonates.[43,128,129] These guidelines may have important implications for the legal liability of physicians and nurses in delivery rooms.

In many cases it is possible to anticipate the need for neonatal resuscitation through improved prenatal care and use of fetal monitoring. These improvements may increase the potential for professional liability. Birth-related problems are the largest single source of malpractice suits against pediatricians.

There are circumstances in which noninitiation or discontinuation of resuscitation in the delivery room may be appropriate. National and local protocols should dictate the procedures to be followed. Ongoing evolution of resuscitation and intensive care interventions and neonatal outcome make it imperative that all such protocols be reviewed regularly and modified as necessary.

The *ECC Guidelines 2000*[55] recommend that after appropriate discussion and with an advance directive from the family, noninitiation of resuscitation may be appropriate for an infant with a confirmed gestation of less than 23 weeks or birthweight less than 400 g, anencephaly, or confirmed specific congenital anomalies.[43] In cases of uncertain prognosis, including uncertain gestational age, the resuscitation options are a trial of therapy or noninitiation or discontinuation of therapy after assessment of the infant. In such cases initiation of resuscitation at delivery does not mandate continued support.

Discontinuation of resuscitative efforts may be appropriate if effective resuscitative interventions for a newly born infant with cardiac arrest do not result in spontaneous circulation after 15 minutes.[43] Lack of response to an intensive resusci-

tation attempt of more than 10 minutes' duration carries an extremely poor prognosis for survival or survival without disability.[130-133] The AHA recommends local discussions to formulate guidelines consistent with local resources and outcome data.

Organ and Tissue Recovery

Successful return of spontaneous circulation does not guarantee successful cerebral resuscitation, and brain death may follow. Patients who meet the neurologic criteria for death may be appropriate candidates for vascular organ recovery. Cadaveric tissue donation is also possible after circulatory function ceases, and this form of recovery does not require that the patient meet neurologic criteria for death. Permission from next of kin or prior consent must be obtained for any tissue or organ donation, and the patient's wishes, if expressed before resuscitation, should be considered.

National "required request" laws require documentation that families of potential donors are offered the option of organ donation and that the local organ procurement organization is notified of potential donors.[134] A controversial proposal has been made for "presumed consent," which would permit the body of every deceased person to be used as a potential organ donor unless that person had declared an objection to being a donor before death or the next of kin declares such an objection immediately upon notification of death.[135] Such measures have been adopted in several countries but not in the United States.

The Ethics of Practicing Resuscitation Skills on the Newly Dead

Many healthcare providers lack sufficient clinical experience in advanced skills used during attempted resuscitation of infants and children (eg, advanced airway management). One suggested training alternative is to practice on newly dead patients, but this option raises important ethical and legal issues. For example, under certain circumstances tracheal intubation of newly deceased infants and children may be performed to improve the healthcare providers' skills. This practice, although controversial, is an effective teaching technique and can improve care delivered to future patients. Ethical discussions about this practice are often influenced more by culture and history than by objective science or clinical outcomes.

The culture and sensibilities of family and staff should be respected, and consent should be obtained from family members before the patient's death. Under some circumstances when the child's death will be investigated by a medical examiner, the tracheal tube should not be removed; therefore, intubation cannot be practiced.

Summary Points

ALS providers should explore the ethical and legal obligations that accompany the provision of pediatric lifesaving skills.

- Children are different from adults, and appropriate management regimens cannot safely be derived simply by scaling down adult versions.

- The performance of PALS trainees will be judged against the content of the pediatric BLS and ALS courses as adapted to individual and community needs.

- Providers should develop an appreciation of the unique rights of parents and children, the limits of parental authority, and the role of the state in protecting the welfare of children.

- The healthcare professional should recognize when the rights of parents and children may conflict, especially when making decisions to withhold CPR. Available institutional and judicial resources should be consulted to ensure that the best interests of the child are protected.

- When there is doubt about the authority or reasonableness of guardian requests to withhold CPR, a presumption that resuscitation is indicated should govern professional conduct until the conflict can be resolved.

- Potential rescuers should undertake good-faith efforts at resuscitation to the limits of their ability, relying on legal protection based on common-law doctrines or Good Samaritan statutes.

- Care after attempted resuscitation is important even when resuscitation is unsuccessful in restoring cerebral and cardiopulmonary function. Respect and sensitivity in dealing with organ recovery, postmortem examinations, and bereavement will ultimately benefit the child's family.

Case Scenario and Review Questions

Introductory Case Scenario

A 2-year-old child is found in the family swimming pool. Bystanders call EMS and provide CPR at the scene until EMS personnel arrive. On initial assessment the child appears lifeless and does not respond to basic and advanced life support interventions. The child is transported to the Emergency Department; CPR efforts continue and epinephrine is administered en route.

On arrival in the ED the child is in cardiac arrest, but after several doses of epinephrine there is a return of spontaneous circulation, and the child is subsequently admitted to the pediatric ICU. Over the next 2 days the child remains hemodynamically unstable, and there is no evidence of return of brain function. Several discussions are held with the family about the next appropriate interventions for the child.

Discussion and Review Questions

1. *Should EMS personnel discontinue CPR at the scene if asked by the parents to do so?*

The rights of parents in making medical decisions for their child are given substantial weight. In the prehospital setting, however, EMS personnel are often obligated to provide CPR until an order is received from a physician to terminate efforts or the child has obvious evidence of death (eg, rigor mortis). In some EMS systems healthcare providers are authorized to terminate resuscitative efforts if the child with no mitigating factors remains asystolic despite provision of basic and advanced life support.

2. *Would it be appropriate for the ED physician to discontinue support after the child arrives in the ED?*

Physicians may decide to discontinue support based on evidence that demonstrates a high likelihood that CPR efforts will be futile. For example, in the absence of hypothermia or drug ingestion, substantial data shows that survival to hospital discharge is very unlikely after cardiac arrest followed by prolonged prehospital ALS interventions. CPR is typically provided in the ED until patient assessment is complete and all potentially reversible causes of cardiac arrest are addressed.

3. *Is the discontinuation of technological support, such as removal of the tracheal tube, ethically or morally different than withholding initiation of that support?*

No. Ethicists agree that there is no ethical or moral difference between withholding CPR and discontinuing CPR once it is started. For example, if a child who had a DNAR order in the hospital subsequently arrests at home, it is possible that EMS would initiate resuscitative interventions before confirmation of advance directives could occur. It is ethically and morally acceptable for the medical team to remove a tracheal tube that may have been inserted by EMS providers once confirmation of advance directives has occurred.

4. In the PICU the child's parents want everything done, but the attending physician realizes that this child's outcome is poor. In the event of sudden cardiac arrest, is a physician order for a "slow code" legally and ethically appropriate?

No. It is inappropriate to write or request a "slow code." This type of order is confusing and puts the healthcare providers at the scene at risk for providing what may be perceived as incompetent resuscitation. Agreement between healthcare professionals and family (legal guardians) must be reached on appropriate resuscitative interventions. Such an agreement is usually based on the perceived best interests of the child. Limitation or withdrawal of specific resuscitative interventions should be listed to make the response as clear as possible. Many healthcare systems consult medical ethics committees or boards to help resolve perceived disagreements or conflicts between healthcare providers and guardians.

5. Death by neurologic criteria ("brain death") is documented using an accepted methodology. Do you now need to obtain parental consent to remove the child from the ventilator?

Once death by neurologic criteria ("brain death") is documented, legal death has occurred. The family should be prepared, supported, and informed. Parental "permission" for removal of technological organ support, however, is not required or appropriate. It is important to fully inform the family of what to expect before and during the evaluation for death by neurologic criteria. They should understand that there is no decision for them to make, other than organ recovery, autopsy, and postmortem care arrangements.

References

1. Kouwenhoven WB, Jude JR, Knickerbocker GG. Closed-chest cardiac massage. *JAMA.* 1960;173:1064-1067.

2. Veatch RM. *A Theory of Medical Ethics.* New York, NY: Basic Books; 1981.

3. *Prosser and Keeton on the Law of Torts.* 5th ed. St. Paul, Minn: West; 1984.

4. Wadlington W, Waltz JR, Dworkin RB. *Cases and Materials on Law and Medicine.* Mineola, NY: Foundation Press; 1980.

5. Rozovsky FA. *Consent to Treatment: A Practical Guide.* Boston, Mass: Little Brown & Co; 1984.

6. *Scholendorff v Society of New York Hospital,* 211 NY 125, 105 NE 92 (1914).

7. President's Commission for the Study of Ethical Problems in Medicine and Biomedical and Behavioral Research. *Making Health Care Decisions: A Report on the Ethical and Legal Implications of Informed Consent in the Patient-Practitioner Relationship.* Washington, DC: US Government Printing Office; 1982:55.

8. *Canterbury v Spence,* 464 F2d 772, 787 (1972).

9. Capron AM. Informed consent in catastrophic disease treatment and research. 123 *U PA L R* 340, 387 (1974).

10. Andrews LB. Informed consent statutes and the decision-making process. *J Leg Med.* 1984;5:163-217.

11. Biros MH, Lewis RJ, Olson CM, Runge JW, Cummins RO, Fost N. Informed consent in emergency research: consensus statement from the coalition conference of acute resuscitation and critical care researchers. *JAMA.* 1995;273:1283-1287.

12. Biros MH, Runge JW, Lewis RJ, Doherty C. Emergency medicine and the development of the Food and Drug Administration's final rule on informed consent and waiver of informed consent in emergency research circumstances. *Acad Emerg Med.* 1998;5:359-368.

13. American Academy of Pediatrics Committee on Bioethics. Ethics and the care of critically ill infants and children. *Pediatrics.* 1996;98: 149-152.

14. *Wisconsin v Yoder,* 406 US 205 (1972).

15. *In Re Green,* 307 A2d 279 (1973).

16. *In Re Seiferth,* 127 NE2d 820 (1955).

17. *Prince v Commonwealth of Massachusetts,* 321 US 158 (1944).

18. Rothman DJ, Rothman SM. The conflict over children's rights. *Hastings Cent Rep.* 1980; 10:7-10.

19. *In Re Sampson,* 278 NE2d 918 (1972).

20. *Custody of a Minor,* 393 NE2d 836 (1979).

21. *Matter of Hofbauer,* 393 NE2d 1009 (1979).

22. American Academy of Pediatrics Committee on Bioethics. Religious exemptions from child abuse statutes. *Pediatrics.* 1988;81: 169-171.

23. President's Commission for the Study of Ethical Problems in Medicine and Biomedical and Behavioral Research. *Deciding to Forego Life-Sustaining Treatment.* Washington, DC: US Government Printing Office; 1983.

24. Pub L 98-457; Fed Reg 45 CFR part 1340. April 15, 1985:14878.

25. Kopelman LM, Irons TG, Kopelman AE. Neonatologists judge the "Baby Doe" regulations. *N Engl J Med.* 1988;318:677-683.

26. Carter BS. Neonatologists and bioethics after Baby Doe. *J Perinatol.* 1993;13:144-150.

27. Weir R. *Selective Nontreatment of Handicapped Newborns: Moral Dilemmas in Neonatal Medicine.* New York, NY: Oxford University Press; 1984.

28. Capron AM. The competence of children as self-deciders in biomedical intervention. In: Gaylin W, Macklin R, eds. *Who Speaks for the Child.* New York, NY: Plenum Publishing Corp; 1982.

29. Gaylin W. Competence, no longer all or nothing. In: Gaylin W, Macklin R, eds. *Who Speaks for the Child.* New York, NY: Plenum Publishing Corp; 1982.

30. Leikin SL. Minors' assent or dissent to medical treatment. *J Pediatr.* 1983;102:169-176.

31. Schowalter JE, Ferholt JB, Mann NM. The adolescent patient's decision to die. *Pediatrics.* 1973;51:97-103.

32. *In Re F.G,* 549 NE2d 322 (1989).

33. American College of Legal Medicine. *Legal Medicine: Legal Dynamics of Medical Encounters.* 2nd ed. St. Louis, Mo: Mosby Year Book; 1991.

34. *Shilkret v The Annapolis Emergency Hospital Association,* 349 A2d 245 (1975)

35. *Proceedings of the National Conference on the Medicolegal Implications of Emergency Medical Care.* Dallas, Tex: American Heart Association; 1975:133, 155.

36. Dalen JE, Howe JP III, Membrino GE. Sounding board: CPR training for physicians. *N Engl J Med.* 1980;303:455-457.

37. Quimby CW Jr, Spies FK. Liability of the hospital cardiac team. *Ark L R.* 1972;26:17, 24.

38. *Guerrero v Copper Queen Hospital,* 537 P2d 1329 (1975).

39. Mancini MR, Gale AT. *Emergency Care and the Law.* Rockville, Md: Aspen Systems Corp; 1981.

40. *Darling v Charleston Community Memorial Hospital,* 211 NE2d 253 (1965).

41. Smith WB. Hospital liability for physician negligence. *JAMA*. 1984;251:447-448.

42. *Sparger v Worley Hospital, Inc,* 547 SW2d 582 (1977).

43. The American Heart Association in collaboration with the International Liaison Committee on Resuscitation. Guidelines 2000 for cardiopulmonary resuscitation and emergency cardiovascular care. Part 11: neonatal resuscitation. *Circulation*. 2000;102:I-343-I-357.

44. Cummins RO, Eisenberg MS. Prehospital cardiopulmonary resuscitation: is it effective? *JAMA*. 1985;253:2408-2412.

45. *Principles of Biomedical Ethics*. 2nd ed. New York, NY: Oxford University Press Inc; 1983.

46. Weinrub EJ. The case for a duty to rescue. *Yale L J*. 1980;90:247, 250.

47. Lipkin RJ. Beyond Good Samaritans and moral monsters: an individualistic justification of the general legal duty to rescue. *UCLA L R*. 1983;31:252-253, 262.

48. *Current Opinion of the Judicial Council of the American Medical Association*. 1984:IX.

49. Helminski FJ. Good Samaritan statutes: time for uniformity. *Wayne L R*. 1980;27:217, 221, 331.

50. Mapel FB III, Weigel C II. Good Samaritan laws—who needs them: the current state of Good Samaritan protection in the United States. *S Tex L J*. 1981;21:327, 351.

51. *Restatement of Torts*, 2d 289, 296, 298 (1965).

52. Sullivan B. Some thoughts on the constitutionality of Good Samaritan statutes. *Am J Law Med*. 1982;8:27-43.

53. Standards and guidelines for cardiopulmonary resuscitation (CPR) and emergency cardiac care (ECC). *JAMA*. 1986;255:2905-2989.

54. Emergency Cardiac Care Committee and Subcommittees, American Heart Association. Guidelines for cardiopulmonary resuscitation and emergency cardiac care. *JAMA*. 1992; 268:2171-2295.

55. American Heart Association in collaboration with International Liaison Committee on Resuscitation. *Guidelines 2000 for Cardiopulmonary Resuscitation and Emergency Cardiovascular Care: International Consensus on Science*. *Circulation*. 2000; 102(suppl 1). Also available as a separate volume.

56. National Association of State Emergency Medical Services Directors (NASEMSD) and the National Association of Emergency Medical Services Physicians (NAEMSP). National guidelines for statewide implementation of EMS "do not resuscitate" (DNR) programs. *Prehospital Disaster Med*. 1994; 9:137-139.

57. Kellermann AL. Criteria for dead-on-arrivals, prehospital termination of CPR, and do-not-resuscitate orders. *Ann Emerg Med*. 1993;22: 47-51.

58. Sirbaugh PE, Pepe PE, Shook JE, Kimball KT, Goldman MJ, Ward MA, Mann DM. A prospective, population-based study of the demographics, epidemiology, management, and outcome of out-of-hospital pediatric cardiopulmonary arrest [published correction appears in *Ann Emerg Med*. 1999;33:358]. *Ann Emerg Med*. 1999;33:174-184.

59. Kuisma M, Suominen P, Korpela R. Paediatric out-of-hospital cardiac arrests—epidemiology and outcome. *Resuscitation*. 1995;30:141-150.

60. Innes PA, Summers CA, Boyd IM, Molyneux EM. Audit of paediatric cardiopulmonary resuscitation. *Arch Dis Child*. 1993;68:487-491.

61. Quan L, Wentz KR, Gore EJ, Copass MK. Outcome and predictors of outcome in pediatric submersion victims receiving prehospital care in King County, Washington. *Pediatrics*. 1990;86:586-593.

62. Zaritsky A. Cardiopulmonary resuscitation in children. *Clin Chest Med*. 1987;8:561-571.

63. Barzilay Z, Somekh E, Sagy M, Boichis H. Pediatric cardiopulmonary resuscitation outcome. *J Med*. 1988;19:229-241.

64. Ronco R, King W, Konley DK, Tilden SJ. Outcome and cost at a children's hospital following resuscitation for out-of-hospital cardiopulmonary arrest. *Arch Pediatr Adolesc Med*. 1995;149:210-214.

65. Torphy DE, Minter MG, Thompson BM. Cardiopulmonary arrest and resuscitation of children. *Am J Dis Child*. 1984;138:1099-1102.

66. Schindler MB, Bohn D, Cox PN, McCrindle BW, Jarvis A, Edmonds J, Barker G. Outcome of out-of-hospital cardiac or respiratory arrest in children. *N Engl J Med*. 1996;335:1473-1479.

67. O'Rourke PP. Outcome of children who are apneic and pulseless in the emergency room. *Crit Care Med*. 1986;14:466-468.

68. Young KD, Seidel JS. Pediatric cardiopulmonary resuscitation: a collective review. *Ann Emerg Med*. 1999;33:195-205.

69. DeBard ML. Cardiopulmonary resuscitation: analysis of six years' experience and review of the literature. *Ann Emerg Med*. 1981;10: 408-416.

70. Council on Ethical and Judicial Affairs, AMA. Guidelines for the appropriate use of do-not-resuscitate orders. *JAMA*. 1991;265:1868-1871.

71. Lantos JD, Berger AC, Zucker AR. Do-not-resuscitate orders in a children's hospital. *Crit Care Med*. 1993;21:52-55.

72. American College of Emergency Physicians. Guidelines for 'do not resuscitate' orders in the prehospital setting. *Ann Emerg Med*. 1988;17:1106-1108.

73. Miles SH, Crimmins TJ. Orders to limit emergency treatment for an ambulance service in a large metropolitan area. *JAMA*. 1985;254: 525-527.

74. *Satz v Perlmutter*, 362 So2d 160 (1978).

75. *Lane v Candura*, 376 NE2d 1232 (1978).

76. *Belchertwon State School v Saikewicz*, 370 NE2d 417, 425 (1977).

77. Drane JF. The many faces of competency. *Hastings Cent Rep*. 1985;15:17-21.

78. Jackson DL, Youngner S. Patient autonomy and "death with dignity": some clinical caveats. *N Engl J Med*. 1979;301:404-408.

79. Bedell SE, Delbanco TL. Choices about cardiopulmonary resuscitation in the hospital: when do physicians talk with patients? *N Engl J Med*. 1984;310:1089-1093.

80. Evans AL, Brody BA. The do-not-resuscitate order in teaching hospitals. *JAMA*. 1985;253: 2236-2239.

81. Eisenberg JM. Sociologic influences on decision-making by clinicians. *Ann Intern Med*. 1979;90:957-964.

82. Youngner S, Jackson DL, Allen M. Staff attitudes towards the care of the critically ill in the medical intensive care unit. *Crit Care Med*. 1979;7:35-40.

83. Spencer SS. Sounding board: "code" or "no code": a nonlegal opinion. *N Engl J Med*. 1979;300:138-140.

84. McPhail A, Moore S, O'Connor J, Woodward C. One hospital's experience with a "do not resuscitate" policy. *Can Med Assoc J*. 1981; 125:830-836.

85. Robertson JA. *The Rights of the Critically Ill: The Basic ACLU Guide to the Rights of Critically Ill and Dying Patients*. Cambridge, Mass: Ballinger; 1983.

86. Farber NJ, Bowman SM, Major DA, Green WP. Cardiopulmonary resuscitation (CPR): patient factors and decision making. *Arch Intern Med*. 1984;144:2229-2232.

87. Hashimoto DM. A structural analysis of the physician-patient relationship in no-code decision making. *Yale L R*. 1983;93:363, 381.

88. *In Re Swan*, 569 A2d 1202 (1990).

89. Wanzer SH, Adelstein SJ, Cranford RE, Federman DD, Hook ED, Moertel CG, Safar P, Stone A, Taussig HB, van Eys J. The physician's responsibility toward hopelessly ill patients. *N Engl J Med*. 1984;310:955-959.

90. *In Re Dinnerstein*, 380 NE2d 134 (1978).

91. Jecker NS, Schneiderman LJ. An ethical analysis of the use of 'futility' in the 1992 American Heart Association guidelines for cardiopulmonary resuscitation and emergency cardiac care. *Arch Intern Med.* 1993; 153:2195-2198.

92. Lo B, Steinbrook RL. Deciding whether to resuscitate. *Arch Intern Med.* 1983;143: 1561-1563.

93. *Matter of Quinlan*, 355 A2d 647 (1976).

94. *Matter of Conroy*, 486 A2d 1209 (1985).

95. *Barber v Superior Court*, 195 Cal Rptr 484 (1983).

96. *Custody of a Minor*, 434 NE2d 601 (1982).

97. Veatch RM. Limits of guardian treatment refusal: a reasonableness standard. *Am J Law Med.* 1984;9:427-468.

98. *In Re Storar*, 52 NY2d 363 (1982).

99. Youngner SJ, Lewandowski W, McClish DK, Juknialis BW, Coulton C, Bartlett ET. 'Do not resuscitate' orders: incidence and implications in a medical-intensive care unit. *JAMA.* 1985;253:54-57.

100. Cranford RE, Doudera AE, eds. *Institutional Ethics Committees and Health Care Decision Making.* Ann Arbor, Mich: Health Administration Press; 1984.

101. Fost N, Cranford RE. Hospital ethics committees: administrative aspects. *JAMA.* 1985;253:2687-2692.

102. AMA Judicial Council. Guidelines for ethics committees in health care institutions. *JAMA.* 1985;253:2698-2699.

103. Smith JP, Bodai BI. The urban paramedic's scope of practice. *JAMA.* 1985;253:544-548.

104. 5 *EMT Legal Bull* 4. 1981.

105. 7 *EMT Legal Bull* 7. 1983.

106. 5 *EMT Legal Bull* 3. 1981.

107. Caroline NL. *Emergency Care in the Streets.* 2nd ed. Boston, Mass: Little Brown & Co; 1983:7.

108. Farrell MM, Levin DL. Brain death in the pediatric patient: historical, sociological, medical, religious, cultural, legal, and ethical considerations. *Crit Care Med.* 1993;21: 1951-1965.

109. President's Commission for the Study of Ethical Problems in Medicine and Biomedical and Behavioral Research. *Defining Death: A Report on the Medical, Legal, and Ethical Issues in the Determination of Death.* Washington, DC: US Government Printing Office; 1983.

110. Guidelines for the determination of death: report of the medical consultants on the diagnosis of death to the President's Commission for the Study of Ethical Problems in Medicine and Biomedical and Behavioral Research. *JAMA.* 1981;246: 2184-2186.

111. Olick RS. Brain death, religious freedom, and public policy: New Jersey's landmark legislative initiative. *Kennedy Inst Ethics J.* 1991;1:275-292.

112. Harrison AM, Botkin JR. Can pediatricians define and apply the concept of brain death? *Pediatrics.* 1999;103:e82.

113. The Hastings Center. *Guidelines on the Termination of Life-Sustaining Treatment and the Care of the Dying: A Report.* Briarcliff Manor, NY: The Center; 1987:85.

114. American Academy of Pediatrics Task Force on Brain Death in Children. Report of special task force: guidelines for the determination of brain death in children. *Pediatrics.* 1987;80:298-300.

115. Mejia RE, Pollack MM. Variability in brain death determination practices in children. *JAMA.* 1995;274:550-553.

116. Freeman JM, Rogers MC. On death, dying, and decisions. *Pediatrics.* 1980;66:637-638.

117. Robinson RO. Brain death in children. *Arch Dis Child.* 1981;56:657-658.

118. Eisner JM, Randell LL, Tilson JQ. Judicial decisions concerning brain death. *Conn Med.* 1982;46:193-194.

119. Cook JW, Hirsch L. *I: Medicine and Law.* New York, NY: Springer International; 1982.

120. Dillon WP, Lee RV, Tronolone MJ, Buckwald S, Foote RJ. Life support and maternal brain death during pregnancy. *JAMA.* 1982; 248:1089-1091.

121. Siegler M, Wikler D. Brain death and live birth [editorial]. *JAMA.* 1982;248:1101-1102.

122. Veatch RM. Maternal brain death: an ethicist's thoughts [editorial]. *JAMA.* 1982;248: 1102-1103.

123. Bowes WA Jr, Selgestad B. Fetal versus maternal rights: medical and legal perspectives. *Obstet Gynecol.* 1981;58:209-214.

124. Omnibus Reconciliation Act of 1990, Public Law No. 101-508 Sec 4206, 4751

125. Wolf SM, Boyle P, Callahan D, Fins JJ, Jennings B, Nelson JL, Barondess JA, Brock DW, Dresser R, Emanuel L, et al. Sources of concern about the Patient Self-Determination Act. *N Engl J Med.* 1991;325:1666-1671.

126. Silverman HJ, Vinicky JK, Gasner MR. Advance directives: implications for critical care. *Crit Care Med.* 1992;20:1027-1031.

127. Jefferson LS, White BC, Louis PT, Brody BA, King DD, Roberts CE. Use of the Natural Death Act in pediatric patients. *Crit Care Med.* 1991;19:901-905.

128. American Academy of Pediatrics, College of Obstetricians and Gynecologists. *Guidelines for Perinatal Care.* 3rd ed. Evanston, Ill/ Washington, DC; 1992.

129. Kattwinkel J, ed. *Textbook of Neonatal Resuscitation.* 4th ed. Elk Grove Village, IL: American Academy of Pediatrics; 2000.

130. Davis DJ. How aggressive should delivery room cardiopulmonary resuscitation be for extremely low birth weight neonates? *Pediatrics.* 1993;92:447-450.

131. Jain L, Ferre C, Vidyasagar D, Nath S, Sheftel D. Cardiopulmonary resuscitation of apparently stillborn infants: survival and long-term outcome. *J Pediatr.* 1991; 118:778-782.

132. Yeo CL, Tudehope DI. Outcome of resuscitated apparently stillborn infants: a ten year review. *J Paediatr Child Health.* 1994;30: 129-133.

133. Casalaz DM, Marlow N, Speidel BD. Outcome of resuscitation following unexpected apparent stillbirth. *Arch Dis Child Fetal Neonatal Ed.* 1998;78:F112-F115.

134. Omnibus Reconciliation Act of 1986 (OBRA), Public Law 99-509.

135. Moskop JC. Organ transplantation in children: ethical issues. *J Pediatr.* 1987;110: 175-180.

Respiratory Failure

Pediatric Advanced Life Support

American Academy
of Pediatrics
DEDICATED TO THE HEALTH OF ALL CHILDREN

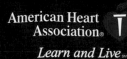

American Heart
Association
Learn and Live

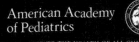

Learning Objectives

At the end of this session the participant will be able to

- Identify prearrest conditions of respiratory distress and respiratory failure
- List the signs and symptoms of upper airway obstruction
- Describe the general approach to the management of a child with respiratory distress or failure
- Describe the potential causes of inadequate improvement or acute deterioration after initiating oxygen therapy and supporting ventilation in the child with respiratory distress or failure
- Describe appropriate technique of primary and secondary confirmation of tracheal tube placement
- List reasons for **sudden deterioration** in an intubated child

---

Recognition of Respiratory Failure

Initial Respiratory Assessment

1. **Airway**
   - Clear
   - Maintainable
   - Unmaintainable without intubation
2. **Breathing**
   - Rate
   - Effort/mechanics: retractions, grunting, nasal flaring, chest movement
   - Air entry/tidal volume
     — Inspiratory stridor
     — Expiratory wheeze
   - Skin color (pulse oximetry)

Classification of Respiratory Failure

4 Categories of Respiratory Problems

- **Upper airway obstruction**
  — Symptoms more apparent during inspiration than expiration
- **Lower airway obstruction**
  — Symptoms more apparent during expiration than inspiration
- **Parenchymal lung disease**
  — Hypoxemia, tachypnea, increased work of breathing
- **Abnormal control of ventilation**
  — Apnea or "funny breathing" (abnormal rhythm)

Management of Respiratory Failure

Initial Management: Respiratory Distress

- Allow child to assume position of comfort
- Administer oxygen as tolerated
- Consider pulse oximetry and ECG monitor
- Maintain NPO if significant distress is present
- Management of upper airway obstruction: consider steroids and aerosolized epinephrine
- Management of lower airway obstruction: consider steroids and β_2-agonists

Initial Management: Respiratory Failure

- Control/secure airway
- Administer Fio_2 of 1.00 (100% oxygen)
- Assist or provide ventilation
- Monitor pulse oximetry and ECG
- Establish vascular access
- Provide nothing by mouth

Potential Explanations for Inadequate Improvement or Acute Deterioration During Positive-Pressure Ventilation

- Inadequate tidal volume
- Excessive leak around the tracheal tube
- Excessive tidal volume or respiratory rate → air trapping and impaired cardiac output
- Failure to compress the pop-off valve on the manual resuscitator
- A leak or disconnection anywhere in the manual resuscitator or ventilator system
- "DOPE" (see below)
- Inadequate PEEP
- Inadequate O_2 flow from gas source

Confirmation of Tracheal Tube Position

- Observation of chest rise
- Auscultation of breath sounds
- Detection of exhaled CO_2
- Direct visualization if needed

Causes of Acute Deterioration in Intubated Patient: DOPE

- **D**isplacement of the tracheal tube
  — Extubation
  — Migration to a mainstem bronchus
- **O**bstruction of the tracheal tube
- **P**neumothorax
- **E**quipment failure

Shock

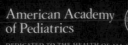

American Academy of Pediatrics
DEDICATED TO THE HEALTH OF ALL CHILDREN™

American Heart Association®
Learn and Live℠

Pediatric Advanced Life Support

Learning Objectives

At the end of the session the participant will be able to
- Describe the clinical signs of shock in infants and children
- Describe the clinical classification of shock
- Differentiate decompensated from compensated shock
- Describe a systematic approach to achieving vascular access for the infant or child in shock
- Describe the intraosseous vascular access technique
- Discuss the clinical signs and initial treatment of hypovolemic, cardiogenic, and distributive (septic) shock in infants and children

Recognition of Shock

Definition: Inadequate systemic perfusion and oxygen delivery

Initial Cardiopulmonary Assessment:

Appearance: Note mental status, tone, and response to stimulation

Airway: Typically open

Breathing: Quiet tachypnea to compensate for metabolic acidosis

Circulation: Check for direct and indirect signs of inadequate perfusion (see below)

Cardiovascular Assessment for Shock

- *Direct* cardiovascular assessment:
  Heart rate
  Pulse quality — proximal and distal
  Blood pressure and pulse pressure
- **Indirect cardiovascular assessment: evaluation of end-organ perfusion**
  Brain — alertness, pupil size, response
  Skin — color, temperature, capillary refill
  Kidneys — urine output

Definition of Hypotension for Age

Age	Systolic BP (mm Hg)
<1 month	≤60
1 month to 1 year	≤70
1 to 10 years	≤70 + (2 × age in y)
>10 years	≤90

Classification of Shock

Classification of Physiologic Status

- Stable
- Respiratory distress
- Respiratory failure
- Shock
  — Compensated
  — Decompensated
- Cardiopulmonary failure
- Cardiopulmonary arrest

Decompensated Shock

- Shock + systolic hypotension

If blood pressure is not available, defined by absent distal pulses, prolonged capillary refill, cool extremities, tachycardia, and decreased level of consciousness/responsiveness

Types of Shock and Key Characteristics

- *Hypovolemic:* most common; peripheral vasoconstriction, narrow pulse pressure
- *Distributive (septic):* wide pulse pressure; hypo- or hyperthermia
- *Cardiogenic:* Systemic or pulmonary edema or both, increased work of breathing; grunting; narrow pulse pressure
- Other (consider special resuscitation circumstances)

Management of Shock

Initial Treatment of Shock

- Ensure adequate **A**irway and **B**reathing. Give oxygen, support ventilation if needed. In cardiogenic shock, early support of ventilation is often important.
- **C**irculation: Establish vascular access. Use IO for decompensated shock.
- Fluid therapy: 10 to 20 mL/kg rapid bolus isotonic crystalloid (may modify if myocardial dysfunction likely).
- Reassess cardiovascular and pulmonary function.
- Administer additional fluid therapy as needed; consider inotropes, vasopressors, and other vasoactive drugs.

Rhythm Disturbances

Pediatric Advanced Life Support

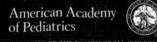American Academy of Pediatrics
DEDICATED TO THE HEALTH OF ALL CHILDREN

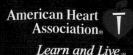American Heart Association.
Learn and Live

Learning Objectives

At the end of the session the participant will be able to

- Recognize and manage bradycardia, tachycardia with poor perfusion, tachycardia with adequate perfusion, and pulseless arrest rhythms (asystole, PEA, VF, and VT)
- Recognize unstable conditions resulting from arrhythmias requiring urgent intervention
- Differentiate SVT from sinus tachycardia
- Stabilize the child with unstable rhythm

- Use vagal maneuvers to treat SVT with adequate perfusion
- Deliver electric shocks safely and for appropriate indications
  — Attempt defibrillation
  — Provide synchronized cardioversion
- Describe indications for and safe use of an **AED**
- Select appropriate medications to treat symptomatic bradycardia, tachycardia, and the arrest rhythms

Recognition and Classification of Arrhythmias

Three Major Categories of Arrhythmias

- Too slow = bradycardia
- Too fast = tachycardia
- Collapse = loss of pulses (arrest rhythm)

Clinical Signs of "Instability" Associated With Arrhythmias

- Shock with hypotension or poor end-organ perfusion
- Altered consciousness
- Sudden collapse

Differentiation of Sinus Tachycardia From Supraventricular Tachycardia

Sinus tachycardia	Supraventricular tachycardia
• History compatible (eg, fever, trauma)	• History incompatible with ST or nonspecific
• P waves present/normal	• P waves absent/abnormal
• HR often varies with activity	• HR not variable with activity
• Variable RR with constant PR	• Abrupt rate changes
• Rate ranges	• Rate ranges:
— Infant: rate usually <220 bpm	— Infant: rate usually >220 bpm
— Child: rate usually <180 bpm	— Child: rate usually >180 bpm

Management of Arrhythmias

General Management

- Administer oxygen, support ventilation as needed
- Perform chest compressions for arrest rhythms and for severe bradycardia (HR <60 bpm associated with poor perfusion) or tachycardia associated with profound hypotension
- Obtain a rhythm strip or ECG if appropriate
- Identify and treat potentially reversible causes (see next column)

Specific Therapies

- **Symptomatic bradycardia:** Epinephrine, consider atropine, consider pacing

- **SVT:** Determine need for electrical vs pharmacologic interventions. Adenosine recommended if IV/IO access available — use rapid 2-syringe technique. Consider vagal maneuvers for SVT with adequate perfusion.

- **Wide-complex tachycardia with pulses:** Consider cardioversion or alternative medications: amiodarone or procainamide or lidocaine

- **VF/Pulseless VT:** Attempt defibrillation immediately (up to 3 × if needed), then drug-shock (or drug-shock-shock-shock); epinephrine; then consider amiodarone or lidocaine; for torsades or hypomagnesemia, give magnesium

Unstable Rhythm: Consider Potentially Reversible Causes

- **H**ypoxemia (bradycardia)
- **H**ypothermia (bradycardia) or **H**yperthermia (tachycardia)
- **H**ypo- or **H**yperkalemia and metabolic disorders (ventricular arrhythmias)
- **H**ypovolemia
- Additional **H**'s for bradycardia: Head injury, Heart block, Heart transplant

- **T**amponade (cardiac) (PEA)
- **T**ension pneumothorax (PEA)
- **T**oxins/poisons/drugs (bradycardia or tachycardia)
- **T**hromboembolism (PEA, tachycardia)

Defibrillation Shocks vs Cardioversion

Attempted Defibrillation	Synchronized Cardioversion
• **Not** synchronized to ECG	• Synchronized to ECG
• Use for **pulseless** rhythms (VF and pulseless VT)	• Use for rhythms **with pulses** (VT and SVT with pulses)
• Initially 2 J/kg × 1, 2 to 4 J/kg × 1, then 4 J/kg	• 0.5 to 1 J/kg (consider sedation)

Suggestions for Instructors

American Academy of Pediatrics
DEDICATED TO THE HEALTH OF ALL CHILDREN

American Heart Association.
Learn and Live

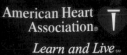

Pediatric Advanced Life Support

Learning Objectives

At the end of the session the instructor candidate will be able to
- State the **goals** of the PALS Course
- List **attributes of a skilled instructor**
- Learn to be a **facilitator** rather than a teacher
- State **instructor Do's and Don'ts**
- List qualities of **effective feedback**
- State 5 steps in **teaching a procedure**

Core Objectives of PALS Training

A PALS provider should demonstrate the following cognitive and psychomotor skills:

1. Provide **pediatric BLS**
2. **Recognize** impending **respiratory failure and shock**
3. Initiate treatment:
   — Open the **airway**
   — Provide **O_2 and ventilation**
   — Obtain **vascular access**
   — Initiate **fluid therapy**
4. Stabilize and evaluate the **trauma** victim
5. Identify and treat **rhythm** disturbances
6. **Initiate the first 10 minutes of resuscitation** (BLS and ALS)
7. **Triage** to definitive care
8. **Provide support** to patients, families, and colleagues

Attributes of a Skilled Instructor

- Enthusiastic
- Establishes rapport
- Knowledgeable
- Facilitator, not lecturer
- Models effectively
- Well prepared
- Admits ignorance
- Provides effective feedback

Instructor "Do's"

- Do read all course material in preparation for the course
- Do adhere to the schedule
- Do encourage participant discussion and action
- Do admit when you don't know an answer
- Do provide positive feedback

Instructor "Don'ts"

- Don't go off course (ie, stick to the objectives)
- Don't lecture or dominate discussion
- Don't present opinion as facts
- Don't read from notes or slides
- Don't neglect eye contact

Effective Feedback

- Immediate
- Clear
- Positive

Five Steps in Teaching a Procedure

1. Orientation: indications and contraindications
2. Instructor "talk-through" — step-by-step description
3. Participant "repeat talk-through"
4. Instructor (or video) demonstration
5. Participant's supervised demonstration
   May compress steps 2 and 3 into 4 and 5

PALS Facilitators

- Instructors are **facilitators**, not lecturers
- Have confidence in most participants: expect precourse preparation
- Support weak participants